Endocrine Disorders in Kidney Disease

Connie M. Rhee
Kamyar Kalantar-Zadeh
Gregory A. Brent
Editors

Endocrine Disorders in Kidney Disease

Diagnosis and Treatment

Springer

Editors
Connie M. Rhee
Division of Nephrology
and Hypertension
Departments of Medicine
and Public Health
University of California Irvine
School of Medicine
Orange, CA
USA

Kamyar Kalantar-Zadeh
Division of Nephrology
and Hypertension
Departments of Medicine,
Pediatrics, Public Health,
and Nursing Sciences
University of California Irvine
School of Medicine
Orange, CA
USA

Gregory A. Brent
Division of Endocrinology,
Diabetes, and Hypertension
Departments of Medicine
and Physiology
David Geffen School of Medicine
at UCLA
Los Angeles, CA
USA

ISBN 978-3-319-97763-8 ISBN 978-3-319-97765-2 (eBook)
https://doi.org/10.1007/978-3-319-97765-2

Library of Congress Control Number: 2018964571

This Springer imprint is published by the registered company Springer Nature Switzerland AG
The registered company address is: Gewerbestrasse 11, 6330 Cham, Switzerland

Preface

This inaugural edition of *Endocrine Disorders in Kidney Disease: Diagnosis and Treatment* is dedicated to examining the complex interplay between endocrine and kidney disorders and how this interrelationship impacts patients with chronic kidney disease, including those receiving renal replacement therapy in the form of dialysis and kidney transplantation. Indeed, chronic kidney disease patients are a unique population among whom a myriad of hormonal derangements may exist. While there has been growing appreciation of this important link between endocrinology and nephrology, many endocrine disorders may remain latent and under-recognized among kidney disease patients.

Hence, this scholarly work is the product of a collaborative effort among experts in areas of endocrinology and nephrology in order to provide a comprehensive overview of the most relevant endocrine disorders observed in the chronic kidney disease population. Part 1 entitled *Diabetes, Insulin, Resistance, and the Metabolic Syndrome* presents a practical overview of areas commonly encountered in the clinical management of diabetic kidney disease patients, as well as kidney transplant recipients who develop new onset diabetes. Part 2 entitled *Thyroid Dysfunction* presents innovative themes pertaining to the high prevalence of thyroid dysfunction in kidney disease, including real-world interpretation of thyroid functional derangements and emerging data on thyroid dysfunction and outcomes in the chronic kidney disease population. Part 3 presents highly pertinent information on *Gonadal Disorders*, which include testosterone deficiency and other testicular conditions, as well as amenorrhea and estrogen disorders in the chronic kidney disease population. Also included in this section is a chapter on pregnancy in kidney disease describing maternal, fetal, and obstetric outcomes, as well as general principles of management. Part 4 entitled *Dyslipidemia* provides valuable insights into the vast spectrum of lipid disorders associated with chronic kidney disease and nephrotic syndrome, as well as a rigorous summary of existing evidence and clinical practice guidelines addressing the management of dyslipidemia in kidney disease. Part 5 provides an extensive overview of the full-spectrum of *Mineral Bone Disorders* encountered in kidney disease, including calcium, phosphate, fibroblast growth factor 23, vitamin D, and parathyroid hormone alterations; osteoporosis and osteomalacia; and mineral bone derangements observed in kidney transplantation. Emerging data on *Obesity and Adipokines* in kidney disease are presented in Part 6. Then in Part 7 entitled *Other Pituitary Disorders*, experts in the field describe pituitary disorders in kidney disease including growth hormone disorders and abnormal stature, as well as prolactin, glucocorticoid, and arginine vasopressin derangements. Finally, Part 8 synthesizes many of the aforementioned themes by describing the Multi-System *Implications of Endocrine Derangements in Kidney Disease*, including endocrine derangements in acute kidney injury, as well as the interaction between nutrition and endocrine disorders in kidney disease.

We hope that the insights provided by this scholarly endeavor will engender greater understanding of the magnitude of impact that endocrine disorders have upon the kidney disease population, as well as identification of persistent gaps in knowledge that point toward future areas of investigation, with the overarching goal of improving the health and survival of chronic kidney disease patients. We thank all of our authors for their extraordinary expertise and valuable contributions, as well as the Springer editorial team for their tremendous support, which made the development of this unique textbook and resource possible.

Orange, CA, USA Connie M. Rhee
Orange, CA, USA Kamyar Kalantar-Zadeh
Los Angeles, CA, USA Gregory A. Brent

Contents

Contributors

Masanori Abe Division of Nephrology, Hypertension, and Endocrinology, Department of Internal Medicine, Nihon University School of Medicine, Tokyo, Japan

Amira Al-Uzri Division of Pediatric Kidney Services and Hypertension, Department of Pediatrics, Oregon Health and Science University, Portland, OR, USA

Hatem Amer Division of Nephrology and Hypertension, Department of Internal Medicine, Mayo Clinic, Rochester, MN, USA

Sivakumar Ardhanari Divisions of Nephrology and Cardiovascular Medicine, Department of Medicine, University of Missouri-Columbia School of Medicine, Columbia, MO, USA

Shalender Bhasin Research Program in Men's Health: Aging and Metabolism, Brigham and Women's Hospital/Harvard Medical School, Boston, MA, USA

Gregory A. Brent Division of Endocrinology, Diabetes, and Hypertension, Departments of Medicine and Physiology, David Geffen School of Medicine at UCLA, Los Angeles, CA, USA

Graziano Ceresini Endocrinology of the Development and Aging Unit, Parma University Medical School, Parma, PR, Italy

Harini Chakkera Division of Nephrology, Mayo Clinic, Scottsdale, AZ, USA

Michel Chonchol Division of Renal Diseases and Hypertension, Department of Medicine, University of Colorado Hospital, Aurora, CO, USA

Deborah A. Chon Division of Diabetes, Endocrinology, and Metabolism, David Geffen School of Medicine at UCLA, VA Greater Los Angeles Healthcare System, Los Angeles, CA, USA

Annabelle N. Chua Department of Pediatrics, Duke University School of Medicine, Durham, NC, USA

Curtiss B. Cook Division of Endocrinology, Mayo Clinic College of Medicine, Scottsdale, AZ, USA

Enrico Fiaccadori Renal Failure Unit, Parma University Medical School, Parma, PR, Italy

Anna L. Goldman Research Program in Men's Health: Aging and Metabolism, Brigham and Women's Hospital/Harvard Medical School, Boston, MA, USA

Irl B. Hirsch Division of Metabolism, Endocrinology, and Nutrition, University of Washington School of Medicine, Seattle, WA, USA

Wenyu Huang Division of Endocrinology, Metabolism and Molecular Medicine, Northwestern University Feinberg School of Medicine, Chicago, IL, USA

Kamyar Kalantar-Zadeh Division of Nephrology and Hypertension, Departments of Medicine, Pediatrics, Public Health, and Nursing Sciences, University of California Irvine School of Medicine, Orange, CA, USA

Jessica Kendrick Division of Renal Diseases and Hypertension, Department of Medicine, Denver Health Medical Center and University of Colorado, Denver, CO, USA

Joel Kopple Division of Nephrology, Department of Medicine, Harbor-UCLA Medical Center, Torrance, CA, USA

Csaba P. Kovesdy Division of Nephrology, Department of Medicine, University of Tennessee Health Science Center, Memphis, TN, USA

Holly Kramer Departments of Public Health Sciences and Medicine, Loyola University Medical Center, Maywood, IL, USA

Rajiv Kumar Division of Nephrology and Hypertension, Departments of Internal Medicine, Biochemistry, and Molecular Biology, Mayo Clinic, Rochester, MN, USA

Michela Marina Endocrinology of the Development and Aging Unit, Parma University Medical School, Parma, PR, Italy

Mark E. Molitch Division of Endocrinology, Metabolism, and Molecular Medicine, Northwestern University Feinberg School of Medicine, Chicago, IL, USA

Hamid Moradi Division of Nephrology and Hypertension, University of California Irvine School of Medicine, Orange, CA, USA

Tibor Rubin Veterans Affairs Medical Center, Long Beach, CA, USA

Rashmi S. Mullur Division of Diabetes, Endocrinology, and Metabolism, David Geffen School of Medicine at UCLA, VA Greater Los Angeles Health System, Los Angeles, CA, USA

Joshua J. Neumiller Department of Pharmacotherapy, Washington State University, Spokane, WA, USA

Sagar U. Nigwekar Division of Nephrology, Department of Medicine, Massachusetts General Hospital, Boston, MA, USA

Yoshitsugu Obi Division of Nephrology and Hypertension, University of California Irvine School of Medicine, Orange, CA, USA

Rachael T. Oxman Division of Diabetes, Endocrinology, and Metabolism, David Geffen School of Medicine at UCLA, VA Greater Los Angeles Healthcare System, Los Angeles, CA, USA

Madeleine V. Pahl Division of Nephrology and Hypertension, University of California Irvine School of Medicine, Orange, CA, USA

Vikram Patney Division of Nephrology, Department of Medicine, University of Missouri-Columbia School of Medicine, Columbia, MO, USA

Stephanie Smooke Praw Division of Endocrinology, Diabetes, and Metabolism, Department of Medicine, David Geffen School of Medicine at UCLA, Los Angeles, CA, USA

Connie M. Rhee Division of Nephrology and Hypertension, Departments of Medicine and Public Health, University of California Irvine School of Medicine, Orange, CA, USA

Alice Sabatino Renal Failure Unit, Parma University Medical School, Parma, PR, Italy

Anuja Shah Division of Nephrology and Hypertension, Harbor-UCLA Medical Center, Torrance, CA, USA

Stuart M. Sprague Division of Nephrology and Hypertension, NorthShore University HealthSystem, Evanston, IL, USA

University of Chicago Pritzker School of Medicine, Chicago, IL, USA

Robert C. Stanton Kidney and Hypertension Section, Department of Medicine, Joslin Diabetes Center, Beth Israel Deaconess Medical Center, Harvard Medical School, Boston, MA, USA

Peter Stenvinkel Division of Renal Medicine, Department of Clinical Science, Intervention and Technology, Karolinska Institutet, Stockholm, Sweden

Karolinska University Hospital, Stockholm, Sweden

Dan A. Streja Department of Medicine, David Geffen School of Medicine at UCLA, VA Greater Los Angeles Health Care System, Los Angeles, CA, USA

Elani Streja Division of Nephrology and Hypertension, University of California Irvine School of Medicine, Orange, CA, USA

Tibor Rubin Veterans Affairs Medical Center, Long Beach, CA, USA

Nosratola D. Vaziri Division of Nephrology and Hypertension, University of California Irvine School of Medicine, Orange, CA, USA

Kavitha Vellanki Department of Medicine, Loyola University Medical Center, Maywood, IL, USA

Bradley A. Warady University of Missouri—Kansas City School of Medicine, Kansas City, MO, USA

Division of Pediatric Nephrology, Department of Pediatrics, Children's Mercy Hospital, Kansas City, MO, USA

Jennifer Sue An Way Division of Endocrinology, Metabolism, and Hypertension, Department of Medicine, David Geffen School of Medicine at UCLA, Los Angeles, CA, USA

Jane Eileen Weinreb Division of Endocrinology, Department of Medicine, David Geffen School of Medicine at UCLA, VA Greater Los Angeles Healthcare System, Los Angeles, CA, USA

Rebecca Weiss Department of Endocrinology, Kaiser Permanente—Woodland Hills, Woodland Hills, CA, USA

Adam Whaley-Connell Division of Nephrology, Department of Medicine, University of Missouri-Columbia School of Medicine, Columbia, MO, USA

Research Service, University of Missouri School of Medicine, Harry S. Truman VA Medical Center, Columbia, MO, USA

Jerry Zhong Yu Nephrology Associates Medical Group, Riverside, CA, USA

Part I

Diabetes, Insulin Resistance, and the Metabolic Syndrome

1 Insulin Resistance and the Metabolic Syndrome in Kidney Disease (e.g., the Cardiorenal Metabolic Syndrome)

Vikram Patney, Sivakumar Ardhanari, and Adam Whaley-Connell

Introduction

The metabolic syndrome is a collection of abnormalities that are risk factors for the development of cardiovascular and chronic kidney disease (CKD). While current dogma suggest that obesity is at the core of this constellation of risk factors, the association between blood pressure and diabetes was described as early as 1921 [1–4]. Then during the 1988 Banting lecture, G.M. Reaven suggested that the clustering of risk factors in an individual including high blood pressure, impaired glucose tolerance, and dyslipidemia was associated with coronary artery disease. At that time he grouped these metabolic disorders and referred to them as "syndrome X." He proposed that resistance to insulin-stimulated glucose uptake and compensatory hyperinsulinemia contributed to the development of non-insulin-dependent diabetes mellitus, hypertension, and coronary artery disease [5]. This interest in "syndrome X" became an area of investigative interest for many in the 1990s and early 2000s that ultimately led to a better understanding of the relationship between obesity, insulin resistance, and cardiovascular and kidney disease.

In modern terms, the "metabolic syndrome" refers to a set of physical and laboratory parameters whose co-occurrence in an individual may help clinicians identify the presence of insulin resistance as a chance to intervene early in the course of cardiovascular disease [6, 7]. In addition to syndrome X, other terms that have been used to describe a similar group of risk factors are "insulin resistance syndrome," "dysmetabolic syndrome X," and also "Reaven's syndrome." Since then, a number of organizations have sought to name and define this syndrome including the National Cholesterol Education Program Adult Treatment Panel III (ATP III), World

V. Patney (✉)
Division of Nephrology and Hypertension, Department of Medicine, University of Missouri-Columbia School of Medicine, Columbia, MO, USA
e-mail: patneyv@health.missouri.edu

S. Ardhanari
Division of Nephrology and Hypertension, Department of Medicine, University of Missouri-Columbia School of Medicine, Columbia, MO, USA

Division of Cardiovascular Medicine, University of Missouri-Columbia School of Medicine, Columbia, MO, USA

A. Whaley-Connell
Division of Nephrology and Hypertension, Department of Medicine, University of Missouri-Columbia School of Medicine, Columbia, MO, USA

Division of Cardiovascular Medicine, University of Missouri-Columbia School of Medicine, Columbia, MO, USA

Research Service, University of Missouri School of Medicine, Harry S. Truman VA Medical Center, Columbia, MO, USA

C. M. Rhee et al. (eds.), *Endocrine Disorders in Kidney Disease*,
https://doi.org/10.1007/978-3-319-97765-2_1

Health Organization, American Association of Clinical Endocrinologists, European Group for the Study of Insulin Resistance, and International Diabetes Federation among others. The common criteria for this syndrome consistently rely on the presence of obesity and insulin resistance. It should be noted the central difference between the various organizations in describing the syndrome is in measurement thresholds of insulin resistance, blood pressure, obesity, and/or the presence of microalbuminuria.

There is a well-described relationship between diabetes and CKD; however, over the past decade, there has been considerable interest in the effects of insulin resistance, distinct from that of diabetes, on CKD. Obesity and the presence of the compensatory hyperinsulinemia from insulin resistance have emerged as important contributors to the development of CKD. Thereby in this chapter, we will focus on the importance of the metabolic syndrome and insulin resistance in kidney disease and then review some of the important mechanisms that underlie this relationship [8–12].

Definition(s) of the Cardiorenal Metabolic Syndrome

Over the years, the diagnostic criteria for the identification of the metabolic syndrome have evolved. There have been a number of diagnostic criteria used in the cardiorenal metabolic syndrome to help identify the heightened risk for diabetes, cardiovascular, and, for our discussion, kidney disease. As per Reaven's original description, syndrome X referred to the following risk factors: glucose intolerance, dyslipidemia, and hypertension [5]. Reaven proposed a causative role for insulin resistance. However, his description did not mention central obesity, which is now viewed by most as the unifying feature of the syndrome.

In 1999, a World Health Organization (WHO) diabetes group proposed a definition that included impaired glucose tolerance or diabetes mellitus and/or insulin resistance together with two or more of the following: raised arterial pressure ≥160/90 mmHg, plasma triglycerides >150 mg/dl, HDL <35 mg/dl in men or <9 mg/dl in women, central obesity suggested by waist/hip ratio of >0.90 in men and >0.85 in women and/or BMI >30 kg/m^2, and/or microalbuminuria ≥20 μg/min or albumin/creatinine ratio ≥20 mg/gm [13]. Subsequently, the European Group for the Study of Insulin Resistance suggested some modifications to the WHO definition of metabolic syndrome. They excluded diabetic individuals as the current thought at that time was that there was no simple way to measure insulin resistance and suggested different cutoffs for other criteria [14]. The NCEP:ATP III proposed a definition that focused on facilitating diagnosis and risk reduction for individuals at high risk for cardiovascular disease [15]. The ATP III suggested the diagnosis of metabolic syndrome with the presence of three or more from the following criteria: waist circumference >40 inches in men or >35 inches in women, triglycerides ≥150 mg/dl, high-density lipoprotein cholesterol <40 mg/dl in men or <50 mg/dl in women, blood pressure ≥130/ ≥85 mmHg, and/or fasting glucose ≥100 mg/dl [15].

The existence of multiple definitions of the syndrome resulted in difficulties with comparison and interpretation of data between studies of the syndrome as well as confusion with application for clinical use [16]. It is important to note these groups did not consider in their recommendations ethnic differences in measurements of obesity and especially in waist circumference [16]. To address these concerns, a consensus group panel meeting arranged by the International Diabetes Federation (IDF) in 2004 proposed a "global" definition for use in clinical practice [17]. The working group of the IDF suggests the presence of obesity as measured by waist circumference that had values with ethnicity in mind in addition to two of the following factors: elevated triglycerides (≥150 mg/dl or on treatment), reduced HDL cholesterol (<50 mg/dl in females and <40 mg/dl in males), raised blood pressure (≥130 mmHg systolic or ≥85 mmHg diastolic or on treatment for hypertension), and fasting plasma glucose (fasting glucose ≥100 mg/dl or diagnosis of diabetes) [17]. Waist circumference cutoffs based on ethnicity included (1) Europoids, sub-Saharan Africans,

Eastern Mediterranean, and Middle East (Arab) populations, ≥94 cm for men and ≥80 cm for women; (2) South Asians, Chinese, Ethnic South, and Central Americans, ≥90 cm for men and ≥80 cm for women; and (3) Japanese, ≥85 cm for men and ≥90 cm for women [17].

Epidemiology of the Cardiorenal Metabolic Syndrome

The prevalence of metabolic syndrome varies with the diagnostic criteria used, region studied, as well as age and ethnicity of the population. In 2010, based on data from the National Health and Nutrition Examination Survey (NHANES), the age-adjusted prevalence of the cardiorenal metabolic syndrome in the adult US population was estimated to be ~23% [18]. The study utilized waist circumference cutoffs of ≥40 inches for men and ≥35 inches for women based on the ATP III definition while utilizing the cutoffs from the IDF definition for the other criteria. The use of more generous cutoffs for defining abdominal obesity may have led to an underestimation of that parameter in the US population. Comparison of the data from 1999 to 2000 and 2009 to 2010 revealed an improving trend for metabolic syndrome, blood pressure, triglycerides, and HDL cholesterol and a worrisome increasing trend in hyperglycemia and waist circumference. The improvement in blood pressure and lipid trends was thought to have corresponded to increases in awareness and incorporation of antihypertensive and lipid-lowering therapies [18]. Hispanic-American adults, especially females, have a higher prevalence compared to other US racial subgroups [18]. In an epidemiological study of 1800 adults in an urban population in India, the prevalence of the syndrome was ~13% [19]. Further, in another population, a cross-sectional study in the Guangdong province of South China using the NCEP:ATP III criteria showed an unadjusted prevalence of ~27% [20]. Along with other risk factors such as hypertension and diabetes, it is important to note the prevalence of the syndrome increases with age until 70 years and then declines [21].

While it is clear the cardiorenal metabolic syndrome is highly prevalent, there is sufficient additional evidence to support an association between insulin resistance and CKD. Observational data from NHANES III support a direct correlational relationship between insulin resistance and both the presence of microalbuminuria and overt CKD [11, 22]. Important in these observational data is the ability to distinguish between insulin resistance or overt diabetes and development of CKD. It is important to note then that insulin resistance has been documented in a nondiabetic population in early stages of CKD as well as in more advanced stages [12]. In one prospective cohort, the Atherosclerosis Risk in Communities (ARIC) study, there was an increased risk for the development of CKD in nondiabetics that met the definition of the syndrome. This occurred independent of baseline confounders such as diabetes and hypertension and even with their development over the duration of the study [9]. Additional data from the Framingham Heart Study support that in a cohort of individuals without diabetes followed over 7 years, insulin resistance was significantly associated with development of CKD following adjustments for confounders [10]. These collective data suggest a trend has emerged between CKD and the cardiorenal metabolic syndrome irrespective of overt diabetes.

The Cardiorenal Metabolic Syndrome and CKD

The syndrome is associated with an increase in risk for myocardial infarction, cardiovascular mortality, and stroke as well as all-cause mortality [23]. The presence of the cardiorenal metabolic syndrome has been associated with a greater risk for type 2 diabetes [24] and independently increases the risk of microalbuminuria and incident CKD [25, 26]. Hence, the presence of metabolic syndrome in one out of every four to five adults provides an opportunity to identify and treat risk factors that predispose to type 2 diabetes, CKD, as well as all-cause CKD-associated mortality. In this context, there has been much interest in the presence of microalbuminuria or albuminuria as a risk predictor or as an actual outcome of the metabolic derangements associated with the cardiorenal metabolic syndrome. There have been a number of population level studies that have included microalbuminuria in nondiabetics with CKD to evaluate risk in this syndrome [27–30]. Further, microalbuminuria is an independent, modifiable predictor of risk and largely considered a marker of generalized endothelial dysfunction [31].

The contribution that visceral adiposity has to these metabolic-induced vascular abnormalities includes insulin resistance, lipoprotein abnormalities, as well as promotion of a pro-inflammatory/pro-oxidative milieu that induces systemic hemodynamic changes [32, 33]. While overweight/obesity status, sedentary lifestyle, as well as genetics predispose to these risks, a unifying mechanism is difficult to elucidate and is likely a conglomerate of factors [34]. Numerous metabolic abnormalities have been suggested that explain the association between obesity, insulin resistance, and albuminuria of which the most significant ones are inappropriate activation of the sympathetic nervous system (SNS) and renin-angiotensin-aldosterone system (RAAS) and the diminishing actions of protective cytokines [35]. Excessive visceral adipose tissue in obese individuals is a well-known source for pro-inflammatory adipokines which promote insulin resistance [35]. The resulting hyperinsulinemic state in addition to obesity-induced kidney structural and functional changes then potentiates glomerulosclerosis and thickening of glomerular basement membrane in animal models [35]. The following are some of the mechanisms thought to contribute to increased risk of CKD in individuals with the metabolic syndrome.

Insulin Resistance/Hyperinsulinemia

Insulin helps control energy homeostasis by facilitating the glucose uptake and glycogen storage in the liver and skeletal muscle tissue. In addition, insulin stimulates the storage of lipids as triglycerides in adipose tissue [36]. Insulin binds and activates the insulin receptor tyrosine kinase in skeletal muscle [36]. This leads to phosphorylation of insulin receptor substrate-1 (IRS-1) which then binds and activates phosphatidylinositol 3-kinase (PI3K) [36]. PI3K then promotes translocation of glucose transporter type 4 (GLUT4) to the plasma membrane, thereby leading to glucose uptake [36]. Impaired insulin metabolic signaling in the skeletal muscle, liver, and adipose tissue due to reduced binding or phosphorylation of its receptor, decreased tyrosine kinase activity, and impaired phosphorylation of IRS proteins contributes to insulin resistance [36]. The persistent excess insulin levels eventually lead to impairments in renal hemodynamics contributing to an elevation of glomerular filtration rate (e.g., hyperfiltration) in experimental studies [37, 38]. The state of hyperinsulinemia in these insulin-resistant individuals also contributes to salt sensitivity and thereby increased glomerular pressure, hyperfiltration, and overtime maladaptive structural remodeling that leads to albuminuria in diabetes [39]. The contribution then of insulin excess to vascular homeostasis is a critical link to understanding the underpinning of insulin resistance to the intrarenal hemodynamic changes that lead to CKD. There is clear data regarding the impact of insulin resistance/hyperinsulinemia in vasoconstriction activity through activation of vascular sympathetic tone through catecholamine secretion [40]. Bioavailable nitric oxide (NO) is regulated, in part, by insulin through stimulation of PI3K signaling pathways in impaired vascular tissue in the insulin-resistant state. The alterations in vascular tone contribute not only to the development of vasoconstriction and hypertension but also lead to glomerular hypertension and albuminuria.

Not only does excess insulin over time contribute to the vascular abnormalities that induce endothelial dysfunction, but excess insulin contributes to vascular cell proliferation, mesangial expansion, along with extracellular matrix deposition that promotes tubulointerstitial fibrosis [41]. The actions of insulin in this capacity can occur either directly by insulin or occur in conjunction with other growth factors such as insulin-like growth factor (IGF)-1 and transforming growth factor-β (TGF-β). IGF-1 has similar effects to insulin on the vasculature but also promotes mesangial cell and glomerular expansion [42]. Insulin has been shown to produce TGF-β in both proximal tubular and mesangial cells which in turn lead to glomerular and tubulointerstitial extracellular matrix expansion and fibrosis [43].

Inflammatory Cytokines

Increased accumulation of macrophages has been seen in adipose tissue of obese individuals. (45) Visceral adipose tissue in obesity expresses increased amounts of pro-inflammatory molecules as well as procoagulant proteins [44]. Further, increased adipocyte macrophages are thought to produce several of these pro-inflammatory molecules and have been shown to decrease insulin sensitivity and increase lipolysis and hepatic triglyceride secretion [45]. Leptin is an adipocyte-derived hormone with structure similar to the cytokine IL-2 and is thought to mediate energy balance through its actions on the hypothalamus [46]. Obese individuals with metabolic syndrome display elevations in circulating leptin and are resistant to the central neurologic effects of leptin that decrease appetite and increase energy expenditure [47]. This promotes maintenance of excess weight and helps amplify the consequences [46]. Findings in the West of Scotland Coronary Prevention Study (WOSCOPS) suggested that elevated leptin levels are independently associated with increased risk of coronary artery disease [48]. In this study higher leptin levels correlated strongly with C-reactive protein (CRP) in individuals who had a coronary event, suggesting then there exists a chronic low-grade inflammation that may increase the risk for cardiovascular disease [48].

A study of data from the third National Health and Nutrition Examination Survey (NHANES III) looked at the presence of inflammation in patients with the syndrome and varying levels of kidney function [49]. This study found that an increase in number of component conditions of metabolic syndrome increased the odds of inflammation as measured by CRP levels at various levels of kidney function [49]. While this suggests an association, direct causation has not been proved. Adiponectin is a polypeptide that is produced by adipose tissue that exhibits properties that are insulin sensitizing along with anti-inflammatory and antioxidant [50]. In this context, low adiponectin levels are associated with insulin resistance, cardiovascular disease, as well as kidney disease in obese individuals [51]. It has been shown that urine albumin excretion is inversely related to adiponectin levels in obese individuals [52] and regulates albuminuria and podocyte function in mice [53]. The MDRD study showed that each 1 μg/ml increase in adiponectin increased risk of cardiovascular mortality by 6% [54]. The cause of this paradoxical relationship in patients with CKD is unclear.

Inappropriate Activation of the RAAS

The RAAS is a complex and widely studied topic well known for its central role in the regulation of blood pressure, kidney blood flow, and sodium and water regulation. The RAAS pathway encompasses several peptides and enzymes. Angiotensin II has long been considered to be the predominant effector peptide of the RAAS to exert its maladaptive effects via the angiotensin II receptor type I. However, recently several other effector molecules have been identified at the tissue level establishing the existence of both circulatory and tissue-based RAAS in several non-kidney tissues including the brain, heart, adipose tissue, and pancreas [55]. Additionally, there have been a number of observations that highlight the tissue level RAAS functions independent of the systemic RAAS.

Angiotensin II levels in the kidneys are several fold higher than the systemic levels [56], and angiotensin receptor blockade contributes to a disproportionately higher vasodilation despite low plasma renin activity [57]. Further, in the obese, insulin-resistant individual, persistently elevated insulin levels lead to activation of SNS and RAAS along with obesity-induced physical compression of kidneys that collectively contribute to increased renal tubular sodium reabsorption, volume expansion, and hypertension [58].

When considering the salt retention and hyperfiltration and the systemic activation of the RAAS, this is then inappropriate.

It is well known angiotensin II increases glomerular pressure and induces intrarenal inflammatory cytokines and growth factors that contribute to development of albuminuria [59, 60]. Angiotensin II is also shown to stimulate proliferation of mesangial cells, glomerular endothelial cells, and fibroblasts [60]. Additionally, there has recent interest in excess aldosterone in promotion of altered insulin signaling and its contribution to hypertension and kidney structural and functional abnormalities independent to that of angiotensin II [61, 62].

Inappropriate activation of the RAAS is associated with cardiovascular and kidney diseases. Recently, an abnormally hyperactive RAAS has also been implicated in pathogenesis of metabolic syndrome [63–66]. Hyperactive systemic RAAS and adipose tissue RAAS has been associated with human obesity and various other animal obesity models [67]. The common link also extends to hyperglycemia, hypertension, and cortisol that are associated with activation of RAAS and also are risk factors for metabolic syndrome [68]. Recently, specific polymorphisms in RAAS have been linked to the development of the syndrome [69].

Patients with diabetes demonstrate hyperglycemia either secondary to impaired secretion of insulin or decreased sensitivity to insulin. The resultant hyperglycemia is associated with activation of RAAS at the tissue level. In rodent models, Singh et al. demonstrated that hyperglycemia is associated with an increase in angiotensinogen and angiotensin I ultimately resulting in an increased mesangial angiotensin II. They also demonstrated other angiotensin-related peptides (angiotensin 1–9, angiotensin 1–7, and angiotensin 3–8) and also that hyperglycemia facilitates the conversion of mesangial angiotensin 1–9 to angiotensin II [70]. Zhang et al. proved that these are mediated through the stimulatory effect of hyperglycemia on angiotensinogen gene expression in the renal proximal tubular cells and on a molecular level at least partly through the activation of protein kinase C independent, p38 mitogen-activated protein kinase signal transduction pathway [71]. There is also a role for succinate stimulating the novel metabolic receptor GPR91 behind the mechanism of RAAS activation in hyperglycemia [72]. Similar observations of increased angiotensin II levels in the cardiac myocytes leading to cardiomyocyte apoptosis and fibrosis have been made [73].

Both animal and human experiments have proven the ability of RAAS inhibition to improve hyperglycemia. In human studies, angiotensin receptor blockade improves beta-cell function and insulin sensitivity and reduces the progression to overt diabetes [74, 75]. In another study, although angiotensin-converting enzyme (ACE) inhibition did not reduce the incidence of diabetes, it demonstrated increased regression to normoglycemia [76]. These observations elucidate the causal link of RAAS in causing hyperglycemia and the ability to regress toward normoglycemia with its inhibition [77].

Increased adipose tissue is the hallmark of obesity, and it is an integral part of metabolic syndrome, impaired glucose tolerance, and diabetes [78]. The decreased insulin sensitivity of obesity has been well known for its association with hyperglycemia, and RAAS inhibition results in decreased incidence of hyperglycemia. There is also strong evidence that obesity activates both systemic and tissue RAAS emphasizing it as a unifying mechanism in the cardiorenal metabolic syndrome. Adipose tissue is regarded as an autocrine organ with presence of all the components of RAAS [79]. Typically angiotensinogen is synthesized by the liver in lean individuals, but in obese individuals adipose tissue is an important source [80]. After the above described cascade of reactions, the final effector molecule angiotensin II acts locally to mediate fat mass expansion via angiotensin II receptor (AT_1R) types 1 and 2, by decreasing lipolysis and increasing lipogenesis, respectively. About one-third of the circulating angiotensinogen is contributed by adipose tissue and is to be considered as an autocrine and more recently an endocrine organ [81].

Patients with obesity demonstrate several abnormalities including increased circulating levels of angiotensinogen, renin, ACE, and angiotensin II and increased adipose tissue levels of renin, ACE, and angiotensin II expression [67, 82]. These abnormalities tend to improve or resolve with weight loss [83]. There is some discrepancy from animal models of obesity that revealed that these relationships could be strain specific. There is also evidence that systemic RAAS stimulation results in weight loss in contrast to the stimulation of the adipose tissue RAAS that causes weight gain [81, 84]. These facts highlight the complexity of the pathology behind the syndrome. Overall, the consensus is that both systemic and tissue RAAS are overactive in humans with obesity. RAAS inhibition has been demonstrated to have reduced obesity in hypertensive obese humans [85].

Endothelial Dysfunction

The endothelium is composed of a single layer of cells lining the luminal surface of the vasculature and plays a central role in vascular tone. This is primarily mediated by the local production of nitric oxide (NO). Endothelial NO synthase, an enzyme, and tetrahydrobiopterin, a cofactor, facilitate the reaction that leads to synthesis of NO from L-arginine. Mechanical shear stress is the most important stimulus for eNOS [86]. Several other chemical mediators like bradykinin and adenosine mediate nonmechanical stimulation of eNOS [87]. NO diffuses into the vascular smooth muscle activating guanylate cyclase and resulting in a c-GMP-mediated vasodilation. Beyond vasomotor regulation, a normal endothelium is important in prevention of atherosclerosis through regulation of smooth muscle cell proliferation and vessel wall inflammation, cellular adhesion, and even resistance to thrombus formation [88]. Endothelial function is assessed by endothelium-dependent vasodilation, markers of activation, and damage [89]. Assessment of endothelium-dependent vasodilation is done by the degree of vasodilation in response to nitric oxide, the local levels of which can be increased pharmacologically or mechanically. Endothelial activation and damage occur with the inflammation of the endothelium with excess circulating levels of factors such as soluble intercellular adhesion molecule, von Willebrand factor, plasminogen activator inhibitor-1 (PAI-1), and CRP [88, 90–93].

The hallmark of a diseased endothelium is decreased NO and impaired vasodilation. This can result from reduced NO production or increased destruction of NO by reactive oxygen species [88]. Diabetes or impaired glucose intolerance, dyslipidemia, and hypertension are independent risk factors for endothelial dysfunction [94–97]. This is explained by the presence of impaired endothelium-dependent vasodilation [94, 98, 99] and increased levels of various markers in circulation as described above [100–102]. Metabolic syndrome is a clinical entity that is a result of clustering of several of the above risk factors. This translates to a proportionally greater magnitude of the biochemical abnormality [103] and greater cardiovascular risk [98]. The overall endothelial dysfunction leads to leaky capillaries in the kidneys giving rise to microalbuminuria that has elevated microalbuminuria as a diagnostic criterion to define metabolic syndrome [13]. In patients with metabolic syndrome, several interventions including dietary alterations, physical exercise, and treatment of diabetes, dyslipidemia, and hypertension are associated with improvement in the markers of endothelial dysfunction [89, 100, 104].

Conclusions and Perspectives

The relationship between diabetes and CKD and CKD-related outcomes is well established. However, the impact that insulin resistance and hyperinsulinemia has on cardiorenal risk and progressive kidney dysfunction is emerging and as important as the effects of hyperglycemia derived from overt diabetes. There is strong population level data to support this association and equally strong experimental data to support this relationship. The various mechanisms that excess insulin has on fat-derived adipokines, inflammation, oxidative stress, and inappropriate activation of the RAAS and SNS collectively lead to impaired renal hemodynamics and downstream vascular proliferation, extracellular matrix deposition, and fibrosis. There is further need to understand the impact of insulin resistance and hyperinsulinemia on kidney disease. While the impact that interruption of the RAAS has on CKD is clear, the effect of non-pharmacological measures such as physical activity and weight reduction, along with pharmacological interventions such as insulin-sensitizing agents, is less clear.

References

1. Sarafadis PA, Nilsson PM. The metabolic syndrome: a glance at its history. J Hypertens. 2006;24(4):621–6.
2. Hitzenberger K. Uber den Blutdruck bei diabetes mellitus. Wiener Arch Innere Med. 1921;2:461–6.
3. Kylin E. Hypertonie and Zuckerkrankheit. Zentralblatt fur Innere Medizin. 1921;42:873–7.
4. Maranon G. Uber Hypertonie and Zuckerkrankheit. Zentralblatt fur Innere Medizin. 1923;43:169–76.
5. Reaven GM. Role of insulin resistance in human disease. Diabetes. 1988;37:1595–607.
6. Facchiini FS, et al. Insulin resistance as a predictor of age-related diseases. J Clin Endocrinol Metab. 2001;86(8):3574–8.
7. Yip J, Facchini FS, Reaven GM. Resistance to insulin-mediated glucose disposal as a predictor of cardiovascular disease. J Clin Endocrinol Metab. 1998;83(8):2773–6.
8. Whaley-Connell A, et al. Overnutrition and the cardiorenal syndrome: use of a rodent model to examine mechanisms. Cardiorenal Med. 2011;1:23–30.
9. Kurella M, Lo JC, Chertow GM. Metabolic syndrome and the risk for chronic kidney disease among nondiabetic adults. J Am Soc Nephrol. 2005;16(7):2134–40.
10. Fox CS, et al. Glycemic status and development of kidney disease: the Framingham heart study. Diabetes Care. 2005;28(10):2436–40.
11. Chen J, Muntner P, Hamm LL, et al. The metabolic syndrome and chronic kidney disease in US adults. Ann Intern Med. 2004;28(10):167–74.
12. Fliser D, Pacini G, Enelleiter R, et al. Insulin resistance and hyperinsulinemia are already present in patients with incipient renal disease. Kidney Int. 1998;53(5):1343–7.
13. Alberti KGMM, ZImmet PZ. Definition, diagnosis and classification of diabetes mellitus and its complications Part 1: diagnosis and classification of diabetes mellitus provisional report of WHO a consultation. Diabet Med. 1998;15:539–53.
14. Balkau B, Charles MA, for the European Group for the Study of Insulin Resistance (EGIR). Comment on the provisional report from the WHO consultation. Diabet Med. 1999;16(5):442–3.
15. Cleeman JI, et al. Executive summary of the third report of the National Cholesterol Education Program (NCEP) expert panel on detection, evaluation, and treatment of high blood cholesterol in adults (adult treatment panel III). J Am Med Assoc. 2001;285(19):2486–97.
16. Alberti K, Zimmet P, Shaw J. The metabolic syndrome- a new worldwide definition. Lancet. 2005;366:1059–61.
17. The International Diabetes Federation. The IDF worldwide definition of the metabolic syndrome. The IDF consensus worldwide definition of the Metabolic Syndrome. [Online] 2005. http://www.idf.org/webdata/docs/IDF_Meta_def_final.pdf.
18. Beltran-Sanchez H, et al. Prevalence and trends of metabolic syndrome in the adult U.S. population, 1999-2010. J Am Coll Cardiol. 2013;62(8):697–703.
19. Gupta A, et al. Prevalence of diabetes, impaired fasting glucose and insulin resistance syndrome in an urban Indian population. Diabetes Res Clin Pract. 2003;61:69–76.
20. Li J-B, et al. Metabolic syndrome: prevalence and risk factors in southern China. J Int Med Res. 2010;38:1142–8.
21. Ford ES, Giles WH, Dietz WH. Prevalence of the metabolic syndrome among US adults. JAMA. 2002;287(3):356–9.
22. Chen J, Muntner P, Hamm LL, et al. Insulin resistance and risk of chronic kidney disease in nondiabetic US adults. J Am Soc Nephrol. 2003;14(2):469–77.
23. Mottillo S, et al. The metabolic syndrome and cardiovascular risk. J Am Coll Cardiol. 2010;56(14):1113–32.
24. Wilson PWF, et al. Metabolic syndrome as a precursor of cardiovascular disease and type 2 diabetes mellitus. Circulation. 2005;112:3066–72.
25. Hoenher CM, et al. Association of the insulin resistance syndrome and microalbuminuria among nondiabetic Native Americans. The Inter-Tribal Heart Project. J Am Soc Nephrol. 2002;13:1626–34.
26. Cheng J, et al. The metabolic syndrome and chronic kidney disease in U.S. adults. Ann Intern Med. 2004;140(3):167–74.
27. Mykannen L, et al. Microalbuminuria is associated with insulin resistance in nondiabetic subjects: the insulin resistance atherosclerosis study. Diabetes. 1998;47(5):793–800.
28. Hoehner CM, et al. Association of the insulin resistance syndrome and microalbuminuria among nondiabetic Native Americans. The Inter-Tribal Heart Project et al. J Am Soc Nephrol. 2002;13(6):1626–34.
29. Palaniappan L, Carnetheon M, Fortmann S. P. Association between microalbuminuria and the metabolic syndrome: NHANES III. Am J Hypertens. 2003;16(11 Pt 1):952–8.
30. Fujikawa R, et al. Insulin resistance precedes the appearance of albuminuria in non-diabetic subjects: 6 year follow up study. Diabetes Res Clin Pract. 2001;53(2):99–106.
31. Abuaisha B, et al. Relationship of elevated urinary albumin excretion to components of the metabolic syndrome in non-insulin-dependent diabetes mellitus. Diabetes Res Clin Pract. 1998;39(2):93–9.

32. Ballantyne CM, et al. Metabolic syndrome risk of cardiovascular disease and diabetes in the ARIC study. Int J Obes. 2008;32(Suppl 2):S21–4.
33. Wahba IM, Mak RH. Obesity and obesity-initiated metabolic syndrome: mechanistic links to chronic kidney disease. Clin J Am Soc Nephrol. 2007;2(3):550–62.
34. Bagby SP. Obesity-initiated metabolic syndrome and the kidney: a recipe for chronic kidney disease. J Am Soc Nephrol. 2004;15(11):2775–91.
35. Whaley-Connell A, Johnson MS, Sowers JR. Aldosterone: role in cardiometabolic syndrome and resistant hypertension. Prog Cardiovasc Dis. 2010;52(5):401–9.
36. Cusumano AM, Bodkin NL, Hansen BC, et al. Glomerular hypertrophy is associated with hyperinsulinemia and precedes overt diabetes in aging rhesus monkeys. Am J Kidney Dis. 2002;40(5):1075–85.
37. Shulman GI. Ectopic fat in insulin resistance, dyslipidemia, and cardiometabolic disease. N Engl J Med. 2014;371(12):1131–41.
38. Morino K, et al. Regulation of mitochondrial biogenesis by lipoprotein lipase in muscle of insulin-resistant offspring of parents with type 2 diabetes. Diabetes. 2012;61:877–87.
39. Shulman GI, et al. Mitochondrial dysfunction in the elderly: possible role in insulin resistance. Science. 2003;300:1140–1.
40. Cohen AJ, McCarthy DM, Stoff JS. Direct hemodynamic effect of insulin in the isolated perfused kidney. Am J Physiol. 1989;257(4 Pt 2):F580–5.
41. Dengel DR, et al. Insulin resistance, elevated glomerular filtration fraction, and renal injury. Hypertension. 1996;28(1):127–32.
42. Catalano C, Muscelli E, Quinones Galvan A, et al. Effect of insulin on systemic and renal handling of albumin in nondiabetic and NIDDM subjects. Diabetes. 1997;46(5):868–75.
43. McFarlane SI, Banerji M, Sowers JR. Insulin resistance and cardiovascular disease. J Clin Endocrinol Metab. 2001;86(2):713–8.
44. Young BA, Johnson RJ, Alpers CE, et al. Cellular events in the evolution of experimental diabetic nephropathy. Kidney Int. 1995;47(3):935–44.
45. Conti FJ, et al. Studies on binding and mitogenic effect of insulin and insulin-like growth factor I in glomerular mesangial cells. Endocrinology. 1988;122(6):2788–95.
46. Anderson PW, Zhang XY, Tian J, et al. Insulin and Angiotensin II are additive in stimulating TGF-beta 1 and matrix mRNAs in mesangial cells. Kidney Int. 1996;50(3):745–53.
47. Weisberg SP, et al. Obesity is associated with macrophage accumulation in adipose tissue. J Clin Invest. 2003;112(12):1796–808.
48. Nonogaki K, et al. Interleukin-6 stimulates hepatic triglyceride secretion in rats. Endocrinology. 1995;136:2143–9.
49. Wisse BE. The inflammatory syndrome: the role of adipose tissue cytokines in metabolic disorders linked to obesity. J Am Soc Nephrol. 2004;15:2792–800.
50. Flier JS. Obesity wars: molecular progress confronts an expanding epidemic. Cell. 2004;116(2):337–50.
51. Lord G. Role of leptin in immunology. Nutr Rev. 2002;60(Suppl):S35–S8.
52. Wallace AM, et al. Plasma leptin and the risk of cardiovascular disease in the west of Scotland coronary prevention study (WOSCOPS). Circulation. 2001;104:3052–6.
53. Beddhu S, et al. Associations of metabolic syndrome with inflammation in CKD: results from the third National Health and nutrition examination survey (NHANES III). Am J Kidney Dis. 2005;46(4):577–86.
54. Maury E, Brichard SM. Adipokine dysregulation, adipose tissue inflammation and metabolic syndrome. Mol Cell Endocrinol. 2010;314:1–16.
55. Sweiss N, Sharma K. Adiponectin effects on the kidney. Best Pract Res Clin Endocrinol Metab. 2014;28:71–9.
56. Yano Y, Hoshide S, Ishikawa J, et al. Differential impacts of adiponectin on low-grade albuminuria between obese and nonobese individuals without diabetes. J Clin Hypertens. 2007;9(10):775–82.
57. Sharma K, Ramachandrarao S, Qiu G, et al. Adiponectin regulates albuminuria and podocyte function in mice. J Clin Invest. 2008;118(5):1645–56.
58. Jia T, et al. The complex role of adiponectin in chronic kidney disease. Biochimie. 2012;94:2150–6.
59. Menon V, et al. Adiponectin and mortality in patients with chronic kidney disease. J Am Soc Nephrol. 2006;17:2599–606.
60. Paul M, Poyan Mehr A, Kreutz R. Physiology of local renin-angiotensin systems. Physiol Rev. 2006;86(3):747–803.
61. Seikaly MG, Arant BS Jr, Seney FD Jr. Endogenous angiotensin concentrations in specific intrarenal fluid compartments of the rat. J Clin Invest. 1990;86(4):1352–7.
62. Price DA, et al. The paradox of the low-renin state in diabetic nephropathy. J Am Soc Nephrol. 1999;10(11):2382–91.
63. Hall JE, Henegar JR, Dwyer TM, et al. Is obesity a major cause of chronic kidney disease? Adv Ren Replace Ther. 2004;11(1):41–54.
64. Ruster C, Wolf G. Renin-angiotensin-aldosterone system and progression of renal disease. J Am Soc Nephrol. 2006;17(11):2985–91.
65. Wolf G, Neilson EG. Angiotensin II induces cellular hypertrophy in cultured murine proximal tubular cells. Am J Physiol. 1990;259(5 Pt 2):F768–77.
66. Rodriguez-Vita J, et al. Angiotensin II activates the Smad pathway in vascular smooth muscle cells by a transforming growth factor-beta-independent mechanism. Circulation. 2005;111(19):2509–17.
67. Sarzani R, et al. Renin-angiotensin system, natriuretic peptides, obesity, metabolic syndrome, and hypertension: an integrated view in humans. J Hypertens. 2008;26(5):831–43.
68. de Kloet AD, Krause EG, Woods SC. The renin angiotensin system and the metabolic syndrome. Physiol Behav. 2010;100(5):525–34.

69. Putnam K, et al. The renin-angiotensin system: a target of and a contributor to dyslipidemias, altered glucose homeostasis, and hypertension of the metabolic syndrome. Am J Physiol Heart Circ Physiol. 2012;302(6):H1219–30.
70. Kishi T, Hirooka Y. Sympathoexcitation associated with renin-angiotensin system in metabolic syndrome. Int J Hypertens. 2013;2013:406897.
71. Kalupahana PS, Moustaid-Moussa N. The renin-angiotensin system: the link between obesity, inflammation and insulin resistance. Obes Rev. 2012;13(2):136–49.
72. Skov J, et al. Tissue renin-angiotensin systems: a unifying hypothesis of metabolic disease. Front Endocrinol. 2014;5:23.
73. Herrera CL, et al. Association of polymorphisms within the renin-angiotensin system with metabolic syndrome in a cohort of Chilean subjects. Arch Endocrinol Metab. 2016;60(3):190–8.
74. Singh R, et al. Mechanism of increased angiotensin II levels in glomerular mesangial cells cultured in high glucose. J Am Soc Nephrol. 2003;14(4):873–80.
75. Zhang SL, et al. High levels of glucose stimulate angiotensinogen gene expression via the p38 mitogen-activated protein kinase pathway in rat kidney proximal tubular cells. Endocrinology. 2000;141(12):4637–46.
76. Peti-Peterdi J. High glucose and renin release: the role of succinate and GPR91. Kidney Int. 2010;78(12):1214–7.
77. Singh VP, et al. High glucose induced regulation of intracellular ANG II synthesis and nuclear redistribution in cardiac myocytes. Am J Physiol Heart Circ Physiol. 2007;293(2):H939–48.
78. van der Zijl NJ, et al. Valsartan improves {Beta}-cell function and insulin sensitivity in subjects with impaired glucose metabolism: a randomized controlled trial. Diabetes Care. 2011;34(4):845–51.
79. The Navigator Study Group. Effect of valsartan on the incidence of diabetes and cardiovascular events. N Engl J Med. 2010;362(16):1477–90.
80. The Dream trial investigators. Effect of ramipril on the incidence of diabetes. N Engl J Med. 2006;355(15):1551–62.
81. Scheen AJ. Renin-angiotensin system inhibition prevents type 2 diabetes mellitus. Part 1. A meta-analysis of randomised clinical trials. Diabetes Metab. 2004;30(6):487–96.
82. Yvan-Charvet L, Quignard-Boulange A. Role of adipose tissue with renin-angiotensin system and inflammatory diseases associated with obesity. Kidney Int. 2011;79(2):162–8.
83. Engeli S, et al. The adipose tissue renin-angiotensin system: role in the metabolic syndrome? Int J Biochem Cell Biol. 2003;35(6):807–25.
84. Yasue S, et al. Adipose tissue-specific regulation of angiotensinogen in obese humans and mice: impact of nutritional status and adipocyte hypertrophy. Am J Hypertens. 2010;23(4):425–31.
85. Massiera F, et al. Adipose angiotensinogen is involved in adipose tissue growth and blood pressure regulation. FASEB J. 2001;15(14):2727–9.
86. Gorzelniak K, et al. Hormonal regulation of the human adipose-tissue angiotensin system: relationship to obesity and hypertension. J Hypertens. 2002;20(5):965–73.
87. Engeli S, et al. Weight loss and the renin-angiotensin-aldosterone system. Hypertension. 2005;45(3):356–62.
88. Cassis S, et al. Angiotensin II regulates oxygen consumption. Am J Physiol Regul Integr Comp Physiol. 2002;282(2):R445–53.
89. Fogari R, et al. Comparison of the effects of valsartan and Felodipine on plasma leptin and insulin sensitivity in hypertensive obese patients. Hypertens Res. 2005;28(3):209–14.
90. Corson MA, et al. Phosphorylation of endothelial nitric oxide synthase in response to fluid shear stress. Circ Res. 1996;79(5):984–91.
91. Govers R, Rabelink TJ. Cellular regulation of endothelial nitric oxide synthase. Am J Physiol Renal Physiol. 2001;280(2):F193–206.
92. Deanfield JE, Halcox JP, Rabelink TJ. Endothelial function and dysfunction: testing and clinical relevance. Circulation. 2007;115(10):1285–95.
93. Tziomalos K, et al. Endothelial dysfunction in metabolic syndrome: prevalence, pathogenesis, and management. Nutr Metab Cardiovasc Dis. 2010;20(2):140–6.
94. Barac A, Campia U, Panza JA. Methods for evaluating endothelial function in humans. Hypertension. 2007;49(4):748–60.
95. Festa A, et al. Relative contribution of insulin and its precursors to fibrinogen and PAI-1 in a study (IRAS). Arterioscler Thromb Vasc Biol. 1999;19(3):562–8.
96. Potter van loon BJ, et al. The cardiovascular risk factor plasminogen activator inhibitor type 1 is related to insulin resistance. Metabolism. 1993; 42(8):945–9.
97. Bahia L, et al. Relationship between adipokines, inflammation, and vascular reactivity in lean controls and obese subjects with metabolic syndrome. Clinics (Sao Paulo). 2006;61(5):433–40.
98. Benjamin EJ, et al. Clinical correlates and heritability of flow-mediated dilation in the community: the Framingham Heart Study. Circulation. 2004;109(5):613–9.
99. McVeigh GE, et al. Impaired endothelium-dependent and independent vasodilation in patients with type 2 (non-insulin-dependent) diabetes mellitus. Diabetologia. 1992;35(8):771–6.
100. Panza JA, et al. Abnormal endothelium-dependent vascular relaxation in patients with essential hypertension. N Engl J Med. 1990;323(1):22–7.
101. Williams SB, et al. Impaired nitric-oxide mediated vasodilation in patients with non-insulin dependent diabetes mellitus. J Am College Cardiol. 1996;27(3):567–74.

102. Hamburg NM, et al. Metabolic syndrome, insulin resistance, and brachial artery vasodilator function in Framingham offspring participants without clinical evidence of cardiovascular disease. Am J Cardiol. 2008;101(1):82–8.
103. Lteif AA, Han K, Mather KJ. Obesity, insulin resistance and the metabolic syndrome: determinants of endothelial dysfunction in whites and blacks. Circulation. 2005;112(1):32–8.
104. Blanco-Colio LM, et al. Elevated ICAM-1, MCP-1 plasma levels in subjects at high cardiovascular risk are diminished by atorvastatin treatment. Atorvastatin on inflammatory markers study: a subsidy of achieve targets fast with atorvastatin stratified titration. Am Heart J. 2007;153(5):881–8.

Diabetic Kidney Disease

2

Robert C. Stanton

Epidemiology

Chronic kidney disease (CKD) is growing at an epidemic rate throughout the world. The major causes are diabetes and hypertension. CKD from both diabetes and hypertension have been increasing for over 20 years, but the increase in diabetic kidney disease (DKD) has been significantly more rapid [1]. The best way to appreciate the epidemic rise is to examine the changes in the numbers of people with end-stage kidney disease (ESKD). The reasons for this are as follows. Chronic kidney disease (CKD) is defined as an estimated glomerular filtration rate (eGFR – as calculated using one of the eGFR formulae) of <60 ml/min and/or an increase in the urine albumin/creatinine ratio of 30 mg/g [1]. By this definition, about 13.6% of the US population has CKD. There is a legitimate argument as to whether everyone at these levels has CKD as, for example, eGFR declines with age. At birth, eGFR ranges from 110 to 140 ml/min. Normal rate of decline is as high as 1 ml/min/year. Hence many people 65 and over may have an eGFR of <60 ml/min/1.73m^2 as a consequence of normal aging. Therefore using the CKD definition, the number of people older than 65 with CKD may be an overestimate. But there is no controversy as to the numbers of people with ESKD (includes all dialysis and transplant) patients. In 1978, there were 41,000 people with ESKD and 307,000 in 1996. By 2015, 700,000 people had ESKD in the United States [1]. This is a 17-fold rise in ESKD patients since 1978. Type 2 diabetes mellitus (DM) is the main cause of ESKD (type 2 DM comprises >90% of all DM cases). In 1996, there were about 99,000 cases of ESKD ascribed to DM, and as of 2015, it was 267, 956 cases in 2015. Forty-five percent of the new cases in 2013 were due to DM, and 28% were due to hypertension.

This dramatic increase in ESKD is especially surprising as it is occurring despite the following facts: (1) Many studies have shown that it is more likely that a person with DM and CKD will die from a cardiovascular event rather than progress to ESKD. For example, decreasing eGFR and/or increasing urine albumin level led to a highly significant increased risk for death from a cardiovascular event [2]. Moreover an important study from 2014 determined that death rates in type 2 DM patients in excess of the age-matched non-DM population were associated with CKD [3]. By analyzing the NHANES database, these researchers found that the presence of albuminuria (>30 mg/g) or a decrease in eGFR led to increased death rates as compared to people with type 2 DM and no evidence of CKD. Furthermore,

R. C. Stanton
Kidney and Hypertension Section, Department of Medicine, Joslin Diabetes Center, Beth Israel Deaconess Medical Center, Harvard Medical School, Boston, MA, USA
e-mail: Robert.stanton@joslin.harvard.edu

C. M. Rhee et al. (eds.), *Endocrine Disorders in Kidney Disease*,
https://doi.org/10.1007/978-3-319-97765-2_2

the combination of increased urine albumin and decreased eGFR was associated with the highest death rates. Of most importance though was that those with type 2 DM and no signs of CKD had death rates similar to the age-matched population who did not have type 2 DM. This finding suggested that all excess deaths in type 2 DM patients were associated with the presence of CKD. (2) The death rates for people on dialysis in the United States are as high as 21% per year [4]. Hence when considering that most people with CKD will die before reaching ESKD and that the yearly death rates for people on dialysis are quite high, the CKD number must be in the millions to maintain the high (and increasing) numbers of people with ESKD. Of note, in addition to the personal costs of increased morbidity and mortality, there are tremendous financial costs. In 2013, the US government spent about 6% of the healthcare budget (31 billion dollars) on ESKD (which is about 0.2% of the population) [1].

This increase in CKD and ESKD is occurring worldwide. China and India have the greatest number of cases, and the rise in both countries is continuing. Interestingly, not all ethnic and racial groups share the same risk. According to the data from the United States, African-Americans, Hispanics, American Indians, and Asians have significantly higher rates of CKD and ESKD [1]. Thus, physicians need to be even more vigilant when caring for people from these ethnic and racial groups.

Pathophysiology

There is no definitive explanation as to why people with diabetes develop DKD. Interestingly most people with DM do not develop DKD. Many studies estimate that the percentage of people who develop DKD vary from 20% to 40% depending on whether one has type 1 or type 2 DM. And of those who develop DKD – diagnosed clinically primarily as a combination of eGFR of <60 ml/min/1.73m^2 and/or an increase in urine albumin level that is associated with a bland urine sediment – most will not progress to ESKD. Indeed major research efforts are focused on determining who is at risk to develop DKD and who is going to progress to ESKD [5–7]. A number of potential markers have been found including the tumor necrosis factor alpha receptor and kidney injury molecule 1 (KIM-1). To date, it is not clear whether any of these markers will offer more clinical utility than following changes in eGFR and the urine albumin level. They may become particularly useful for research studies since it is very challenging to do clinical DKD studies. This is because only a subset of DM patients will ever develop DKD and it takes years to develop DKD. Knowing who will develop DKD and knowing who will progress to ESKD will make it possible to use fewer patients in clinical studies for shorter periods of time, greatly increasing research productivity.

There are a number of mechanisms that likely play a role in the development and progression of DKD. The exact importance of each of these mechanisms is unclear. A major reason for all of this uncertainty is that the animal models of human DKD are generally not reflective of human DKD and it is difficult to do pathophysiological studies in humans as development and progression of DKD occur over many years. In this section, some of the relevant mechanisms will be discussed.

At the molecular and cellular level, a number of deleterious pathways have been implicated from cell culture and animal studies. The principal inciting cause for these pathways is elevated glucose. For all mechanisms described, drugs have been developed or are being developed:

1. Reactive oxygen species (ROS). ROS have been shown to be elevated in both animals and humans [8–10]. In many studies the elevation of ROS has been shown to be due to a combination of increased ROS production and decreased antioxidant function [8, 10]. Increased ROS leads to oxidation of lipids, proteins, and carbohydrates and deleterious cellular changes that may lead to cellular dysfunction and cell death. To date, antioxidant treatment has not been effective. This is likely due to the lack of specificity of current antioxidant treatments. Drug development aimed at targeting specific enzymes or pathways known to play a role in

the development of ROS is either in development or in clinical trials and will hopefully have significant therapeutic benefits.

2. Transforming growth factor β (TGFβ). TGFβ has a number of normal as well as abnormal functions [11]. In DKD, many studies have shown that increased TGFβ plays a significant role in the fibrosis seen in DKD and in a process called endothelial to mesenchymal transformation that is also part of DKD pathophysiology. There are no specific inhibitors of TGFβ, but studies in animals have demonstrated that blocking TGFβ (e.g., with an antibody) prevents the development of DKD. There have been small studies using a non-specific anti-fibrosis medication (pirfenidone) that have appeared intriguing but to date have not been shown to be useful [12]. There are ongoing efforts to find drugs that specifically block TGFβ.
3. Protein kinase C β (PKCβ). There is a large family of PKC proteins [13]. Although a variety of isoforms have been implicated in the pathogenesis of DKD, in particular, PKCβ has been seen shown to be increased in DKD leading to multiple cellular defects [13]. A specific inhibitor of PKCβ has been developed and studied in human clinical trials [14]. No clear benefit for DKD was observed in these studies.
4. Advanced glycation end products (AGEs). AGEs are proteins that are glycated through nonenzymatic processes [15, 16]. These proteins accumulate as blood sugar levels rise and lead to altered cell membranes, increased ROS, and other pathophysiological processes [15, 16]. Unfortunately, to date trials of drugs designed to prevent AGE formation and to prevent or treat DKD have not been successful in humans [16].

There are a number of other possible mechanisms [17, 18]. To date, drugs targeting these pathways have either not been effective or not yet tried in humans. Some have speculated that perhaps a combination pill or medication cocktail that consists of drugs against all or a combination of these targets would be effective. Others speculate that some of these mechanisms are relevant for development but not progression of DKD such that particular drugs may have not been given at their optimal effective time. Whatever the role these play, more work is needed to define importance, timing, and how these mechanisms interact with each other so that better treatments are developed and delivered at the optimal time.

In addition to the cellular pathophysiology, there are very important hemodynamic mechanisms. First, systemic high blood pressure is a clear factor both in the development and progression of DKD [19–22]. As vascular damage occurs in DKD (due to the effects of hyperglycemia on endothelial cells), hypertension likely leads to more damage of already susceptible endothelial cells leading to loss of nephrons. Many studies have demonstrated that control of hypertension is important for both prevention and progression of DKD [19–22]. Second, glomerular hyperfiltration has been shown to play a likely central role in the progression of DKD [23]. Glomerular hyperfiltration, which was mechanistically delineated using micropuncture studies in rats, is manifested as increased GFR [24]. Treating glomerular hyperfiltration in animal models of DKD has been demonstrated to prevent development and slow progression of DKD [25]. There are two approaches to decreasing glomerular hyperfiltration in animals, using medications that block the action of angiotensin II and low-protein diets [26]. Both approaches appear to work by decreasing glomerular hyperfiltration. Angiotensin II regulates glomerular filtration by causing vasoconstriction of the efferent arteriole and because of the increased resistance to outflow from the glomerulus, increased glomerular pressures, and, as a result, increased GFR [26]. Hence blocking the actions of angiotensin II leads to lower glomerular pressures. Low-protein diets also lower glomerular hyperfiltration via changes in renal blood flow. These diets are effective treatment in animals with DKD. On the other hand, high-protein diets in animals greatly accelerate DKD. In humans drugs that decrease the actions (via decreasing production or blocking action) of angiotensin II appear to be most beneficial for slowing progression in people with increased albumin levels in the urine but do not appear to be beneficial for preventing the development of DKD. In humans the benefit of a low protein diet is much less clear and most nephrologists are not recommending a low protein diet [27–31]. But there may well be a risk for progression of DKD from high-protein diets in humans.

Natural History

Natural history studies for DKD are difficult for already mentioned reasons: only a subset of DM patients will develop DKD, and it takes years to develop DKD (typically 5–15 years after the onset of type 1 diabetes). It is even more difficult to study the natural history of DKD in type 2 DM patients as the typical person with type 2 DM has it for years before it is diagnosed. Nevertheless, the classic view of the natural history of DKD is as follows [32]. The earliest sign is glomerular hyperfiltration (eGFR >140 ml/min/1.73m^2), followed by an elevated urine albumin level, followed by a progressive increase in the urine albumin level, and followed by a progressive decline in GFR. It is clear now that even though this construct does fit a subset of patients with DKD (at least in people with DKD due to type 1 DM), there are many variations for the majority of patients whether they have type 1 or type 2 DM [32]. For example, the decline in eGFR that has been thought to occur in following the development of increased urine albumin level does not always occur. Indeed, there are a variety of patterns that occur after developing an increased urine albumin level. Some people revert to normal urine albumin levels, some stay at the same level, and some have increases in the urine albumin level [5, 33–35]. And the association of GFR decline with albuminuria is variable as well. GFR may stay stable or decline completely independent of the urine albumin level [5, 33–35]. In general, the higher the urine albumin level, the more likely the GFR will decrease. And the best current marker of future decline in GFR is a continuously rising urine albumin level. Of note though GFR may decline even in the absence of elevated urine albumin [5, 33–35]. Hence the development of increased urine albumin should raise the concern that the GFR might decline in the future, but it is not definite that GFR will decline. Also the absence of an increase in urine albumin should not lead to complacency that there is no DKD in a particular patient. One should be following eGFR as well as the urine albumin level. Hence health-care professionals should be vigilant in searching for DKD and not assume that there is a clear pattern that any particular patient will follow.

Diagnosis

Diagnosis of DKD is done by measuring the urine albumin levels and by measuring the serum creatinine and calculating eGFR (the formulae are accurate within 10–20% of true GFR). The diagnostic signs for DKD in a person with DM are an elevated urine albumin and/or decreased eGFR associated with a relatively bland urinalysis (Table 2.1). The urine albumin level should be measured at least once per year using the albumin/creatinine ratio preferably by collecting a spot urine and measuring the ratio of albumin/creatinine as this method has been shown to closely reflect the

Table 2.1 Diagnosis of diabetic kidney disease

1. Either increased urine albumin/creatinine ratio (>30 mg/g) or decreased eGFR (<60 ml/min/1.73m^2) in a person with diabetes
2. Relatively unremarkable urine sediment analysis. None to few red blood cells or white blood cells
3. Pathology: increased glomerular basement membrane thickening, tubular basement membrane thickening, and mesangial expansion
4. Reasons to consider kidney diseases other than DKD:
   (a) Development of kidney disease in a person with type 1 DM of less than 5-year duration
   (b) Active urinary sediment (e.g., many white or red blood cells or many casts)
   (c) Lack of diabetic retinopathy especially in a person with type 1 DM
   (d) Rapidly declining eGFR or a change in pattern from a slow rate of decline to a rapid rate of decline in eGFR
   (e) Normal urine albumin level in a person with decreased eGFR
   (f) Long-term well-controlled blood sugar

24-hour urine albumin level [36]. Normal is <30 mg/g. If the level is elevated, it should be repeated in about 1 month as there are reasons for transient elevations such as exercise, pregnancy, urinary tract infection, congestive heart failure, sudden rise in blood pressure, and high blood sugar (Table 2.2). It is important to remember that measuring urine albumin level by urine dipstick is not an adequate screening test as it is a qualitative (not quantitative) test, and it is not sensitive enough to detect a low-level increase in the urine albumin level. One should always use the urine albumin/creatinine ratio test. It is also critical to calculate eGFR using one of the GFR formulae. Of note the Chronic Kidney Disease Epidemiology Collaboration eGFR formula (CKD-EPI) has been shown to predict cardiovascular and renal outcomes better than other formulae [37].

It is important to remember that just because a person has DM and kidney disease does not mean that they have diabetic kidney disease (Table 2.1). Reasons to consider other causes of kidney disease in diabetic patients include:

1. Short duration of DM. Kidney disease in a person with type 1 DM of less than 5 years duration.
2. No diabetic retinopathy. In general (especially in people with type 1 diabetes), diabetic retinopathy is diagnosed prior to the development of DKD. Although there are many patients with DKD and no retinopathy, it should raise a concern for another kidney disease if there is no retinopathy.
3. Active urinary sediment. Usually DKD has a bland urinary sediment or just a few red blood cells. If there are many red blood cells, white blood cells, or other substances in the urine, there should be concern that there is another cause of the kidney disease.
4. Rapidly declining eGFR or rapidly rising urine albumin level. The usual rate of decline in eGFR for DKD patients is 2–5 ml/min/year, so if there is a very rapid rate, there may be another etiology of kidney disease. Similarly, urine albumin levels usually rise gradually in DKD patients and do not get to very high levels.
5. Normal urine albumin level. Most patients with DKD have increased urine albumin level. But, as previously noted, this is not always seen, and people may have very advanced disease with low or normal urine albumin levels [33, 38].
6. Excellent blood sugar control. If a DM patient has had long-term excellent blood sugar control (hemoglobin A1c of 6–8%), then that should raise the concern that there is another cause of kidney disease.

When should a patient see a nephrologist for diagnosis and possible kidney biopsy? A referral to a nephrologist for diagnosis need only be done if the primary care doctor or endocrinologist are concerned that a diagnosis other than DKD is responsible for the kidney disease. Hence there needs to be a clear understanding of the signs as noted above that would alert the physician to these other causes. The nephrologist would likely do a detailed history, urinary sediment analysis, possibly a kidney ultrasound, and possibly a number of serologic and other lab tests. The nephrologist will also consider whether a kidney biopsy should be done. Hypertension is the most common cause of kidney disease other than diabetes in people with DM, but studies have shown that all types of kidney disease have been diagnosed in people with DM [39]. Classic findings on biopsy for DKD are glomerular basement membrane thickening, mesangial expansion, and tubular basement membrane thickening followed

Table 2.2 Screening and monitoring of DKD

1. Measurement of urine albumin level with spot urine albumin/creatinine ratio (normal <30 mg/g) at least yearly for screening. Repeat 1 month later if abnormal. Reasons for transient change in urine albumin level:
(a) Strenuous exercise
(b) Pregnancy
(c) Urinary tract infection
(d) Congestive heart failure
(e) Rapid elevation in blood pressure
(f) Hyperglycemia
2. At least yearly measurement of serum creatinine and calculation of eGFR using preferably the CKD-EPI equation to screen for DKD
3. Monitoring of DKD includes checking the urine albumin/creatinine ratio and calculating eGFR at each visit

by glomerulosclerosis and tubular-interstitial fibrosis [40].

Prevention and Treatment

Proven treatments for primary prevention of DKD are glucose control and blood pressure control (Table 2.3). Many studies have clearly demonstrated a lower incidence of the development of DKD in people with better glucose control. The Diabetes Control and Complications Trial (DCCT) study [41] followed 1441 patients for a mean of 6.5 years who were assigned to conventional or intensive treatment. Conventionally treated people had an average hemoglobin A1c of 9.1%, and intensively treated people had an average hemoglobin A1c of 7.2%. Intensive treatment decreased the development of microalbuminuria by 39%. The original cohort has been followed since then, and the 25-year follow-up Epidemiology of Diabetes Interventions and Complications (EDIC) study was reported recently [42]. After the original 6.5 years, both groups were treated the same with an average hemoglobin A1c of 7.9%. Thus in the EDIC study, the only difference between the two groups occurred during the first 6.5 years. The original intensively treated group had 50% less development of microalbuminuria and 50% less development of an eGFR of <60 ml/min/1.73m^2 as compared to the original conventional group 25 years later. Hence tight control of blood glucose as early as possible has long-term benefits for the prevention of DKD in people with type 1 DM. Similar findings have been found for people with type 2 DM in studies such as the United Kingdom Prospective of Diabetes Study (UKPDS) [43].

Table 2.3 Prevention and treatment of diabetic kidney disease

1. Prevention
(a) Blood glucose control – aim for a hemoglobin A1c of <7%
(b) Blood pressure control – aim for 130/80
(c) No clear unique role for RAAS inhibitors
2. Treatment
(a) Blood glucose control – goal for hemoglobin A1c of 7%
(b) Blood pressure control – goal is 130/80
(c) Use RAAS inhibitors if urine albumin level is elevated. Goal is to lower urine albumin level to at least <300 mg/g
(d) Consider using combination of ACE-I with aldosterone antagonist or ARB with aldosterone antagonist
(e) Routine use of low-protein diets has unclear benefit (<0.8 g/kg/day)
(f) Avoid high-protein diets (>1.5–2.0 g/kg/day)
(g) Smoking cessation and weight loss also may slow progression of DKD

Blood pressure control is also very important for the primary prevention of DKD. As has been well documented, hypertension alone causes kidney disease [44]. At the time of writing of this chapter, there is much debate as to the best blood pressure levels for prevention and for treatment of DKD. Since 2008, influential, large hypertension and diabetes studies have been published. The Action to Control Cardiovascular Risk in Diabetes study is typical of these studies in that they were primarily focused on cardiovascular risk in people already at high risk for cardiovascular disease [45]. In ACCORD and other studies, it appeared that a systolic blood pressure of 120 mm Hg was not better than 135 mm Hg for reducing cardiovascular outcomes. Moreover a systolic blood pressure of <115 mm Hg appeared to lead to worse cardiovascular outcomes in some of the studies [46]. Hence many guideline committees changed their recommendations for optimal blood pressure control from <130/80 to <140/80 or <140/90, but these studies were not DKD studies. Studies in DKD suggest that lower blood pressure is better both for prevention and treatment [20, 47, 48]. Hence, 130/80 seems to be a better goal than 140/80 as it is possibly more protective for the development of DKD. Moreover in ACCORD and other studies, although there was not a cardiovascular benefit for lower blood pressures, there was a significant stroke prevention benefit. So it seems that 130/80 is an excellent blood pressure goal that can prevent many diabetic complications in addition to providing cardiovascular protection and stroke protection. In the future, it is likely that the guideline committees will be again recommending a blood pressure of 130/80 for prevention of DKD.

Some have proposed that blockers of angiotensin II, specifically ACE inhibitors (ACE-I) or angiotensin receptor blockers (ARBs), should be used to prevent the development of DKD. Although there is very clear evidence for activation of the renin-angiotensin-aldosterone system (RAAS) in people with DM, there is little to no evidence that using these medications prevents the development of DKD. An excellent study on type 1 DM patients (where ACE-Is and ARBs were compared to placebo for prevention of DKD over 5 years) observed no benefit for ACE-Is or ARBs for the either the development of albuminuria but more importantly for the prevention of pathological changes in the kidney as determined by kidney biopsy at the start of the study and at the end of the study [49]. In type 2 DM, some studies reported prevention of DKD using an ACE-I or ARB [50, 51]. But the studies that seemed to show prevention using RAAS inhibition had higher starting blood pressures than large studies that showed no benefit [52]. Thus the studies reporting a beneficial effect may have been due more to a blood pressure lowering effect rather than due to a unique effect of the RAAS inhibitors. At this time, the main treatments to prevent development of DKD are blood glucose control (aim for a hemoglobin A1c of 7%) and blood pressure control (aim for 130/80), and there is no unique role for RAAS inhibitors for the primary prevention of DKD.

For treatment of DKD, there are three major goals: blood sugar control, blood pressure control, and lowering of the urine albumin level (Table 2.3). Many studies have validated the importance of blood sugar control for people with DKD [42, 53]. In general the hemoglobin A1c goal is 7%. Although there are no specific medications that lower blood sugar that are uniquely beneficial for treating DKD, there are trials of newer agents being done. Studies are ongoing for DPP-4 inhibitors (CARMELINA study – Cardiovascular and Renal Microvascular Outcome Study With Linagliptin in Patients With Type 2 Diabetes Mellitus) and for SGLT-2 inhibitors (CREDENCE study – Evaluation of the Effects of Canagliflozin on Renal and Cardiovascular Outcomes in Participants with Diabetic Nephropathy) to determine if these classes of medications slow progression of DKD that are likely to be reported on in the years 2018–2020. Recently the EMPA-REG trial reported dramatic reductions in cardiovascular mortality in participants taking the SGLT-2 inhibitor, empagliflozin [54]. Intriguingly analysis of the kidney data from the same study showed significant decreases in rate of decline of eGFR in the participants [55]. Most of the participants in this study had normal eGFR so this may indicate that empagliflozin may have a role in prevention, but it is not clear yet if empagliflozin has a role in treatment of established DKD. The CREDENCE study is a combined renal and cardiovascular study and includes patients with lower eGFRs.

As with primary prevention of DKD, blood pressure control is of great importance for the treatment of DKD. As previously noted for primary prevention, the blood pressure goal is controversial and based on studies primarily designed to assess cardiovascular risk. But some recent analyses have offered new insights on the best blood pressure for DKD. For example, the VA NEPHRON-D (Diabetes in Nephropathy Study) study suggests that at least <140 mm Hg and likely <130/80 mm Hg lead to better outcomes for DKD patients [47]. Analysis of the slope of decline in eGFR as a factor of the blood pressure showed that rate of eGFR declined as systolic blood pressure declined. Clearly 130–139 mm Hg was better than >140 mm Hg, but there was also a clear trend for slowing of eGFR decline below 130 mm Hg. Although current recommendations are to aim for <140/80 mm Hg if there are low levels of urine albumin/creatinine ratio (<300 mg/g) and <125/75 mm Hg if there are higher levels of the urine albumin/creatinine ratio, it seems that 130/80 mm Hg or better is the more appropriate target for DKD patients.

Although RAAS inhibitors do not have a unique role for prevention of DKD, there are many studies showing a major benefit for slowing progression if the patient has high levels of urine albumin/creatinine ratio (>300 mg/g) [56]. Lowering urine albumin appears to not only slow progression of DKD but is likely to lower the risk of cardiovascular events [2]. Indeed all patients with increased urine albumin level may well benefit from being on an RAAS inhibitor. In addition to ACE-Is and ARBs, the renin inhibitor, aliskiren, has been shown to be effective in lowering urine albumin level [57]. Of great interest is aldosterone blockade, as elevated aldosterone has many deleterious side effects [58] and blocking aldosterone has both cardiovascular and kidney benefits. There is an ongoing trial with a new aldosterone blocker called finerenone that will determine whether the addition of finerenone to ACE-I or ARB will improve cardiovascular and/or kidney outcomes in people with diabetes [59]. This trial is likely to be reported in 2019 or 2020.

There has also been much interest in combining RAAS agents for greater effect. Large studies have suggested that the combination is not more effective than these agents alone and may be more dangerous in combination [60, 61]. But there are questions about the inclusion criteria in these studies, and there still may be a role for combining these medications to help treat DKD. For example, a recent meta-analysis determined that the combination of ACE-I and ARB was more protective than either agent alone with respect to progression to end-stage kidney disease [62]. And there is also a study called Preventing ESRD in Overt Nephropathy of Type 2 Diabetes (VALID), which is evaluating benazepril and valsartan in combination that is to be reported on in 2017. At this time it is not clear what recommendation to make with regard to combining ACE-Is and ARBs. Hopefully VALID and other studies will provide more insight. One other class of antihypertensives that have been shown to have a modest albumin-lowering effect is the non-dihydropyridine medications diltiazem and verapamil [63]. Hence if a patient cannot take a RAAS inhibitor (e.g., high potassium, allergy, etc.), one of these agents may be considered.

Many have suggested that low-protein diets are of use in slowing progression of DKD based on the animal studies. A low-protein diet is often defined as <0.8 g/kg/day. Studies in humans have not been impressive or compelling, and often there is another explanation for the positive effect such as lowering salt intake and lowering blood pressure [30]. Hence routine use of a low-protein diet cannot be recommended. Studies will never be done on the possible risks of a high-protein diet, but there is enough evidence from animal studies and from very few human studies that a high-protein diet in people with DKD may accelerate decline in eGFR [64]. Thus it is best to avoid a high-protein diet which may be defined as >1.5–2.0 g/kg/day although the exact level of what constitutes a high-protein diet is not clearly defined.

Complications of Chronic Kidney Disease

Chronic kidney disease including DKD has a number of associated co-morbidities. The presence of chronic kidney disease and DM leads to even higher prevalence of these comorbidities. As previously noted, there is a very strong association between the development of DKD and cardiovascular disease [2]. Many studies have shown that even a small increase in the urine albumin level leads to increased cardiovascular events and cardiovascular mortality. In addition, decreasing eGFR is also associated with highly significant increases in cardiovascular events and death [3]. The combination of increased urine albumin level and decreased eGFR has an additive and possibly synergistic effect leading to even a higher incidence of cardiovascular events. As previously noted, most CKD patients (even more so in DKD patients) have a much higher chance of dying a cardiovascular death than getting to dialysis.

Anemia [65] and possibly secondary hyperparathyroidism occur at higher eGFRs in DKD patients as compared to nondiabetic CKD patients (Table 2.4). This is likely due to the combined effect in people with DM of loss of kidney tissue (primary cause of these complications seen in all CKD patients) and the deleterious effect of hyperglycemia on the enzymes in the remaining cells that impairs these metabolic processes.

Table 2.4 Complications of diabetic kidney disease

These may occur at higher eGFR levels in patients with DKD as compared to those with other types of chronic kidney disease
1. Anemia
(a) Caused, in part, by decreased production of erythropoietin and increased levels of hepcidin leading to decreased iron absorption
(b) Treated by increasing iron stores, controlling blood sugar, and possibly giving erythropoietin
2. Secondary hyperparathyroidism
(a) Caused mainly by decreased activity of the 1-a hydroxylase enzyme in the proximal tubular cell. In later-stage chronic kidney disease, increasing serum phosphate level plays a significant role
(b) Treated primarily by increasing vitamin D levels (goal is >30 ng/ml) using precursors to 1,25 dihydroxyvitamin D (such as vitamin D2 or D3). Use 1,25 dihydroxyvitamin D or analogs if vitamin D levels are >30 ng/ml and parathyroid hormone levels are still elevated. Limit phosphate in diet and/or use phosphate binders if elevated phosphate

Anemia occurs due to a combination of less production of erythropoietin (red blood cell growth factor that is produced in the kidney) and to decreased absorption of iron in part due to increased hepcidin levels [66]. Secondary hyperparathyroidism occurs for a variety of reasons, but a major one is decreased number and function of the 1-α-hydroxylase proteins in the kidney proximal tubule cells that activate vitamin D and regulate parathyroid hormone [67]. The decreased number of 1-α-hydroxylase is due to loss of kidney tissue and decreased function due to the effects of hyperglycemia [67]. Hence in a patient with DKD, it is very important to screen for cardiovascular disease, anemia, and hyperparathyroidism and treat as indicated.

Conclusions

There is an epidemic rise in the number of people with DKD. All physicians caring for diabetic patients need to understand how to optimally manage these patients to help prevent the development of DKD. It is also critical to screen for DKD and to aggressively implement treatments. Early and aggressive treatments do not cure DKD, but current treatments can significantly slow both the development of DKD and slow progression of DKD.

References

1. Survey USRD. www.usrds.org. 2016.
2. Ninomiya T, Perkovic V, de Galan BE, Zoungas S, Pillai A, Jardine M, et al. Albuminuria and kidney function independently predict cardiovascular and renal outcomes in diabetes. J Am Soc Nephrol (JASN). 2009;20(8):1813–21.
3. Afkarian M, Sachs MC, Kestenbaum B, Hirsch IB, Tuttle KR, Himmelfarb J, et al. Kidney disease and increased mortality risk in type 2 diabetes. J Am Soc Nephrol (JASN). 2013;24(2):302–8.
4. Foley RN, Hakim RM. Why is the mortality of dialysis patients in the United States much higher than the rest of the world? J Am Soc Nephrol (JASN). 2009;20(7):1432–5.
5. Krolewski AS, Niewczas MA, Skupien J, Gohda T, Smiles A, Eckfeldt JH, et al. Early progressive renal decline precedes the onset of microalbuminuria and its progression to macroalbuminuria. Diabetes Care. 2014;37(1):226–34.
6. Niewczas MA, Gohda T, Skupien J, Smiles AM, Walker WH, Rosetti F, et al. Circulating TNF receptors 1 and 2 predict ESRD in type 2 diabetes. J Am Soc Nephrol (JASN). 2012;23(3): 507–15.
7. Nowak N, Skupien J, Niewczas MA, Yamanouchi M, Major M, Croall S, et al. Increased plasma kidney injury molecule-1 suggests early progressive renal decline in non-proteinuric patients with type 1 diabetes. Kidney Int. 2016;89(2):459–67.
8. Forbes JM, Coughlan MT, Cooper ME. Oxidative stress as a major culprit in kidney disease in diabetes. Diabetes. 2008;57(6):1446–54.
9. Kashihara N, Haruna Y, Kondeti VK, Kanwar YS. Oxidative stress in diabetic nephropathy. Curr Med Chem. 2010;17(34):4256–69.
10. Singh DK, Winocour P, Farrington K. Oxidative stress in early diabetic nephropathy: fueling the fire. Nat Rev Endocrinol. 2011;7(3):176–84.
11. Zhu Y, Usui HK, Sharma K. Regulation of transforming growth factor beta in diabetic nephropathy: implications for treatment. Semin Nephrol. 2007;27(2):153–60.
12. RamachandraRao SP, Zhu Y, Ravasi T, McGowan TA, Toh I, Dunn SR, et al. Pirfenidone is renoprotective in diabetic kidney disease. J Am Soc Nephrol (JASN). 2009;20(8):1765–75.

13. Geraldes P, King GL. Activation of protein kinase C isoforms and its impact on diabetic complications. Circ Res. 2010;106(8):1319–31.
14. Bakris GL. Protein kinase C-beta inhibition: a promise not yet fulfilled. Clin J Am Soc Nephrol (CJASN). 2007;2(4):619–20.
15. Goldin A, Beckman JA, Schmidt AM, Creager MA. Advanced glycation end products: sparking the development of diabetic vascular injury. Circulation. 2006;114(6):597–605.
16. Singh VP, Bali A, Singh N, Jaggi AS. Advanced glycation end products and diabetic complications. Korean J Physiol Pharmacol. 2014;18(1):1–14.
17. Gnudi L. Cellular and molecular mechanisms of diabetic glomerulopathy. Nephrol Dial Transplant. 2012;27(7):2642–9.
18. Reidy K, Kang HM, Hostetter T, Susztak K. Molecular mechanisms of diabetic kidney disease. J Clin Invest. 2014;124(6):2333–40.
19. Bakris GL, Weir MR, Shanifar S, Zhang Z, Douglas J, van Dijk DJ, et al. Effects of blood pressure level on progression of diabetic nephropathy: results from the RENAAL study. Arch Intern Med. 2003;163(13):1555–65.
20. Emdin CA, Rahimi K, Neal B, Callender T, Perkovic V, Patel A. Blood pressure lowering in type 2 diabetes: a systematic review and meta-analysis. JAMA. 2015;313(6):603–15.
21. Ettehad D, Emdin CA, Kiran A, Anderson SG, Callender T, Emberson J, et al. Blood pressure lowering for prevention of cardiovascular disease and death: a systematic review and meta-analysis. Lancet. 2016;387(10022):957–67.
22. Schrier RW, Estacio RO, Esler A, Mehler P. Effects of aggressive blood pressure control in normotensive type 2 diabetic patients on albuminuria, retinopathy and strokes. Kidney Int. 2002;61(3):1086–97.
23. Palatini P. Glomerular hyperfiltration: a marker of early renal damage in pre-diabetes and pre-hypertension. Nephrol Dial Transplant. 2012;27(5):1708–14.
24. Zatz R, Meyer TW, Rennke HG, Brenner BM. Predominance of hemodynamic rather than metabolic factors in the pathogenesis of diabetic glomerulopathy. Proc Natl Acad Sci U S A. 1985;82(17):5963–7.
25. Zatz R, Dunn BR, Meyer TW, Anderson S, Rennke HG, Brenner BM. Prevention of diabetic glomerulopathy by pharmacological amelioration of glomerular capillary hypertension. J Clin Invest. 1986;77(6):1925–30.
26. Brenner BM, Lawler EV, Mackenzie HS. The hyperfiltration theory: a paradigm shift in nephrology. Kidney Int. 1996;49(6):1774–7.
27. Bellizzi V, Di Iorio BR, De Nicola L, Minutolo R, Zamboli P, Trucillo P, et al. Very low protein diet supplemented with ketoanalogs improves blood pressure control in chronic kidney disease. Kidney Int. 2007;71(3):245–51.
28. Brenner BM, Meyer TW, Hostetter TH. Dietary protein intake and the progressive nature of kidney disease: the role of hemodynamically mediated glomerular injury in the pathogenesis of progressive glomerular sclerosis in aging, renal ablation, and intrinsic renal disease. N Engl J Med. 1982;307(11):652–9.
29. Levey AS, Greene T, Beck GJ, Caggiula AW, Kusek JW, Hunsicker LG, et al. Dietary protein restriction and the progression of chronic renal disease: what have all of the results of the MDRD study shown? Modification of Diet in Renal Disease Study group. J Am Soc Nephrol (JASN). 1999;10(11):2426–39.
30. Otoda T, Kanasaki K, Koya D. Low-protein diet for diabetic nephropathy. Curr Diab Rep. 2014;14(9):523.
31. Pan Y, Guo LL, Jin HM. Low-protein diet for diabetic nephropathy: a meta-analysis of randomized controlled trials. Am J Clin Nutr. 2008;88(3):660–6.
32. Pugliese G. Updating the natural history of diabetic nephropathy. Acta Diabetol. 2014;51(6):905–15.
33. Krolewski AS. Progressive renal decline: the new paradigm of diabetic nephropathy in type 1 diabetes. Diabetes Care. 2015;38(6):954–62.
34. Perkins BA, Ficociello LH, Ostrander BE, Silva KH, Weinberg J, Warram JH, et al. Microalbuminuria and the risk for early progressive renal function decline in type 1 diabetes. J Am Soc Nephrol (JASN). 2007;18(4):1353–61.
35. Perkins BA, Ficociello LH, Silva KH, Finkelstein DM, Warram JH, Krolewski AS. Regression of microalbuminuria in type 1 diabetes. N Engl J Med. 2003;348(23):2285–93.
36. Schwab SJ, Christensen RL, Dougherty K, Klahr S. Quantitation of proteinuria by the use of protein-to-creatinine ratios in single urine samples. Arch Intern Med. 1987;147(5):943–4.
37. Matsushita K, Mahmoodi BK, Woodward M, Emberson JR, Jafar TH, Jee SH, et al. Comparison of risk prediction using the CKD-EPI equation and the MDRD study equation for estimated glomerular filtration rate. JAMA. 2012;307(18):1941–51.
38. Dwyer JP, Parving HH, Hunsicker LG, Ravid M, Remuzzi G, Lewis JB. Renal dysfunction in the presence of Normoalbuminuria in type 2 diabetes: results from the DEMAND study. Cardiorenal Med. 2012;2(1):1–10.
39. Sharma SG, Bomback AS, Radhakrishnan J, Herlitz LC, Stokes MB, Markowitz GS, et al. The modern spectrum of renal biopsy findings in patients with diabetes. Clin J Am Soc Nephrol (CJASN). 2013;8(10):1718–24.
40. Fioretto P, Mauer M. Histopathology of diabetic nephropathy. Semin Nephrol. 2007;27(2):195–207.
41. Group DER, de Boer IH, Sun W, Cleary PA, Lachin JM, Molitch ME, et al. Intensive diabetes therapy and glomerular filtration rate in type 1 diabetes. N Engl J Med. 2011;365(25):2366–76.
42. de Boer IH, Group DER. Kidney disease and related findings in the diabetes control and complications trial/epidemiology of diabetes interventions and complications study. Diabetes Care. 2014;37(1):24–30.
43. Intensive blood-glucose control with sulphonylureas or insulin compared with conventional treatment and

risk of complications in patients with type 2 diabetes (UKPDS 33). UK Prospective Diabetes Study (UKPDS) Group. Lancet. 1998;352(9131):837–53.
44. Thomas MC, Atkins RC. Blood pressure lowering for the prevention and treatment of diabetic kidney disease. Drugs. 2006;66(17):2213–34.
45. Group AS, Cushman WC, Evans GW, Byington RP, Goff DC Jr, Grimm RH Jr, et al. Effects of intensive blood-pressure control in type 2 diabetes mellitus. N Engl J Med. 2010;362(17):1575–85.
46. Cooper-DeHoff RM, Gong Y, Handberg EM, Bavry AA, Denardo SJ, Bakris GL, et al. Tight blood pressure control and cardiovascular outcomes among hypertensive patients with diabetes and coronary artery disease. JAMA. 2010;304(1):61–8.
47. Leehey DJ, Zhang JH, Emanuele NV, Whaley-Connell A, Palevsky PM, Reilly RF, et al. BP and renal outcomes in diabetic kidney disease: the veterans affairs nephropathy in diabetes trial. Clin J Am Soc Nephrol (CJASN). 2015;10(12):2159–69.
48. Lipman ML, Schiffrin EL. What is the ideal blood pressure goal for patients with diabetes mellitus and nephropathy? Curr Cardiol Rep. 2012;14(6):651–9.
49. Mauer M, Zinman B, Gardiner R, Suissa S, Sinaiko A, Strand T, et al. Renal and retinal effects of enalapril and losartan in type 1 diabetes. N Engl J Med. 2009;361(1):40–51.
50. Jermendy G, Ruggenenti P. Preventing microalbuminuria in patients with type 2 diabetes. Diabetes Metab Res Rev. 2007;23(2):100–10.
51. Remuzzi G, Macia M, Ruggenenti P. Prevention and treatment of diabetic renal disease in type 2 diabetes: the BENEDICT study. J Am Soc Nephrol (JASN). 2006;17(4 Suppl 2):S90–7.
52. Bilous R, Chaturvedi N, Sjolie AK, Fuller J, Klein R, Orchard T, et al. Effect of candesartan on microalbuminuria and albumin excretion rate in diabetes: three randomized trials. Ann Intern Med. 2009;151(1):11–20. W3-4
53. Writing Team for the Diabetes C, Complications Trial/Epidemiology of Diabetes I, Complications Research G. Sustained effect of intensive treatment of type 1 diabetes mellitus on development and progression of diabetic nephropathy: the Epidemiology of Diabetes Interventions and Complications (EDIC) study. JAMA. 2003;290(16):2159–67.
54. Zinman B, Wanner C, Lachin JM, Fitchett D, Bluhmki E, Hantel S, et al. Empagliflozin, cardiovascular outcomes, and mortality in type 2 diabetes. N Engl J Med. 2015;373(22):2117–28.
55. Wanner C, Inzucchi SE, Lachin JM, Fitchett D, von Eynatten M, Mattheus M, et al. Empagliflozin and progression of kidney disease in type 2 diabetes. N Engl J Med. 2016.
56. Gnudi L, Goldsmith D. Renin angiotensin aldosterone system (RAAS) inhibitors in the prevention of early renal disease in diabetes. F1000 Med Rep 2010;2:18 (https://doi.org/10.3410/M2-18)
57. Persson F, Rossing P, Parving HH. Direct renin inhibition in chronic kidney disease. Br J Clin Pharmacol. 2012;
58. Briet M, Schiffrin EL. Aldosterone: effects on the kidney and cardiovascular system. Nat Rev Nephrol. 2010;6(5):261–73.
59. Bakris GL, Agarwal R, Chan JC, Cooper ME, Gansevoort RT, Haller H, et al. Effect of finerenone on albuminuria in patients with diabetic nephropathy: a randomized clinical trial. JAMA. 2015;314(9).884–94.
60. Investigators O, Yusuf S, Teo KK, Pogue J, Dyal L, Copland I, et al. Telmisartan, ramipril, or both in patients at high risk for vascular events. N Engl J Med. 2008;358(15):1547–59.
61. Pham JT, Schmitt BP, Leehey DJ. Effects of dual blockade of the renin-angiotensin system in diabetic kidney disease: a systematic review and meta-analysis. J Nephrol Ther. 2012;S2:1–8.
62. Palmer SC, Mavridis D, Navarese E, Craig JC, Tonelli M, Salanti G, et al. Comparative efficacy and safety of blood pressure-lowering agents in adults with diabetes and kidney disease: a network meta-analysis. Lancet. 2015;385(9982):2047–56.
63. Bakris GL, Copley JB, Vicknair N, Sadler R, Leurgans S. Calcium channel blockers versus other antihypertensive therapies on progression of NIDDM associated nephropathy. Kidney Int. 1996;50(5):1641–50.
64. Cirillo M, Lombardi C, Chiricone D, De Santo NG, Zanchetti A, Bilancio G. Protein intake and kidney function in the middle-age population: contrast between cross-sectional and longitudinal data. Nephrol Dial Transplant. 2014;29(9):1733–40.
65. Bosman DR, Winkler AS, Marsden JT, Macdougall IC, Watkins PJ. Anemia with erythropoietin deficiency occurs early in diabetic nephropathy. Diabetes Care. 2001;24(3):495–9.
66. Babitt JL, Lin HY. Mechanisms of anemia in CKD. J Am Soc Nephrol (JASN). 2012;23(10):1631–4.
67. Saliba W, El-Haddad B. Secondary hyperparathyroidism: pathophysiology and treatment. J Am Board Fam Med. 2009;22(5):574–81.

Glucose Homeostasis and the Burnt-Out Diabetes Phenomenon in Patients with Kidney Disease

3

Masanori Abe, Csaba P. Kovesdy, and Kamyar Kalantar-Zadeh

Introduction

Maintenance dialysis patients, with or without diabetes, may experience both hypo- and hyperglycemia through multifactorial mechanisms related to kidney dysfunction, the uremic environment, and dialysis [1–4].

In many chronic kidney disease (CKD) patients with established diabetes mellitus, a decline in insulin requirements and even spontaneous hypoglycemia can occur [5]. The reasons for alterations in glucose homeostasis involve various mechanisms related to both decreased kidney function and dialysis therapies. Maintaining consistent glycemic control is difficult in end-stage kidney disease (ESKD), specifically because of altered glucose metabolism, fluctuating insulin resistance, impaired insulin secretion, and decreased insulin degradation; the effects of dialysis on drug metabolism further complicate glycemic management. In addition, it is also not uncommon to observe wide intra-patient variability on a day-to-day basis with regard to food intake, adherence to glycemic control drugs, and cognitive function relative to the dialysis schedule. These factors create unique challenges for glycemic control, as well as increase the risk of hypoglycemia in ESKD. Factors associated with hypo- and hyperglycemia in patients with ESKD are shown in Fig. 3.1 [1]. The focus of this chapter is to summarize these aspects of the management of hypoglycemia and hyperglycemia in patients with kidney disease.

M. Abe (✉)
Division of Nephrology, Hypertension, and Endocrinology, Department of Internal Medicine, Nihon University School of Medicine, Tokyo, Japan
e-mail: abe.masanori@nihon-u.ac.jp

C. P. Kovesdy
Division of Nephrology, Department of Medicine, University of Tennessee Health Science Center, Memphis, TN, USA

K. Kalantar-Zadeh
Division of Nephrology and Hypertension, Departments of Medicine, Pediatrics, Public Health, and Nursing Sciences, University of California Irvine School of Medicine, Orange, CA, USA

Glucose Homeostasis in Kidney Disease

Clearance of Insulin

The renal clearance of insulin significantly exceeds the glomerular filtration rate (GFR), indicating the significant uptake and degradation of insulin in the peritubular epithelial and endothelial cell membranes. The renal clearance of insulin changes minimally until the GFR is less than 40 mL/min and is significantly diminished once the GFR declines below 15–20 mL/min [5].

The impaired degradation of insulin in nonrenal tissues, such as the liver and muscle, contributes to the prolonged half-life of insulin in uremia. The metabolic clearance rate of insulin is prolonged in ESKD but can be normalized by

C. M. Rhee et al. (eds.), *Endocrine Disorders in Kidney Disease*,
https://doi.org/10.1007/978-3-319-97765-2_3

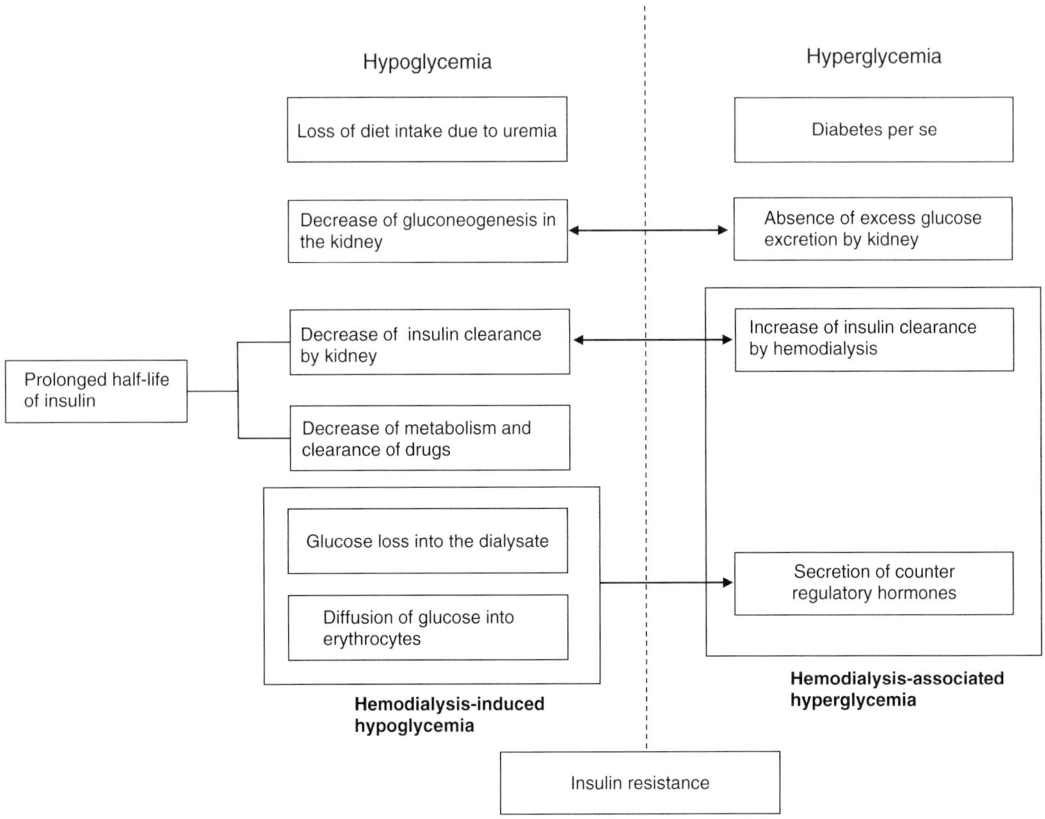

Fig. 3.1 The factors associated with the alteration of glucose homeostasis in dialysis patients. (Reproduced from Abe and Kalanter-Zadeh [1], with permission of Nature Publishing Group)

hemodialysis. The accumulation of dialyzable uremic toxins due to the progressive loss of renal function may inhibit the insulin degradation system, especially by the liver, which normally removes ~50% of the insulin secreted into the portal circulation [6]. Therefore, patients with impaired kidney function are prone to hypoglycemia because of the delay in the metabolism and excretion of both insulin and oral hypoglycemic agents.

Hypoglycemia Due to Antidiabetic and Other Agents

Among the oral hypoglycemic agents, sulfonylureas stimulate insulin secretion and tend to induce hypoglycemia, which upon development is prolonged. Accordingly, some of them are contraindicated in dialysis patients [7–9]. Therefore, the adjustment of antidiabetic agent doses is recommended in patients with CKD.

Exogenous insulin is primarily excreted by the kidney, while endogenously secreted insulin is degraded by the liver (18). After being freely filtered by the glomerulus, insulin is reabsorbed principally by the proximal tubule and to a lesser extent by the peritubular endothelial cells, where it is degraded into peptide fragments. Intensive insulin therapy can help to achieve target glycemic control but also increases the risk of severe hypoglycemia in patients with kidney impairment. Total insulin requirements decrease by 25% when the estimated GFR (eGFR) falls below 50 mL/min/1.73m^2 and by a further 50% when it falls below 10 mL/min/1.73m^2 [10–12]. Moreover, rapid glycemic control through intensive insulin therapy may worsen retinopathy and neuropathy [13]. To prevent hypoglycemia, education in the self-monitoring of blood glucose should be provided to patients in addition to appropriate hypoglycemia management [14].

In addition to antidiabetic medications, agents such as propranolol, salicylates, and disopyramide are common causes of hypoglycemia [15]. Additional triggering events include alcohol consumption, sepsis, chronic malnutrition, acute caloric deprivation, gastroparesis, concomitant liver disease, and congestive heart failure. The risk of hypoglycemia is increased in diabetic patients receiving β-blocking medication, which impairs gluconeogenesis.

Decreased Gluconeogenesis in the Kidney

Although diet is usually the main source of glucose, it can be produced endogenously by glycogenolysis and gluconeogenesis during fasting to maintain plasma glucose levels [16–18]. Glycogenolysis involves the breakdown of glycogen to glucose-6-phosphate and its subsequent hydrolysis by glucose-6-phosphatase to glucose; gluconeogenesis involves the formation of glucose-6-phosphate from a variety of precursors such as lactate, glycerol, and amino acids and its subsequent hydrolysis by glucose-6-phosphatase to glucose. However, activities of gluconeogenic enzymes and glucose-6-phosphatase sufficient to contribute significant amounts of glucose via endogenous production are present only in the liver and kidney. Because the kidney usually stores modest quantities of glycogen and the renal cells that store glycogen lack the glucose-6-phosphatase required for glycogenolysis, renal glucose production is thought to be principally due to gluconeogenesis [19]. Furthermore, the kidney is responsible for up to 20% of all glucose production by contributing to ~40% of gluconeogenesis [20].

The early findings of neutral glucose production by the kidney were likely because the kidney regulates glucose metabolism in the medulla and cortex differentially [21]. In this organ, the poorly vascularized, and hence relatively hypoxic medulla is a site of considerable glycolysis, whereas the cortex is the site for gluconeogenesis. Therefore, the net organ equilibrium of glucose does not represent a lack of glucose production but rather the difference between the renal glucose release by the cortex and the renal glucose uptake by the medulla (Fig. 3.2) [18].

Renal gluconeogenesis varies in response to various stimuli including fasting, hypoglycemia, and diabetes. Renal gluconeogenesis is more

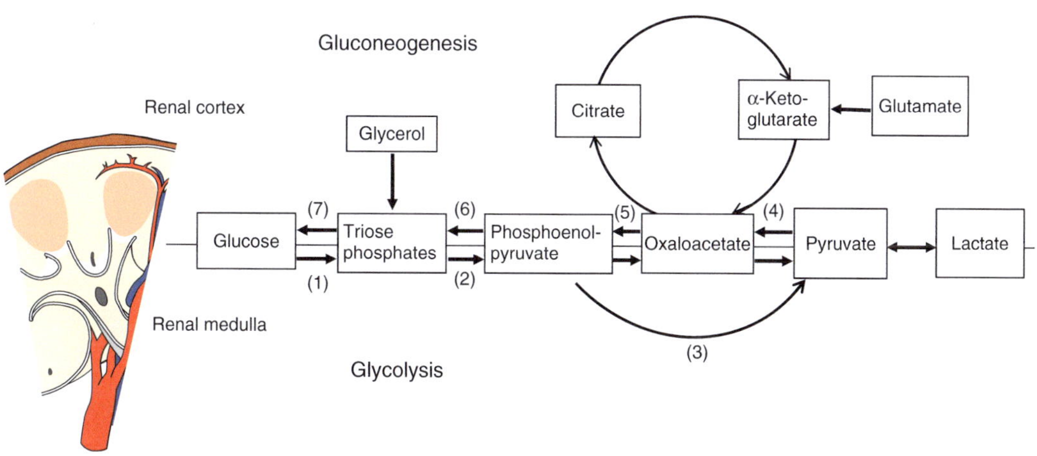

Fig. 3.2 Mechanisms underlying renal glycolysis and gluconeogenesis. The glycolytic enzymes (1) hexokinase, (2) phosphofructokinase, and (3) pyruvate kinase are predominantly localized in cells of the renal medulla. The key enzymes of gluconeogenesis, (4) pyruvate carboxylase, (5) phosphoenol pyruvate carboxykinase, (6) fructose-1,6-biphosphatase, and (7) glucose 6-phosphatase, are found mainly in the renal cortical cells. (Adapted from Stumvoll et al. [21], copyright Springer-Verlag)

sensitive to the presence of insulin and catecholamines than is hepatic gluconeogenesis, whereas glucagon has little to no effect on renal gluconeogenesis but increases the hepatic production of glucose [22–24]. Unlike the liver, the kidney increases its release of glucagon after glucose ingestion, potentially contributing to postprandial hyperglycemia in diabetic patients [22]. Hypoglycemia promotes renal gluconeogenesis by increasing the renal uptake of circulating gluconeogenic substrates.

Renal gluconeogenesis is therefore important not only for its contribution to maintaining normal glucose in the fasting state but also for its role in inducing diabetic postprandial hyperglycemia and the counteractive increase in glucose production seen in patients with diabetes. However, in many ESKD patients, the thinning of the renal cortex continues and gluconeogenesis is reduced. Therefore, when they experience hypoglycemic episodes, the episodes tend to be prolonged due to reduced gluconeogenesis by the renal cortex.

Insulin Secretion and Insulin Resistance

Insulin resistance, as evidenced by the reduced sensitivity to the hypoglycemic action of exogenous insulin, is common in patients with ESKD [25]. However, hepatic glucose production is normally suppressed in response to insulin in patients with ESKD. This suggests a peripheral site for insulin resistance in ESKD. Since the adipose tissue accounts for the disposal of <2% of the glucose load, muscle tissue is likely to be the primary site of such resistance [26]. Furthermore, the accumulation of uremic toxins may cause or contribute to insulin resistance in ESKD. A peptide in the middle molecule range that induces insulin resistance in adipose cells has been partially characterized from uremic serum and appears to be specific to uremia [27]. There is evidence that pseudouridine, which accumulates in the circulation of patients with renal failure, could be the uremic toxin that impairs insulin-mediated glucose utilization at the level of calcium required to modulate signal transduction of the insulin receptor [28].

Another contributing factor to insulin resistance in ESKD patients may be poor physical fitness [29]. Improved tissue oxygen supply and exercise tolerance in erythropoietin-corrected anemia have been shown to normalize hyperglycemia and glucose intolerance [30–32]. Insulin secretion appears to improve after the treatment of hyperparathyroidism and after the administration of active vitamin D [33]. The consequences of insulin resistance and deficiency in ESKD are complex and may influence patient outcomes beyond glucose homeostasis. Some studies showed that they were associated with muscle protein breakdown through the ubiquitin-proteasome pathway via the suppression of phosphatidylinositol-3 kinase [34–36]. It suggests that insulin resistance and deficiency may contribute to protein-energy wasting (PEW) leading to higher mortality in the dialysis population [37].

Both chronic inflammation and malnutrition have been reported in patients on maintenance hemodialysis [37–40]. In particular, the link between inflammation and malnutrition and atherosclerosis has enabled the identification of the malnutrition-inflammation-complex syndrome (MICS), which is associated with poor outcomes [41]. Increased insulin resistance and hyperinsulinemia may also cause accelerated atherosclerosis in uremic patients and possibly contribute to the pathogenesis of hypertension [42]. Insulin resistance, as measured by the homeostasis model assessment for insulin resistance (HOMA-IR), independently predicts cardiovascular mortality in hemodialysis patients [43]. Therefore, inflammation is the common factor in insulin resistance, MICS, and the pathogenesis of atherosclerosis.

The elevated levels of C-reactive protein often observed in hemodialysis patients reflect the enhanced release of proinflammatory cytokines such as interleukin-6 and tumor necrosis factor-alpha (TNF-α), both of which promote cardiovascular disease through their role in endothelial dysfunction, oxidative stress, insulin resistance, and stimulation of adhesive molecules [44–46]. Furthermore, the cytokines secreted by adipocytes (adipocytokines) play important roles in insulin resistance; in fact, TNF-α and leptin have been shown to induce insulin resistance [47]. Diabetic patients on hemodialysis with MICS exhibit lower response to erythropoietin and higher resistance to insulin [48]. This may explain the poor outcomes observed in these patients and demonstrates the importance of diagnosis and therapeutic management. Although insulin resistance leads to hyperglycemia in the general type 2 diabetes population, insulin resistance with PEW or MICS tends to result in hypoglycemia in the dialysis population.

Recent evidence of the links between fibroblast growth factor 23 (FGF23) levels and inflammation in CKD [49] implicates the regulation of FGF23 in preventing inflammation and insulin resistance. Therefore, in view of the relatively few established treatments for insulin resistance at this time, it is important to consider the optimal frequency, duration, dose, and modality of dialysis treatment and the use of biocompatible membranes and ultrapure dialysate as well as the nutritional status of the patients.

Table 3.1 Causes of PEW in diabetic dialysis patients

Causes of PEW in both diabetic and nondiabetic ESKD patients
1. Inflammation
2. Illness or trauma that anteceded ESKD and that may be unrelated to CKD
3. Inadequate nutrient intake
4. Losses of nutrients during the dialysis procedure
5. Acidemia
6. Hormonal disorders (e.g., resistance to insulin, growth hormone and IGF-I, hyperparathyroidism, hyperglucagonemia, low 1,25-dihydroxycholecalciferol)
7. Decreased physical conditioning
8. Oxidative and carbonyl stress
Specific contribution of diabetes mellitus to PEW in ESKD patients
1. Increased comorbidity of the diabetic ESKD patient
2. Hyperglycemia
3. Gastroparesis and other autonomic gastrointestinal disorders
4. Deficiency of insulin
5. Resistance to insulin
6. Increased serum levels of the counter-regulatory hormones, glucagon, epinephrine, and cortisol

Adapted from Noori and Kopple [51], with permission of Wiley

CKD chronic kidney disease, *ESKD* end-stage kidney disease, *PEW* protein-energy wasting

Protein-Energy Wasting (PEW)

PEW is characterized by the loss of somatic protein stores (as reflected by the reduced low fat-free and edema-free mass and measures of muscle mass such as urinary or serum creatinine levels), decreased visceral protein levels (as indicated by low serum albumin, transthyretin, transferrin, and cholesterol), and decreased energy stores (e.g., total body fat and/or glycogen) [50]. PEW occurs commonly in patients with diabetes mellitus who have ESKD and are undergoing maintenance hemodialysis therapy. Some, but not all, studies indicate that PEW is more prevalent in diabetic when compared with nondiabetic dialysis patients. The possible causes of PEW are listed in Table 3.1 [51]. The factors that induce PEW are linked to insulin resistance, including inflammation, acidemia, hormonal disorders, decreased physical conditioning, and oxidative stress. In particular, hormonal disorders in CKD can contribute to PEW in at least three ways: resistance to certain anabolic hormones including insulin, growth hormone, and insulin-like growth factor-I [33, 52]; increased serum levels of some catabolic hormones, including glucagon and parathyroid hormone [53]; and the deficiency of some anabolic hormones such as the deficiency of 1,25-dihydroxycholecalciferol, a common sequelae of CKD, which may induce muscle wasting [53].

Since diabetic patients are more likely to sustain catabolic events such as cardiovascular diseases, the likelihood that they will develop PEW and that their PEW may be more severe in comparison with the nondiabetic ESKD patients is increased. It is possible that hyperglycemia in the ESKD patient may in and of itself promote PEW. Diabetic ESKD patients are also more likely to develop gastroparesis with episodes of anorexia, nausea, or vomiting [50].

Insulin is a strong anabolic hormone for protein, fat, and glycogen accrual, and deficiency or resistance to insulin may also promote PEW [54–56]. Insulin deprivation in patients with insulin-dependent diabetes mellitus is associated with the elevated levels of plasma amino acids, increased protein turnover and protein oxidation, and negative nitrogen balance [57, 58]. Serum levels of the counter-regulatory hormones, glucagon, growth hormone, epinephrine, and cortisol, may increase during insulin deprivation [59]. Studies in healthy subjects have shown that, during insulin deficiency, glucagon increases the energy expenditure, protein breakdown, and leucine oxidation and is catabolic during a protein meal [60, 61]. Although epinephrine can produce long-term elevations of metabolic rate, its effects on protein metabolism are minimal beyond the acute changes affecting amino acid levels [62]. Increases in the circulating levels of cortisol within the physiologic range may increase protein breakdown and leucine oxidation, but the serum cortisol levels are typically unchanged during short-term insulin deficiency [63]. Growth hormone stimulates protein synthesis, antagonizes the antiproteolytic activity of insulin, and inhibits leucine oxidation [64].

Burnt-Out Diabetes Phenomenon

In diabetic dialysis patients with a presumptive diagnosis of diabetic nephropathy, glycemic control improves spontaneously with the progression of CKD, loss of residual kidney function, and the initiation of dialysis therapy, leading to normal-to-low levels of glycated hemoglobin (HbA1c) and glucose irrespective of treatment; this phenomenon is commonly observed and is referred to as "burnt-out diabetes" [1–4]. In a study of 23,618 diabetic dialysis patients from a large US dialysis organization, up to one-third were observed to have HbA1c levels <6% (Fig. 3.3) [65, 66]. Although many of those patients usually have full-blown sequelae of diabetes mellitus such as proliferative retinopathy, polyneuropathy, and peripheral vascular disease or other cardiovascular disorders, frequent hypoglycemic episodes may result in the discontinuation of insulin and oral antidiabetic agents [3, 4]. In this cohort, although higher HbA1c values were incrementally associated with increased death risk after controlling for demographics and other confounders, low HbA1c, especially <5%, was also associ-

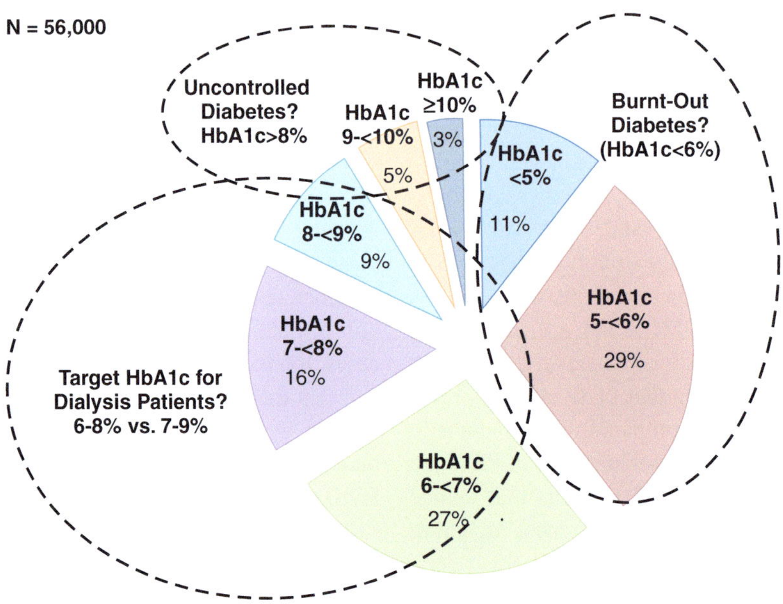

Fig. 3.3 Approximately one-third of diabetic dialysis patients have an average HbA1c level < 6%, referred to as "burnt-out diabetes." (Adapted from Rhee et al. [92], with permission of Wiley)

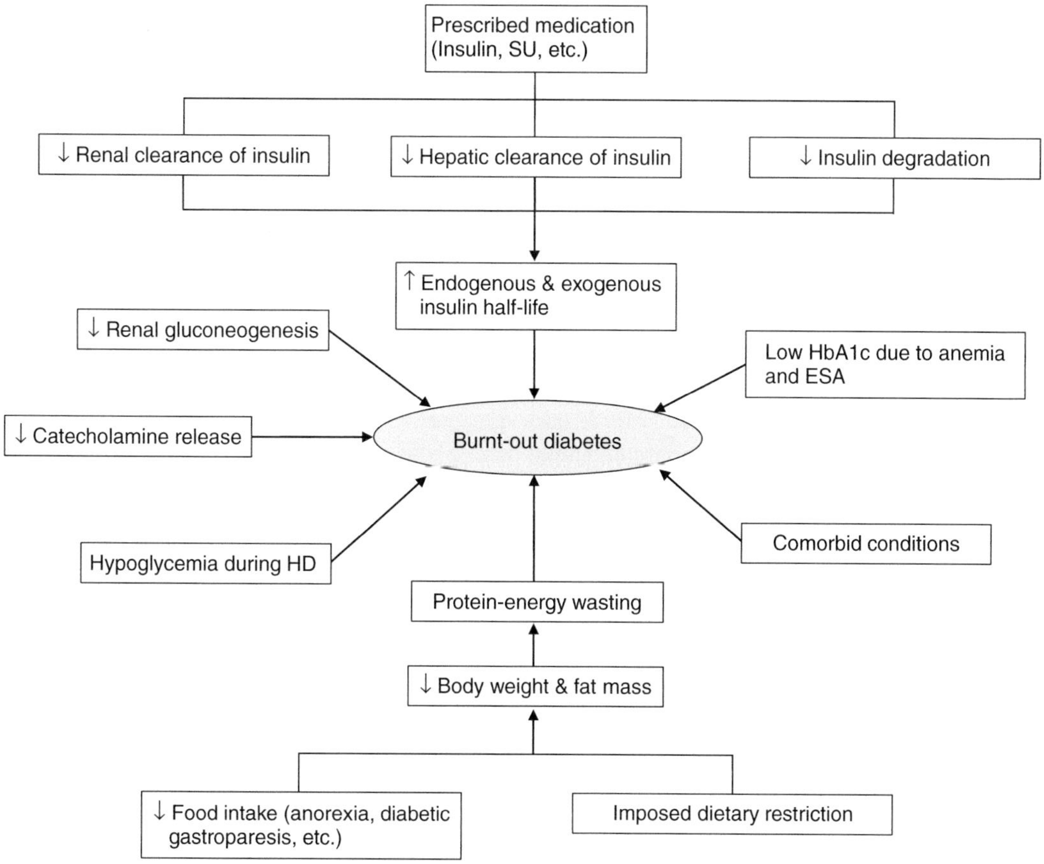

Fig. 3.4 Diagram showing the potential contributors to the "burnt-out diabetes" phenomenon in dialysis patients

ated with poor survival. Others reported that about 40% of 23,504 patients had HbA1c levels <6% and 37% of these patients were not administered insulin or oral hypoglycemic agents [67].

The reasons for those alterations in glucose homeostasis are multifactorial and involve various mechanisms related to decreased kidney function and dialytic therapies (Fig. 3.4).

In dialysis patients, the life span of red blood cells is shorter (approximately 60 days), and blood loss and hemorrhage may occur during dialysis; by increasing the proportion of young erythrocytes in the blood, both anemia- and erythropoiesis-stimulating agents can falsely lower the HbA1c level, which can lead to hyperglycemia being missed. Therefore, dialysis patients tend to show low HbA1c levels, which may underestimate glycemic control. Indeed, this phenomenon may be one of the causes of "burnt-out diabetes." In contrast, the glycated albumin level is not significantly associated with the life span of red blood cells, hemoglobin level, or erythropoiesis-stimulating agent dose in diabetic patients undergoing hemodialysis [68–70]. Therefore, glycated albumin might be a better indicator of glycemic control than HbA1c in diabetic hemodialysis patients. Several studies have shown that higher glycated albumin levels are associated with all-cause or cardiovascular mortality in diabetic hemodialysis patients [71–74]. Notably, there was no significant association between the average HbA1c levels and mortality in these subjects. It is important to note that glycated albumin is not widely available and outcome studies are limited. Therefore, further clinical trials are needed to strengthen the basis of these suggestions, since many of the recommendations for the treatment of diabetes in dialysis patients are based on longer-term studies of HbA1c levels.

Hemodialysis-Related Hypoglycemia and Hyperglycemia

Hemodialysis-Induced Hypoglycemia

Hypoglycemia occurs frequently in patients with ESKD, especially during hemodialysis treatment sessions, and is even more common in patients with diabetes mellitus [75, 76]. Asymptomatic hypoglycemia, which was defined as a serum glucose level below 72 mg/dL, occurs in approximately 40% of patients with or without diabetes, when using glucose-free dialysate [75]. It has been reported that 100 mg/dL glucose-containing dialysate solutions were preferable to glucose-free dialysate solutions for preventing acute hemodialysis-induced hypoglycemia and maintaining good glycemic control in hemodialysis patients with and without diabetes. Currently, the use of 100 mg/dL glucose-containing dialysate is the standard procedure in many dialysis clinics. Typically, if the plasma glucose level exceeds 100 mg/dL with the dialysate containing 100 mg/dL glucose, the plasma glucose is expected to diffuse from the blood to the dialysate across the concentration gradient. However, in reality, the glucose level at the post-dialyzer site decreases to <100 mg/dL in many hemodialysis patients due to the countercurrent passage of plasma through the dialyzer [77]. This decrease in blood glucose levels may be caused by diffusion of plasma glucose into erythrocytes, probably due to the glucose consumption resulting from the accelerated anaerobic metabolism, which was induced by changes in the cytoplasmic pH of erythrocytes during hemodialysis [78]. Thus, the use of glucose-free or low glucose dialysate is associated with a greater risk of developing hypoglycemia than that with a high (≥100 mg/dL) glucose-containing dialysate.

Metabolic Effects Associated with Glucose-Free Dialysate

Significant increases in β-hydroxybutyrate and acetoacetate are more likely after dialysis with a glucose-free dialysate than with a glucose-containing one [79]; this implies that the body tries to maintain an adequate blood glucose concentration when a glucose-free dialysate is used and does this by changing to a more catabolic state of gluconeogenesis and glycogenolysis. This is why levels of lactate and pyruvate, substances important for gluconeogenesis, are lower under such circumstances. The energy for gluconeogenesis is provided by the subsequent significant increases in the β-hydroxybutyrate and acetoacetate levels that occur secondary to fatty acid oxidation [79]. Several studies investigating the association between the metabolic effects of glucose-free dialysate solutions have revealed that patients enter a catabolic state similar to a fasting state [80]. During a glucose-free dialysis session, 15–30 g of glucose is removed from patients, and this can result in clinically evident or undiagnosed hypoglycemia [81–83]. This drop in glucose concentration is counteracted by endogenous glucose production that occurs through gluconeogenesis and glycogenolysis. Patients without diabetes can usually tolerate this state, whereas those with malnutrition or a weakened physical state often cannot, which increases their hypoglycemic risk. Diabetic dialysis patients are at higher risk for hypoglycemia, particularly those who have been receiving long-acting insulin or oral hypoglycemic agents. Therefore, the use of a dialysate fluid that contains glucose reduces anaerobic metabolism and interrupts the vicious cycle that eventually leads to hypoglycemia in the short term and neurological deficits in the long term [84–86].

Hemodialysis-Associated Hyperglycemia

Anuric ESKD patients are vulnerable to postprandial hyperglycemia, since they cannot excrete excess plasma glucose in the urine.

Insulin Removal by Hemodialysis

Theoretically, plasma insulin can be removed by diffusion and/or convection because insulin is a small peptide hormone (molecular weight, 6.2 kDa) and the protein binding rate of plasma insulin is 1%. Accordingly, the concentration gradient in hemodialysis may be responsible for the removal of plasma insulin. In 1976, it was reported that a small amount of insulin crossed the membrane during hemodialysis [87], suggesting that insulin might be dialyzed to a certain extent when the gradient is exceedingly high. The study used a cuprophane membrane dialyzer as a low-flux membrane. However, when high-flux membranes were used, studies report that the plasma insulin level after leaving the dialyzer was significantly decreased compared with the level before entering it and that the clearance of insulin differed with different types of membranes [88, 89]. Furthermore, whether the removal mechanism is diffusion, convection, or adsorption remains to be elucidated. Recently, plasma insulin clearance by hemodialysis has been shown to be mainly due to adsorption, which involves electrostatic as well as hydrophobic interactions between the membranes and insulin [90]. Plasma insulin removal is therefore highly significant in the case of diabetic hemodialysis patients with low C-peptide levels, particularly in those with type 1 or 2 diabetes and deteriorated β-cell function [89].

Hemodialysis-Associated Hyperglycemia Resembling the Somogyi Effect

In humans with a tendency toward a hypoglycemic state, plasma glucose levels are maintained by the decreased secretion of insulin and the increased secretion of counter-regulatory hormones such as glucagons, adrenocorticotropic hormone, and cortisol [91]. During hemodialysis, plasma glucose diffuses across the concentration gradient from blood to the dialysate. In addition, the plasma glucose level at the post-dialyzer site decreases to less than the glucose concentration of the dialysate, possibly as a result of diffusion of plasma glucose into erythrocytes. A decrease in endogenous insulin secretion in response to the decrease in plasma glucose level together with the adsorption of insulin by the dialyzer results in a decrease in plasma insulin level during hemodialysis. Counter-regulatory hormones are secreted in response to the hypoglycemic state resulting from the hemodialysis session. The combination of a relative and absolute lack of insulin after hemodialysis, the counter-regulatory hormone response, and the postprandial state leads to hemodialysis-associated hyperglycemia [1]. This phenomenon is similar to the Somogyi effect. Therefore, to maintain good glycemic control in diabetic hemodialysis patients, hypoglycemia during hemodialysis should be avoided by using a glucose-containing dialysate; this prevents the counter-regulatory hormones from being secreted and decreases the blood glucose levels pre-dialysis so as to minimize fluctuation during hemodialysis.

References

1. Abe M, Kalanter-Zadeh K. Haemodialysis-induced hypoglycaemia and glycaemic disarrays. Nat Rev Nephrol. 2015;11:302–13.
2. Kalantar-Zadeh K, Derose SF, Nicholas S, Benner D, Sharma K, Kovesdy CP. Burnt-out diabetes: impact of chronic kidney disease progression on the natural course of diabetes mellitus. J Ren Nutr. 2009;19:33–7.
3. Kovesdy CP, Park JC, Kalantar-Zadeh K. Glycemic control and burnt-out diabetes in ESRD. Semin Dial. 2010;23:148–56.
4. Park J, Lertdumrongluk P, Molnar MZ, Kovesdy CP, Kalantar-Zadeh K. Glycemic control in diabetic dialysis patients and the burnt-out diabetes phenomenon. Curr Diab Rep. 2012;12:432–9.
5. Mak RHK. Impact of end-stage renal disease and dialysis on glycemic control. Semin Dial. 2000;13:4–8.
6. Mak RHK. Renal disease, insulin resistance and glucose intolerance. Diabetes Rev. 1994;2:19–28.
7. Yale JF. Oral antihyperglycemic agents and renal disease: new agents, new concepts. J Am Soc Nephrol. 2005;16:7–10.
8. Abe M, Okada K, Soma M. Antidiabetic agents in patients with chronic kidney disease and end-stage renal disease on dialysis: metabolism and clinical practice. Curr Drug Metab. 2011;12:57–69.
9. Tuttle KR, Bakris GL, Bilous RW, et al. Diabetic kidney disease: a report from an ADA consensus conference. Am J Kidney Dis. 2014;64:510–33.
10. Charpentier G, riveline JP, Varroud-Vial M. Management of drugs affecting blood glucose in diabetic patients with renal failure. Diabetes Metab. 2000;26:73–85.
11. Snyder RW, Berns JS. Use of insulin and oral hypoglycemic medications in patients with diabetes mellitus and advanced kidney disease. Semin Dial. 2004;17:365–70.

12. Reilly JB, Berns JS. Selection and dosing of medications for management of diabetes in patients with advanced kidney disease. Semin Dial. 2010;23:163–8.
13. The Diabetes Control and Complication Trial (DCCT) Research Group. The early worsening of diabetic retinopathy in the diabetes control and complication trial. Arch Ophthalmol. 1998;116:874–86.
14. Ohkubo Y, Kishikawa H, Araki E, et al. Intensive insulin therapy prevents the progression of diabetic microvascular complications in Japanese patients with non-insulin-dependent diabetes mellitus: a randomized prospective 6-year study. Diabetes Res Clin Pract. 1995;28:103–17.
15. Abe M, Maruyama T, Fujii Y, et al. Disopyramide-induced hypoglycemia in a non-diabetic patient with hemodialysis: a case report and review of the literature. Clin Nephrol. 2011;76:401–6.
16. Boden G. Gluconeogenesis and glycogenolysis in health and diabetes. J Investig Med. 2004;52:375–8.
17. Gerich JE. Physiology of glucose homeostasis. Diabetes Obes Metabol. 2000;2:345–50.
18. Mather A, Pollock C. Glucose handling by the kidney. Kidney Int. 2011;79:S1–6.
19. Gerich JE, Meyer C, Woerle HJ, et al. Renal gluconeogenesis: its importance in human glucose homeostasis. Diabetes Care. 2001;24:382–91.
20. Meyer C, Stumvoll M, Dostou J, et al. Renal substrate exchange and gluconeogenesis in normal postabsorptive humans. Am J Phys. 2002;282:E428–34.
21. Stumvoll M, Meyer C, Mitrakou A, et al. Renal glucose production and utilization: new aspects in humans. Diabetologia. 1997;40:749–57.
22. Cersosimo E, Garlick P, Ferretti J. Renal substrate metabolism and gluconeogenesis during hypoglycemia in humans. Diabetes. 2000;49:1186–93.
23. Cersosimo E, Garlick P, Ferretti J. Renal glucose production during insulin-induced hypoglycemia in humans. Diabetes. 1999;48:261–6.
24. Meyer C, Dostou JM, Gerich JE. Role of the human kidney in glucose counterregulation. Diabetes. 1999;48:943–8.
25. Mak RHL. Renal disease, insulin resistance and glucose intolerance. Diabetes Rev. 1994;2:19–28.
26. DeFronzo RA, Alvestrand A, Smith D, et al. Insulin resistance in uremia. J Clin Invest. 1981;67:563–72.
27. McCaleb ML, Izzo MS, Lockwood DH. Characterization and partial purification of a factor from uremic serum that induces insulin resistance. J Clin Invest. 1985;75:391–6.
28. Dzuric R, Spustova V, Lajdova I. Inhibition of glucose utilization is isolated rat soleus muscle by pseudouridine: implications for renal failure. Nephron. 1993;65:108–10.
29. Eidmak I, Feldt-Rasmussen B, Kanstrup IL, Nielsen SL, Schmitz O, Strangaard S. Insulin resistance and hyperinsulinemia in mild to moderate progressive chronic renal failure and its association with aerobic work capacity. Diabetologia. 1995;38:565–72.
30. Goldberg A, Hagberg J, Delmez J, Haynes ME, Harter HR. The metabolic effects of exercise training in hemodialysis patients. Kidney Int. 1989;18:754–61.
31. Mak RHK. Correction of anemia by erythropoietin reverses insulin resistance and hyperinsulinemia in uremia. Am J Phys. 1996;270:F839–94.
32. Abe M, Okada K, Soma M, Matsumoto K. Relationship between insulin resistance and erythropoietin responsiveness in hemodialysis patients. Clin Nephrol. 2011;75:49–58.
33. Fouque D. Insulin-like growth factor 1 resistance in chronic renal failure. Miner Electrolyte Metab. 1996;22:133–7.
34. Ikizler TA. Effects of glucose homeostasis on protein metabolism in patients with advanced chronic kidney disease. J Ren Nutr. 2007;17:13–6.
35. Cusi K, Maezono K, Osman A, et al. Insulin resistance differentially affects the PI 3-kinase- and MAP kinase-mediated signaling in human muscle. J Clin Invest. 2000;105:311–20.
36. Lee SW, Dai G, Hu Z, et al. Regulation of muscle protein degradation: coordinated control of apoptotic and ubiquitin-proteasome systems by phosphatidylinositol 3 kinase. J Am Soc Nephrol. 2004;15:1537–45.
37. Fouque D, Kalantar-Zadeh K, Kopple J, et al. A proposed nomenclature and diagnostic criteria for protein-energy wasting in acute and chronic kidney disease. Kidney Int. 2008;73:391–8.
38. Stenvinkel P, Heimburger O, Lindholm B, et al. Are there two types of malnutrition in chronic renal failure? Evidence for relationship between malnutrition, inflammation and atherosclerosis (MIA syndrome). Nephrol Dial Transplant. 2000;15:953–60.
39. Kalantar-Zadeh K, Block G, McAllister CJ, et al. Appetite and inflammation, nutrition, anemia, and clinical outcome in hemodialysis patients. Am J Clin Nutr. 2004;80:299–307.
40. Filho RP, Lindholm B, Stenvinkel P. The malnutrition, inflammation, and atherosclerosis (MIA) syndrome – the heart of the matter. Nephrol Dial Transplant. 2002;17:28–31.
41. Kalantar-Zadeh K, Ikizler A, Block G, et al. Malnutrition-inflammation complex syndrome in dialysis patients: causes and consequences. Am J Kidney Dis. 2003;42:864–81.
42. Shoji T, Kawagishi T, Emoto M, et al. Additive impacts of diabetes and renal failure on carotid atherosclerosis. Atherosclerosis. 2000;153:257–8.
43. Shinohara K, Shoji T, Emoto M, et al. Insulin resistance as an independent predictor of cardiovascular mortality in patients with end-stage renal disease. J Am Soc Nephrol. 2002;13:1894–900.
44. Stenvinkel P, Ketteler M, Johnson RJ, et al. IL-10, IL-6, and TNF-alpha: central factors in the altered cytokine network of uremia-the good, the bad, and the ugly. Kidney Int. 2005;67:1216–33.
45. Sande FM, Kooman JP, Leunissen KML. The predictive value of C-reactive protein in end-stage renal disease: is it clinically significant? Blood Purif. 2006;24:335–41.
46. Zimmermann J, Herrlinger S, Pruy A, Metzeger T, Wanner C. Inflammation enhances cardiovascular risk and mortality in hemodialysis patients. Kidney Int. 1999;55:648–58.

47. Zoccali C, Mallamaci F, Tripepi G, et al. Adiponectin, metabolic risk factors, and cardiovascular events among patients with end-stage renal disease. J Am Soc Nephrol. 2002;13:134–41.
48. Abe M, Okada K, Maruyama T, et al. Relationship between erythropoietin responsiveness, insulin resistance, and malnutrition-inflammation-atherosclerosis (MIA) syndrome in hemodialysis patients with diabetes. Int J Artif Organs. 2011;34:16–25.
49. Munoz Mendoza J, Isakova T, Ricardo AC, et al. Fibroblast growth factor 23 and inflammation in CKD. Clin J Am Soc Nephrol. 2012;7:1155–62.
50. Dukkipati R, Kopple JD. Causes and prevention of protein-energy wasting in chronic kidney failure. Semin Nephrol. 2009;29:39–49.
51. Noori N, Kopple JD. Effect of diabetes mellitus on protein-energy wasting and protein wasting in end-stage renal disease. Semin Dial. 2010;23:178–84.
52. Siew ED, Pupim LB, Majchrzak KM, Shintani A, Flakoll PJ, Ikizler TA. Insulin resistance is associated with skeletal muscle protein breakdown in non-diabetic chronic hemodialysis patients. Kidney Int. 2007;71:146–52.
53. Brickman AS, Coburn JW, Massry SG, Norman AW. 1,25 Dihydroxy-vitamin D3 in normal man and patients with renal failure. Ann Intern Med. 1974;80:161–8.
54. Bennet WM, Rennie MJ. Protein anabolic actions of insulin in the human body. Diabet Med. 1991;8:199–207.
55. Ikeoka D, Krusinova E. Insulin resistance and lipid metabolism. Rev Assoc Med Bras. 2009;55:234.
56. Goley A, Munger R, Assimacopoulos-Jeannet F, Bobbioni-Harsch E, Habicht F, Felber JP. Progressive defect of insulin action on glycogen synthase in obesity and diabetes. Metabolism. 2002;51:549–53.
57. Bennet WM, Connacher AA, Jung RT, Stehle P, Rennie MJ. Effects of insulin and amino acids on leg protein turnover in IDDM patients. Diabetes. 1991;40:499–508.
58. Nair KS, Ford GC, Halliday D. Effects of intravenous insulin treatment on in vivo whole body leucine kinetics and oxygen consumption in insulin-deprived type 1 diabetic patients. Metabolism. 1987;36:491–5.
59. Charlton M, Nair KS. Protein metabolism in insulin-dependent diabetes. J Nutr. 1998;128:323S–7S.
60. Nair KS. Hyperglucagonemia increases resting metabolic rate in man during insulin deficiency. J Clin Endocrinol Metab. 1987;64:896–901.
61. Charlton MR, Adey DB, Nair KS. Evidence for a catabolic role of glucagon during an amino acid load. J Clin Invest. 1996;98:90–9.
62. Matthews DE, Pesola G, Campbell RG. Effect of epinephrine on amino acid and energy metabolism in humans. Am J Phys. 1990;258:E948–56.
63. Beaufrere B, Horber FF, Schwenk WF, Marsh HM, Matthews D, Gerich JE, Haymond MW. Glucocorticosteroids increase leucine oxidation and impair leucine balance in humans. Am J Phys. 1989;257:E712–21.
64. Horber FF, Haymond MW. Human growth hormone prevents the protein catabolic side effects of prednisone in humans. J Clin Invest. 1990;86:265–72.
65. Kalantar-Zadeh K, Kopple JD, Regidor DL, et al. A1C and survival in maintenance hemodialysis patients. Diabetes Care. 2007;30:1049–55.
66. Ricks J, Molnar MZ, Kovesdy CP, et al. Glycemic control and cardiovascular, mortality in hemodialysis patients with diabetes: a 6-year cohort study. Diabetes. 2012;61:708–15.
67. Williams ME, Lacson E Jr, Teng M, Ofsthun N, Lazarus JM. Hemodialyzed type I and type II diabetic patients in the US: characteristics, glycemic control, and survival. Kidney Int. 2006;70:1503–9.
68. Inaba M, Okuno S, Kumeda Y, et al. Glycated albumin is a better glycemic indicator than glycated hemoglobin values in hemodialysis patients with diabetes: effect of anemia and erythropoietin injection. J Am Soc Nephrol. 2007;18:896–903.
69. Abe M, Matsumoto K. Glycated hemoglobin or glycated albumin for assessment of glycemic control in dialysis patients with diabetes? Nat Clin Pract Nephrol. 2008;4:482–3.
70. Peacock TP, Shihabi ZK, Bleyer AJ, et al. Comparison of glycated albumin and hemoglobin A1c levels in diabetic subjects on hemodialysis. Kidney Int. 2008;73:1062–8.
71. Fukuoka K, Nakao K, Morimoto H, et al. Glycated albumin levels predict long–term survival in diabetic patients undergoing haemodialysis. Nephrology. 2008;13:278–83.
72. Okada T, Nakao T, Matsumoto H, et al. Association between markers of glycemic control, cardiovascular complications and survival in type 2 diabetic patients with end-stage renal disease. Intern Med. 2007;46:807–14.
73. Inaba M, Maekawa K, Okuno S, et al. Impact of atherosclerosis on the relationship of glycemic control and mortality in diabetic patients on hemodialysis. Clin Nephrol. 2012;78:273–80.
74. Isshiki K, Nishio T, Isono M, et al. Glycated albumin predicts the risk of mortality in type 2 diabetic patients on hemodialysis: evaluation of a target level for improving survival. Ther Apher Dial. 2014;18:434–42.
75. Jackson MA, Holland MR, Nichols J, et al. Hemodialysis-induced hypoglycemia in diabetic patients. Clin Nephrol. 2000;54:30–4.
76. Simic-Ogrizovic S, Backus G, Mayer A, et al. The influence of different glucose concentrations in hemodialysis solutions on metabolism and blood pressure stability in diabetic patients. Int J Artif Organs. 2001;24:863–9.
77. Abe M, Kaizu K, Matsumoto K. Plasma insulin is removed by hemodialysis: evaluation of the relation between plasma insulin and glucose by using a dialysate with or without glucose. Ther Apher Dial. 2007;11:280–7.
78. Takahashi A, Kubota T, Shibahara N, et al. The mechanism of hypoglycemia caused by hemodialysis. Clin Nephrol. 2004;62:362–8.

79. Wathen RL, Keshaviah P, Hommeyer P, et al. The metabolic effects of hemodialysis with and without glucose in the dialysate. Am J Clin Nutr. 1978;31:1870–5.
80. Borah M, Schoenfeld PY, Gotch FA, et al. Nitrogen balance during intermittent dialysis therapy of uremia. Kidney Int. 1978;14:491–500.
81. Ward RA, Wathen RL, Williams TE, et al. Hemodialysate composition and intradialytic metabolic, acidbase and potassium changes. Kidney Int. 1987;32:129–35.
82. Gutierrez A, Bergstrom J, Alvestrand A. Hemodialysis-associated protein catabolism with and without glucose in the dialysate fluid. Kidney Int. 1994;46:814–22.
83. Skutches CL, Sigler MH. Plasma glucose turnover and oxidation during hemodialysis: nutritional effect of dialysis fluid. Am J Clin Nutr. 1997;65:128–35.
84. DeFeo P, Gallai V, Mazzotta G, et al. Modest decrements in plasma glucose concentration cause early impairment in cognitive function and later activation of glucose counterregulation in the absence of hypoglycemic symptoms in normal man. J Clin Incest. 1988;82:436–44.
85. Heller SR, Macdonald IA. Physiological disturbances in hypoglycemia: effect on subjective awareness. Clin Sci. 1991;81:1–9.
86. Maran A, Lomas J, Macdonald IA, et al. Lack of preservation of higher brain function during hypoglycemia in patients with intensively treated IDDM. Diabetologia. 1995;38:1412–8.
87. Avram MM, Lipner HI, Sadiqali R, Iancu M, Gan AC. Metabolic changes in diabetic uremic patients on hemodialysis. Trans Amer Soc Artif Int Organs. 1976;22:412–9.
88. Abe M, Kikuchi F, Kaizu K, et al. The influence of hemodialysis membranes on the plasma insulin level of diabetic patients on maintenance hemodialysis. Clin Nephrol. 2008;69:354–60.
89. Abe M, Okada K, Maruyama T, et al. Comparison of the effects of polysulfone and polyester-polymer alloy dialyzers on glycemic control in diabetic patients undergoing hemodialysis. Clin Nephrol. 2009;71:514–20.
90. Abe M, Okada K, Ikeda K, et al. Characterization of insulin adsorption behavior of dialyzer membranes used in hemodialysis. Artif Organs. 2011;35:398–403.
91. Abe M, Kaizu K, Matsumoto K. Evaluation of the hemodialysis-induced changes in plasma glucose and insulin concentrations in diabetic patients: comparison between the hemodialysis and non-hemodialysis days. Ther Apher Dial. 2007;11:288–95.
92. Rhee CM, Leung AM, Kovesdy CP, Lynch KE, Brent GA, Kalantar-Zadeh K. Updates on the management of diabetes in dialysis patients. Semin Dal. 2014;27(2):135–45.

Glycemic Metrics and Targets in Kidney Disease

4

Joshua J. Neumiller and Irl B. Hirsch

Introduction

The growing incidence and prevalence of diabetes mellitus (DM) has made a notable impact on the development of diabetic kidney disease (DKD) [1]. Comorbid DM and chronic kidney disease (CKD) are common, with DM contributing to a large proportion of cases of end-stage renal disease (ESRD) in developed countries [2]. While "intensive" glycemic management has been shown to delay the onset and progression of increased urinary albumin excretion and reduced eGFR in DM patients [3], conservative dose selection and adjustment of antidiabetic medications is necessary to balance achievement of glycemic goals with risks of overtreatment. Patients with stage 3–5 CKD (eGFR levels <60 ml/min/1.73 m^2) are well established as having a higher risk for experiencing hypoglycemic events. Factors that may contribute to this increased risk can include slowed elimination of hypoglycemic agents, acute caloric deprivation, chronic malnutrition, and decreased renal gluconeogenesis as kidney function declines, among other potential contributing factors [4–6]. In terms of antihyperglycemic therapies, many currently available agents are dose adjusted in the setting of kidney disease due to altered drug pharmacokinetics or other disease-specific factors [4]. Renal safety profiles of individual antihyperglycemic agents are additional factors that must be considered. To further complicate glycemic management in DKD, the accuracy of glycemic control metrics is to a large degree unclear as are optimal glycemic targets. This article will review currently available indices of glycemic control, consideration related to their use in DKD, and associated considerations when setting glycemic goals in patients with diabetes and kidney disease.

J. J. Neumiller (✉)
Department of Pharmacotherapy, Washington State University, Spokane, WA, USA
e-mail: jneumiller@wsu.edu

I. B. Hirsch
Division of Metabolism, Endocrinology, and Nutrition, University of Washington School of Medicine, Seattle, WA, USA
e-mail: ihirsch@u.washington.edu

Glycemic Metrics and Their Role in Kidney Disease

A variety of factors associated with kidney disease and/or the uremic state can impact the accuracy and interpretation of indices of glycemic control. The following provides a discussion of measures such as glycated hemoglobin, glycated albumin, fructosamine, 1,5-anhydroglucitol, and continuous glucose monitoring with an emphasis on considerations pertinent in the setting of DKD (see Table 4.1).

C. M. Rhee et al. (eds.), *Endocrine Disorders in Kidney Disease*,
https://doi.org/10.1007/978-3-319-97765-2_4

Table 4.1 Comparison and contrast of glycemic control measures in DKD [7, 8]

Glycemic measure	Approximate period of assessment	Key strengths	Potential limitations
Glycated hemoglobin (A1C)	2–3 months	Routinely available in clinic laboratories Scientific evidence on association with diabetes-related outcomes	Values can be falsely altered depending on erythrocyte turnover and other factors (see Table 4.1)
Glycated albumin (GA)	2–3 weeks	Not influenced by altered hemoglobin levels or altered erythropoiesis	Limited data on relationship to outcomes Not widely available in clinic laboratories
Fructosamine	10–14 days	Not influenced by altered hemoglobin levels or altered erythropoiesis	Limited data on relationship to outcomes Not widely available in clinic laboratories
1,5-anhydroglucitol (1,5-AG)	1–2 weeks	Sensitive to day-to-day fluctuations in glucose Relatively accessible in clinic laboratories	Limitations for use in subjects with renal tubular acidosis and advanced kidney disease
Continuous glucose measurement (CGM)	Continuous	Theoretical best measure of glycemic control Allows for examination of short-term glycemic changes around the time of dialysis	Limited data

Glycated Hemoglobin (A1C)

Glycated hemoglobin (A1C) represents the fraction of hemoglobin bound to glucose. A1C values have been the "gold standard" marker of glycemic control for several decades, yet it has significant limitations related to precision and interpretation in the DKD population [9]. Variability in erythrocyte turnover is a major cause of A1C imprecision in the setting of kidney disease (see Table 4.2). Erythrocyte survival times become shorter as estimated glomerular filtration rate (eGFR) falls, resulting in a reduction in measured A1C. Treatment with erythrocyte-stimulating agents (ESAs) can also contribute to a lowering of A1C, perhaps due to a combination of an overall "younger" erythrocyte pool and associated changes in hemoglobin concentrations [11, 12]. Iron replacement therapy has additionally been linked with a decrease in A1C, with ESA- and iron replacement-associated A1C declines occurring independent of changes in glycemic control [13, 14]. On the contrary, decreased erythropoiesis due to a deficiency in iron or vitamin B12 can lead to a relative increase in circulating aged erythrocytes, thus resulting in

Table 4.2 Key factors known to influence glycated hemoglobin (A1C) levels[a]

Physiological states	Aging
	Pregnancy
Hematological conditions	Anemia
	Accelerated erythrocyte turnover
	Thalassemia
	Sickle cell disease
	Reticulocytosis
	Hemolysis
Drugs/medications	Alcohol
	Opioids
	Vitamin C
	Vitamin E
	Aspirin
	Erythropoietin
	Dapsone
	Ribavirin
Other disease states	HIV infection
	Uremia
	Hyperbilirubinemia
	Dyslipidemia
	Cirrhosis
	Hypothyroidism
Medical therapies	Blood transfusion
	Hemodialysis

[a]Adapted from Hirsch et al. [10]

a rise in measured A1C independent of glycemia [15]. Additional factors relevant to the kidney disease population that may contribute to an artificial fall in A1C include the uremic environment, blood pH, and receipt of blood infusions. When assessed in patients receiving peritoneal dialysis, the association between A1C and blood glucose was found to differ from that expected in patients with normal kidney function [16], with the potential for A1C levels to measure falsely low in patients receiving either hemodialysis or peritoneal dialysis [13].

Further complicating the use of A1C in general is the finding that certain patients considered to have "good" glycemic control per generally accepted A1C targets still develop complications, while other individuals with poorer A1C values remain free of complications [17]. While the landmark Diabetes Control and Complications Trial (DCCT) did find that intensified control in patients with type 1 diabetes mellitus (T1DM) reduced the risk of progression of retinopathy by 76%, A1C and duration of diabetes explained only about 11% of the variation in retinopathy risk observed in the study population [18–20]. This finding begs the question of what factor or factors contribute the remaining 89%. These findings may additionally be driven by the fact that a given A1C value may reflect very different average glucose values from one individual to the next. Table 4.3 summarized data obtained from an analysis of the A1c-Derived Average Glucose (ADAG) Study [9]. As can be appreciated in the table when considering the 95% confidence intervals established for each A1C value (these subjects had normal renal and hepatic function and did not have anemia or iron deficiency), an individual with an average glucose of 170 mg/dL could have an A1C of 9%, while another person with the same average glucose could have an A1C of 7%. These collective findings underscore not only the limitations of A1C in patients with DKD due to issues related to erythrocyte turnover and other disease-specific considerations but also a potential lack of reliability even when comparing individuals in the general diabetes population without kidney disease. One could speculate that with all of the issues noted above with red blood cell lifespan and ESAs in DKD, these 95% confidence intervals would only be wider in this population.

Table 4.3 Average glucose values versus glycated hemoglobin (A1C)[a]

A1C (%)	Average glucose [mg/dL (95% CI)]
5	97 (76–120)
6	126 (100–152)
7	154 (123–185)
8	183 (147–217)
9	212 (170–249)
10	249 (192–282)
11	269 (217–314)
12	298 (240–347)

[a]Adapted from Nathan et al. [9]

Glycated Albumin (GA)

An emerging marker for glycemia is glycated albumin (GA), a ketoamine formed via nonenzymatic glycation of albumin. Because the half-life of albumin is approximately 15 days, GA is a reflection of mean glycemia over the previous 2–3 weeks. Unlike A1C, GA measurements are not influenced by erythrocyte lifespan or use of ESAs [13]. GA levels can, however, be influenced by age and nutritional status [21]. While outcome studies are limited, initial data suggests GA is associated with mortality and hospitalization [22]. Freedman et al. [22] followed 444 patients with DKD over a median 2.3 years. The study found no association between glycemic control as measured by A1C or casual serum glucose levels and survival. Higher GA levels in this study, however, were found to predict hospitalization and reduced survival in DKD patients receiving dialysis. Studies evaluating the utility of GA measurement in patients undergoing dialysis have reported the measure to more accurately reflect recent glycemic control when compared to A1C [13, 22, 23] which was additionally reported to be the case in a study of pre-dialysis patients with DKD [24].

Unfortunately, GA is not generally available in the clinical setting in the United States. Notably, there exists a lack of clinical outcome studies assessing GA levels with microvascular or macrovascular complications in diabetes, and the relationship between GA and A1C is not linear [4]. Therefore, GA levels cannot be extrapolated to corresponding A1C levels to assess risks of complications.

Fructosamine

Fructosamine has been proposed as an alternate glycemic biomarker in settings where A1C is less reliable, such as in DKD. Whereas GA is a measure of glycated albumin, fructosamine is a measure reflecting total serum protein glycation and is considered to correlate best with the average glucose levels occurring in the preceding 10–14 days. Because fructosamine is a measure of nonenzymatic glycation of proteins present in the same compartment as plasma glucose, fluctuations in measured fructosamine are believed to reflect plasma glucose fluctuations [25]. While fructosamine is not altered by disorders of hemoglobin metabolism, factors that may influence fructosamine levels include plasma concentrations of bilirubin, urea, and uric acid, as well as serum protein concentration and profiles [26]. With the most abundant serum protein being albumin, hypoalbuminemia will result in low measured fructosamine levels, constituting a potential limitation in the setting of DKD [4]. Studies correlating fructosamine and mean glucose concentrations have found that calculated estimated average glucose (eAG) from fructosamine may underestimate mean blood glucose levels in patients with CKD stages 3–4 [27] and that fructosamine and glycated plasma proteins correlated poorly with glycemic control in hemodialysis patients [28]. Findings from the Choices for Healthy Outcomes in Caring for ESRD (CHOICE) study linked levels of fructosamine and GA with mortality and first cardiovascular event in a subgroup of DKD patients receiving dialysis [29]. Studies to date have included relatively small cohorts, however, with additional investigation of the role of fructosamine in patients with kidney disease warranted.

1,5-Anhydroglucitol (1,5-AG)

1,5-anhydroglucitol (1,5-AG) is a sugar alcohol obtained via the diet that undergoes minimal degradation or metabolism within the body [30]. 1,5-AG is lost via the urine with glucose and is dependent on the renal tubular threshold for glucose reclamation. 1,5-AG is structurally very similar to glucose (see Fig. 4.1), and its reabsorption in the kidney competes with that of glucose. In turn, the renal reabsorption of 1,5-AG is inhibited in the presence of glucosuria, resulting in a reduction of serum 1,5-AG concentration with repeated states of hyperglycemia [30]. This marker can be measured every 1–2 weeks, with a reduction in 1,5-AG indicative of increased hyperglycemic peaks during the day [30]. One limitation of A1C is that it cannot differentiate between individuals reaching target mean glucose levels in the presence of considerable glycemic variability and those with less pronounced glycemic excursions. 1,5-AG levels may provide an important measure of glycemic variability, which may predict hypoglycemia risk and contribute to the development of long-term vascular complications [19, 31]. While there are no long-term data correlating 1,5 AG levels with micro- or macrovascular diabetes complications, there is a suggestion that abnormal levels in pregnant women with diabetes impact fetal outcomes, particularly macrosomia, which is not surprising given the known detrimental effects of postprandial spikes on the fetus [32].

Serum 1,5-AG levels can decline in the setting of DKD due to decreases in reabsorption that occur independent of urinary glucose excretion.

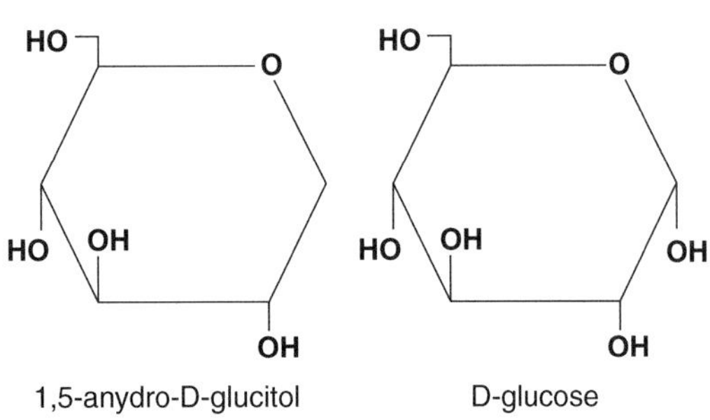

Fig. 4.1 Structures of 1,5-anhydroglucitol and glucose

Several small studies have reported that 1,5-AG may be affected by conditions associated with disturbed and/or impaired renal function [33, 34]. A cross-sectional study assessing the use of 1,5-AG in various stages of CKD showed that eGFR levels did not influence 1,5-AG in subjects with mild or moderate renal dysfunction but did identify an effect in those with severe renal dysfunction or ESRD [35]. In line with these findings, the manufacturer of the currently available 1,5-AG assay notes that artificially low levels can occur in the setting of stage 4 or 5 kidney disease [36]. While 1,5-AG provides a short-term measure of glycemic variability that can be useful in augmenting A1C results, this measure does have limitations in the setting of advanced kidney disease.

Continuous Glucose Monitoring (CGM)

Continuous glucose monitoring (CGM) is a promising tool for evaluating glycemic trends [7]. The role and use of CGM in DKD patients is an area of significant interest. CGM use in dialysis patients has been shown to be unaffected by urea levels and erythrocyte levels or lifespan, with CGM proving useful in measuring glycemic patterns around the time of dialysis [37]. While the use of CGM in the setting of dialysis is of particular interest, CGM has promise in terms of preventing hypoglycemic events and associated morbidity and mortality in all patients with DKD. Ongoing trials, such as Continuous Glucose Monitoring to Assess Glycemia in Chronic Kidney Disease – Changing Glucose Management [CANDY-CANE] [38] and others, will continue to provide insight on the role of CGM in this population.

Glycemic Targets in Kidney Disease

The American Diabetes Association (ADA) currently recommends a target A1C of <7.0% or as close to that target as possible that can be achieved without the occurrence of unacceptable hypoglycemia [3]. This general goal, which should be modified based on individualized factors, is largely based on studies demonstrating the benefits of "tight" glycemic control on the progression of microvascular complications [18, 39]. It should be noted, however, that the landmark trials highlighting the benefits of glycemic control on prevention of microvascular complications excluded patients with significant kidney disease and in fact focused on those soon after the diagnosis of their diabetes. The ideal glycemic targets in this population are therefore unknown given the current lack of data from prospective randomized trials to evaluate the impact of specific glycemic targets on outcomes. It should emphasized that the three trials published in 2008 with more advanced type 2 diabetes as cardiovascular disease as a primary endpoint did not show any benefit of tight glycemic control but did all show benefits in microvascular outcomes [40–42], a secondary endpoint. Follow-up of one trial, however, did show a significant improvement in cardiovascular events with intensive glucose control 10 years after the study ended [43].

As noted in Table 4.3, the most recent update of the National Kidney Disease Outcomes Quality Initiative (KDOQI) guidelines, like the ADA guidelines, suggests a general target of 7% in patients with or without diabetes [6], with an extension of this recommendation to a target above 7% for those with comorbidities or limited life expectancy. This is consistent with the ADA recommendation for a goal of approximately 8% for patients with established vascular complications [3]. While management of glycemia is a cornerstone of DM management, intensification of glycemic control carries with it the risk of added hypoglycemia when sulfonylureas or insulin is required. The Action to Control Cardiovascular Risk in Diabetes (ACCORD) study findings highlight the potential cardiovascular risk associated with hypoglycemia [40], with the risk of hypoglycemia known to be considerably higher in patients with renal dysfunction when compared to those without [44]. Notably, when compared to patients with normal renal function, those with baseline serum creatinine of 1.3–1.5 mg/dL had a 66% increased risk of severe hypoglycemia in ACCORD [45].

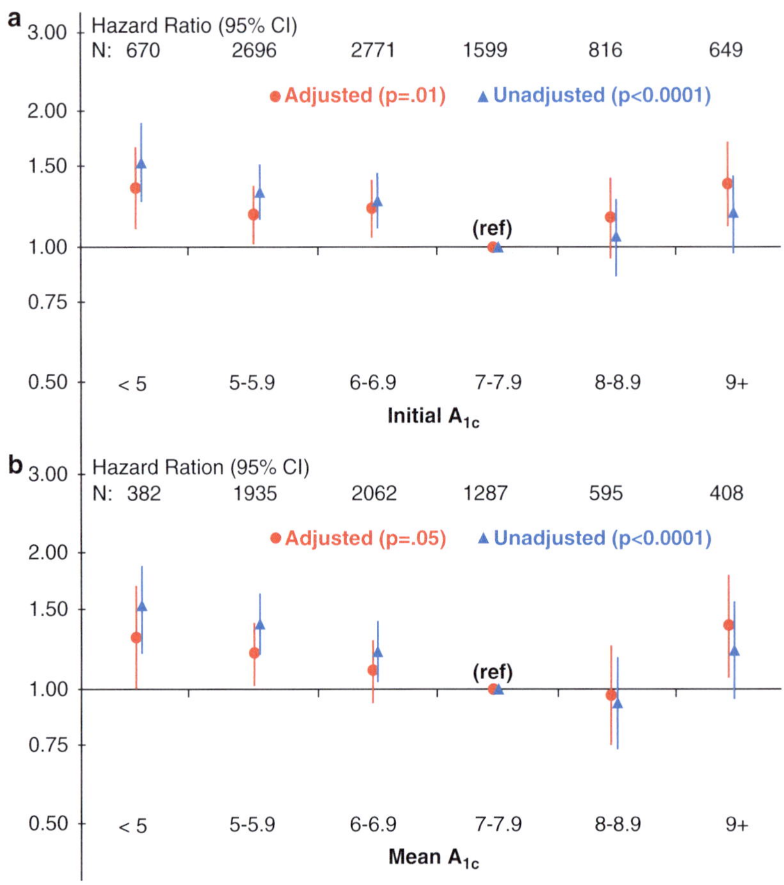

Fig. 4.2 (**a**) Risk of mortality by initial glycated hemoglobin (A1C), adjusted for age, sex, race, body mass index (BMI), years of dialysis, albumin, creatinine, ten comorbid conditions, insulin use, hemoglobin, HDL cholesterol, country, and study phase. (**b**) Risk of mortality by mean A1C, adjusted for age, sex, race, BMI, years of dialysis, albumin, creatinine, ten comorbid conditions, insulin use, hemoglobin, HDL cholesterol, country, and study phase. (Reproduced from Ramirez et al. [49], with permission from the ADA)

The role of improved glycemic control in mitigating the exceedingly high mortality risk in dialysis patients with DM is additionally unclear. Management of hyperglycemia in DKD patients is challenging, given changes in glucose homeostasis, the questionable accuracy of glycemic biomarkers previously discussed, and the altered pharmacokinetics of glucose-lowering drugs [46, 47]. An observational study in non-dialysis DM patients with eGFR <60 ml/min/1.73m^2 identified a "U-shaped" relationship between mortality and A1C levels, with A1C values above 9% and below 6.5% associated with an increased mortality risk [48]. A similar "U-shaped" relationship between A1C and mortality has been demonstrated in studies examining patients undergoing either form of dialysis (see Fig. 4.2) [49–51]. It has been suggested that hypoglycemia may be one reason for higher mortality rates observed in those with A1C levels below 6.5% in these observational studies [48, 49, 52]. This is a compelling argument given the increased awareness of ventricular arrhythmias from hypoglycemia in type 2 diabetes, which could potentially be even more deadly in those with DKD [53]. A meta-analysis by Hill et al. investigated the relationship between A1C and risk of death in DKD patients receiving hemodialysis [54]. The meta-analysis included nine observational studies and one secondary analysis of a randomized trial. When analyzed, baseline A1C values greater than 8.5% were associated with a 29% increase in the adjusted risk of death when compared to patients with an A1C ranging from 6.5% to 7.4%. Mean A1C levels below 5.4% were additionally associated with a small, but nonsignificant, increase in mortality [54]. Pretransplant glycemic control is also associated with posttransplant outcomes in kidney transplant recipients with diabetes [55].

Table 4.4 Select glycemic target recommendations for patients with kidney disease

Guideline/consensus report	Recommendations/suggestions
Diabetic kidney disease: A report from an ADA consensus conference [4]	A1C <8% when GFR <60 mL/min/1.73m^2 due to increased hypoglycemia risk Reliance on SMBG in making treatment decisions due to imprecision of A1C
ADA standards of medical care in diabetes – 2016 [3]	Less stringent A1C goals (such as <8%) may be appropriate for patients with advanced complications
KDOQI clinical practice guideline for diabetes and CKD: 2012 update [6]	Recommend not treating to an A1C of <7.0% in patients at risk of hypoglycemia Suggest that target A1C be extended above 7.0% in individuals with comorbidities or limited life expectancy and risk of hypoglycemia

While targeting lower A1C values is known to convey increased risk of hypoglycemia, A1C is not the best indicator of acute hypoglycemia risk. A follow-up analysis of DCCT (which were all patients with type 1 diabetes) using A1C and seven-point capillary glucose profile data showed that mean blood glucose and glycemic variability, as defined by within-day standard deviation (SD) of glucose measurements, when used together or individually signaled hypoglycemia risk independent of A1C [56]. To further support the importance of glycemic variability, an observational study using CGM analysis over a 2-day period in patients with type 2 DM demonstrated that the risk of asymptomatic hypoglycemia was drastically reduced when the SD surrounding the mean glucose value was reduced below a threshold of approximately 30 mg/dL [31]. Interestingly, one retrospective analysis of patients receiving hemodialysis reported higher A1C values and greater glucose variability as risk factors for severe hypoglycemia, as defined as hypoglycemia requiring hospitalization [57]. As a general rule, the more insulin deficient the patient, the greater the glycemic variability, independent of pharmacologic therapies.

A recent report from an ADA consensus conference provides some guidance on glycemic goal setting in patients with DKD [4]. As highlighted in Table 4.4, the report recommends a modified A1C goal to less than 8% once eGFR falls below 60 mL/min/1.73m^2 with the goal of hypoglycemia avoidance. The report additionally advocates for a strengthened reliance on SMBG in making treatment decisions, especially when considering the imprecision of A1C in such individuals. Indeed, SMBG has been called out as a crucial tool to consolidate individualized therapeutic goals [10] and as noted above can be utilized to modify treatment to prevent unnecessary hypoglycemia-associated morbidity and mortality. Many clinicians and patients prefer more specific targets which are quite reasonable but have not been specifically tested. Due to the concerns about hypoglycemia, reasonable pre-meal targets would be between 100 and 140 mg/dL with 2-hour postprandial goals of less than 220 mg/dL. Recall that for those without DKD, an A1C of 8% would equate to an estimated average glucose of 183 mg/dL so these specific glycemic targets seem reasonable [9].

While SMBG and A1C largely remain the cornerstone of glycemic monitoring, other indices of glycemic control may play an important role of identifying aspects of glycemic dysregulation that are not otherwise captured with SMBG and A1C measurement alone [10]. This includes increased use of CGM, particularly for those with hypoglycemia unawareness, and more utilization and research into the use of glycated albumin.

Conclusion

Glycemic control is the centerpiece of good diabetes care. However, the effects of intensive control in DKD are less clear than in those without kidney disease. Those with low eGFR are at a high risk for hypoglycemia, an immediate and serious adverse event. DM management is further complicated by limitations of currently available measures of glycemic control. Despite the inherent limitations of A1C measurement as a surrogate marker of glycemic control, it remains a key monitoring parameter in the glycemic management of people with DKD [52]. At the current time, A1C results should be interpreted carefully in conjunction with SMBG data to achieve glycemic goals and mitigate hypoglycemia risk. Better tools for glycemic assessment and more definitive research on glycemic targets would be welcomed.

References

1. de Boer IH, Rue TC, Hall YN, Heagerty PJ, Weiss NS, Himmelfarb J. Temporal trends in the prevalence of diabetic kidney disease in the United States. JAMA. 2011;305:2532–9.
2. U.S. Renal Data System. USRDS 2015 Annual Data Report: Atlas of Chronic Kidney Disease and End-Stage Renal Disease in the United States, National Institutes of Health, National Institute of Diabetes and Digestive and Kidney Diseases, Bethesda, MD. Available at: http://www.usrds.org/adr.aspx. Accessed January 4, 2016.
3. American Diabetes Association. Standards of medical Care in Diabetes – 2016. Diabetes Care. 2016;39(Suppl. 1):S1–112.
4. Tuttle KR, Bakris GL, Bilous RW, Chiang JL, de Boer IH, Goldstein-Fuchs J, et al. Diabetic kidney disease: a report from an ADA consensus conference. Diabetes Care. 2014;37:2864–83.
5. Gerich JE, Meyer C, Woerle HJ, Stumvoll M. Renal gluconeogenesis: its importance in human glucose homeostasis. Diabetes Care. 2001;24(2):382–91.
6. National Kidney Foundation. KDOQI clinical practice guideline for diabetes and CKD: 2012 update. Am J Kidney Dis. 2012;60(5):850–86.
7. Speeckaert M, van Biesen W, Delanghe J, Slingerland R, Wiecek A, Heaf J, et al. Are there better alternative than haemoglobin A1c to estimate glycaemic control in the chronic kidney disease population? Nephrol Dial Transplant. 2014;29:2167–77.
8. Rhee CM, Leung AM, Kovesdy CP, Lynch KE, Brent GA, Kalantar-Zadeh K. Updates on the Management of Diabetes in Dialysis patients. Semin Dial. 2014;27(2):135–45.
9. Nathan DM, Kuenen J, Borg R, Zheng H, Schoenfeld D, Heine RJ, et al. Translating the A1C assay into estimated average glucose values. Diabetes Care. 2008;31(8):1473–8.
10. Hirsch IB, Amiel SA, Blumer IR, Bode BW, Edelman SV, Seley JJ, et al. Using multiple measures of glycemia to support individualized diabetes management: recommendations for clinicians, patients, and payers. Diabetes Technol Ther. 2012;14(11):973–83.
11. Vos FE, Schollum JB, Coulter CV, Doyle TC, Duffull SB, Walker RJ. Red blood cell survival in long- term dialysis patients. Am J Kidney Dis. 2011;58(4):591–8.
12. Nakao T, Matsumoto H, Okada T, Han M, Hidaka H, Yoshino M, et al. Influence of erythropoietin treatment on hemoglobin A1c levels in patients with chronic renal failure on hemodialysis. Intern Med. 1998;37(10):826–30.
13. Inaba M, Okuno S, Kumeda Y, Yamada S, Imanishi Y, Tabata T, et al. Glycated albumin is a better glycemic indicator than glycated hemoglobin values in hemodialysis patients with diabetes: effect of anemia and erythropoietin injection. JASN. 2007;18(3):896–903.
14. Ng JM, Jennings PE, Laboi P, Jayagopal V. Erythropoetin treatment significantly alters measured glycated haemoglobin (HbA1c). Diabet Med. 2008;25(2):239–40.
15. Gallagher EJ, Le Roith D, Bloomgarden Z. Review of hemoglobin A(1c) in the management of diabetes. J Diabetes. 2009;1:9–17.
16. Hoshino J, Mehrotra R, Rhee CM, Yamagata K, Ubara Y, Takaichi K, et al. Using hemoglobin A1c to derive mean blood glucose in peritoneal dialysis patients. Am J Nephrol. 2013;37(5):413–20.
17. Zhang L, Krzentowski G, Albert A, Lefebvre PJ. Risk of developing retinopathy in diabetes control and complications trial type 1 diabetic patients with good or poor metabolic control. Diabetes Care. 2001;24:1275–9.
18. The Diabetes Control and Complications Trial Research Group. The effect of intensive treatment of diabetes on the development and progression of long-term complications in insulin-dependent diabetes mellitus. NEJM. 1993;329(14):977–86.
19. Hirsch IB, Brownlee M. Beyond hemoglobin A1c-need for additional markers of risk for diabetic microvascular complications. JAMA. 2010;303:2291–2.
20. Lachin JM, Genuth S, Nathan DM, Zinman B, Rutledge BN, DCCT/EDIC Research Group. Effect of glycemic exposure on the risk of microvascular complications in the diabetes control and complications trial-revisited. Diabetes. 2008;57:995–1001.
21. Okada T, Nakao T, Matsumoto H, Yamanaka T, Nagaoka Y, Tamekuni T. Influence of age and nutritional status on glycated albumin values in hemodialysis patients. Intern Med. 2009;48(17):1495–9.
22. Freedman BI, Andries L, Shihabi ZK, Rocco MV, Byers JR, Cardona CY, et al. Glycated albumin and risk of death and hospitalizations in diabetic dialysis patients. CJASN. 2011;6(7):1635–43.
23. Peacock TP, Shihabi ZK, Bleyer AJ, Dolbare EL, Byers JR, Knovich MA, et al. Comparison of glycated albumin and hemoglobin A(1c) levels in diabetic subjects on hemodialysis. Kidney Int. 2008;73(9):1062–8.
24. Kim IY, Kim MJ, Lee DW, Lee SB, Rhee H, Song SH, et al. Glycated albumin is a more accurate glycaemic indicator than haemoglobin A1c in diabetic patients with pre-dialysis chronic kidney disease. Nephrology. 2015;20:715–20.
25. Cohen RM, Holmes YR, Chenier TC, Joiner CH. Discordance between HbA1c and fructosamine: evidence for a glycosylation gap and its relation to diabetic nephropathy. Diabetes Care. 2003;26(1):163–7.

26. Goldstein DE, Little RR, Lorenz RA, Malone JI, Nathan D, Peterson CM, et al. Tests of glycemia in diabetes. Diabetes Care. 2004;27(7):1761–73.
27. Chen HS, Wu TE, Lin HD, Jap TS, Hsiao LC, Lee SH, et al. Hemoglobin A(1c) and fructosamine for assessing glycemic control in diabetic patients with CKD stage 3 and 4. Am J Kidney Dis. 2010;55(5):867–74.
28. Joy MS, Cefalu WT, Hogan SL, Nachman PH. Long-term glycemic control measurements in diabetic patients receiving hemodialysis. Am J Kidney Dis. 2002;39(2):297–307.
29. Shafi T, Sozio SM, Plantinga LC, Jaar BG, Kim ET, Parekh RS, et al. Serum fructosamine and glycated albumin and risk of mortality and clinical outcomes in hemodialysis patients. Diabetes Care. 2013;36(6):1522–33.
30. Yamanouchi T, Ogata N, Tagaya T, Kawasaki T, Sekino N, Funato H, et al. Clinical usefulness of serum 1,5-anhydroglucitol in monitoring glycaemic control. Lancet. 1996;347(9014):1514–8.
31. Monnier L, Wojtusciszyn A, Colette C, Owens D. The contribution of glucose variability to asymptomatic hypoglycemia in persons with type 2 diabetes. Diabetes Technol Ther. 2011;13:813–8.
32. Wright L, Hirsch IB, Gooley T, Brown Z. 1, 5-Anhydroglucitol and neonatal complications in pregnancy complicated by diabetes. Endocr Pract. 2015;21(7):725–33.
33. Fujisawa T, Ikegami H, Tsutsui T, Kawaguchi Y, Ueda H, Shintani M, et al. Renal tubular function affects glycosuria-related urinary excretion of 1,5-anhydroglucitol. Diabetes Care. 1999; 22(5):863–4.
34. Emoto M, Tabata T, Inoue T, Nishizawa Y, Morii H. Plasma 1,5-anhydroglucitol concentration in patients with end-stage renal disease with and without diabetes mellitus. Nephron. 1992;61(2):181–6.
35. Kim WJ, Park C-Y, Lee KB, Park SE, Rhee EJ, Lee WY, et al. Serum 1,5-anhydroglucitol concentrations are a reliable index of glycemic control in type 2 diabetes with mild or moderate renal dysfunction. Diabetes Care. 2012;35(2):281–6.
36. GlycoMark, Inc. Clinical Guide: 1,5-anhydroglucitol (1,5-AG) blood test. Available at: http://www.glycomark.com/wp-content/uploads/2015/10/GlycoMark_Clinical_Guide.pdf. Accessed January 4, 2016.
37. Jung HS, Kim HI, Kim MJ, Yoon JW, Ahn HY, Cho YM, et al. Analysis of hemodialysis-associated hypoglycemia in patients with type 2 diabetes using a continuous glucose monitoring system. Diabetes Tehcnol Ther. 2010;12(10):801–7.
38. Continuous Glucose Monitoring to Assess Glycemia in Chronic Kidney Disease – Changing Glucose Management (CANDY-CANE). Available at: ClinicialTrials.gov. Accessed January 4, 2016.
39. U.K. Prospective Diabetes Study Group. Intensive blood-glucose control with sulphonylureas or insulin compared with conventional treatment and risk of complications in patients with type 2 diabetes (UKPDS 33). Lancet. 1998;352(9131):837–53.
40. Action to Control Cardiovascular Risk in Diabetes (ACCORD) Study Group. Effects of intensive glucose lowering in type 2 diabetes. N Engl J Med. 2008;358:2545–59.
41. ADVANCE Collaborative Group. Intensive blood glucose control and vascular outcomes in patients with type 2 diabetes. N Engl J Med. 2008;358(24):2560–72.
42. Duckworth W, Abraira C, Moritz T, Reda D, Emanuele N, Reaven PD, et al. Glucose control and vascular complications in veterans with type 2 diabetes. N Engl J Med. 2009;360:129–39.
43. Hayward RA, Reaven PD, Emanuele VN, VADT Investigators. Follow-up glycemic control and cardiovascular outcomes in type 2 diabetes. N Engl J Med. 2015;373(10):978.
44. Moen MJ, Zhan M, Hsu VD, Walker LD, Einhorn LM, Seliger SL, et al. Frequency of hypoglycemia and its significance in chronic kidney disease. Clin J Am Soc Nephrol. 2009;4:1121–7.
45. Miller ME, Bonds DE, Gerstein HC, Seaquist ER, Bergenstal RM, Calles-Escandon J, et al. The effects of baseline characteristics, glycaemia treatment approach, and glycated haemoglobin concentration on the risk of severe hypoglycaemia: post hoc epidemiological analysis of the ACCORD study. BMJ. 2010;340:b5444. https://doi.org/10.1136/bmj.b5444.
46. Kalantar-Zadeh K, Block G, Humphreys MH, Kopple JD. Reverse epidemiology of cardiovascular risk factors in maintenance dialysis patients. Kidney Int. 2003;63(3):793–808.
47. Neumiller JJ, Hirsch IB. Management of hyperglycemia in diabetic kidney disease. Diabetes Spectr. 2015;28(3):214–9.
48. Shurraw S, Hemmelgarn B, Lin M, Majumdar SR, Klarenbach S, Manns B, et al. Association between glycemic control and adverse outcomes in people with diabetes mellitus and chronic kidney disease: a population-based cohort study. Arch Intern Med. 2011;171(21):1920–7.
49. Ramirez SP, McCullough KP, Thumma JR, Nelson RG, Morgenstern H, Gillespie BW, et al. Hemoglobin A(1c) levels and mortality in the diabetic hemodialysis population: findings from the Dialysis Outcomes and Practice Patterns Study (DOPPS). Diabetes Care. 2012;35(12):2527–32.
50. Ricks J, Molnar MZ, Kovesdy CP, Shah A, Nissenson AR, Williams M, et al. Glycemic control and cardiovascular mortality in hemodialysis patients with diabetes: a 6-year cohort study. Diabetes. 2012;61(3):708–15.
51. Duong U, Mehrotra R, Molnar MZ, Noori N, Kovesdy CP, Nissenson AR, et al. Glycemic control and survival in peritoneal dialysis patients with diabetes mellitus. Clin J Am Soc Nephrol (CJASN). 2011;6(5):1041–8.
52. Kalantar-Zadeh K. A critical evaluation of glycated protein parameters in advanced nephropathy: a matter of life or death: A1C remains the gold standard outcome predictor in diabetic dialysis patients. Counterpoint. Diabetes Care. 2012;35(7):1625–8.

53. Chow E, Bernjak A, Williams S, Fawdry RA, Hibbert S, Freeman J, et al. Risk of cardiac arrhythmias during hypoglycemia in patients with type 2 diabetes and cardiovascular risk. Diabetes. 2014;63:1738–47.
54. Hill CJ, Maxwell AP, Cardwell CR, Freedman BI, Tonelli M, Emoto M, et al. Glycated hemoglobin and risk of death in diabetic patients treated with hemodialysis: a meta-analysis. Am J Kidney Dis. 2014;63(1):84–94.
55. Molnar MZ, Kovesdy CP, Bunnapradist S, Streja E, Mehrotra R, Krishnan M, et al. Associations of pretransplant serum albumin with post-transplant outcomes in kidney transplant recipients. Am J Transplant. 2011;11(5):1006–15.
56. Kilpatrick ES, Rigby AS, Goode K, Atkin SL. Relating mean blood glucose and glucose variability to the risk of multiple episodes of hypoglycemia in type 1 diabetes. Diabetologia. 2007;50:2553–61.
57. Williams ME, Garg R, Wang W, Lacson R, Maddux F, Lacson E Jr. High hemoglobin A1c levels and glycemic variability increase risk of severe hypoglycemia in diabetic hemodialysis patients. Hemodial Int. 2014;18(2):423–32.

Diabetic Pharmacotherapies in Kidney Disease

5

Deborah A. Chon, Rachael T. Oxman, Rashmi S. Mullur, and Jane Eileen Weinreb

Introduction

The pharmacokinetics of antihyperglycemic medications are altered in chronic kidney disease (CKD) in several ways including reduced renal clearance, uremic alterations of hepatic and GI drug metabolism, and increased levels of unbound drug in hypoalbuminemia [1]. These alterations predispose to hypoglycemic events. Unfortunately, patients with CKD are less able to compensate for hypoglycemic events because of reduced renal gluconeogenesis [2, 3] as well as decreased food intake due to poor appetite and dietary restrictions [4]. This can be a dangerous combination. For this reason, treatment of diabetes in CKD requires attention to drug interactions, cautious dose titration, and close glucose monitoring. As renal disease progresses, patients often require dose reductions of insulin and/or oral antihyperglycemic medications to avoid hypoglycemic events. Once patients initiate dialysis therapy, drug pharmacokinetics are altered again with increased drug and urea clearance [2, 3]. As a result, treatment of diabetes in CKD requires frequent reassessment to meet the patient's changing drug response and needs.

D. A. Chon · R. T. Oxman · R. S. Mullur ·
J. E. Weinreb (✉)
Division of Diabetes, Endocrinology, and Metabolism, David Geffen School of Medicine at UCLA, VA Greater Los Angeles Healthcare System, Los Angeles, CA, USA
e-mail: jane.Weinreb@va.gov

Biguanides

Metformin is recommended as first-line medical therapy for type 2 diabetes in all treatment guidelines and is the most widely used diabetes medication. It is affordable, has been extensively studied, is weight neutral, and does not increase the risk of hypoglycemia. The glucose-lowering effect is via activation of adenosine monophosphate protein kinase (AMPK) in hepatocytes and myocytes, thereby suppressing hepatic gluconeogenesis and promoting glucose uptake in skeletal muscle [5]. Metformin lowers fasting plasma glucose in a dose-related manner with a dose of 2000 mg daily resulting in a 2% lowering of HbA1c compared with placebo [6]. Moreover, metformin is associated with additional benefits such as a lipid-lowering effect and a significant risk reduction in myocardial infarction and all-cause mortality [5, 7]. The most common side effects are initial gastrointestinal disturbance, such as nausea, bloating, flatulence, and diarrhea.

Metformin is renally cleared, and when renal function is impaired, clearance decreases in parallel to the decrease in eGFR. There is concern that accumulation of the drug could precipitate lactic acidosis as was frequently seen with its predecessor, phenformin. Hence, metformin carried an

C. M. Rhee et al. (eds.), *Endocrine Disorders in Kidney Disease*,
https://doi.org/10.1007/978-3-319-97765-2_5

FDA boxed warning stating it is contraindicated with renal disease or dysfunction, as defined by a serum creatinine of ≥1.5 mg/dL in men and ≥1.4 mg/dL in women [8]. The original prescribing label was intended to provide a margin of safety to minimize the risk of lactic acidosis [9], but the prevalence of metformin causing lactic acidosis is low. Salpeter et al. pooled data from 347 studies with type 2 diabetics, and the true incidence of lactic acidosis per 100,000 patient-years was 4.3 cases with metformin and 5.4 cases in the non-metformin group [10]. Moreover, a recent review by Inzucchi et al. showed that while metformin clearance is decreased in the setting of renal dysfunction, drug levels remain within the therapeutic range when estimated glomerular filtration rate (eGFR) is >30 mL/min/1.73 m^2 and lactate levels are not significantly increased [9]. Further support for metformin use in patients with mild to moderate renal impairment comes from an observational study of nearly 20,000 type 2 diabetic patients with known atherosclerotic disease; mortality was reduced with metformin therapy in patients with a creatinine clearance of 30–60 mL/min/1.73 m^2 [11].

Thus, Inzucchi et al. proposed a strategy of prescribing metformin in patients with mild to moderate CKD that is endorsed by the American Diabetes Association. He suggested that maximal effective dose (2000 mg daily) could be used in patients with an eGFR of 45–60 mL/min/1.73 m^2 (CKD 3a), whereas a reduced dose of up to 1000 mg daily could be used in patients with an eGFR of 30–45 mL/min/1.73 m^2 (CKD 3b) if they were already on the medication, but not to initiate therapy at this stage [9]. These dose adjustments require more cautious follow-up of renal function, and avoiding metformin therapy is advised if kidney function is expected to be unstable. This plan for metformin use in chronic kidney disease is now formally endorsed by the FDA [12].

Sulfonylureas

Sulfonylureas (SUs) are insulin secretagogues. The potency of different SUs varies, but their efficacy is generally equivalent, reducing HbA1c by ~1.25–1.5%. SUs are primarily metabolized in the liver and predominantly excreted by the kidneys [13, 14]. SUs act by binding to the sulfonylurea receptor, a subunit of the ATP-dependent potassium channels on beta cells, triggering channel closure and prompting cell depolarization; this allows calcium influx which stimulates insulin secretion in a non-glucose-dependent manner. This mechanism inherently increases risk of hypoglycemia, especially in populations who may have blunted gluconeogenesis, inconsistent nutrition, or malnutrition as may be seen in CKD patients. Relative hypoglycemic risk among individual SUs in CKD depends on drug half-life, the extent of hepatic metabolism, and the hypoglycemic activity of hepatic metabolites. However, all SUs should be used with caution, initiated at low doses, and titrated slowly.

First-generation SUs include chlorpropamide, acetohexamide, tolazamide, and tolbutamide. All first-generation SUs have active hepatic metabolites which accumulate in CKD prolonging drug half-life and predisposing to hypoglycemia. These agents should be avoided in CKD because of concerns for accumulation and poor side effect profile in comparison to second-generation SUs [9, 10].

Second-generation SUs include glyburide, glipizide, and glimepiride. In general, second-generation SUs are better tolerated in CKD than first-generation agents. *Glyburide* is the exception. Glyburide has a long half-life of ~10 h, an active hepatic metabolite (4-hydroxyglibenclamide), and has been associated with severe, prolonged, and more frequent hypoglycemia [15–18]. Hence, glyburide should not be used in CKD.

Glimepiride has limited use in CKD because it is hepatically metabolized, and one of its metabolites, M1, retains partial hypoglycemic activity of ~33% of glimepiride's original potency [14, 19]. M1 progressively accumulates with declining renal clearance and likely accounts for higher rates of hypoglycemia compared to SUs such as gliclazide, which, like glipizide, does not accumulate in renal disease [19, 20]. Glimepiride may be used with caution in CKD at a starting dose of 1 mg/day but should be avoided in dialysis patients [1, 2, 21, 22].

Glipizide is the preferred SU in CKD because it is hepatically metabolized to inactive metabolites, less than 10% is excreted unmetabolized, and it has a short half-life of 2–4 h [1, 2, 14, 23]. Glipizide can be used in all CKD stages and dialysis without dose adjustment though conservative initial dosing of 2.5–5 mg/daily is recommended [2, 21, 24].

Meglitinides

Meglitinides are rapid-onset, short-acting insulin secretagogues administered at mealtimes which reduce postprandial hyperglycemia. Meglitinides act through a unique binding site on beta cells separate from sulfonylureas, closing potassium channels and thereby prompting insulin release. In general, it is not recommended to use meglitinide and SU therapy simultaneously because these agents have a similar mechanism of action and the combination has not been studied, while combination therapy with other agents such as metformin, TZDs, and acarbose is known to have additive effect in lowering HbA1c [25]. When choosing between meglitinide and SU therapy, it is important to note that meglitinides target postprandial hyperglycemia rather than basal hyperglycemia addressed by SUs. Meglitinides also have a lower incidence of hypoglycemia. This reduced hypoglycemia is likely multifactorial including shorter half-life, mealtime administration, and, in the case of nateglinide, glucose-dependent insulin secretion [26–29]. Furthermore, HbA1c lowering with repaglinide can be equivalent to SU therapy, but this is not the case for nateglinide which is less efficacious [26, 29].

Repaglinide can reduce HbA1c by 1.0–1.5% [26, 30]. Repaglinide is metabolized in the liver by P450 cytochrome enzymes to three inactive metabolites (M1, M2, M7), has a short half-life of ~1 h, and 90% is excreted in bile with only 8% excreted renally [31]. Severe renal impairment (eGFR <30 mL/min) increases repaglinide's half-life and/or area under the curve (AUC) though it is unaffected in mild to moderate kidney disease [32, 33]. Despite these pharmacokinetic changes, hypoglycemic risk is equivalent in patients with and without kidney disease. Overall, repaglinide is a safe and effective therapeutic diabetic treatment option in kidney disease [32, 34]. However patients with advanced kidney disease may require lower doses, and it should be initiated at a dose of 0.5 mg with meals especially if eGFR is <30 mL/min [2, 34]. Additionally, there is potential for drug interactions if administered concurrently with P450 cytochrome inhibitors including gemfibrozil which can cause an eightfold greater repaglinide AUC and threefold longer half-life [1, 29, 31].

Nateglinide therapy can lower HbA1C by 0.5–1.0% and is associated with less weight gain (0.7 kg vs 1.8 kg) than repaglinide therapy [26, 30]. Nateglinide is similarly metabolized in the liver with a short half-life of ~1 h, but in contrast to repaglinide, it has active metabolites, and 83% of the drug is cleared by the kidneys [35, 36]. While the pharmacokinetics after 120 mg single-dose administration seems to be equivalent across all stages of CKD and normal renal function patients, there is suggestion by case report that nateglinide's metabolites can accumulate in CKD with prolonged hypoglycemic effect [37, 38]. Nateglinide may be initiated at low dose (60 mg with meals TID) in patients with CKD [2]. However, given the differences in metabolite activity and clearance between the meglitinides, it seems reasonable for repaglinide to be the meglitinide of choice in CKD.

Glucagon-Like Peptide 1 Receptor Agonists (GLP-1 RAs)

GLP-1 and gastric inhibitory peptide (GIP) are known as incretins, intestinal peptides released in response to nutrients in the gut that promote glucose-dependent insulin secretion, suppress glucagon release, slow gastric emptying, and centrally inhibit appetite [39]. Type 2 diabetics have a small but significant reduction in meal-stimulated levels of GLP-1 [39]. GLP-1 RAs serve as incretin analogs, targeting both postprandial glucose excursions in addition to fasting glucose levels. This class of drugs is safe as it achieves its glucose-lowering effects without hypoglycemia and also has the added benefit of dose-dependent progressive weight loss [39–41]. Two drugs in this class, liraglutide and semaglutide, result in a significant decrease in three-point major adverse cardiovascular outcomes (MACE) (fatal and nonfatal MI and stroke) in patients with known cardiovascular (CV) disease or high CV risk [42, 43]. Liraglutide additionally decreased death due to CV disease by 22% as well as all-cause mortality, whereas semaglutide decreases MACE mostly due to decrease in nonfatal stroke.

The most common side effects of these injectable medications are gastrointestinal in nature, predominantly nausea, but this usually decreases over time [39–41]. Of note, there is a boxed warning by the FDA stating that GLP-1 RAs have been shown to cause dose-dependent and treatment duration-dependent thyroid C-cell tumors in rats and mice [44–47]. Thus, this class of medications is contraindicated in patients with personal or family history of medullary thyroid carcinoma and multiple endocrine neoplasia syndrome type 2 [44–47]. Also, there is concern regarding incretin-based medications and their association with acute pancreatitis and potential for pancreatic cancer, given the stimulation of beta-cell proliferation and inhibition of apoptosis [48]. Although other studies have not confirmed this increased risk [49], it is recommended that an alternative medication class be used in patients with a history of pancreatitis.

Exenatide is administered as 5–10 mcg subcutaneous (SC) injection twice daily within 60 min prior to a meal. In phase III trials, exenatide was added to ongoing therapy with oral hypoglycemic agents in patients with suboptimal control and was found to reduce HbA1c concentrations by 0.8–1.0% over 30 weeks with a weight loss of 1.5–3 kg [40, 50, 51]. Patients who continued in an open-label extension lost 4–5 kg after 80 weeks [52]. The kidney is the primary route of elimination and degradation. Linnebjerg et al. evaluated the pharmacokinetics of exenatide in renal impairment. In subjects with mild to moderate renal impairment (CrCl 30–80 mL/min), exenatide clearance was decreased, but tolerability was unchanged [53]. However, exenatide clearance was significantly decreased (84%) in ESRD patients, and even low-dose exenatide of 5 mcg was not well tolerated due to gastrointestinal side effects [53]. Thus, there are no recommendations for dosing adjustments in mild to moderate renal impairment, but use is not recommended for CrCl <30 mL/min or in ESRD [44]. A long-acting formulation of exenatide, exenatide extended release (Bydureon®), was approved by the FDA in 2012. It is administered as 2 mg SC injection weekly. In the DURATION-5 comparator trial, this formulation resulted in greater glycemic improvements (1.6% from baseline A1c of 8.5%) as monotherapy or in addition to one or more oral diabetic agents at 24 weeks with a weight loss of 2.3 kg and less nausea *(Blevins)*. Patients taking extended release exenatide 2 mg weekly had a 62% and 33% increase in exposure in moderate and mild renal impairment compared to those with normal renal function *(package insert)*. Caution is advised in patients with moderate renal impairment (CrCl 30–50 mL/min). No studies have been done in severe renal impairment or ESRD *(package insert)*.

Liraglutide is administered as a once daily 0.6–1.8 mg SC injection. In a placebo-controlled, double-blind trial evaluating liraglutide as add-on therapy in patients with moderate renal impairment, there was a significant decrease in HbA1c by 0.66% from a baseline of about 8% compared to placebo at 26 weeks [54]. There was also a significant weight loss of 1.32 kg compared to placebo with maximum-dose liraglutide [54]. Elimination occurs via endogenous dipeptidyl peptidase IV (DPP-4) enzyme degradation, and there is no significant renal clearance. In a single dosing study of liraglutide 0.75 mg daily, there was no significant effect of decreasing creatinine clearance on the pharmacokinetics of liraglutide nor any associated increased risk of adverse events [55]. Per the package insert, there are no current recommended dosage adjustments in mild to severe renal impairment, but caution is suggested with initiating or escalating doses [45].

Dulaglutide is a long-acting GLP-1 RA administered as a 0.75–1.5 mg SC once weekly injection. The AWARD (Assessment of Weekly

Administration of Dulaglutide) trials assessed the efficacy and safety of dulaglutide as monotherapy and as add-on diabetes therapy. Dulaglutide was shown to have greater reductions in HbA1c in comparison to metformin, exenatide, glargine, sitagliptin, among others and found to be noninferior to liraglutide [56, 57]. In a randomized, double-blind, placebo-controlled monotherapy trial, HbA1c was significantly reduced by 1.0% from a baseline of 7.6–7.8% compared with placebo at 12 weeks on dulaglutide 1.5 mg weekly [58]. Dulaglutide is degraded by general protein catabolism. Thus, the pharmacokinetics are not expected to be affected by renal impairment, and there is no dosage adjustment necessary [59]. Per the package insert, there are no current recommended dosage adjustments in mild to severe renal impairment, but caution is suggested with initiating or escalating doses [46].

Lixisenatide is a once daily 10–20 mcg SC injection. The GetGoal trials were randomized, double-blind, placebo-controlled trials in patients with type 2 diabetes evaluating efficacy of lixisenatide as monotherapy or as add-on therapy to metformin, pioglitazone, sulfonylurea, or basal insulin. In the monotherapy trial, HbA1c was significantly reduced by 0.85% from a baseline of about 8% compared with placebo at 12 weeks [60]. Mean decrease of body weight in the trials was 0.2–2 kg [60–64]. Elimination occurs via glomerular filtration and proteolytic degradation (*package insert*). No dose adjustment is necessary in patients with mild renal impairment (eGFR 60–89 mL/min/1.73 m^2) or moderate renal impairment (eGFR 30 to <60 mL/min/1.73 m^2), but close monitoring of gastrointestinal reactions that may lead to dehydration and changes in renal function is recommended [65]. Clinical experience is limited in severe renal impairment (eGFR 15 to <30 mL/min/1.73 m^2), but exposure was higher and close monitoring is advised (*package insert*). Use in ESRD is not recommended given lack of experience (*package insert*).

Semaglutide is a weekly injectable GLP-1 RA dosed as 0.25–1.0 mg SC weekly [66]. The SUSTAIN clinical trials demonstrated clinical efficacy and safety of semaglutide as monotherapy or add-on diabetes therapy. Semaglutide has been found to have a superior reduction in A1c as compared to sitagliptan, exanatide, and dulaglutide, and it is noninferior to basal insulin [67–70]. The SUSTAIN 1 trial demonstrated that 30 weeks of 0.5 mg semaglutide monotherapy reduced HbA1c by 1.45%, and 1.0 mg semaglutide monotherapy reduced HbA1c 1.55% from a baseline HbA1c of 8.05% as compared to placebo [71]. The SUSTAIN 5 trial confirmed similar reductions among uncontrolled type 2 diabetics on basal insulin with or without metformin showing a 1.4% A1c reduction with 0.5 mg and a 1.8% A1c reduction with 1.0 mg semaglutide add-on therapy [72]. Semaglutide is degraded by general protein catabolism, which is followed by beta-oxidation. It is excreted in urine and feces. Only 3% of semaglutide is excreted intact through the urine. There is no dose adjustment recommended for renal impairment [66]. However, it should be noted that pharmacokinetic studies after single dose of 0.5 mg semaglutide did note a 22% higher mean exposure in non-dialysis patients with severe renal impairment (eGFR <30 mL/min) and higher rates of nausea in this same group [73]. SUSTAIN 6 found a positive cardiovascular benefit to semaglutide therapy with a 26% risk reduction in the composite outcome of nonfatal myocardial infarction, nonfatal stroke, and cardiovascular death. However, the composite outcome was driven by improvements in nonfatal MI and stroke, as there was no significant difference in rates of cardiovascular death between semaglutide and placebo-treated participants [42].

Dipeptidyl Peptidase IV (DPP-4) Inhibitors

Endogenous incretins are rapidly inactivated by the enzyme DPP-4. Selective DPP-4 inhibitors limit the degradation of GLP-1 and thus potentiate endogenous incretin hormone activity. Thus, this class of medications has similar actions as the GLP-1 receptor agonists, including glucose-dependent stimulation of insulin secretion and inhibition of glucagon secretion. However, DPP-4 inhibitors are generally not associated with slowing of gastric emptying [39], and their use is not commonly associated with nausea or weight loss as occurs with the GLP-1 receptor agonists. These agents have the benefit of once daily oral dosing. Moreover, they have been studied in dialysis patients and while they may need dose adjustments, they are safe for use in these patients for whom diabetic treatment options are limited [74].

There is similar concern for acute pancreatitis and potential risk for pancreatic cancer as with GLP-1 receptor agonists [48]. Also, the FDA issued a warning in August 2015 that all four DPP-4 inhibitors may cause joint pain that is severe and disabling, based on 33 cases of severe arthralgia reported from 2006 to 2013 [75]. The onset of symptoms appeared within a month following initiation in a majority of the cases but ranged between a day and years. Symptoms resolved after medication was discontinued, but some patients had recurrent symptoms with reinitiation or switch to another DPP-4 inhibitor.

Sitagliptin is administered as a once daily oral dose of 100 mg. It is primarily eliminated via renal excretion. Various studies have demonstrated efficacy and safety of sitagliptin use in patients with renal impairment. Following a 50 mg oral dose of sitagliptin, subjects with moderate renal insufficiency (CrCl 30–50 mL/min), severe renal insufficiency (<30 mL/min but not on dialysis), or ESRD on dialysis had approximately 2.3-fold, 3.8-fold, or 4.5-fold higher plasma concentrations compared to those with normal renal function or mild renal impairment [76]. Thus, dose adjustments are recommended in renal insufficiency to keep plasma concentrations comparable to those with normal renal function, as follows: 50 mg once daily for CrCl 30 to 50 mL/min and 25 mg once daily for CrCl <30 mL/min, ESRD, or on dialysis [76, 77]. Chan et al. studied the safety of dose-adjusted therapy with sitagliptin as per the recommendations noted above in patients with moderate and severe renal insufficiency, including patients with ESRD on dialysis [78]. At 12 weeks, there was a significant reduction of HbA1c by 0.4% from a baseline of 7.6–7.8% compared to placebo and a mean reduction in HbA1c by 0.7% at 54 weeks in the sitagliptin group [78]. Sitagliptin can be administered irrespective of hemodialysis timing [76].

Saxagliptin is administered orally as 2.5–5 mg once daily. In a multicenter phase 3 trial of type 2 diabetic patients with moderate or severe renal impairment or ESRD on dialysis randomized to saxagliptin 2.5 mg daily or placebo, there was a significant decrease in mean HbA1c by 0.73% from a baseline of 8.1–8.5% compared to placebo at 52 weeks [79]. Reductions in adjusted mean HbA1c were numerically greater with saxagliptin than placebo in patients with renal impairment rated as moderate (0.94% vs 0.19%, respectively) or severe (0.81% vs 0.49%) but similar to placebo for those with ESRD (1.13% vs 0.99%) [79]. Hepatic metabolism produces an active metabolite that is 50% less potent than saxagliptin, and elimination occurs predominantly via renal route [14]. Saxagliptin and its major metabolite were 1.2- and 1.7-fold higher in mild renal impairment, 1.4- and 2.9-fold higher in moderate renal impairment, and 2.1- and 4.5-fold higher in severe renal impairment in comparison to normal renal function [80]. There are currently no dosage adjustment recommendations until moderate to severe impairment (CrCl ≤50 mL/min), when dose should be decreased to 2.5 mg once daily [81]. In dialysis patients, a single 4-h session removes 23% of a saxagliptin dose and thus should be taken after the dialysis session [14]. Of note, a study by Scirica et al. evaluated the effect of saxagliptin versus placebo in type 2 diabetic patients at risk for cardiovascular events [82]. There was no effect found on the rate of ischemic events; however, the rate of hospitalizations for heart failure was increased. There are currently no specific recommendations in the package insert regarding saxagliptin use for patients with heart failure. We would lean toward the use of an alternative agent for a patient with significant heart failure.

Linagliptin is administered as 5 mg orally once daily. In a pooled analysis of three phase 3 trials, linagliptin 5 mg was compared to placebo or as add-on therapy in type 2 diabetic subjects with normal, mild, and moderate renal impairment [83]. At 24 weeks, there was a significant placebo-corrected mean HbA1c reduction of

0.63% in normal renal function, 0.67% in mild renal impairment, and 0.53% in moderate renal impairment from a baseline of 8.0–8.2% with no inter-group difference [83]. McGill et al. found a reduction in HbA1c of 0.6% from a baseline of 7–10% in type 2 diabetic subjects with severe renal impairment taking linagliptin 5 mg compared to placebo at 12 weeks that was sustained at 1 year [84]. Eighty-five percent of the ingested dose is fecally eliminated, while only 5% of the dose is excreted renally [85]. Plasma concentrations were similar in type 2 diabetic subjects with mild, moderate, and severe renal impairment after a 5 mg dose of linagliptin [86]. As there was no indication that even severe renal impairment prolongs the elimination of linagliptin, there is no dosage adjustment necessary [87].

Alogliptin is administered as a once daily oral dose of 25 mg. A number of phase 3 clinical trials have shown the efficacy of alogliptin as add-on therapy. HbA1c reduction ranged from 0.5% to 0.78% compared to placebo from a baseline of about 7–10% with alogliptin 25 mg daily added on therapies such as metformin and pioglitazone [88, 89]. Elimination is primarily via renal excretion. After a 50 mg oral dose of alogliptin, exposure was increased by 1.7-, 2.1-, 3.2-, and 3.8-fold in patients with mild, moderate, and severe renal impairment and ESRD, respectively [90]. Thus, no dosage adjustment is necessary with CrCl ≥60 mL/min, but daily dose should be reduced to 12.5 mg for CrCl 30–60 mL/min and 6.25 mg for CrCl <30 mL/min or dialysis patients [91]. In a prospective, open-label study of 30 type 2 diabetic patients on hemodialysis, alogliptin 6.25 mg daily administered regardless of timing of dialysis improved glycemic control as monotherapy or add-on therapy and was generally well tolerated [92].

Thiazolidinediones

Thiazolidinediones (TZDs) are peroxisome proliferator-activated receptor gamma (PPARγ) agonists which improve glycemic control via improved insulin sensitivity. PPARγ is a nuclear transcription factor which regulates gene transcription; it is expressed most strongly in adipose tissue but also has lower expression in the liver, heart, and muscle [93]. The antihyperglycemic effect of PPARγ stimulation is largely indirect through reduction in free fatty acids with increased subcutaneous adipogenesis as well as effects on adipokine expression. TZDs also have a direct antihyperglycemia effect by upregulating the expression of GLUT4 which is the insulin-sensitive glucose transporter in muscle and adipose tissue [94]. These indirect and direct effects culminate to enhance peripheral insulin sensitivity at the liver and muscle by decreasing hepatic glucose production, increasing glycogen synthesis, and increasing muscle glucose disposal [14, 93, 95].

Clinically, TZDs have multiple beneficial effects including improved fasting and postprandial hyperglycemia, reduced fat accumulation in the liver, improved lipid profiles with lower fatty acid levels and higher HDL, and also reduced average blood pressure by a small but statistically significant amount [14, 93, 95–97]. There is also growing literature that TZDs have a renoprotective effect; this is expounded upon in section "Impact of Antihyperglycemic Agents on Renal Function".

Unfortunately, TZD therapy has been associated with multiple adverse side effects. Most prominently TZD therapy is associated with weight gain and fluid retention with complications of peripheral edema and increased frequency of CHF exacerbations [93, 98–100]. TZD-induced fluid retention may be less responsive to diuretics and be especially severe when TZDs are used in combination therapy with insulin [93, 98, 100]. TZDs are contraindicated in patients with NYHA Class III and IV heart failure and were given a black-box warning in 2007 [98]. TZDs can be used as insulin sensitizers in patients with CKD who are not candidates for metformin use. However, CKD patients are high risk for volume overload as well as comorbid heart disease, and hence, some feel these agents are better avoided [21, 101]. When TZD therapy is used in CKD, patients require close monitoring for evidence of fluid retention. In addition, TZD therapy is also associated with hepatotoxicity and increased appendicular fracture risk, which has been attributed to PPARγ2 inhibition of osteoblastogenesis leading to decreased bone mineral density in men and women. This increased risk of fracture has been clearly documented in women only [98, 102–104]. Finally, in 2010 rosiglitazone was placed under prescribing and dispensing restrictions for potential increased cardiovascular mortality. To fully evaluate this concern, the FDA performed a comprehensive readjudication of the RECORD trial as well as independent expert review by the Duke Clinical Research Institute (DCRI) which concluded that rosiglitazone had equivalent cardiovascular risk as compared to other standard DM therapies (metformin and sulfonylurea), and the distribution restrictions were subsequently removed in 2013 [105].

Pioglitazone can reduce HbA1c by 1.0–1.6% in monotherapy depending on dose [98]. Pioglitazone undergoes hepatic hydroxylation and oxidation to two active metabolites (M-III & M-IV) which retain ~40–60% of the potency of the original compound. Peak serum levels occur ~ 2 h after administration. Pioglitazone half-life is variable (3–7 h) as is the half-life of its metabolites, ranging 16–24 h. Drug clearance is primarily through bile and feces with negligible renal contribution [98]. Pharmacokinetic studies show that both parent pioglitazone and its metabolites have increased drug clearance in moderate and severe renal disease which results in shorter half-lives and peak concentrations compared to subjects with normal renal function. It has been postulated that this increased clearance is secondary to reduced protein binding in CKD resulting in higher proportions of unbound or free forms facilitating greater hepatic clearance [106]. Ultimately, no dose adjustment is necessary in patients with CKD, and a starting dose of 15 mg daily can be considered. In hemodialysis patients, a dose of 30 mg has been tolerated [1].

Rosiglitazone can reduce HbA1c by 0.8–1.5% in monotherapy depending on dose with maximum efficacy at 4 mg twice daily dosing in the general population [107]. Rosiglitazone undergoes hepatic metabolism through N-demethylation, hydroxylation, and then conjugation into inactive metabolites [107–109]. Metabolism is specifically mediated by CYP2C8, a cytochrome P450 enzyme; this enzyme is clinically relevant because gemfibrozil is a CYP2C8 inhibitor which can increase rosiglitazone concentrations when used concurrently [110]. Rosiglitazone has excellent oral bioavailability at 99% with peak serum levels at ~1 h after oral administration, and a half-life between 3 and 4 h. Clearance of drug metabolites is 64% through urine and 23% by feces [107]. Rosiglitazone pharmacokinetics in regard to AUC and maximum plasma concentration are unchanged in all stages of CKD including hemodialysis but increased 2–3 times in patients with Child-Pugh Class B or C liver disease [107, 108]. No dose adjustment is necessary in CKD, and a starting dose of 4 mg daily can be considered.

Sodium-Glucose Co-transporter 2 (SGLT2) Inhibitors

SGLT2 inhibitors are the newest oral hypoglycemic agents approved by the FDA for type 2 diabetes. The mechanism of action is based on the competitive inhibition of SGLT2, a tubular carrier protein that reabsorbs 90% of the glucose filtered in the glomerulus, leading to enhanced loss of glucose through the urine [111]. Studies have shown an improvement in glycemic control with low risk of hypoglycemia and other benefits such as weight loss and potential lowering of blood pressure [112]. Moreover, a recent study showed that type 2 diabetic patients at high risk of cardiovascular events who received empagliflozin had significantly lower rates of three-point MACE (fatal and nonfatal MI and stroke) and death from cardiovascular causes and all-cause mortality versus placebo [113]. Canagliflozin similarly reduced three-point MACE in a high-risk population [114]. Common side effects of therapy are an increase in urinary tract and genital infections. Since SGLT2 inhibitors depend on glomerular filtration for their primary mechanism of action, impaired renal function can reduce the glucose-lowering efficacy of these agents [115]. Thus, these medications are not expected to be efficacious in patients with severe renal insufficiency with an eGFR <30 mL/min/1.73 m^2 or in dialysis patients.

Of note, the FDA issued a warning of an increased risk of euglycemic diabetic ketoacidosis (DKA) with the use of all approved SGLT2 inhibitors, based on 20 reported cases requiring hospitalization between March 2013 and June 2014 in the FDA Adverse Event Reporting System database [116]. DKA occurs mostly in insulin-deficient patients. This is thought to be due to an alteration in the balance of glucagon to insulin, with resultant increase in fatty acid oxidation and ketone production [117]. Normally DKA is associated with marked hyperglycemia, osmotic diuresis, and dehydration; however, SGLT2 inhibitors can lower BG to less than 200 mg/dl, allowing euglycemic DKA to be easily missed based on clinical signs alone [118]. Some of these cases occurred in type 1 diabetic patients, for whom the FDA has not approved the use of SGLT2 inhibitors despite increasing off-label use. A commentary in Diabetes Care noted that based on evaluation of limited clinical data that exists, the risk for DKA is likely to be low in type 2 diabetic patients [119]. Further, this drug class may still be useful even in the type 1 diabetic population, for whom adjunctive therapies are limited, as long as appropriate precautions are given [119]. The FDA additionally recently issued a warning of increased risk of necrotizing fasciitis, based upon 12 such episodes reported, all of which required antibiotics and surgery and one of which resulted in death. They warn that patients seek immediate medical help if they experience any symptoms of tenderness, redness or swelling of the genitals together with a fever above 100.4 F. (www.fda.gov/safety/medwatch/safetyinformation/safety/alertsforhumanmedicalproducts/ucm618908.htm).

Canagliflozin is administered once daily at a dose of 100–300 mg, usually before the first meal of the day. Metabolism is primarily via O-glucuronidation in the liver with metabolites excreted in the urine. In a phase 3 trial of type 2 diabetic subjects with stage 3 CKD (restricted in this study to eGFR 30 to <50 mL/min/1.73 m^2), there was a significant decrease in HbA1c with canagliflozin (100 mg and 300 mg) versus placebo and overall adverse events were similar between all groups [115]. HbA1c decreased 0.3% with 100 mg dosing compared to placebo at 26 weeks from a baseline of about 8% [115]. Current dosing recommendation guidelines advise a dose reduction to 100 mg/day with an eGFR of 45–59 mL/min/1.73 m^2, and use is contraindicated in eGFR <45 mL/min/1.73 m^2, ESRD, and dialysis [120]. Of note, canagliflozin carries a warning for increased fracture risk. A significant increase in fractures was seen with canagliflozin (4%) versus placebo (2.6%) in a subset of patients who were older, with prior history/risk of cardiovascular disease, lower baseline eGFR, and higher baseline diuretic use, thought to be mediated by falls [121]. The incidence, however, was similar in pooled studies of patients without high cardiovascular risk.

Dapagliflozin is administered at a dose of 5–10 mg once daily. In a study of type 2 diabetics with moderate renal impairment (mean eGFR 45 mL/min/1.73 m^2), there was no significant reduction in HbA1c with both dapagliflozin 5 mg and 10 mg versus placebo at 24 weeks [122]. Metabolism is both hepatic and renal. Kasichayanula et al. showed that plasma concentrations of the drug are increased incrementally with declining renal function, with steady-state peak serum concentration 4%, 6%, and 9% higher in patients with mild, moderate, and severe renal impairment [123]. Also, the glucose-lowering effect was attenuated with a renal glucose clearance reduction of 42%, 83%, and 84% in patients with mild, moderate, or severe renal impairment, respectively [123]. Thus, use is not recommended with eGFR <60 mL/min/1.73 m^2 and contraindicated in eGFR <30 mL/min/1.73 m^2, ESRD, and dialysis [122]. Of note, dapagliflozin carries a warning regarding bladder cancer—concerns were raised in the new drug application submitted to the FDA due to the numerical imbalance of bladder cancer reports in the treatment group versus control [124]. A causal relationship could not be established, but use is not advised in patients with active bladder cancer.

Empagliflozin is administered once daily at a dose of 10–25 mg in the morning. A phase 3 multinational study revealed that empagliflozin was effective in patients with stage 2 and 3 CKD, significantly lowering HbA1c by 0.68% in stage 2 CKD and 0.42% in stage 3 CKD from a baseline of about 8% compared to placebo with 25 mg dosing at 24 weeks [125]. Metabolism is primarily via glucuronidation in the liver. Macha et al. studied the effect of renal impairment on the pharmacodynamics and pharmacokinetics of empagliflozin [126]. The pharmacokinetic properties were largely unaltered by renal impairment, and there was no difference in adverse events, suggesting that no dose adjustments are required. However, in the study by Barnett et al., there were a limited number of subjects with stage 4 CKD evaluated in the study with higher rates of adverse events than those with stage 2 or 3 CKD [125]. Current dosing guidelines suggest use is not recommended with eGFR <45 mL/min/1.73 m^2, and use is contraindicated in eGFR <30 mL/min/1.73 m^2, ESRD, and dialysis [127].

Ertugliflozin is a once daily SGLT-2 inhibitor dosed as 5 or 15 mg daily (Steglatro package insert). It has been studied as monotherapy and in combination with metformin or sitagliptin, as well as on therapy with either a sulfonylurea or a dipeptidyl peptidase 4 (DPP-4) inhibitor. In the VERTIS-MONO trial, patients randomized to ertugliflozin had significantly greater reductions in A1C, FPG, body weight, and 2-h PPG and were significantly more likely to have an A1C <7.0% when compared to placebo. Additionally, ertugliflozin treatment was associated with a trend toward lower blood pressure [128]. In the VERTIS-MET trial, ertugliflozin was studied in T2DM participants inadequately controlled on metformin monotherapy. After 26 weeks, ertugliflozin significantly reduced A1c in a dose-dependent fashion, −0.7% and −0.9% for ertugliflozin 5 and 15 mg, respectively [129]. In the VERTIS-SU Trial, ertugliflozin or glimepiride was added on to patients already taking on metformin ≥1500 mg/day. Designed as a non-inferiority study, the primary hypothesis was that ertugliflozin 15 mg was noninferior to glimepiride. After 52 weeks, mean change (95% CI) from baseline in HbA1c was – 0.6%, – 0.6%, and – 0.7% in the ertugliflozin 15 mg, ertugliflozin 5 mg, and glimepiride groups, respectively. The between-group difference for ertugliflozin 15 mg and glimepiride of 0.1% met the prespecified non-inferiority criterion [130]. In the VERTIS-SITA trial, the safety of initial combination therapy of ertugliflozin and sitagliptin was compared to that of placebo. After 26 weeks, significantly greater reductions from baseline were observed in HbA1c, FPG, 2-h PPG, body weight, and systolic blood pressure in patients receiving combination therapy compared with placebo [131]. In the VERTIS-SITA2 trial, ertugliflozin was added to patients receiving combination therapy with metformin and sitagliptin. Greater reductions in HbA1c, FPG, body weight, and systolic blood pressure and a greater proportion of patients with an HbA1c <7.0% were observed with ertugliflozin compared with placebo [132]. Finally, in the VERTIS RENAL study, ertugliflozin was studied in patients with hemoglobin A1c 7.0–10.5% and stage 3 CKD [estimated glomerular filtration rate (eGFR) ≥30 to <60 mL/min/1.73 m^2] who were undergoing treatment with standard diabetes therapy including insulin and/or sulfonylureas. At week 26, there was no significant reduction from baseline in A1C of ertugliflozin versus placebo. Per the authors, metformin use was precluded in 17% of patients and impacted the primary endpoint [133]. At the time of this publication, no clinical trials of ertugliflozin have shown any reduction or benefit in primary cardiovascular endpoints outside of improvements in blood pressure. Ertugliflozin is primarily cleared via metabolism with glucuronidation and is excreted in the feces and urine (Steglatro package insert). Use of ertugliflozin is contraindicated in patients with an eGFR less than 30 mL/min/1.73 m^2. Initiation and persistent use of ertugliflozin are not recommended in patients with an eGFR of 30 to less than 60 mL/min/1.73 m^2. No dose adjustments are required for patients with mild renal impairment.

Alpha-Glucosidase Inhibitors

Alpha-glucosidase inhibitors are antidiabetic medications which disrupt complex carbohydrate absorption at the intestinal lining, thereby slowing glucose absorption and lowering postprandial glycemic excursions [1, 134, 135]. Alpha-glucosidase inhibitors do not augment insulin secretion and therefore have low hypoglycemic potential as sole therapy. However, when paired with insulin secretagogues or insulin therapy, the hypoglycemic risk is increased. Notably, when hypoglycemia does occur in patients on acarbose therapy, treatment specifically requires either pure dextrose (glucose tablets) or lactose (milk) [134, 136, 137]; lactose is digested by lactase, a beta-glucosidase enzyme. The absorption of sucrose, fructose, and carbohydrates are inherently delayed in alpha-glucosidase inhibitor therapy and are thus not effective in acute hypoglycemia treatment [137]. Patients can also be treated emergently with glucagon injection or dextrose infusion [134, 136].

Acarbose can reduce HbA1c by ~0.5–1.00% in monotherapy depending on dose with average reduction of 0.77% [26, 134, 135]. Acarbose is itself a complex carbohydrate which reversibly and competitively inhibits both pancreatic alpha-amylase and alpha-glucosidase hydrolase enzymes at the intestinal brush border. Acarbose is metabolized exclusively in the gut, but ~35% of acarbose dose is absorbed predominantly in the form of 13 metabolites with less than 2% of the dose absorbed in parent drug form. Once absorbed, acarbose and metabolites are cleared renally with a half-life of ~2 h. Unfortunately, in severe renal insufficiency (GFR <25 mL/min/1.73 m^2) there is significant accumulation with peak plasma levels five times higher than patients with normal renal function. There is also a trend toward higher peak levels in elderly patients [134]. There is a paucity of research as to the effects of higher acarbose levels acutely or long term in CKD patients. However, there is concern for potential rare occurrence of hepatic injury, and it is generally avoided in patients with underlying liver disease [134, 138]. Presumably, patients with comorbid CKD and cirrhosis could be at especially high risk. Primary side effects include flatulence and diarrhea [139]. Acarbose may be used without dose adjustment in early stages of CKD but should be avoided once eGFR <25 mL/min or in dialysis [2, 14]. Acarbose may be initiated at a dose of 25 mg TID AC; the FDA-approved maximum dose is 100 mg TID AC, but a Cochran meta-analysis suggests a maximum effective dose of 50 mg TID AC because of increased side effects without increased glycemic efficacy [134, 138]. Acarbose may have additional benefit in reducing myocardial infarction and hypertension in prediabetics although this has not been explicitly studied in CKD [140]. Further, its cardioprotective effect is likely inferior to that of metformin [141].

Miglitol can reduce HbA1c by 0.26–0.81% in monotherapy depending on dose with average reduction of 0.68% [135, 136]. Miglitol is also an oligosaccharide which competitively inhibits alpha-glucosidase hydrolase enzymes. However unlike acarbose, miglitol is not metabolized but rather is absorbed in parent drug form. The degree of absorption is dose dependent with near complete absorption of a 25 mg tablet versus 50–70% of a 100 mg tablet. Once absorbed, serum drug levels peak at 2–3 h, half-life is short at 2 h, and greater than 95% of miglitol is excreted renally. While systemic miglitol does not have hypoglycemic effect, there is twofold serum drug accumulation when eGFR falls below 25 mL/min on low-dose miglitol (25 mg TID AC), and there is limited long-term clinical trial data in patients with comorbid CKD. For these reasons, miglitol use is not recommended in patients with GFR <25 mL/min [136].

Bromocriptine

Bromocriptine-QR (BQR) is a quick release formula of the ergot alkaloid bromocriptine mesylate, a sympatholytic dopamine D2 receptor agonist. Bromocriptine is unique in that it acts via resetting of the dopaminergic and sympathetic tone within the central nervous system. There is a circadian rhythm to insulin sensitivity, with a decrease in early morning dopamine levels leading to increased sympathetic activity at the level of the suprachiasmatic nucleus (SCN) and the ventromedial hypothalamus (VMH). Animal studies have shown that dopamine levels are low in an insulin-resistant state and high norepinephrine causes severe insulin resistance, glucose intolerance, and accelerated lipolysis in hamsters and rats [142, 143]. Bromocriptine administration leads to a decrease in VMH noradrenergic levels and subsequent decline in hepatic glucose production, reduced lipolysis, and improved insulin sensitivity [144, 145].

BQR is available as a 0.8 mg tablet that is administered within 2 h of waking and can be titrated to a maximum of 4.8 mg/day. Phase 3 trials have evaluated BQR efficacy as monotherapy and as adjunctive therapy to oral antidiabetic agents, demonstrating a decline in HbA1c of about 0.55% with BQR 4.8 mg daily versus placebo at 24 weeks [146]. BQR significantly reduced the fasting and postprandial glucose concentrations, free fatty acid concentrations, and triglyceride concentrations. There was no change in body weight. Of note, a 3070-subject randomized trial demonstrated a significant 40% reduction in cardiovascular events among BQR-treated subjects [147]. Analyzing the data for hard endpoints of myocardial infarction, stroke, and cardiovascular death, there was a significant 52% reduction in relative risk with BQR therapy [148].

There is extensive hepatic first-pass metabolism via the cytochrome CYP450 system, and only 2–6% appears in the urine [149]. The main side effects are nausea, asthenia, constipation, and dizziness [146]. Although these side effects were generally mild and transient, 13% of BQR-treated subjects withdrew because of adverse events compared with 3–5% of placebo-treated subjects ($P < 0.01$) [146]. There was no difference in serious adverse events and hypoglycemia between both groups. There has only been one study evaluating the safety of BQR in patients with reduced eGFR. In this trial, cardiovascular and renal effects were evaluated in 14 type 2 diabetic patients with stage 4 CKD on BQR titrated up to 7.5 mg daily versus placebo [150]. CrCl remained statistically unchanged in the BQR-treated group while it declined significantly in the placebo group; thus, it was postulated that BQR prevented the progression of CKD, but clearly additional data are needed [150].

Bile Acid Resins

Bile acid resins are most frequently used in the management of hyperlipidemia. However, they can also improve glycemic control in combination therapy with one or more other antidiabetic agents. Colesevelam is the only bile acid resin FDA approved specifically for glycemic control. *Colesevelam* has been studied in multidrug therapy including metformin, insulin, SU, and TZDs with significant and consistent reductions in HbA1c of 0.5–0.54% [151, 152].

Bile acid resins lower LDL levels by complexing with bile acids within the gastrointestinal tract preventing reabsorption into the enterohepatic circulation and promoting bile acid excretion [153]. The wasting of bile acids decreases absorption of dietary lipids and promotes conversion of serum cholesterol into new bile acids. This effectively reduces LDL but can increase HDL as well as triglyceride levels [153]. The mechanism of glycemic improvement, however, is not well established. Some studies have suggested that reduced bile acid levels may decrease stimulation of farnesoid X receptor (FXR), a nuclear transcription factor that regulates hepatic gluconeogenesis, potentially by modulating the expression of PEPCK, a rate-limiting enzyme in gluconeogenesis [153–155]. Other studies have shown that colosevelam therapy can increase postprandial GLP-1 and GIP though without concomitant greater insulin secretion [154, 156]. Clinically, colosevelam reduces both fasting and postprandial hyperglycemia [154]. It is associated with a low rate of hypoglycemia and does not cause weight gain [151]. Colesevelam can be considered as add-on therapy, especially in patients with comorbid LDL elevations [152]. It is unknown if bile acid resins have antihyperglycemic benefit when paired with incretin therapies (DPP4 inhibitors or GLP-1 agonists) [152]. Additionally it should be avoided in patients with hypertriglyceridemia with serum triglyceride levels greater than 500 or in patients with history of triglyceride-induced pancreatitis [157]. Finally, it is avoided in patients with history of small bowel obstruction or bowel motility disorders including gastroparesis because of its constipating effect [157].

Colesevelam is a water-insoluble polymer that is neither digested nor absorbed in the GI tract. No dose adjustment is necessary in renal disease. It is both efficacious and safe in CKD, including hemodialysis-dependent patients [157, 158]. A starting dose of 3.75 gm daily or 1.875 gm twice daily can be considered [157].

Insulin

Fifty percent of endogenously secreted insulin is removed from the portal circulation by the liver via the first-pass effect [159]. Conversely, exogenous insulin enters the bloodstream directly, and a higher proportion is eliminated by the kidneys than with endogenous insulin. Renal clearance and degradation of insulin occurs via two mechanisms. First, insulin is freely filtered at the glomerulus, then reabsorbed from the tubular lumen by proximal tubular cells via endocytosis, and degraded into smaller peptides [160, 161]. Second, the remaining insulin not cleared by the first route diffuses from peritubular capillaries into the tubular lumen with uptake and degradation by tubular cells [160, 162].

With progressive renal failure and consequent decrease in glomerular filtration, the first mechanism of clearance is reduced. Peritubular insulin uptake increases, compensating for the decline in degradation of filtered insulin until the eGFR decreases to less than about 20 mL/min/1.73 m^2 [161]. At this point, insulin clearance falls dramatically [159]. Impairment of kidney function leads to increased maximal concentration of insulin levels and prolonged duration of action [163].

Accordingly, the risk of hypoglycemia is increased in patients with CKD due to decreased insulin clearance but also due to impaired renal gluconeogenesis [3]. In a retrospective study, type 1 diabetics with significant creatinine elevations (mean 2.2 mg/dL) had a fivefold higher incidence of severe hypoglycemic episodes than those with normal creatinine levels at comparable levels of HbA1c [164]. Thus, it is critical to anticipate hypoglycemia in CKD patients using insulin, especially as renal function declines over time, and intensively monitor blood glucose and reduce doses as needed.

The basic principles of insulin therapy in CKD are the same for any diabetic patient, with basal insulin coverage (NPH, glargine, detemir, degludec) and nutritional coverage with rapid-acting insulin (lispro, aspart, glulisine, inhaled insulin) or short-acting insulin (regular). Unfortunately, the pharmacokinetics of the various insulin preparations have not been well studied in varying degrees of renal dysfunction.

The prescribing information for detemir indicates no change in pharmacokinetics in renal impairment [165]; however, detemir binds to serum albumin in the circulation and may be less predictable in patients with nephrotic syndrome and hypoalbuminemia [166]. Pharmacokinetics for glargine and NPH have not been studied in renal impairment [167, 168]. Degludec is a new-generation basal insulin with ultra-long duration of action. Kiss et al. found that pharmacokinetic properties were similar for patients with normal renal function; mild, moderate, severe renal impairment; and ESRD on dialysis.

For rapid-acting insulin analogs, package inserts reveal no difference in pharmacokinetics in renal impairment for aspart or lispro [169, 170]. However, Rave et al. suggested a 30–40% reduction in the clearance of regular and lispro insulins in patients with a mean eGFR of 54 mL/min/1.73 m^2 [163]. Glulisine has also been noted to have reduced clearance of 20% in moderate renal impairment (CrCl 30–50 mL/min) and 25% in severe renal impairment (<30 mL/min) with subsequent 29% and 40% increase in insulin exposure, respectively, compared to normal renal function [171]. The effect of renal impairment on pharmacokinetics of inhaled insulin has not been studied [172]. However, the carrier molecule, fumaryl diketopiperazine, appears to have an 18–25% higher AUC in the setting of mild and moderate renal impairment, respectively, a longer half-life, and a 52% greater overall exposure compared to subjects with normal renal function [173].

There are no specific guidelines outlining dosing adjustments based on the level of eGFR. However, Biesenbach et al. found that insulin requirements were reduced by 51% in type 2 diabetes as eGFR deteriorated from 80 to 10 mL/min/1.73 m^2 [174]. One recommendation is that insulin dosage be reduced by 25% when eGFR decreases to between 10 and 50 mL/min/1.73 m^2 and that insulin dosage be reduced by 50% when eGFR decreases to <10 mL/min/1.73 m^2 [166]. For prandial insulin coverage, rapid-acting insulin analogs may be of benefit given their quick onset, shorter duration of action compared to regular insulin, and the possibility of being administered after meals in patients with unreliable oral intake [175].

For patients on multiple daily injections (MDI), an insulin pump infusing rapid-acting insulin continuously and a continuous glucose monitor may allow for fine-tuning of dose adjustments and improve quality of life. There are no studies to show a lower risk of hypoglycemia or better glycemic control with the use of insulin pumps or continuous glucose monitoring in CKD patients. However, these may be good options in patients who are challenged in achieving glycemic control on MDI, under the management of an endocrinologist.

With the initiation of dialysis, peripheral insulin resistance improves with clearance of uremic toxins, and patients will likely require further insulin dose reductions [159]. Sobngwi et al. demonstrated at 15% decrease in the daily insulin needs on the day after hemodialysis compared to that of the day prior and a significant reduction of basal hourly insulin requirements by 25% in a 24-h euglycemic clamp study of type 2 diabetic patients on maintenance hemodialysis [176]. In light of this, we recommend evaluation of glycemic patterns in relation to dialysis time and day to determine if the insulin regimen needs to be varied.

In contrast, patients undergoing peritoneal dialysis (PD) are exposed to high concentrations of glucose in the dialysate. Generally 60–80% of glucose from PD solution instilled in the peritoneal cavity is absorbed, though the daily amount depends on the glucose concentration in the solution [177]. Blood sugars can be difficult to manage and may require a combination of insulin (SC or intraperitoneal (IP)), oral hypoglycemic agents, and minimally absorbed non-glucose-based solutions (icodextrin). IP insulin passes directly into the portal vein and allows for more rapid absorption, better insulin sensitivity, and minimization of blood glucose fluctuations compared to SC administration [159, 177]. Dosing for IP insulin is twofold higher than with SC insulin [178], in part due to 14% ± 5% of insulin added to dialysate being adsorbed onto the dialysate delivery system [179]. Some disadvantages are higher cost due to larger dose of insulin required, increased risk of peritonitis, worsening lipid profile, and hepatic steatosis [177].

Management of diabetic patients with CKD and ESRD on dialysis can be very complex. These patients would benefit from tailored individual therapy, and optimization of care will likely require a partnership between a nephrologist and an endocrinologist.

Amylin Analog

Amylin is a neuroendocrine hormone that is co-secreted from beta cells with insulin. Beta-cell deficiency in type 1 and in advanced type 2 diabetes leads to loss of both insulin and amylin. Amylin improves postprandial glycemic control by slowing gastric emptying, centrally increasing satiety, and suppressing glucagon secretion, thereby suppressing hepatic glucose production [180, 181].

Pramlintide is an amylin analog which differs from amylin at three sites of phosphorylation rendering it biochemically stable for pharmacologic use while maintaining the glycemic-lowering effects of amylin [181,

182]. In type 1 and type 2 diabetic patients with suboptimal control on insulin therapy, pramlintide can be considered as add-on therapy. The addition of pramlintide to insulin can reduce HbA1c 0.25–0.34% in type 1 diabetics and 0.30–0.34% in type 2 diabetics in comparison to placebo and insulin after 6 months of treatment [183]. It also has the benefit of mild weight loss and reduction in the total daily dose of insulin [181].

Unfortunately, pramlintide has multiple adverse effects and can be clinically difficult to implement. Pramlintide is a subcutaneous injection which cannot be combined with insulin because of differences in pH precipitation [182, 183]; patients therefore require two separate injections prior to meals. Pramlintide additionally causes a significant increase in the incidence of severe hypoglycemia when used in combination with insulin therapy, and it is contraindicated in patients with hypoglycemic unawareness [183]. To increase safety, all patients initiating pramlintide therapy should preemptively reduce their mealtime insulin by 50% and should have a history of good medication compliance, glucose monitoring, and clinic attendance [183, 184]. It is also contraindicated in patients with known gastroparesis because of its effect on gastric emptying and the frequent incidence of nausea. Of note, the slowed gastric emptying that occurs with pramlintide can affect absorption of oral medications. To avoid this, oral medications should be given either 1 h before or 2 h after pramlintide injection [184].

Pramlintide is metabolized in the kidney into an active metabolite (2,37 pramlintide). The half-life of pramlintide is 50 min, peak serum levels occur at 20 min, and it is predominantly cleared within 3 h of administration [183]. Pramlintide may be safe in patients with eGFR >30 and may be used without dose adjustment as there has been no increase in AUC or peak serum levels noted [21, 183]. However, it has not been studied in ESRD and should be avoided [21, 183]. A starting dose of 15 mcg for type 1 diabetics and a starting dose of 30 mcg for type 2 diabetic can be considered [183].

Impact of Antihyperglycemic Agents on Renal Function

Several classes of agents have now been shown to have positive impact on proteinuria and/or eGFR. This may be considered when choosing antihyperglycemic therapy. TZD activity on the kidney is not entirely understood but likely multifactorial and overall positive. TZDs have been shown to reduce capillary and glomerular pressures, inflammatory markers (IL-1, TNF-alpha, IL-6) in tubular and mesangial cells, and the contractility of mesangial cells; mechanistically it appears that some of these changes may be related to inhibition of angiotensin II receptor expression leading to general suppression of the renin-angiotensin system [96, 97]. TZD-induced changes result in decreased glomerular hyperfiltration and its sequela [95]. In clinical studies, TZD therapy reduces albuminuria in both mono- and combination therapies when compared to insulin, SU, alpha-glucosidase, and metformin therapies despite similar HbA1c reductions reinforcing that improvement is not from better glycemic control alone [95, 185]. Animal studies suggest that TZDs could have equivalent if not superior renoprotective effect in reducing proteinuria compared with angiotensin-converting enzyme (ACE) inhibitors [95, 186]. Whether or not reduced proteinuria in TZD therapy results in slowing of CKD progression or improved GFR is less well established. Due to lack of long-term clinical data at this time, TZD therapy should not be explicitly chosen for renoprotection.

SGLT2 inhibition appears to slow decline in renal function as well as death from renal disease. In the EMPA-REG OUTCOME trial, microvascular disease was a prespecified secondary outcome; empagliflozin reduced incident or worsening nephropathy (defined by progression to macroalbuminuria, doubling of creatinine, initiation of renal replacement therapy, or death from renal disease) by 39% (12.7 vs 18.8%), and reduced progression to macroalbuminuria by a similar degree (11.2 vs 16.2%) [111, 113]. These renal benefits were even seen in patients with eGFR 30–45 mL/min/1.73m^2, even though these patients did not achieve glycemic benefit. Similarly, in the CANVAS program, canagliflozin reduced progression of albuminuria, and a post hoc exploratory analysis revealed reduction in the composite outcome of sustained 40% reduction in eGFR, need for renal replacement therapy, or death from renal causes [114, 187]. As described earlier for TZDs, it is thought that the renal benefits of the SGLT2 inhibitors are likely due to lowering of blood pressure, decrease in intraglomerular pressure, reduction in albuminuria, and amelioration of volume overload [188]. It is notable that there have also been reports of acute kidney injury with use of canagliflozin (www.accessdata.fda.gov/drugsatfda_docs/label/2016/204042s015s019lbl.pdf accessed 9-26-18) and dapagliflozin (http://www.fda.gov/Drugs/DrugSafety/ucm505860.htm, accessed 9-26-18), including patients requiring hospitalization and dialysis. It is postulated that perhaps this occurred in patients who were dehydrated, hypotensive or on additional medications which may have contributed to renal dysfunction when started on these agents. As with the TZDs, definitive long-term renal outcomes regarding the effects of SGLT2 inhibitors are likely to be further elucidated when the results of ongoing studies are published.

Similarly, cardiovascular outcome studies for the GLP-1 receptor agonists often explored renal impact of these agents as secondary endpoints. Liraglutide resulted in significant 22% reduction in the combined endpoint of new-onset persistent macroalbuminuria, persistent doubling of the serum creatinine, end-stage renal disease, or death due to renal disease; results were driven by lower incidence of new-onset persistent macroalbuminuria [189]. Semaglutide similarly reduced new or worsening nephropathy defined by new macroalbuminuria [42]. This reduction in the development of macroalbuminuria may be due to observed reduction in systolic blood pressure in treated patients [42]. This cannot be clearly delineated as a class effect as it was not observed with lixisenatide [190]. In contrast, exenatide has been noted to be associated with acute renal failure, and this was most prominently described in patients with nausea, vomiting, reduced fluid intake, and concomitant use of an ACE inhibitor (www.fda.gov/Safety/MedWatch/SafetyInformation/SafetyAlertsforHumanMedicalProducts/ucm188703.htm accessed 9-26-18); its use is contraindicated in the setting of significant renal dysfunction, i.e., eGFR <30 mL/min/1.73m^2. As with the other agents, further data are needed to elucidate long-term renal effects of these agents.

A small study exploring renal benefits of the DPP-4 inhibitor linagliptin failed to show change in eGFR or albuminuria despite improved glycemic control [191]. Over the next several years, it is expected that additional data to shed light on renal benefits of antihyperglycemic agents and their clinical applications will be forthcoming.

Conclusion

Management of diabetes in CKD requires an understanding of the alterations in the pharmacokinetics of antihyperglycemic medications due to reduced renal clearance, increased levels of unbound drug, and uremic disruption of hepatic and GI drug metabolism. In addition, reduced renal gluconeogenesis and decreased food intake limit the ability of patients with CKD to adequately compensate for hypoglycemia. As a result, attention to drug interactions and cautious dose titration become increasingly important as renal disease progresses. Patients will require close glucose monitoring and dose reductions of insulin and/or oral antihyperglycemic medications to prevent hypoglycemic events. Ideally, treatment of diabetes in CKD should involve a close partnership between the patient's primary care physician, an endocrinologist, and the nephrologist (Table 5.1).

Table 5.1 Dosing adjustments for non-insulin hypoglycemic agents in CKD

Drug class	Medications	HbA1c reduction	Initial – max dosing	Hypoglycemia	Recommendations in CKD
Biguanides					
	Metformin (Glucophage®, Glumetza®, Riomet®, Fortamet®)	2% with 2 gm/day	500 mg daily – 1000 mg PO BID	No	eGFR 45–60 mL/min/1.73m²: 2 gm/day acceptable eGFR 30–45 mL/min/1.73m²: 1 gm/day if already on. Do not initiate therapy at this stage
Sulfonylureas					
	Glyburide (Diaßeta®, Glynase®)	1.25–1.5%	1.25–20 mg daily	Yes, severe	Avoid in CKD and dialysis patients
	Glimepiride (Amaryl®)		1–4 mg[a] daily	Yes	Use with caution in CKD. Avoid in dialysis patients
Sulfonylurea of choice in CKD	Glipizide (Glucorol®)		2.5 mg daily – 10 mg BID[a]	Yes	No dose adjustment in CKD or dialysis patients
Meglitinides					
Meglitinide of choice in CKD	Repaglinide (Prandin®)	1.0–1.5%	0.5–4 mg AC TID	Yes	Initiate at low dose 0.5 mg if eGFR <30 mL/min/1.73m²; limited information in dialysis patients but no direct contraindications
	Nateglinide (Starlix®)	0.5–1.0%	60–120 mg AC TID	Yes	Initiate at low dose 60 mg if eGFR <30 mL/min/1.73m²; avoid in dialysis patients given limited information and greater potential for metabolite accumulation than repaglinide
GLP-1 receptor agonists					
	Exenatide (Byetta®)	0.78–0.86% on 10 mcg BID as add-on therapy (normal renal function)	5–10 mcg SC BID	No	Mild to moderate CKD: No dosage adjustments eGFR <30 mL/min/1.73m² or ESRD: Not recommended
	Extended release Exenatide (Bydureon®)	1.6% on 2 mg weekly as mono- or add-on therapy (normal renal function)	2 mg SC weekly	No	Mild to moderate CKD: No dosage adjustments. Caution in moderate CKD Not studied in severe CKD or ESRD (use not recommended)
	Liraglutide (Victoza®)	0.66% on 1.8 mg daily as add-on therapy (moderate renal impairment)	0.6–1.8 mg SC daily	No	Mild to severe CKD: No dosage adjustments per package insert but caution suggested with initiating or escalating doses

(continued)

Table 5.1 (continued)

Drug class	Medications	HbA1c reduction	Initial – max dosing	Hypoglycemia	Recommendations in CKD
	Dulaglutide (Trulicity®)	1% on 1.5 mg weekly as monotherapy (normal renal function)	0.75–1.5 mg SC weekly	No	Mild to severe CKD: No dosage adjustments per package insert but caution suggested with initiating or escalating doses
	Lixisenatide (Adlyxin®)	0.6–1.0% on 20 mcg daily as add-on therapy (normal renal function)	10–20 mcg SC daily	No	eGFR ≥30 mL/min/1.73 m^2: No dosage adjustment necessary; monitor closely eGFR 15–29 mL/min/1.73m^2: No dosage adjustment provided in manufacturer labeling but exposure increased. Monitor closely eGFR <15 mL/min/1.73 m^2: Not recommended (not studied)
	Semaglutide (Ozempic®)	1.4–1.8% on 0.5–1.0 mg weekly as add-on therapy (normal renal function)	0.5–1.0 mg SC weekly	No	Mild to severe CKD: No dosage adjustments per package insert
DPP-4 inhibitors					
	Sitaglitin (Januvia®)	0.4% on 25–50 mg daily as monotherapy (moderate CKD, severe CKD, ESRD on HD)	25–50 mg PO daily	No	CrCl 30–50 mL/min: 50 mg daily CrCl <30 mL/min, ESRD or on HD: 25 mg daily (administer irrespective of HD timing)
	Saxagliptin (Onglyza®)	0.73% on 2.5 mg daily as monotherapy (moderate CKD, severe CKD, ESRD on HD)	2.5 mg PO daily	No	Moderate to severe CKD (CrCl ≤50 mL/min): 2.5 mg daily (administer after HD session)
DPP-4 of choice in CKD	Linagliptin (Tradjenta®)	0.67% mild CKD, 0.53% moderate CKD, 0.6% severe CKD on 5 mg daily as monotherapy or add-on therapy	5 mg PO daily	No	No dosage adjustment necessary
	Alogliptin (Nesina®)	0.5–0.78% on 25 mg daily as add-on therapy (normal renal function)	6.25–12.5 mg PO daily	No	CrCl 30–60 mL/min: 12.5 mg daily CrCl <30 mL/min, ESRD or on HD: 6.25 mg daily (administer irrespective of HD timing)
Thiazolidinediones					
	Pioglitazone (Actos®)	1.0–1.6%	15–45 mg daily (max dose of 30 mg studied in dialysis patients)	No	No dose adjustment in CKD. Note maximum dose of 30 mg daily studied in dialysis patients. May cause edema and volume overload
	Rosiglitazone (Avandia®)	0.8–1.5%	4 mg daily – 4 mg BID	No	No dose adjustment in CKD or dialysis patients. May cause edema and volume overload

SGLT2 inhibitors					
	Canagliflozin (Invokana®)	0.3% on 100 mg daily as monotherapy (eGFR 30 to <50 mL/min/1.73m^2)	100 mg PO daily	No	eGFR 45–59 mL/min/1.73m^2: 100 mg daily eGFR <45 mL/min/1.73m^2, ESRD, and HD: Contraindicated
	Dapagliflozin (Farxiga®)	No efficacy with 5 or 10 mg in moderate CKD (mean eGFR 45 mL/min/1.73m^2)	N/A	No	eGFR <60 mL/min/1.73m^2: Not recommended eGFR <45 mL/min/1.73m^2, ESRD and HD: Contraindicated
	Empagliflozin (Jardiance®)	0.68% in CKD2, 0.42% in CKD3 on 25 mg daily as monotherapy	10–25 mg PO daily	No	eGFR <45 mL/min/1.73m^2: Not recommended eGFR <30 mL/min/1.73m^2, ESRD and HD: Contraindicated
	Ertugliflozin (Steglatro®)	0.6–0.9% as add-on therapy; efficacy may be significantly less in CKD3	5–15 mg PO daily	No	eGFR <60 mL/min/1.73m^2: Not recommended eGFR <30 mL/min/1.73m^2: Contraindicated
Alpha-glucosidase inhibitors					
	Acarbose (PRECOSE®)	0.5–1.0%	25–50 mg TID AC	No	No dose adjustment when eGFR >25 mL/min/1.73m^2. Avoid when eGFR <25 mL/min/1.73m^2 and in dialysis patients
	Miglitol (Glyset®)	0.26–0.81%	25–100 mg TID AC	No	No dose adjustment when eGFR >25 mL/min/1.73m^2. Avoid when eGFR <25 mL/min/1.73m^2 and in dialysis patients
Bile acid resins					
	Colesevelam (WelChol®)	0.5–0.54%	3.75 gm daily or 1.875 gm BID	No	No dose adjustment in CKD or dialysis patients
D2-dopamine agonist					
	Bromocriptine-QR (Cycloset®)	0.55% on 4.8 mg daily as monotherapy or add-on therapy (normal renal function)	0.8–4.8 mg PO daily[a]	No	No dosage adjustments included in package insert
Amylin analog					
	Pramlintide in type 1 diabetics	0.25–0.34%	15–60 mcg SC TID	Yes	No dose adjustment when eGFR >30 mL/min/1.73m^2. Avoid when eGFR <30 mL/min/1.73m^2 and in dialysis patients
	Pramlintide in type 2 diabetics	0.30–0.34%	30–120 mcg SC TID		

[a]Maximum dosing may be lower than approved FDA maximums based on known maximum efficacy and/or the author's clinical experience

References

1. Abe M, Okada K, Soma M. Antidiabetic agents in patients with chronic kidney disease and end-stage renal disease on dialysis: metabolism and clinical practice. Curr Drug Metab. 2011;12(1):57–69.
2. National Kidney Foundation. KDOQI clinical practice guideline for diabetes and CKD: 2012 update. Am J Kidney Dis Off J Natl Kidney Found. 2012;60(5):850–86.
3. Gerich JE, Meyer C, Woerle HJ, Stumvoll M. Renal gluconeogenesis: its importance in human glucose homeostasis. Diabetes Care. 2001;24(2):382–91.
4. Carrero JJ, Stenvinkel P, Cuppari L, Ikizler TA, Kalantar-Zadeh K, Kaysen G, et al. Etiology of the protein-energy wasting syndrome in chronic kidney disease: a consensus statement from the International Society of Renal Nutrition and Metabolism (ISRNM). J Ren Nutr Off J Counc Ren Nutr Natl Kidney Found. 2013;23(2):77–90.
5. Zhou G, Myers R, Li Y, Chen Y, Shen X, Fenyk-Melody J, et al. Role of AMP-activated protein kinase in mechanism of metformin action. J Clin Invest. 2001;108(8):1167–74.
6. Garber AJ, Duncan TG, Goodman AM, Mills DJ, Rohlf JL. Efficacy of metformin in type II diabetes: results of a double-blind, placebo-controlled, dose-response trial. Am J Med. 1997;103(6):491–7.
7. Holman RR, Paul SK, Bethel MA, Matthews DR, Neil HAW. 10-year follow-up of intensive glucose control in type 2 diabetes. N Engl J Med. 2008;359(15):1577–89.
8. Glucophage (R) [package insert]. Princeton: Bristol-Myers Squibb Company; 2015.
9. Inzucchi SE, Lipska KJ, Mayo H, Bailey CJ, McGuire DK. Metformin in patients with type 2 diabetes and kidney disease: a systematic review. JAMA. 2014;312(24):2668–75.
10. Salpeter SR, Greyber E, Pasternak GA, Salpeter EE. Risk of fatal and nonfatal lactic acidosis with metformin use in type 2 diabetes mellitus. Cochrane Database Syst Rev. 2010;4:CD002967.
11. Roussel R, Travert F, Pasquet B, Wilson PWF, Smith SC, Goto S, et al. Metformin use and mortality among patients with diabetes and atherothrombosis. Arch Intern Med. 2010;170(21):1892–9.
12. FDA Drug Safety Communication. FDA revises warnings regarding use of the diabetes medicine metformin in certain patients with reduced kidney function. https://www.fda.gov/Drugs/DrugSafety/ucm493244.htm. Accessed 2016.
13. Harrower AD. Pharmacokinetics of oral antihyperglycaemic agents in patients with renal insufficiency. Clin Pharmacokinet. 1996;31(2):111–9.
14. Arnouts P, Bolignano D, Nistor I, Bilo H, Gnudi L, Heaf J, et al. Glucose-lowering drugs in patients with chronic kidney disease: a narrative review on pharmacokinetic properties. Nephrol Dial Transplant Off Publ Eur Dial Transpl Assoc – Eur Ren Assoc. 2014;29(7):1284–300.
15. Krepinsky J, Ingram AJ, Clase CM. Prolonged sulfonylurea-induced hypoglycemia in diabetic patients with end-stage renal disease. Am J Kidney Dis Off J Natl Kidney Found. 2000;35(3):500–5.
16. Rydberg T, Jönsson A, Røder M, Melander A. Hypoglycemic activity of glyburide (glibenclamide) metabolites in humans. Diabetes Care. 1994;17(9):1026–30.
17. Holstein A, Plaschke A, Egberts EH. Lower incidence of severe hypoglycaemia in patients with type 2 diabetes treated with glimepiride versus glibenclamide. Diabetes Metab Res Rev. 2001;17(6):467–73.
18. van Staa T, Abenhaim L, Monette J. Rates of hypoglycemia in users of sulfonylureas. J Clin Epidemiol. 1997;50(6):735–41.
19. Rosenkranz B, Profozic V, Metelko Z, Mrzljak V, Lange C, Malerczyk V. Pharmacokinetics and safety of glimepiride at clinically effective doses in diabetic patients with renal impairment. Diabetologia. 1996;39(12):1617–24.
20. Schernthaner G, Grimaldi A, Di Mario U, Drzewoski J, Kempler P, Kvapil M, et al. GUIDE study: double-blind comparison of once-daily gliclazide MR and glimepiride in type 2 diabetic patients. Eur J Clin Investig. 2004;34(8):535–42.
21. Tuttle KR, Bakris GL, Bilous RW, Chiang JL, de Boer IH, Goldstein-Fuchs J, et al. Diabetic kidney disease: a report from an ADA Consensus Conference. Diabetes Care. 2014;37(10):2864–83.
22. Amaryl(R) [package insert]. Bridgewater: Sanofi-aventis U.S., LLC.
23. Balant L, Zahnd G, Gorgia A, Schwarz R, Fabre J. Pharmacokinetics of glipizide in man: influence of renal insufficiency. Diabetologia. 1973:331–8.
24. Yale J-F. Oral antihyperglycemic agents and renal disease: new agents, new concepts. J Am Soc Nephrol. 2005;16(3 suppl 1):S7–10.
25. Riddle M. Combining sulfonylureas and other oral agents. Am J Med. 2000;108(6., Supplement 1):15–22.
26. Cheng AYY, Fantus IG. Oral antihyperglycemic therapy for type 2 diabetes mellitus. CMAJ Can Med Assoc J. 2005;172(2):213–26.
27. Hu S, Wang S, Dunning BE. Glucose-dependent and glucose-sensitizing insulinotropic effect of nateglinide: comparison to sulfonylureas and repaglinide. Int J Exp Diabetes Res. 2001;2(1):63–72.
28. Dornhorst A. Insulinotropic meglitinide analogues. Lancet. 2001;358(9294):1709–16.
29. Moses R. A review of clinical experience with the prandial glucose regulator, repaglinide, in the treatment of Type 2 diabetes. Expert Opin Pharmacother. 2000;1(7):1455–67.
30. Rosenstock J, Hassman DR, Madder RD, Brazinsky SA, Farrell J, Khutoryansky N, et al. Repaglinide versus nateglinide monotherapy a randomized, multicenter study. Diabetes Care. 2004;27(6):1265–70.
31. Prandin(R) [package insert]. Princeton: Novo Nordisk, Inc.; 2003–2009.

32. Schumacher S, Abbasi I, Weise D, Hatorp V, Sattler K, Sieber J, et al. Single- and multiple-dose pharmacokinetics of repaglinide in patients with type 2 diabetes and renal impairment. Eur J Clin Pharmacol. 2001;57(2):147–52.
33. Marbury TC, Ruckle JL, Hatorp V, Andersen MP, Nielsen KK, Huang WC, et al. Pharmacokinetics of repaglinide in subjects with renal impairment. Clin Pharmacol Ther. 2000;67(1):7–15.
34. Hasslacher C. Safety and efficacy of repaglinide in type 2 diabetic patients with and without impaired renal function. Diabetes Care. 2003;26(3):886–91.
35. Weaver ML, Orwig BA, Rodriguez LC, Graham ED, Chin JA, Shapiro MJ, et al. Pharmacokinetics and metabolism of nateglinide in humans. Drug Metab Dispos Biol Fate Chem. 2001;29(4 Pt 1):415–21.
36. Starlix(R) [package insert]. East Hanover: Novartis Pharmaceuticals Corporation, Inc.; 2011.
37. Devineni D, Walter YH, Smith HT, Lee JS, Prasad P, McLeod JF. Pharmacokinetics of nateglinide in renally impaired diabetic patients. J Clin Pharmacol. 2003;43(2):163–70.
38. Nagai T, Imamura M, Iizuka K, Mori M. Hypoglycemia due to nateglinide administration in diabetic patient with chronic renal failure. Diabetes Res Clin Pract. 2003;59(3):191–4.
39. Drucker DJ, Nauck MA. The incretin system: glucagon-like peptide-1 receptor agonists and dipeptidyl peptidase-4 inhibitors in type 2 diabetes. Lancet Lond Engl. 2006;368(9548):1696–705.
40. Buse JB, Henry RR, Han J, Kim DD, Fineman MS, Baron AD, et al. Effects of exenatide (exendin-4) on glycemic control over 30 weeks in sulfonylurea-treated patients with type 2 diabetes. Diabetes Care. 2004;27(11):2628–35.
41. Nauck MA, Hompesch M, Filipczak R, Le TDT, Zdravkovic M, Gumprecht J, et al. Five weeks of treatment with the GLP-1 analogue liraglutide improves glycaemic control and lowers body weight in subjects with type 2 diabetes. Exp Clin Endocrinol Diabetes Off J Ger Soc Endocrinol Ger Diabetes Assoc. 2006;114(8):417–23.
42. Marso SP, Bain SC, Consoli A. Semaglutide and cardiovascular outcomes in patients with type 2 diabetes. N Engl J Med. 2016;375(19):1834–44.
43. Marso SP, Daniels GH, Brown-Frandsen K, et al. Liraglutide and cardiovascular outcomes in type 2 diabetes. New Engl J Med. 2016;375:311–22.
44. Byetta(R) [package insert]. San Diego: Amylin Pharmaceuticals, Inc.; 2009.
45. Victoza (R) [package insert]. Princeton: Novo Nordisk, Inc.; 2010.
46. Trulicity (R) [package insert]. Indianapolis: Eli Lilly and Company; 2015.
47. Tanzeum (R) [package insert]. Wilmington: GlaxoSmithKline LLC; 2015.
48. Butler PC, Elashoff M, Elashoff R, Gale EAM. A critical analysis of the clinical use of incretin-based therapies: are the GLP-1 therapies safe? Diabetes Care. 2013;36(7):2118–25.
49. Giorda CB, Nada E, Tartaglino B, Marafetti L, Gnavi R. A systematic review of acute pancreatitis as an adverse event of type 2 diabetes drugs: from hard facts to a balanced position. Diabetes Obes Metab. 2014;16(11):1041–7.
50. DeFronzo RA, Ratner RE, Han J, Kim DD, Fineman MS, Baron AD. Effects of exenatide (exendin-4) on glycemic control and weight over 30 weeks in metformin-treated patients with type 2 diabetes. Diabetes Care. 2005;28(5):1092–100.
51. Zinman B, Hoogwerf BJ, Durán García S, Milton DR, Giaconia JM, Kim DD, et al. The effect of adding exenatide to a thiazolidinedione in suboptimally controlled type 2 diabetes: a randomized trial. Ann Intern Med. 2007;146(7):477–85.
52. Riddle MC, Henry RR, Poon TH, Zhang B, Mac SM, Holcombe JH, et al. Exenatide elicits sustained glycaemic control and progressive reduction of body weight in patients with type 2 diabetes inadequately controlled by sulphonylureas with or without metformin. Diabetes Metab Res Rev. 2006;22(6):483–91.
53. Linnebjerg H, Kothare PA, Park S, Mace K, Reddy S, Mitchell M, et al. Effect of renal impairment on the pharmacokinetics of exenatide. Br J Clin Pharmacol. 2007;64(3):317–27.
54. Davies MJ, Bain SC, Atkin SL, Rossing P, Scott D, Shamkhalova MS, et al. Efficacy and safety of liraglutide versus placebo as add-on to glucose-lowering therapy in patients with type 2 diabetes and moderate renal impairment (LIRA-RENAL): a randomized clinical trial. Diabetes Care. 2016;39(2):222–30.
55. Jacobsen LV, Hindsberger C, Robson R, Zdravkovic M. Effect of renal impairment on the pharmacokinetics of the GLP-1 analogue liraglutide. Br J Clin Pharmacol. 2009;68(6):898–905.
56. Umpierrez G, Tofé Povedano S, Pérez Manghi F, Shurzinske L, Pechtner V. Efficacy and safety of dulaglutide monotherapy versus metformin in type 2 diabetes in a randomized controlled trial (AWARD-3). Diabetes Care. 2014;37(8):2168–76.
57. Gurung T, Shyangdan DS, O'Hare JP, Waugh N. A novel, long-acting glucagon-like peptide receptor-agonist: dulaglutide. Diabetes Metab Syndr Obes Targets Ther. 2015;8:363–86.
58. Grunberger G, Chang A, Garcia Soria G, Botros FT, Bsharat R, Milicevic Z. Monotherapy with the once-weekly GLP-1 analogue dulaglutide for 12 weeks in patients with Type 2 diabetes: dose-dependent effects on glycaemic control in a randomized, double-blind, placebo-controlled study. Diabet Med J Br Diabet Assoc. 2012;29(10):1260–7.
59. Geiser JS, Heathman MA, Cui X, Martin J, Loghin C, Chien JY, et al. Clinical pharmacokinetics of dulaglutide in patients with type 2 diabetes: analyses of data from clinical trials. Clin Pharmacokinet. 2016;55(5):625–34.
60. Fonseca VA, Alvarado-Ruiz R, Raccah D, et al. Efficacy and safety of the once-daily GLP-1 receptor agonist lixisenatide in monotherapy: a randomized, double-blind, placebo-controlled trial in patients

with type 2 diabetes (GetGoal-Mono). Diabetes Care. 2012;35(6):1225–31.
61. Ahren B, Dimas AL, Miossec P, et al. Efficacy and safety of lixisenatide once-daily morning or evening injections in type 2 diabetes inadequately controlled on metformin (GetGoal-M). Diabetes Care. 2013;36(9):2543–50.
62. Pinget M, Goldenberg R, Niemoeller E, et al. Efficacy and safety of lixisenatide once daily versus placebo in type 2 diabetes insufficiently controlled on pioglitazone (GetGoal-P). Diabetes Obes Metab. 2013;15(11):1000–7.
63. Rosenstock J, Hanefeld M, Shamanna P, et al. Beneficial effects of once-daily Lixisenatide on overall and postprandial glycemic levels without significant excess of hypoglycemia in Type 2 diabetes inadequately controlled on a sulfonylurea with or without metformin (GetGoal-S). J Diabetes Complicat. 2014;28(3):386–92.
64. Riddle MC, Forst T, Aronson R, et al. Adding once-daily lixisenatide for type 2 diabetes inadequately controlled with newly initiated and continuously titrated basal insulin glargine: a 24-week, randomized, placebo-controlled study (GetGoal-Duo-1). Diabetes Care. 2013;36(9):2497–503.
65. Hanefeld M, Arteaga JM, Leiter LA, et al. Efficacy and safety of lixisenatide in patients with type 2 diabetes and renal impairment. Diabetes Obes Metab. 2017;19(11):1594–601.
66. Ozempic [package insert]. Plainsboro: Novo Nordisk Inc.; 2017.
67. Ahrén B, Masmiquel L, Kumar H, et al. Efficacy and safety of once-weekly semaglutide versus once-daily sitagliptin as an add-on to metformin, thiazolidinediones, or both, in patients with type 2 diabetes (SUSTAIN 2): a 56-week, double-blind, phase 3a, randomised trial. Lancet Diabetes Endocrinol. 2017;5(5):341–54.
68. Ahmann AJ, Capehorn M, Charpenier G, et al. Efficacy and safety of once-weekly semaglutide versus exenatide ER in subjects with type 2 diabetes (SUSTAIN 3): a 56-week, open-label, randomized clinical trial. Diabetes Care. 2018;41(2):258–66.
69. Aroda VR, Bain SC, Cariou B, et al. Efficacy and safety of once-weekly semaglutide versus once-daily insulin glargine as add-on to metformin (with or without sulfonylureas) in insulin-naive patients with type 2 diabetes (SUSTAIN 4): a randomised, open-label, parallel-group, multicentre, multinational, phase 3a trial. Lancet Diabetes Endocrinol. 2017;5(5):355–66. do.
70. Pratley RE, Aroda VR, Lingvay I, et al. Semaglutide versus dulaglutide once weekly in patients with type 2 diabetes (SUSTAIN 7): a randomised, open-label, phase 3b trial. Lancet Diabetes Endocrinol. 2018;6(4):275–86.
71. Soreli C, et al. Efficacy and safety of once-weekly semiglutide monotherapy versus placebo in patients with type 2 diabetes (SUSTAIN 1): a double-blund, randomized, placebo-controlled, parellel-group, multinational, multicentre phase 3a trial. Lancet Diabetes Encodinol. 2017;5(4):251–60.
72. Rodbard HW, Lingavay I, Reed J, et al. Semaglutide added to basal insulin in type 2 diabetes (SUSTAIN 5): a randomized, controlled trial. J Clin Endocrinol Metab. 2018;103(6):2291–301.
73. Marbury TC, Flint A, Jacobsen JB, et al. Pharmacokinetics and tolerability of a single dose of semaglutide, a human glucagon-like peptide-1 analog, in subjects with and without renal impairment. Clin Pharmacokinet. 2017;56(11):1381–90.
74. Nakamura Y, Hasegawa H, Tsuji M, Udaka Y, Mihara M, Shimizu T, et al. Diabetes therapies in hemodialysis patients: dipeptidase-4 inhibitors. World J Diabetes. 2015;6(6):840–9.
75. FDA Drug Safety Communication. FDA warns that DPP-4 inhibitors for type 2 diabetes may cause severe joint pain. 2015.
76. Bergman AJ, Cote J, Yi B, Marbury T, Swan SK, Smith W, et al. Effect of renal insufficiency on the pharmacokinetics of sitagliptin, a dipeptidyl peptidase-4 inhibitor. Diabetes Care. 2007;30(7):1862–4.
77. Januvia (R) [package insert]. Whitehouse Station: Merck & Co., Inc.; 2010.
78. Chan JCN, Scott R, Arjona Ferreira JC, Sheng D, Gonzalez E, Davies MJ, et al. Safety and efficacy of sitagliptin in patients with type 2 diabetes and chronic renal insufficiency. Diabetes Obes Metab. 2008;10(7):545–55.
79. Nowicki M, Rychlik I, Haller H, Warren M, Suchower L, Gause-Nilsson I, et al. Long-term treatment with the dipeptidyl peptidase-4 inhibitor saxagliptin in patients with type 2 diabetes mellitus and renal impairment: a randomised controlled 52-week efficacy and safety study. Int J Clin Pract. 2011;65(12):1230–9.
80. Boulton DW, Li L, Frevert EU, Tang A, Castaneda L, Vachharajani NN, et al. Influence of renal or hepatic impairment on the pharmacokinetics of saxagliptin. Clin Pharmacokinet. 2011;50(4):253–65.
81. Onglyza (R) [package insert]. Princeton: Bristol-Myers Squibb Company; 2009.
82. Scirica BM, Bhatt DL, Braunwald E, Steg PG, Davidson J, Hirshberg B, et al. Saxagliptin and cardiovascular outcomes in patients with type 2 diabetes mellitus. N Engl J Med. 2013;369(14):1317–26.
83. Groop P-H, Del Prato S, Taskinen M-R, Owens DR, Gong Y, Crowe S, et al. Linagliptin treatment in subjects with type 2 diabetes with and without mild-to-moderate renal impairment. Diabetes Obes Metab. 2014;16(6):560–8.
84. McGill JB, Sloan L, Newman J, Patel S, Sauce C, von Eynatten M, et al. Long-term efficacy and safety of linagliptin in patients with type 2 diabetes and severe renal impairment: a 1-year, randomized, double-blind, placebo-controlled study. Diabetes Care. 2013;36(2):237–44.
85. Blech S, Ludwig-Schwellinger E, Gräfe-Mody EU, Withopf B, Wagner K. The metabolism and disposition of the oral dipeptidyl peptidase-4 inhibitor,

linagliptin, in humans. Drug Metab Dispos Biol Fate Chem. 2010;38(4):667–78.
86. Graefe-Mody U, Friedrich C, Port A, Ring A, Retlich S, Heise T, et al. Effect of renal impairment on the pharmacokinetics of the dipeptidyl peptidase-4 inhibitor linagliptin(*). Diabetes Obes Metab. 2011;13(10):939–46.
87. Tradjenta (R) [package insert]. Ridgefield: Boehringer Ingelheim Pharmaceuticals, Inc.; 2012.
88. Nauck MA, Ellis GC, Fleck PR, Wilson CA, Mekki Q, Alogliptin Study 008 Group. Efficacy and safety of adding the dipeptidyl peptidase-4 inhibitor alogliptin to metformin therapy in patients with type 2 diabetes inadequately controlled with metformin monotherapy: a multicentre, randomised, double-blind, placebo-controlled study. Int J Clin Pract. 2009;63(1):46–55.
89. Kaku K, Itayasu T, Hiroi S, Hirayama M, Seino Y. Efficacy and safety of alogliptin added to pioglitazone in Japanese patients with type 2 diabetes: a randomized, double-blind, placebo-controlled trial with an open-label long-term extension study. Diabetes Obes Metab. 2011;13(11):1028–35.
90. Pratley RE. Alogliptin: a new, highly selective dipeptidyl peptidase-4 inhibitor for the treatment of type 2 diabetes. Expert Opin Pharmacother. 2009;10(3):503–12.
91. Nesina (R) [package insert]. Deerfield: Takeda Pharmaceuticals America, Inc.; 2013.
92. Fujii Y, Abe M, Higuchi T, Mizuno M, Suzuki H, Matsumoto S, et al. The dipeptidyl peptidase-4 inhibitor alogliptin improves glycemic control in type 2 diabetic patients undergoing hemodialysis. Expert Opin Pharmacother. 2013;14(3):259–67.
93. Yki-Järvinen H. Thiazolidinediones. N Engl J Med. 2004;351(11):1106–18.
94. Armoni M, Kritz N, Harel C, Bar-Yoseph F, Chen H, Quon MJ, et al. Peroxisome proliferator-activated receptor-γ represses GLUT4 promoter activity in primary adipocytes, and rosiglitazone alleviates this effect. J Biol Chem. 2003;278(33):30614–23.
95. Tontonoz P, Spiegelman BM. Fat and beyond: the diverse biology of PPARgamma. Annu Rev Biochem. 2008;77:289–312.
96. Sarafidis PA, Bakris GL. Protection of the kidney by thiazolidinediones: an assessment from bench to bedside. Kidney Int. 2006;70(7):1223–33.
97. Sugawara A, Uruno A, Kudo M, Matsuda K, Yang CW, Ito S. Effects of PPARγ on hypertension, atherosclerosis, and chronic kidney disease. Endocr J. 2010;57(10):847–52.
98. Actos(R) [package insert]. Deerfield: Takeda Pharmaceuticals America, Inc.; 2009–2011.
99. Nissen SE, Wolski K. Rosiglitazone revisited: an updated meta-analysis of risk for myocardial infarction and cardiovascular mortality. Arch Intern Med. 2010;170(14):1191–201.
100. Nesto RW, Bell D, Bonow RO, Fonseca V, Grundy SM, Horton ES, et al. Thiazolidinedione use, fluid retention, and congestive heart failure a consensus statement from the American Heart Association and American Diabetes Association. Diabetes Care. 2004;27(1):256–63.
101. Rocco MV, Berns JS. KDOQI clinical practice guideline for diabetes and CKD: 2012 update. Am J Kidney Dis. 2012;60(5):850–86.
102. Yaturu S, Bryant B, Jain SK. Thiazolidinedione treatment decreases bone mineral density in type 2 diabetic men. Diabetes Care. 2007;30(6):1574–6.
103. Schwartz AV, Sellmeyer DE, Vittinghoff E, Palermo L, Lecka-Czernik B, Feingold KR, et al. Thiazolidinedione use and bone loss in older diabetic adults. J Clin Endocrinol Metab. 2006;91(9):3349–54.
104. Habib ZA, Havstad SL, Wells K, Divine G, Pladevall M, Williams LK. Thiazolidinedione use and the longitudinal risk of fractures in patients with type 2 diabetes mellitus. J Clin Endocrinol Metab. 2010;95(2):592–600.
105. FDA Drug Safety Communication. FDA requires removal of some prescribing and dispensing restrictions for rosiglitazone-containng diabetes medicines [Internet]. 2013 [cited 2015 Dec 15]. Available from: http://www.fda.gov/downloads/Drugs/DrugSafety/UCM381108.pdf.
106. Budde K, Neumayer H-H, Fritsche L, Sulowicz W, Stompôr T, Eckland D. The pharmacokinetics of pioglitazone in patients with impaired renal function. Br J Clin Pharmacol. 2003;55(4):368–74.
107. Avandia(R) [package insert]. Research Triangle Park: GlaxoSmithKline, Inc.; 2007.
108. Thompson-Culkin K, Zussman B, Miller AK, Freed MI. Pharmacokinetics of rosiglitazone in patients with end-stage renal disease. J Int Med Res. 2002;30(4):391–9.
109. Cox PJ, Ryan DA, Hollis FJ, Harris A-M, Miller AK, Vousden M, et al. Absorption, disposition, and metabolism of rosiglitazone, a potent thiazolidinedione insulin sensitizer, in humans. Drug Metab Dispos. 2000;28(7):772–80.
110. Niemi M, Backman JT, Granfors M, Laitila J, Neuvonen M, Neuvonen PJ. Gemfibrozil considerably increases the plasma concentrations of rosiglitazone. Diabetologia. 2003;46(10):1319–23.
111. Idris I, Donnelly R. Sodium-glucose co-transporter-2 inhibitors: an emerging new class of oral antidiabetic drug. Diabetes Obes Metab. 2009;11(2):79–88.
112. Paisley AN, Paisley AJ, Yadav R, Younis N, Rao-Balakrishna P, Soran H. Dapagliflozin: a review on efficacy, clinical effectiveness and safety. Expert Opin Investig Drugs. 2013;22(1):131–40.
113. Zinman B, Wanner C, Lachin JM, Fitchett D, Bluhmki E, Hantel S, et al. Empagliflozin, cardiovascular outcomes, and mortality in type 2 diabetes. N Engl J Med. 2015;373(22):2117–28.
114. Neal B, Perkovic V, Mahaffey KW, et al. Canagliflozin and cardiovascular and renal events in type 2 diabetes. N Engl J Med. 2017;377:644–57.
115. Yale J-F, Bakris G, Cariou B, Yue D, David-Neto E, Xi L, et al. Efficacy and safety of canagliflozin in

subjects with type 2 diabetes and chronic kidney disease. Diabetes Obes Metab. 2013;15(5):463–73.
116. FDA Drug Safety Communication. FDA warns that SGLT2 inhibitors for diabetes may result in a serious condition of too much acid in the blood. 2015.
117. Abdul-Ghani MA, Norton L, DeFronzo RA. Renal sodium-glucose cotransporter inhibition in the management of type 2 diabetes mellitus. Am J Physiol Renal Physiol. 2015;309(11):F889–900.
118. Ogawa W, Sakaguchi K. Euglycemic diabetic ketoacidosis induced by SGLT2 inhibitors: possible mechanism and contributing factors. J Diabetes Investig. 2016;7(2):135–8.
119. Rosenstock J, Ferrannini E. Euglycemic diabetic ketoacidosis: a predictable, detectable, and preventable safety concern with SGLT2 inhibitors. Diabetes Care. 2015;38(9):1638–42.
120. Invokana (R) [package insert]. Titusville: Janssen Pharmaceuticals, Inc.; 2013.
121. Watts NB, Bilezikian JP, Usiskin K, Edwards R, Desai M, Law G, et al. Effects of canagliflozin on fracture risk in patients with type 2 diabetes mellitus. J Clin Endocrinol Metab. 2016;101(1):157–66.
122. Farxiga (R) [package insert]. Princeton: Bristol-Myers Squibb Company; 2014.
123. Kasichayanula S, Liu X, Pe Benito M, Yao M, Pfister M, LaCreta FP, et al. The influence of kidney function on dapagliflozin exposure, metabolism and pharmacodynamics in healthy subjects and in patients with type 2 diabetes mellitus. Br J Clin Pharmacol. 2013;76(3):432–44.
124. FDA Briefing Document. New drug application for dapagliflozin. 2013.
125. Barnett AH, Mithal A, Manassie J, Jones R, Rattunde H, Woerle HJ, et al. Efficacy and safety of empagliflozin added to existing antidiabetes treatment in patients with type 2 diabetes and chronic kidney disease: a randomised, double-blind, placebo-controlled trial. Lancet Diabetes Endocrinol. 2014;2(5):369–84.
126. Macha S, Mattheus M, Halabi A, Pinnetti S, Woerle HJ, Broedl UC. Pharmacokinetics, pharmacodynamics and safety of empagliflozin, a sodium glucose cotransporter 2 (SGLT2) inhibitor, in subjects with renal impairment. Diabetes Obes Metab. 2014;16(3):215–22.
127. Jardiance (R) [package insert]. Ridgefield: Boehringer Ingelheim Pharmaceuticals, Inc.; 2014.
128. Terra S, Frias J, Goldman A, Aronson R, Darekar A, Huyck S, Terra S, et al. Long-term efficacy and safety of ertugliflozin monotherapy in patients with inadequately controlled type 2 diabetes despite diet and exercise: the 52-week VERTIS MONO study. Diabetologia. 2017;60(1 Supplement 1). Springer Verlag):S408.
129. Rosenstock J, Frias J, Páll D, Charbonnel B, Pascu R, Saur D, Darekar A, Huyck S, Shi H, Lauring B, Terra SG. Effect of ertugliflozin on glucose control, body weight, blood pressure and bone density in type 2 diabetes mellitus inadequately controlled on metformin monotherapy (VERTIS MET). Diabetes Obes Metab. 2018;20:520–9.
130. Hollander P, Liu J, Hill J, Johnson J, Jiang ZW, Golm G, Huyck S, Terra SG, Mancuso JP, Engel SS, Lauring B. Ertugliflozin compared with glimepiride in patients with type 2 diabetes mellitus inadequately controlled on metformin: the VERTIS SU randomized study. Diabetes Ther. 2018;9:193–207.
131. Lauring B, Miller SS, Krumins T, Zhou HJ, Huyck S, Johnson J, Golm G, Terra SG, Mancuso JP, Engel SS. Safety and efficacy of ertugliflozin in combination with sitagliptin in patients with type 2 diabetes inadequately controlled on diet and exercise: the VERTIS SITA trial. Diabetologia. 2017.
132. Eldor R, Liu J, Dagogo-Jack S, Amorin G, Johnson J, Liao Y, Huyck S, Golm G, Terra SG, Mancuso JP, Engel SS, Lauring B. Safety and efficacy of ertugliflozin after 52 weeks in patients with type 2 diabetes inadequately controlled on metformin and sitagliptin: VERTIS SITA2 trial extension. Conference: 53rd Annual Meeting of the European Association for the Study of Diabetes, EASD 2017. Portugal. Diabetologia. 2017;60(1 Supplement 1):S21.
133. Grunberger G, Camp S, Johnson J, Huyck S, Terra SG, Mancuso JP, Jiang ZW, Golm G, Engel SS, Lauring B. Ertugliflozin in patients with stage 3 chronic kidney disease and type 2 diabetes mellitus: the VERTIS RENAL randomized study. Diabetes Ther. 2018;9(1):49–66.
134. Precose(R) [package insert]. Wayne: Bayer HealthCare Pharmaceuticals, Inc.; 2008.
135. Van de Laar FA, Lucassen PLBJ, Akkermans RP, Van de Lisdonk EH, Rutten GEHM, Van Weel C. Alpha-glucosidase inhibitors for type 2 diabetes mellitus. Cochrane Database Syst Rev. 2005;2:CD003639.
136. Glyset (R) [package insert]. Leverkusen: Bayer HealthCare AG, Inc.; 2008.
137. Woo TM, Wynne AL. Pharmacotherapeutics for nurse practitioner prescribers: F.A. Davis; 2011. p. 1517.
138. van de Laar FA. Alpha-glucosidase inhibitors in the early treatment of type 2 diabetes. Vasc Health Risk Manag. 2008;4(6):1189–95.
139. Chiasson J-L, Josse RG, Gomis R, Hanefeld M, Karasik A, Laakso M, et al. Acarbose for prevention of type 2 diabetes mellitus: the STOP-NIDDM randomised trial. Lancet Lond Engl. 2002;359(9323):2072–7.
140. Chiasson J-L, Josse RG, Gomis R, Hanefeld M, Karasik A, Laakso M, et al. Acarbose treatment and the risk of cardiovascular disease and hypertension in patients with impaired glucose tolerance: the STOP-NIDDM trial. JAMA. 2003;290(4):486–94.
141. Chang C-H, Chang Y-C, Lin J-W, Chen S-T, Chuang L-M, Lai M-S. Cardiovascular risk associated with acarbose versus metformin as the first-line treatment in patients with type 2 diabetes: a nationwide cohort study. J Clin Endocrinol Metab. 2015;100(3):1121–9.
142. Cincotta AH, Luo S, Zhang Y, Liang Y, Bina KG, Jetton TL, et al. Chronic infusion of norepinephrine into the VMH of normal rats induces the obese

glucose-intolerant state. Am J Physiol Regul Integr Comp Physiol. 2000;278(2):R435–44.
143. Luo S, Luo J, Meier AH, Cincotta AH. Dopaminergic neurotoxin administration to the area of the suprachiasmatic nuclei induces insulin resistance. Neuroreport. 1997;8(16):3495–9.
144. Luo S, Meier AH, Cincotta AH. Bromocriptine reduces obesity, glucose intolerance and extracellular monoamine metabolite levels in the ventromedial hypothalamus of Syrian hamsters. Neuroendocrinology. 1998;68(1):1–10.
145. Cincotta AH, Meier AH. Bromocriptine inhibits in vivo free fatty acid oxidation and hepatic glucose output in seasonally obese hamsters (Mesocricetus auratus). Metabolism. 1995;44(10):1349–55.
146. Cincotta AH, Meier AH, Cincotta M Jr. Bromocriptine improves glycaemic control and serum lipid profile in obese Type 2 diabetic subjects: a new approach in the treatment of diabetes. Expert Opin Investig Drugs. 1999;8(10):1683–707.
147. Gaziano JM, Cincotta AH, O'Connor CM, Ezrokhi M, Rutty D, Ma ZJ, et al. Randomized clinical trial of quick-release bromocriptine among patients with type 2 diabetes on overall safety and cardiovascular outcomes. Diabetes Care. 2010;33(7):1503–8.
148. Gaziano JM, Cincotta AH, Vinik A, Blonde L, Bohannon N, Scranton R. Effect of bromocriptine-QR (a quick-release formulation of bromocriptine mesylate) on major adverse cardiovascular events in type 2 diabetes subjects. J Am Heart Assoc. 2012;1(5):e002279.
149. Defronzo RA. Bromocriptine: a sympatholytic, d2-dopamine agonist for the treatment of type 2 diabetes. Diabetes Care. 2011;34(4):789–94.
150. Mejía-Rodríguez O, Herrera-Abarca JE, Ceballos-Reyes G, Avila-Diaz M, Prado-Uribe C, Belio-Caro F, et al. Cardiovascular and renal effects of bromocriptine in diabetic patients with stage 4 chronic kidney disease. Biomed Res Int. 2013;2013:104059.
151. Handelsman Y. Role of bile acid sequestrants in the treatment of type 2 diabetes. Diabetes Care. 2011;34(Supplement 2):S244–50.
152. Fonseca VA, Handelsman Y, Staels B. Colesevelam lowers glucose and lipid levels in type 2 diabetes: the clinical evidence. Diabetes Obes Metab. 2010;12(5):384–92.
153. Staels DB, Kuipers F. Bile acid sequestrants and the treatment of type 2 diabetes mellitus. Drugs. 2012;67(10):1383–92.
154. Beysen C, Murphy EJ, Deines K, Chan M, Tsang E, Glass A, et al. Effect of bile acid sequestrants on glucose metabolism, hepatic de novo lipogenesis, and cholesterol and bile acid kinetics in type 2 diabetes: a randomised controlled study. Diabetologia. 2011;55(2):432–42.
155. Claudel T, Staels B, Kuipers F. The Farnesoid X receptor: a molecular link between bile acid and lipid and glucose metabolism. Arterioscler Thromb Vasc Biol. 2005;25(10):2020–30.
156. Smushkin G, Sathananthan M, Piccinini F, Man CD, Law JH, Cobelli C, et al. The effect of a bile acid sequestrant on glucose metabolism in subjects with type 2 diabetes. Diabetes. 2013;62(4):1094–101.
157. Welchol(R) [package insert]. Parsippany: Daiichi Sankyo, Inc.; 2000.
158. Harper CR, Jacobson TA. Managing dyslipidemia in chronic kidney disease. J Am Coll Cardiol. 2008;51(25):2375–84.
159. Mak RH. Impact of end-stage renal disease and dialysis on glycemic control. Semin Dial. 2000;13(1):4–8.
160. Scheen AJ. Pharmacokinetic considerations for the treatment of diabetes in patients with chronic kidney disease. Expert Opin Drug Metab Toxicol. 2013;9(5):529–50.
161. Rabkin R, Ryan MP, Duckworth WC. The renal metabolism of insulin. Diabetologia. 1984;27(3):351–7.
162. Rubenstein AH, Spitz I. Role of the kidney in insulin metabolism and excretion. Diabetes. 1968;17(3):161–9.
163. Rave K, Heise T, Pfützner A, Heinemann L, Sawicki PT. Impact of diabetic nephropathy on pharmacodynamic and pharmacokinetic properties of insulin in type 1 diabetic patients. Diabetes Care. 2001;24(5):886–90.
164. Mühlhauser I, Toth G, Sawicki PT, Berger M. Severe hypoglycemia in type I diabetic patients with impaired kidney function. Diabetes Care. 1991;14(4):344–6.
165. Levemir (R) [package insert]. Princeton: Novo Nordisk, Inc.; 2005.
166. Reilly JB, Berns JS. Selection and dosing of medications for management of diabetes in patients with advanced kidney disease. Semin Dial. 2010;23(2):163–8.
167. Lantus (R) [package insert]. Bridgewater: Sanofi-Aventis US LLC; 2007.
168. Novolin N (R) [package insert]. Princeton: Novo Nordisk, Inc.; 2005.
169. Novolog (R) [package insert]. Princeton: Novo Nordisk, Inc.; 2015.
170. Humalog (R) [package insert]. Indianapolis: Eli Lilly and Company; 2015.
171. Apidra (R) [package insert]. Bridgewater: Sanofi-aventis U.S., LLC; 2009.
172. Afrezza (R) [package insert]. Danbury: MannKind Corporation; 2014.
173. Potocka E, Cassidy JP, Haworth P, Heuman D, van Marle S, Baughman RA. Pharmacokinetic characterization of the novel pulmonary delivery excipient fumaryl diketopiperazine. J Diabetes Sci Technol. 2010;4(5):1164–73.
174. Biesenbach G, Raml A, Schmekal B, Eichbauer-Sturm G. Decreased insulin requirement in relation to GFR in nephropathic Type 1 and insulin-treated Type 2 diabetic patients. Diabet Med J Br Diabet Assoc. 2003;20(8):642–5.

175. Williams ME, Garg R. Glycemic management in ESRD and earlier stages of CKD. Am J Kidney Dis Off J Natl Kidney Found. 2014;63(2 Suppl 2):S22–38.
176. Sobngwi E, Enoru S, Ashuntantang G, Azabji-Kenfack M, Dehayem M, Onana A, et al. Day-to-day variation of insulin requirements of patients with type 2 diabetes and end-stage renal disease undergoing maintenance hemodialysis. Diabetes Care. 2010;33(7):1409–12.
177. Huang C-C. Treatment targets for diabetic patients on peritoneal dialysis: any evidence? Perit Dial Int J Int Soc Perit Dial. 2007;27(Suppl 2):S176–9.
178. Almalki MH, Altuwaijri MA, Almehthel MS, Sirrs SM, Singh RS. Subcutaneous versus intraperitoneal insulin for patients with diabetes mellitus on continuous ambulatory peritoneal dialysis: meta-analysis of non-randomized clinical trials. Clin Investig Med Médecine Clin Exp. 2012;35(3):E132–43.
179. Fine A, Parry D, Ariano R, Dent W. Marked variation in peritoneal insulin absorption in peritoneal dialysis. Perit Dial Int J Int Soc Perit Dial. 2000;20(6):652–5.
180. Verspohl EJ. Novel pharmacological approaches to the treatment of type 2 diabetes. Pharmacol Rev. 2012;64(2):188–237.
181. Edelman SV, Schroeder BE, Frias JP. Pramlintide acetate in the treatment of Type 2 and Type 1 diabetes mellitus. Expert Rev Endocrinol Metab. 2007;2(1):9–18.
182. Schmitz O, Brock B, Rungby J. Amylin agonists: a novel approach in the treatment of diabetes. Diabetes. 2004;53(Suppl 3):S233–8.
183. Symlin(R) [package insert]. Wilmington: AstraZenecaPharmaceuticals, Inc.; 2014.
184. Alrefai HA, Latif KA, Hieronymus LB, Weakley CR, Moss RJ. Pramlintide: clinical strategies for success. Diabetes Spectr. 2010;23(2):124–30.
185. Bolignano D, Zoccali C. Glitazones in chronic kidney disease: potential and concerns. Nutr Metab Cardiovasc Dis. 2012;22(3):167–75.
186. Hall PM. Prevention of progression in diabetic nephropathy. Diabetes Spectr. 2006;19(1):18–24.
187. Wanner C, et al. N Engl J Med. 2016;375:323–34.
188. Vallianou NG, Geladari E, Kazazis CE. SGLT-2 inhibitors: their pleiotropic properties. Diabetes Metab Syndr. 2017;11:311–5.
189. Mann JFE, Orsted DD, Brown-Frandsen K, et al. Liraglutide and renal outcomes in type 2 diabetes. New Engl J Med. 2017;377:839–48.
190. Pfeffer MA, Claggett B, Diaz R, et al. Lisixenatide in patients with type 2 diabetes and acute coronary syndrome. N Engl J Med. 2015;373:2247–57.
191. Groop PH, Cooper ME, Perkovic V, et al. Linagliptin and its effects on hyperglycemia and albuminuria in patients with type 2 diabetes and renal dysfunction: the randomized MARLINA-T2D trial. Diabetes Obes Metab. 2017;19:1610–9.
192. Nauck MA, Stewart MW, Perkins C, Jones-Leone A, Yang F, Perry C, et al. Efficacy and safety of once-weekly GLP-1 receptor agonist albiglutide (HARMONY 2): 52 week primary endpoint results from a randomised, placebo-controlled trial in patients with type 2 diabetes mellitus inadequately controlled with diet and exercise. Diabetologia. 2016;59(2):266–74.
193. Baylis C, Atzpodien E-A, Freshour G, Engels K. Peroxisome proliferator-activated receptor γ agonist provides superior renal protection versus angiotensin-converting enzyme inhibition in a rat model of type 2 diabetes with obesity. J Pharmacol Exp Ther. 2003;307(3):854–60.
194. Adlyxin ® [package insert]. Bridgewater: Sanofi-Aventis US LLC; 2016.

Diabetes Mellitus and Renal Transplantation

6

Curtiss B. Cook and Harini Chakkera

Introduction

Chronic kidney disease (CKD) continues to be a leading cause of morbidity and mortality in the United States (USA). It is estimated that nearly 26 million people nationally have renal disease, and kidney disease is the ninth leading cause of death in the USA. More than 661,000 Americans have end-stage renal disease (ESRD). Of these, 468,000 individuals are on dialysis. Approximately 193,000 live with a functioning kidney transplant, and more than 100,000 await a transplant [1]. Among the causes of ESRD in the USA, a substantial portion (44%) are due to diabetes mellitus (DM) [2].

Changes in Glucose Homeostasis During Peri-Kidney Transplantation

Hyperglycemia is a well-known complication after solid organ transplantation, even among those without DM [3–8]. Among kidney transplant patients, hyperglycemia is of particular concern because approximately 23% of kidney transplant recipients have ESRD as a result of DM [9], and maintaining good glucose control after transplantation is necessary to prevent recurrent diabetic nephropathy [10]. However, hyperglycemia may also occur de novo (i.e., among patients without known diabetes). DM developing following transplant is often termed new-onset diabetes after transplantation (NODAT). NODAT has been shown to adversely affect long-term graft and patient outcomes [11, 12]. This chapter summarizes current knowledge of NODAT and ends with a discussion about possible prevention strategies.

Changes in Glucose Homeostasis During the Immediate Posttransplant Period

Concerns over hyperglycemia in the renal transplant patient begin right after surgery. The authors have previously defined the immediate posttransplant period as the days occurring while the patient is still hospitalized postoperatively [13]. Using this definition, patients have been stratified into two hyperglycemic subpopulations: (1) individuals with known (or preexisting) DM and (2) persons without preexisting DM but who develop high glucose levels while inpatients. The stress of surgery and use of immunosuppressive

C. B. Cook
Division of Endocrinology, Mayo Clinic College of Medicine, Scottsdale, AZ, USA
e-mail: cook.curtiss@mayo.edu

H. Chakkera (✉)
Division of Nephrology, Mayo Clinic, Arizona, Phoenix, AZ, USA
e-mail: chakkera.harini@mayo.edu

C. M. Rhee et al. (eds.), *Endocrine Disorders in Kidney Disease*,
https://doi.org/10.1007/978-3-319-97765-2_6

medications, in particular glucocorticoids, can cause hyperglycemia in persons without pretransplant DM or exacerbate hyperglycemia in those with known DM.

Hyperglycemia in the hospital is associated with poorer patient outcomes (such as higher mortality or greater costs). Current standards of care emphasize the need to optimize inpatient glycemic control, with a goal of 140–180 mg/dL in non-critically ill patients, including those who are postoperative [14–17]. Thus, strategies to monitor and treat hyperglycemia apply to renal transplant patients in the immediate posttransplant period as they would be for any other inpatient.

In a study cohort of 424 renal transplant recipients (25% with pretransplant DM), all patients with and 87% without pretransplant DM had evidence of hyperglycemia, whereas the prevalence of hypoglycemia was low (4.5%) [18]. Hyperglycemia persisted until hospital discharge. All patients with pretransplant DM and 66% without known pretransplant DM required insulin therapy at hospital discharge. Patients with pretransplant DM were managed primarily with short-acting insulin during the first 24 h postoperatively but eventually required a long-acting insulin as the hospital stay progressed to better control hyperglycemia. Moreover, glycemic control varied throughout the hospital stay. The middle 24-h period of the 4-day median hospital stay exhibited the highest glucose values, likely corresponding to the peak effect of steroids because all transplant patients received high doses of steroids for the first 4–5 days after transplantation [18].

The above data underscores the need for inpatient care teams to monitor glucose levels vigilantly throughout the hospital stay and to be prepared to institute, review, and modify insulin therapy daily. Identification of hyperglycemia during the immediate posttransplant period and optimization of inpatient glycemic control while the patient is still hospitalized would assure a smoother transition to the outpatient setting and potentially decrease readmissions due to glucose-related problems. Moreover, given the high frequency of hyperglycemia and need for insulin, even among those without pretransplant DM, resources must be made available to provide education in self-monitoring of blood glucose and insulin administration to patients since effective inpatient DM education can reduce hospital readmissions [19].

New-Onset Diabetes After Kidney Transplantation

A recent analysis demonstrated that among patients without a pretransplant history of DM, hyperglycemia following hospital discharge can be both remitting and relapsing. Hyperglycemia with glucose values meeting criteria for DM that either persists or which recurs and does not resolve would then be defined as NODAT [20]. NODAT is a common complication of kidney transplantation. Prior studies show that approximately 15–30% of nondiabetic kidney transplant recipients develop NODAT in the first posttransplant year [7, 21, 22]. Many more develop impaired glucose regulation, not quite meeting diagnostic criteria for diabetes. Additionally, it has been reported that among the cohort of nondiabetics who required insulin therapy during hospitalization posttransplant, there was a fourfold increase in NODAT at 1 year after transplant (relative risk [RR] 4.01; confidence interval [CI], 1.49–10.7; $P = 0.006$) [23].

Clinical and Economic Significance of NODAT

Kidney transplantation is the best therapy for ESRD [24], but subsequent development of impaired glucose regulation or NODAT undermines the many benefits of kidney transplantation by lowering allograft and patient survival and impairing quality of life [12, 25]. In a United States Renal Data System (USRDS) study of 11,659 patients transplanted between 1996 and 2000, NODAT was associated with a >60% increased incidence of graft failure (hazard rate (HR) ratio = 1.63, 1.46–1.84) and an almost 90% increased mortality rate (HR ratio = 1.87, 1.60–2.18) [7]. Another analysis of USRDS data demonstrated frequent occurrence of diabetic complications, including ketoacidosis, hyperosmolarity, ophthalmic complications, neurologic complications, and hypoglycemic shock, in patients with NODAT [26]. NODAT also increases the annual cost of posttransplant care from $15,000 to $36,500 annually [22].

It Is Important to Decrease the Incidence of NODAT

Compelling reasons to develop clinical intervention strategies that decrease the incidence of NODAT include (1) avoidance of chronic complications of DM in the transplant recipient, (2) protection of the patient's personal and also the social investment made in the transplant recipient, and (3) optimization of the distribution of a scarce resource (a kidney) so that allografts have good outcomes and recipients do not rejoin the list of those waiting for a kidney. Understanding the pathophysiology of NODAT may point to interventions that may help to decrease its incidence.

Timing of NODAT

During the first year after transplantation, there is a five- to sixfold higher incidence of new-onset DM than in patients who remain on the transplant waiting list, with a decline after the first transplant year to an annual incidence of 4–6% [22]. One retrospective observational study of Medicare beneficiaries estimated the incidence of NODAT occurring in the majority of patients within the first 3–6 months after transplant [11, 27]. Earlier development of NODAT, usually within 1 year after transplant, can occur among patients with seemingly normal glucose metabolism before transplantation. The risks for earlier development relative to those who develop NODAT after the first year are not well understood. One hypothesis is that NODAT and type 2 DM share a common pathophysiology. If so, then NODAT results from similar risk factors for type 2 DM that then interact with transplant-related factors that then accelerate NODAT development.

Pathogenesis of NODAT

Traditional type 2 risk factors (older age, obesity, minority race/ethnicity, family history of type 2 DM, hepatitis C seropositivity) increase the chances of developing DM. Additionally, characteristics unique to transplant recipients (immunosuppressants and cytomegalovirus [CMV] infection) that are associated with NODAT [7, 28, 29] place the renal transplant patient at greater risk of developing DM. Immunosuppressive drugs, including glucocorticoids, calcineurin inhibitors (tacrolimus and cyclosporine), and mTOR inhibitors (sirolimus and everolimus) [30, 31] are other variables associated with higher odds of NODAT.

The mechanism of impaired glucose metabolism caused by immunosuppressive agents varies according to the drug. Glucocorticoids lead to an increase in insulin resistance, enhanced gluconeogenesis in the liver, and decreased glucose uptake and glycogen synthesis in skeletal muscle. Calcineurin inhibitors (CNIs) also cause increased insulin resistance but also impaired insulin secretion [31–33]. CNIs inhibit the activation of a nuclear factor of activated T-cells (NFAT), the transducer of regulated cAMP response element binding (CREB) protein 2 (TORC2), and the P13K/Akt pathway. These mechanisms lead to diminished pancreatic beta cell survival in murine models [33]. Studies in mouse models indicate that calcineurin signaling may indirectly affect the insulin sensitivity of skeletal muscle. Additional studies of the effects of calcineurin inhibition on beta cell survival and/or insulin resistance in humans are warranted. Initially believed to be devoid of diabetogenic effects [34], single-center and large registry studies later found mammalian targets of rapamycin (mTOR) inhibitors such as sirolimus to be associated with higher risk for NODAT independent of the effects of CNI [30, 35]. Proposed pathogenic mechanisms of mTOR-induced glucose intolerance include impaired insulin-mediated suppression of hepatic glucose production, ectopic triglyceride deposition leading to insulin resistance, and direct pancreatic beta cell toxicity.

Can Lifestyle Modification Be Adapted for Prevention of NODAT?

Randomized clinical trials have confirmed that intensive lifestyle interventions that incorporate dietary changes, exercise, and modest weight loss can delay or prevent the onset of type 2 DM [36–38]. It would seem reasonable to translate such strategies to the population with CKD or those that underwent renal transplantation. Several compelling lines of evidence support the idea that lifestyle intervention, implemented before and immediately after transplantation might lower the incidence of NODAT. As noted above, type 2 DM and NODAT share similar risk factors. The prevalence of obesity (body mass index [BMI] $\geq$30 kg/m^2) at the time of transplantation in the USA has doubled between 1987 and 2001 [39]. Since higher BMI pretransplant correlates with insulin resistance after transplantation, lifestyle interventions that promote weight loss seem reasonable interventions. For the purpose of decreasing the incidence of NODAT, reduction of fat mass might best begin in patients awaiting transplantation. Prevention efforts could be beneficial following transplant, especially since there is an observed weight gain of 10% during the first year after transplant [40].

The timing of a lifestyle intervention program remains uncertain in the renal transplant population. Prior studies documented a survival benefit associated with increased BMI in patients on dialysis [41, 42]. However, BMI in these studies could represent either higher muscle mass or greater fat mass. Recent reports suggest that greater BMI is associated with higher muscle mass, rather than higher fat mass [43, 44]. Furthermore, in a longitudinal study of 121,762 hemodialysis patients, declining serum creatinine (a surrogate for muscle mass) over time was a stronger predictor of mortality vs. weight loss, also suggesting that the protective effect of high BMI is a result of muscle mass rather than fat mass [44]. Thus, an intervention aimed at increasing lean body mass before transplantation may decrease the incidence of NODAT [45, 46] as well as conferring improved allograft and patient survival [13]. Further clinical studies are needed to confirm this hypothesis.

Patients with CKD self-report low levels of physical activity [47] and the time-intensive requirements of in-center hemodialysis (i.e., three times per week for 3–4 h per treatment) lead to prolonged periods of inactivity. Studies have shown that hemodialysis patients have lower physical activity on dialysis days than in non-dialysis days, and a majority of the reduced activity is explained by less movement recorded during dialysis treatment [48]. Other factors, such as anemia, hypervolemia, and uremic cachexia, may contribute to decreased physical activity in patients on chronic hemodialysis.

Thus, due to a number of patient-related factors, a type 2 DM-like prevention program may not be possible during the pretransplant period. Since current antirejection therapies are well-established risk factors for NODAT but have few effective alternatives, the potential effectiveness of lifestyle changes may be the only modifiable NODAT risk factors and assume even greater importance in the posttransplant period. The feasibility and efficacy of a lifestyle intervention program to lower the incidence of NODAT requires additional study.

Drugs for Preventing NODAT

Previous studies have reported a high incidence of hyperglycemia during the immediate post-renal transplant period [18, 23]. During this phase of care, the patient is exposed to several stressors including the surgical procedure itself, high-dose corticosteroids, and initiation of CNIs that promote hyperglycemia. While lifestyle changes are most effective in reducing risk of developing type 2 DM [36–38], pharmacological approaches have also shown promise.

Resting the beta cell with basal insulin and optimizing beta cell protection with tighter control to near-normoglycemic levels could further reduce the number of patients with future impaired glucose tolerance and NODAT. For instance, a recent study of nondiabetic subjects randomized two groups in the immediate postoperative period. The first was the basal insulin group where basal insulin treatment was initiated with a morning dose of 6, 8, or 10 IU of isophane insulin for previous evening blood glucose >140–180, >180–240, or >240 mg/dL, respectively, with doses adjusted to reach a target glucose of 110–120 mg/dL (treatment group). Short-acting insulin was used for corrections of hyperglycemia when needed. The control arm received short-acting insulin and/or oral agent therapy for hyperglycemia for blood glucose levels ≥180 mg/dL. Results demonstrated that the treatment group had a significantly lower odds of NODAT (OR = 0.27, CI = 0.10–0.72) compared to the control group, with an average HbA1C 0.38% lower in the treatment group [49].

Other pharmacological agents, especially metformin [36] and pioglitazone [50] have also been shown to be effective in the prevention of type 2 DM. Due to their adverse effects, their use in CKD and ESRD is restricted. Acarbose [51] and rosiglitazone [52] also reduce the risk of developing type 2 DM, but after transplantation, metformin or pioglitazone are prescribed off-label for treatment of preexisting type 2 DM or NODAT in patients with good allograft function [53]; however, no study has investigated a role for either of these agents in the prevention of NODAT.

Conclusion

Kidney transplantation is the best therapy for ESRD; however, patients receiving a new kidney are at risk for developing NODAT, and NODAT affects allograft and patient survival. With the rise in obesity among patients waiting for a kidney transplant, an anticipated increase in the number of patients with NODAT can be expected. Studies to test safe and effective interventions to reduce the incidence of NODAT are needed. Evidence supporting successful prevention of type 2 DM strongly suggests that similar interventions should be tried in the kidney transplant population and perhaps should even be introduced into the pretransplant period. Clinical trials of interventions to prevent NODAT are needed to determine the best timing for such interventions and to determine their long-term effects on graft and patient survival. If successful, lifestyle interventions might ultimately improve quality of life, reduce morbidity and mortality, and decrease the economic impact of NODAT on the renal transplant population.

References

1. National Kidney Foundation. National Kidney Foundation: Available at: https://www.kidney.org/search-results?solr-keywords=statistics&=search. Date accessed 03/24/2016. 2016; Available from.
2. Centers for Disease Control and Prevention. National Diabetes Statistics Report 2014. Available at: http://www.cdc.gov/diabetes/pubs/statsreport14/national-diabetes-report-web.pdf. Date accessed: 03/24/2016. Available from.
3. Baid S, Cosimi AB, Farrell ML, Schoenfeld DA, Feng S, Chung RT, et al. Posttransplant diabetes mellitus in liver transplant recipients: risk factors, temporal relationship with hepatitis C virus allograft hepatitis, and impact on mortality. Transplantation. 2001;72(6):1066–72.
4. Davidson J, Wilkinson A, Dantal J, Dotta F, Haller H, Hernandez D, et al. New-onset diabetes after transplantation: 2003 International consensus guidelines. Proceedings of an international expert panel meeting. Barcelona, Spain, 19 February 2003. Transplantation. 2003;75(10 Suppl):SS3–24.
5. Hur KY, Kim MS, Kim YS, Kang ES, Nam JH, Kim SH, et al. Risk factors associated with the onset and progression of posttransplantation diabetes in renal allograft recipients. Diabetes Care. 2007;30(3):609–15.
6. John PR, Thuluvath PJ. Outcome of patients with new-onset diabetes mellitus after liver transplantation compared with those without diabetes mellitus. Liver Transpl. 2002;8(8):708–13.
7. Kasiske BL, Snyder JJ, Gilbertson D, Matas AJ. Diabetes mellitus after kidney transplantation in the United States. Am J Transplant. 2003;3(2):178–85.
8. Reisaeter AV, Hartmann A. Risk factors and incidence of posttransplant diabetes mellitus. Transplant Proc. 2001;33(5A Suppl):8S–18S.
9. US Renal Data System. USRDS 2007 annual data report: atlas of end-stage renal disease in the United States. Bethesda: National Institutes of Health, National Institute of Diabetes and Digestive and Kidney Diseases; 2007.
10. Fioretto P, Steffes MW, Sutherland DE, Goetz FC, Mauer M. Reversal of lesions of diabetic nephropathy after pancreas transplantation. N Engl J Med. 1998;339(2):69–75.

11. Cosio FG, Kudva Y, van der Velde M, Larson TS, Textor SC, Griffin MD, et al. New onset hyperglycemia and diabetes are associated with increased cardiovascular risk after kidney transplantation. Kidney Int. 2005;67(6):2415–21.
12. Sharif A, Baboolal K. Complications associated with new-onset diabetes after kidney transplantation. Nat Rev Nephrol. 2012;8(1):34–42.
13. Meier-Kriesche HU, Arndorfer JA, Kaplan B. The impact of body mass index on renal transplant outcomes: a significant independent risk factor for graft failure and patient death. Transplantation. 2002;73(1):70–4.
14. American Diabetes Association. Glycemic targets. Diabetes Care 2016;39 Suppl 1:S39–46.
15. American Association of Clinical Endocrinologists. AACE Inpatient Glycemic Control Resource Center Available at: http://resources.aace.com/. Date accessed 03/25/2016; Available from.
16. Moghissi ES, Korytkowski MT, DiNardo M, Einhorn D, Hellman R, Hirsch IB, et al. American Association of Clinical Endocrinologists and American Diabetes Association consensus statement on inpatient glycemic control. Endocr Pract. 2009;15(4):353–69.
17. Society of Hospital Medicine. Glycemic control resource room. Available at: http://www.hospitalmedicine.org/ResourceRoomRedesign/GlycemicControl.cfm. Date accessed: 03/25/2016; Available from.
18. Chakkera HA, Weil EJ, Castro J, Heilman RL, Reddy KS, Mazur MJ, et al. Hyperglycemia during the immediate period after kidney transplantation. Clin J Am Soc Nephrol. 2009;4(4):853–9.
19. Healy SJ, Black D, Harris C, Lorenz A, Dungan KM. Inpatient diabetes education is associated with less frequent hospital readmission among patients with poor glycemic control. Diabetes Care. 2013;36(10):2960–7.
20. Boloori A, Saghafian S, Chakkera HA, Cook CB. Characterization of remitting and relapsing hyperglycemia in post-renal-transplant recipients. PLoS One. 2015;10(11):e0142363.
21. Cosio FG, Pesavento TE, Kim S, Osei K, Henry M, Ferguson RM. Patient survival after renal transplantation: IV. Impact of post-transplant diabetes. Kidney Int. 2002;62(4):1440–6.
22. Woodward RS, Schnitzler MA, Baty J, Lowell JA, Lopez-Rocafort L, Haider S, et al. Incidence and cost of new onset diabetes mellitus among U.S. wait-listed and transplanted renal allograft recipients. Am J Transplant. 2003;3(5):590–8.
23. Chakkera HA, Knowler WC, Devarapalli Y, Weil EJ, Heilman RL, Dueck A, et al. Relationship between inpatient hyperglycemia and insulin treatment after kidney transplantation and future new onset diabetes mellitus. Clin J Am Soc Nephrol. 2010;5(9):1669–75.
24. Wolfe RA, Ashby VB, Milford EL, Ojo AO, Ettenger RE, Agodoa LY, et al. Comparison of mortality in all patients on dialysis, patients on dialysis awaiting transplantation, and recipients of a first cadaveric transplant. N Engl J Med. 1999;341(23):1725–30.
25. Wauters RP, Cosio FG, Suarez Fernandez ML, Kudva Y, Shah P, Torres VE. Cardiovascular consequences of new-onset hyperglycemia after kidney transplantation. Transplantation. 2012;94(4):377–82.
26. Burroughs TE, Swindle J, Takemoto S, Lentine KL, Machnicki G, Irish WD, et al. Diabetic complications associated with new-onset diabetes mellitus in renal transplant recipients. Transplantation. 2007;83(8):1027–34.
27. Ghisdal L, Van Laecke S, Abramowicz MJ, Vanholder R, Abramowicz D. New-onset diabetes after renal transplantation: risk assessment and management. Diabetes Care. 2012;35(1):181–8.
28. Cosio FG, Pesavento TE, Osei K, Henry ML, Ferguson RM. Post-transplant diabetes mellitus: increasing incidence in renal allograft recipients transplanted in recent years. Kidney Int. 2001;59(2):732–7.
29. Cruzado JM, Bestard O, Grinyo JM. Impact of extrahepatic complications (diabetes and glomerulonephritis) associated with hepatitis C virus infection after renal transplantation. Contrib Nephrol. 2012;176:108–16.
30. Johnston O, Rose CL, Webster AC, Gill JS. Sirolimus is associated with new-onset diabetes in kidney transplant recipients. J Am Soc Nephrol. 2008;19(7):1411–8.
31. Ozbay LA, Smidt K, Mortensen DM, Carstens J, Jorgensen KA, Rungby J. Cyclosporin and tacrolimus impair insulin secretion and transcriptional regulation in INS-1E beta-cells. Br J Pharmacol. 2011;162(1):136–46.
32. Chakkera HA, Mandarino LJ. Calcineurin inhibition and new-onset diabetes mellitus after transplantation. Transplantation. 2013;95(5):647–52.
33. Soleimanpour SA, Crutchlow MF, Ferrari AM, Raum JC, Groff DN, Rankin MM, et al. Calcineurin signaling regulates human islet {beta}-cell survival. J Biol Chem. 2010;285(51):40050–9.
34. Tsang CK, Qi H, Liu LF, Zheng XF. Targeting mammalian target of rapamycin (mTOR) for health and diseases. Drug Discov Today. 2007;12(3–4):112–24.
35. Yang SB, Lee HY, Young DM, Tien AC, Rowson-Baldwin A, Shu YY, et al. Rapamycin induces glucose intolerance in mice by reducing islet mass, insulin content, and insulin sensitivity. J Mol Med (Berl). 2012;90(5):575–85.
36. Knowler WC, Barrett-Connor E, Fowler SE, Hamman RF, Lachin JM, Walker EA, et al. Reduction in the incidence of type 2 diabetes with lifestyle intervention or metformin. N Engl J Med. 2002;346(6):393–403.
37. Lindstrom J, Ilanne-Parikka P, Peltonen M, Aunola S, Eriksson JG, Hemio K, et al. Sustained reduction in the incidence of type 2 diabetes by lifestyle intervention: follow-up of the Finnish Diabetes Prevention Study. Lancet. 2006;368(9548):1673–9.
38. Ramachandran A, Snehalatha C, Mary S, Mukesh B, Bhaskar AD, Vijay V. The Indian Diabetes Prevention Programme shows that lifestyle modification and metformin prevent type 2 diabetes in Asian Indian subjects with impaired glucose tolerance (IDPP-1). Diabetologia. 2006;49(2):289–97.

39. Hasse J. Pretransplant obesity: a weighty issue affecting transplant candidacy and outcomes. Nutr Clin Pract. 2007;22(5):494–504.
40. Cashion AK, Sanchez ZV, Cowan PA, Hathaway DK, Lo Costello A, Gaber AO. Changes in weight during the first year after kidney transplantation. Prog Transplant. 2007;17(1):40–7.
41. Leavey SF, McCullough K, Hecking E, Goodkin D, Port FK, Young EW. Body mass index and mortality in 'healthier' as compared with 'sicker' haemodialysis patients: results from the Dialysis Outcomes and Practice Patterns Study (DOPPS). Nephrol Dial Transplant. 2001;16(12):2386–94.
42. Salahudeen AK. Obesity and survival on dialysis. Am J Kidney Dis. 2003;41(5):925–32.
43. Beddhu S, Pappas LM, Ramkumar N, Samore M. Effects of body size and body composition on survival in hemodialysis patients. J Am Soc Nephrol 2003;14(9):2366–72.
44. Kalantar-Zadeh K, Streja E, Molnar MZ, Lukowsky LR, Krishnan M, Kovesdy CP, et al. Mortality prediction by surrogates of body composition: an examination of the obesity paradox in hemodialysis patients using composite ranking score analysis. Am J Epidemiol. 2012;175(8):793–803.
45. Molnar MZ, Kovesdy CP, Mucsi I, Bunnapradist S, Streja E, Krishnan M, et al. Higher recipient body mass index is associated with post-transplant delayed kidney graft function. Kidney Int. 2011;80(2):218–24.
46. Weissenbacher A, Jara M, Ulmer H, Biebl M, Bosmuller C, Schneeberger S, et al. Recipient and donor body mass index as important risk factors for delayed kidney graft function. Transplantation. 2012;93(5):524–9.
47. Painter P, Ward K, Nelson RD. Self-reported physical activity in patients with end stage renal disease. Nephrol Nurs J. 2011;38(2):139–47. quiz 148
48. Majchrzak KM, Pupim LB, Chen K, Martin CJ, Gaffney S, Greene JH, et al. Physical activity patterns in chronic hemodialysis patients: comparison of dialysis and nondialysis days. J Ren Nutr. 2005;15(2):217–24.
49. Hecking M, Haidinger M, Doller D, Werzowa J, Tura A, Zhang J, et al. Early basal insulin therapy decreases new-onset diabetes after renal transplantation. J Am Soc Nephrol. 2012;23(4):739–49.
50. DeFronzo RA, Tripathy D, Schwenke DC, Banerji M, Bray GA, Buchanan TA, et al. Pioglitazone for diabetes prevention in impaired glucose tolerance. N Engl J Med. 2011;364(12):1104–15.
51. Chiasson JL, Josse RG, Gomis R, Hanefeld M, Karasik A, Laakso M. Acarbose for prevention of type 2 diabetes mellitus: the STOP-NIDDM randomised trial. Lancet. 2002;359(9323):2072–7.
52. Gerstein HC, Yusuf S, Bosch J, Pogue J, Sheridan P, Dinccag N, et al. Effect of rosiglitazone on the frequency of diabetes in patients with impaired glucose tolerance or impaired fasting glucose: a randomised controlled trial. Lancet. 2006;368(9541):1096–105.
53. Kurian B, Joshi R, Helmuth A. Effectiveness and long-term safety of thiazolidinediones and metformin in renal transplant recipients. Endocr Pract. 2008;14(8):979–84.

Part II

Thyroid Dysfunction

Evaluating Thyroid Function Tests in Patients with Kidney Disease

7

Stephanie Smooke Praw, Jennifer Sue An Way, and Rebecca Weiss

Introduction

Disorders of thyroid function, especially hypothyroidism, are more prevalent in patients with chronic kidney disease (CKD) and end-stage renal disease (ESRD), compared to the general population [1]. While tests for thyroid function are among the most common hormonal tests ordered, the interpretation of thyroid function tests can be obscured by multiple entities in patients with renal disease, including nonthyroidal illness syndrome (NTI), malnutrition, inflammation, iodine retention, metabolic acidosis, medications, mineral deficiencies, and dialysis. Several studies have shown that both hypothyroidism and hyperthyroidism are associated with increased cardiovascular morbidity and mortality in CKD and ESRD [1]. It is important, then, to understand which thyroid function test results represent authentic thyroid dysfunction, rather than changes secondary to renal disease.

S. S. Praw (✉) · J. S. A. Way
Division of Endocrinology, Diabetes, and Metabolism, Department of Medicine, David Geffen School of Medicine at UCLA, Los Angeles, CA, USA
e-mail: ssmooke@mednet.ucla.edu

R. Weiss
Department of Endocrinology, Kaiser Permanente—Woodland Hills, Woodland Hills, CA, USA

In this chapter, we will review commonly ordered tests of thyroid function, alterations associated with renal disease, testing for thyroid autoimmunity, and the impact of medications on thyroid hormone measurements and thyroid hormone absorption, relevant for the many kidney disease patients that take levothyroxine therapy.

TSH Measurement

Thyroid-stimulating hormone (TSH) is produced in the pituitary gland and released in response to feedback from thyroxine (T4) and triiodothyronine (T3). In the general population, TSH is used for screening for thyroid dysfunction because it is an exquisitely sensitive test for assessing thyroid status since there is a negative logarithmic association between serum TSH with T4 (small changes in T4 result in exponential changes in TSH) [2].

Measurement of thyroid-stimulating hormone (TSH) has changed dramatically over the past 70 years. McKenzie developed the first sensitive assay to measure TSH in 1958 and could detect elevated TSH in mice, but there was significant variability in the assay, up to 25% [3]. Over the next several decades, more accurate methods for measuring TSH were established. Radioimmunoassays (RIA) were developed, which used radiolabeled isotopes (usually with I^{125}) of TSH to bind to an antibody in a sample. When mixed with the patient's serum, the

C. M. Rhee et al. (eds.), *Endocrine Disorders in Kidney Disease*,
https://doi.org/10.1007/978-3-319-97765-2_7

patient's TSH competes with the radiolabeled TSH, decreasing the amount of known radiolabeled TSH in the sample, thus giving an indirect measurement of TSH. Although RIA, which was mostly used between the 1960s and 1985, was superior to prior methods, it still had limited functional sensitivity and could not detect levels below 1.0 mIU/L, so the TSH test was useful only for assessing hypothyroidism, when the TSH level was elevated [4].

The discovery of monoclonal antibodies led to the development of the more modern and sensitive "sandwich" immunometric assay (IMA) in the mid-1980s. In this test, a patient's serum is mixed with two antibodies of TSH. Antibodies are sequentially added to bind TSH, one contained in a solid support (tube, bead, adsorption gel, or magnetic microparticle), and the other TSH antibody, to a different epitope, binds the TSH at a different site [3, 4]. With the advent of IMA using isotopic signals (I I^{125}), there was a tenfold improvement in sensitivity compared to RIA methods (~0.1mIU/L). Further advances in IMA using non-isotopic signals, such as immunochemiluminometric assays and immunoenzymometric assays, are now able to detect levels as low as 0.01 mIU/L and are the standard of care [4, 5]. These assays, with the sensitivity to separate normal from abnormally reduced values, allowed for assessment of patients with hyperthyroidism.

TSH Levels in Chronic Kidney Disease Patients

In CKD and end-stage renal disease (ESRD), TSH alterations may be observed due to impaired pulsatility, reduced renal clearance of TSH, diminished response to thyrotropin-releasing hormone (TRH), or due to non-thyroidal illness (NTI) [1, 6]. The diurnal variation in TSH production, the reverse of the cortisol cycle that drives TSH, is characterized by a TSH rise in the evening, when cortisol is at its nadir, and is reduced in the early morning as cortisol rises. This variation of TSH is diminished or absent in chronic hemodialysis patients and the periodicity of TSH is shorter [6]. Renal clearance of TSH appears to be reduced by about 57% in patients with CKD compared to normal subjects [6, 7]. In patients with acute renal failure who were given TRH, all had a blunted TSH response, which returned to normal after resolution of acute renal failure [8]. Responses to TRH are also blunted in patients with ESRD both before and after hemodialysis [6].

CKD has been associated with a rise in serum TSH based on multiple cross-sectional studies [9–11]. In a study of the Third National Health and Nutrition Examination Survey (NHANES III) respondents, there was a higher prevalence of hypothyroidism (defined as TSH >4.5 mIu/l or treatment with thyroid hormone replacement therapy) in patients with lower estimated glomerular filtration rates (eGFRs). Patients with eGFR of <30 ml/min/1.73m^2 had a prevalence of hypothyroidism of 23% as compared to patients with normal GFR of >90 ml/min/1.73m^2 who had only a 5% prevalence of hypothyroidism [9]. In a cross-sectional analysis of almost 30,000 patients in Norway, a rise of serum TSH by 1-mIU/mL was associated with a reduction of eGFR by 1.9% (95% CI 1.5–2.3%) [10]. In this same study, TSH levels in the lower quartile (subclinical or overt hyperthyroidism) were associated with higher eGFRs.

At least one study has found a higher proportion of progressive CKD in patients with lower TSH [9–12]. The Rotterdam Study followed 5013 patients from several regions in the Netherlands. Thyroid function (using electrochemiluminescence assays to measure TSH and T4) and serum creatinine levels were determined over time. In the cross-sectional analysis, patients with hypothyroidism (defined as TSH >4.0 IU/L) were noted to have lower eGFR, whereas patients with overt hyperthyroidism (defined as TSH <0.4 IU/L and free T4 >25 pmol/L) had a higher baseline eGFR. In a longitudinal analysis, eGFR declined less in the hypothyroid group than in patients with lower TSH levels [12].

Most of the studies examining the relationship between CKD and hypothyroidism found in the literature are retrospective or cross-sectional. However, in a recently published prospective study of more than 100,000 euthyroid Korean patients, there was a positive correlation between higher serum TSH and incident CKD, with a hazard ratio of 1.59 (95% CI 1.29 to 2.95; $p < 0.001$) of developing CKD comparing the highest and the lowest quintiles of TSH [13].

Although TSH may be higher in CKD patients, it is difficult to differentiate between true thyroid dysfunction and changes that occur with nonthyroidal illness (NTI) in this population. Nonthyroidal illness is a state of dysregulation of thyrotropic feedback control during times of acute or chronic stress or critical illnesses such as sepsis, trauma, heart failure, starvation, cirrhosis, or diabetic ketoacidosis. NTI or "euthyroid sick syndrome" is characterized by a wide variety of measured thyroid hormone abnormalities, but the hallmark is the absence of primary thyroid disease, and the changes are only seen due to the stress of illness. Thyroid abnormalities encountered during NTI may include elevated, normal, or low TSH with low T4 and T3. Total T3 and total T4 levels are low, in part, due to decreased binding protein concentrations or impaired T4 or T3 binding [14]. While in most hospitalized patients, repeating thyroid testing after the stress or illness is resolved will help to differentiate between true thyroid dysfunction and NTI, CKD is by nature chronic and progressive, making the distinction between true thyroid dysfunction and NTI more challenging.

In a meta-analysis which included five studies of patients with CKD and thyroid function measurements, patients with CKD were noted to have elevated TSH with a normal free T4 in 1.6 to 28% of patients [15]. In a prospective study of patients on dialysis, patients with transient elevations in TSH were monitored over 14 months, and none of the patients progressed to overt hypothyroidism [17]. However in one cross-sectional analysis of 64 patients on hemodialysis, 82% of patients who had elevated TSH also had low free T4, with symptoms consistent with hypothyroidism, rather than NTI [16].

In several studies of patients with ESRD on dialysis, patients with elevated TSH were noted to have normal total and free T4 [5, 18, 19], consistent with NTI. However, in one of these studies of 1689 patients with various stages of CKD, while there were 39.4% of patients noted to have NTI based on elevated TSH and normal FT4, 22% of patients did have evidence of hypothyroidism based on elevated TSH and low FT4 [19]. In the cohort of patients with CKD stage 5 (eGFR <15 ml/min/1.73m^2, $n = 18$), 50% of these patients were noted to have NTI, while only 11.1% ($n = 2$) had hypothyroidism.

Although TSH has been shown to be elevated in patients with CKD, it is still unclear whether this is due to true thyroid dysfunction, changes in renal clearance leading to elevations in TSH, decreased responsiveness to TRH, or related to chronic illness, as is seen in other NTIs. Retrospective studies showing increased adverse cardiovascular outcomes and mortality in CKD and dialysis patients with even modestly elevated serum TSH suggest that these changes are likely significant. Prospective studies are needed, including evaluation for improvements in outcome with levothyroxine treatment, to determine causality of thyroid dysfunction or whether the TSH changes are markers of more severe disease. It is clear, though, that thyroid function affects kidney function, and kidney function appears to affect measurements of thyroid function.

Measuring Free Thyroxine and Free Triiodothyronine

The majority of thyroxine (T4) and triiodothyronine (T3) circulate bound to plasma proteins, 99.97% and 99.7%, respectively. While T4 is bound to thyroid-binding globulin (TBG) (60–75%), transthyretin (15–30%), and albumin (10%), T3 is primarily bound to TBG [3]. Free T4 (FT4) and free T3 (FT3) may be measured by various methodologies including indirect index methods, two-step labeled immunoassays, one-step labeled hormone methods, and direct free T4 (FT4) or FT3 assays using equilibrium dialysis with liquid chromatography-tandem mass spectrometry or ultrafiltration [20, 21].

An older method of determining FT4 is the T4 index, which measures total T4 and thyroid-binding globulin (TBG) or resin uptake as an estimate of protein binding and then uses this to calculate FT4 Index. These measurements are quite accurate, but cannot be performed on an automated platform and are not available in most laboratories. The index measurements based on only TBG do not account for the changes in albumin and transthyretin, as can be seen in CKD, which may make this a less reliable tool [4, 20]. Additionally, there is some data to suggest that FT4 Index, as determined by indices, may be lower in uremic patients with CKD due to interfering substances [8].

In one-step labeled hormone assays, a proprietary labeled hormone analog (manufacturers use different labels) competes with thyroid hormone (T4 or T3) for a solid-phase antihormone antibody. These assays are intended to minimize interaction with thyroid hormone-binding proteins, but may differ in altered protein states such as CKD and ESRD due to difficulties with ensuring that the analog hormone is "inert" with respect to binding proteins [4, 21]. Two-step immunoassays, which measure hormone in serum by FT4 binding to an immobilized labeled immunoglobulin, which is then washed with the serum to remove proteins, may also be altered in CKD [15]. Analog methods are albumin dependent; if more tracers are available in the sample because of low albumin, as is seen in CKD, this will lead to lower apparent FT4 values [22]. The gold standard for measuring FT4 to remove antibody or protein interference is equilibrium dialysis [14, 21]. However, the equilibrium dialysis method typically takes longer to result than immunoassays, and are more expensive and are generally available only in a reference laboratory.

Thyroxine (T4) Changes with CKD

Low FT4 levels were observed in a wide range, 4.5–9%, of patients with ESRD in one study examining nine different FT4 immunoassays [23]. Due to changes in thyroid-binding globulin (TBG) and other changes which may falsely lower FT4 estimates using immunoassays, measuring FT4 by ultrafiltration or direct equilibrium dialysis with liquid chromatography-tandem mass spectrometry may be more reliable in patients with CKD [15]. Using equilibrium dialysis methods, FT4 levels were normal in 87–97% of patients with ESRD [6]. Similarly, a study examining ESRD patients' sera pre-dialysis using both equilibrium dialysis and an immunoassay found that measured FT4 was similar to normal controls when using equilibrium dialysis, whereas FT4 was significantly lower in 6 of the 27 patients' samples using the immunoassay [24].

Other factors may also influence T4 levels in CKD and ESRD patients. CKD and ESRD patients often have chronic metabolic acidosis, which has been shown to reduce levels of serum FT4 and FT3 and increase TSH [1, 25]. In one study, eliminating the metabolic acidosis corrected the low free T3 [25].

Albuminuria in CKD has also been positively correlated to T4 levels: In a study of 1689 patients with no history of thyroid dysfunction, after adjusting for multiple factors including age, sex, serum albumin, and smoking status, a higher albumin-to-creatinine ratio was associated with both higher FT4 and total T4 levels (p = 0.013) in patients with either CKD and ESRD [19].

Retained organic acids and lipids may also alter measurements of FT4. Retained organic acids and non-esterified fatty acids (NEFA) can displace tracer from albumin [2]. In a study of 35 uremic patients, FT4 was measured by an analog radioimmunoassay and labeled antibody immunoassay both before and after the hemodialysis session [22]. Independent of the assay used, free thyroid hormone levels (both FT3 and FT4) were lower than in healthy subjects. FT3 and FT4 levels both increased after hemodialysis. The most significant increases were observed with the analog RIA method. In the same study, 22 samples from 11 of the patients were used to compare FT4 measurements of equilibrium dialysis to the analog RIA and labeled antibody assay. Using the equilibrium dialysis method, FT4 concentrations were higher than with the other assays [22]. Similarly, in a study of 27 chronic dialysis patients, sera were exposed to non-esterified fatty acids (NEFA) in vitro and then FT4 measured by both equilibrium dialysis and an immunoassay. FT4 measured after hemodialysis was significantly higher when measured by equilibrium dialysis and with the immunoassay [24].

In CKD patients, assays measuring serum FT4 may also be altered due to the presence of medications commonly used, such as furosemide and heparin, which are addressed later in the chapter [1, 25, 26].

Triiodothyronine and Reverse Triiodothyronine in CKD

The most commonly observed thyroid function abnormality seen in CKD patients is low T3 [1]. Low T3 levels in CKD may be due to decreased peripheral deiodinase conversion of T4 to T3 caused by chronic metabolic acidosis and protein malnutrition seen in CKD [6, 27]. Even though levels of T3 are low, ESRD patients with reduced serum FT3 are clinically euthyroid [6].

In a retrospective study of 279 patients with CKD and no history of hypothyroidism, 47% of patients had "low T3 syndrome," defined as normal TSH and low total T3 (reference range 0.87–1.7 ng/ml), using an electrochemiluminescence assay. The prevalence of low T3 syndrome appeared to increase with decreasing GFR; 22% of patients with CKD stage 2 had low T3, as compared to 76% of patients with CKD stage 5 [28]. Similar results were noted in a larger study of 2284 patients in which 11% of patients with CKD stage 2, and 79% of patients with CKD stage 5 were noted to have low T3 but normal TSH [1, 29]. In another cross-sectional analysis which compared 96 patients on hemodialysis to 39 healthy volunteers, hemodialysis patients were noted to have lower FT3 and total T3 as compared to controls [30]. The low T3 levels seen in dialysis patients may be related to nutrition, systemic acidosis, time on dialysis, and inflammation [28].

While reverse T3 (rT3) is elevated in many cases of NTI, rT3 levels have been shown to be normal in ESRD [6, 31]. The clinical significance of this has yet to be defined. In a prospective study of 167 patients with ESRD on hemodialysis, only 9.9% of the cohort had elevated rT3 levels. After 1 year of follow-up, 48 patients (28.7%) had died. Although there was no significant difference in either T3 or rT3 levels from the rest of the cohort, patients who died at any time point during the follow-up period were noted to have lower T3 levels and higher rT3 levels than those who survived, suggesting perhaps that these patients had more severe NTIs [32].

In conclusion, interpretation of thyroid function tests in patients with CKD and ESRD is complicated by a myriad of factors including reduced renal clearance of thyroid hormone, blunted responses of TSH to thyrotropin, assay interference due to the presence of altered binding proteins, and non-thyroidal illness. Laboratory evaluation should be undertaken knowing that the results may be difficult to interpret and should be evaluated in the context of patients' clinical presentations and symptoms. Although measuring serum FT4 by dialysis is considered to be the "gold standard," it is often expensive, has a slow turnaround, and usually needs to be sent to a reference laboratory. The next best alternative may be the T4 and T3 indices, which may be falsely low in setting of low albumin or transthyretin states, but are more widely available. All of the available testing methods may have some inherent error in CKD. Thus, it may be best to use whichever test

Table 7.1 Changes in thyroid function tests with kidney disease

	No CKD	CKD	ESRD
TSH	Normal	Normal or increased	Normal or increased
T4	Normal	Normal to low	Normal to low
T3	Normal	Normal to low	Normal to low
Reverse T3	Normal	Normal	Normal

is the most readily available and account for the fact that T4/T3 may be altered depending on the method used, while also considering the clinical context when interpreting results. Table 7.1 shows changes in thyroid function tests with kidney disease.

Thyroid Autoantibody Measurements

There are three types of thyroid autoantibodies that are commonly used in clinical practice to diagnose autoimmune thyroid diseases. These include antibodies to thyroid-stimulating hormone receptor, thyroglobulin (Tg, formerly colloid antigen), and thyroid peroxidase (TPO, formerly referred to as microsomal antigen). All of these thyroid autoantigens are involved in thyroid hormone synthesis. The TSH receptor is a G protein-coupled receptor that generates cyclic adenosine monophosphate (cAMP) when TSH binds. This in turn stimulates the growth and function of the thyroid follicular cells. Tg is a glycoprotein produced by the thyroid follicular cells and is the substrate for thyroid hormone synthesis. Tyrosine residues on Tg are iodinated to form monoiodotyrosine (MIT) and diiodotyrosine (DIT). The coupling of two DIT moieties forms T_4, while the coupling of one DIT and one MIT forms T_3. TPO is the enzyme that catalyzes the oxidation of iodine and its transfer onto tyrosine residues. TPO also catalyzes the coupling of DIT and MIT [33].

Thyroid Peroxidase Antibodies and Thyroglobulin Antibodies

Autoimmune hypothyroidism includes Hashimoto's thyroiditis (goitrous form) and primary myxedema (atrophic, nongoitrous form). Thyroid peroxidase antibodies (TPO Ab) and Tg antibodies (Tg Ab) are found in the majority of patients with autoimmune hypothyroidism, with TPO Ab being more sensitive than Tg Ab. TPO Ab may play a direct role in immune destruction of the thyroid cell through antibody-dependent cell-mediated cytotoxicity and complement fixation. TPO Ab is also present in about 80% of individuals with Graves' disease. However, approximately 10% of the population without apparent thyroid disease has elevated TPO Ab [2]. TPO Ab is measured via a sequential two-step immunoenzymatic (sandwich) assay. The majority of assays report in international units, using the standard preparation MRC 66/387 as a reference [2].

Patients with autoimmune hypothyroidism may have elevated titers of Tg Ab. However, low titers of Tg Ab are found in up to 27% of individuals without evidence of autoimmune thyroid disease, particularly in the elderly or following viral infections [2]. Tg Ab assay is also a two-step immunoenzymatic (sandwich) assay. In general, it is difficult to standardize Tg Ab measurements between laboratories, due to the great variability of Tg preparations [2].

TSH Receptor Antibody

Thyroid-stimulating hormone receptor antibodies (TRAb) can be stimulating, blocking, or neutral. Thyroid-stimulating immunoglobulins (TSI) are the key pathogenic mechanisms in Graves' disease. They stimulate the thyroid gland to produce thyroid hormone. TSH receptor-blocking antibodies can be found in a minority of patients with autoimmune hypothyroidism and can cause hypothyroidism without long-term tissue destruction [2]. Specifically, TSH receptor-blocking antibodies were detected in 8 of 50 (16%) patients with autoimmune hypothyroidism [34].

There are two types of assays used to detect TRAb, a binding assay and a bioassay. The binding assay is a competitive assay in which the presence of patient's TRAb inhibits the binding of labeled monoclonal TRAb (third-generation assay) or labeled bovine TSH (second-generation assay) to TSH receptor. Thus, this assay is known as the TSH-binding inhibitor immunoglobulin (TBII) assay. While this assay cannot distinguish between TSH receptor stimulating and blocking antibodies, the clinical context guides the interpretation of positive TBII [35]. For example, the presence of TBII in a thyrotoxic patient indicates that the antibody is stimulating and that the patient has Graves' disease. In hyperthyroid patients, the third-generation TBII assay has a sensitivity of 97% and specificity of 99% for Graves' disease [36].

The TRAb bioassay, known as thyroid-stimulating immunoglobulin (TSI) assay, only detects stimulating TRAb. It detects cAMP that is produced when the patient's TRAb binds to TSH receptor. It is highly sensitive and specific. While testing for TSI is available, it may not be necessary in the evaluation of hyperthyroidism, due to the availability of other effective and less expensive tests. It can be useful in rare cases such as Graves' disease in pregnancy if maternal thyroid status cannot be assessed due to previous RAI ablation or thyroidectomy [2].

Thyroid Autoantibody Measurements in Chronic Kidney Disease

There is scant literature regarding the effect of CKD on the interpretation of thyroid autoantibodies. One study from 1991 found that the sera of seven hemodialysis patients had dialyzable "unknown substances" that interfered with the hemagglutination assay of TPO Ab and Tg Ab, creating false-positive results [37]. Since that time, hemagglutination assays have been replaced with immunoassays. Additional studies regarding the measurement of thyroid autoantibodies in CKD would be useful since patients with CKD have higher rates of thyroid disorders than the general population and the mechanism of this is poorly understood [9]. For example, patients with eGFR <30 mL/min/1.73m^2 have a twofold greater risk of hypothyroidism than patients with eGFR ≥90 mL/min/1.73m^2 [9].

Current literature suggests that rates of both autoimmune and nonautoimmune primary hypothyroidism are higher in CKD patients. One study of 915 outpatients (excluding those on dialysis and with overt hyper- or hypothyroidism) found that compared to patients with eGFR ≥90 mL/min/1.73m^2, patients with eGFR <60 mL/min/1.73m^2 had significantly higher rates of subclinical hypothyroidism (26% vs 8%), elevated TPO Ab (28% vs 15%), and elevated Tg Ab (26% vs 10%), even after adjusting for age and sex [38]. In a smaller study comparing 32 diabetic and 31 nondiabetic patients with CKD not on HD, there were significantly higher rates of primary hypothyroidism (including subclinical and overt) in patients with diabetes than without diabetes (38% vs 10%). None of the 63 patients had elevated titers of TPO Ab or Tg Ab, suggesting a nonautoimmune mechanism. Furthermore, thyroid histology in six of the eight patients who had overt hypothyroidism showed no interstitial lymphocytic infiltration. As mentioned earlier, a proposed mechanism for nonautoimmune hypothyroidism in CKD patients is impaired renal excretion of iodine leading to elevated serum iodine and the prolongation of the Wolff-Chaikoff effect. In summary, rates of both autoimmune and nonautoimmune thyroid disease are more common in patients with CKD than those without. Further study is needed to better understand the underlying etiology of thyroid dysfunction in this patient cohort.

Common Medications in Chronic Kidney Disease and Their Impact on Thyroid Function Tests

Thyroid function tests (TFTs) are among the most commonly ordered laboratory hormonal evaluation. While interpretation is usually straightforward, medication and supplement usage may cause alterations in TFTs via a variety of mechanisms as well as impact thyroid medication absorption. We will explore some commonly used medications and supplements and their impact on TFT testing here.

Displacement of Thyroid Hormone from Thyroid Hormone-Binding Proteins

Several drugs cause the displacement of thyroid hormone from thyroid hormone-binding proteins such as thyroid-binding globulin (TBG), albumin, and transthyretin. This results in transiently elevated FT4 and FT3, but if the thyroid axis is functioning normally, production should be proportionately reduced, and the TSH remains in the normal range. Furosemide, heparin, nonsteroidal anti-inflammatory agents, and phenytoin have all been associated with this phenomenon.

Furosemide

Furosemide, particularly intravenous doses of over 80 mg per day, is known to displace thyroid hormone from its binding sites, transiently elevating free thyroid hormone levels. It is quickly cleared from the bloodstream, with 86–97% removed after 4 h. Once the drug is out of the bloodstream, its effect on thyroid hormone binding dissipates. The degree of dissociation of thyroid hormone from its binding sites can be exacerbated in vitro, depending on the assay [39].

Heparin

Unfractionated heparin and low molecular weight heparin cause artifactual increases in free thyroid hormone via displacement of thyroid hormone from its binding proteins in vitro. Heparin activates endothelial lipoprotein lipase in vivo, which acts on triglycerides to release free fatty acids (FFA) in vitro. When high concentrations of FFA exceed their usual binding sites on albumin, they compete with thyroid hormone for TBG binding sites. The FFA-to-albumin molar ratio must exceed approximately five before a significant effect on the serum FT4 concentration occurs. This molar ratio is unlikely to be exceeded in vivo, but occurs in vitro, especially with assays that require long incubation periods [40]. This effect is more pronounced in hypertriglyceridemia and hypoalbuminemia. It has been observed with both intravenous and subcutaneous heparin and with a variety of assay platforms, including equilibrium dialysis, ultracentrifugation, and direct immunoassay. Therefore, for patients receiving heparin, measurements of total thyroid hormone levels are more accurate than free thyroid hormone levels. If serum FT4 and FT3 levels are needed, the sample should be obtained at least 10 h after the last injection of heparin and analyzed without delay [14].

Nonsteroidal Anti-inflammatory Drugs

Select nonsteroidal anti-inflammatory drugs including aspirin and salicylates also inhibit the binding of T4 and T3 to TBG. This results in a transient increase in circulating free thyroid hormone levels, which, in turn, causes temporary TSH suppression and reduced endogenous thyroid hormone secretion. In a study of 25 healthy patients, 1 week of aspirin (4 g per day) administration caused total T4, total T3, and free T3 to decrease by approximately 30% from baseline. Similarly, after 1 week of salicylates (4 g per day), free and total thyroid hormone levels decreased by 40–50% from baseline. With both medications, TSH decreased by more than 30%, but remained within the normal range. The other NSAIDs studied – ibuprofen, naproxen, and indomethacin – had no effect on thyroid hormone levels [41].

Common Medications in Chronic Kidney Disease and Their Interaction with Levothyroxine

Oral levothyroxine (synthetic T4) is the most common form of thyroid hormone replacement used to treat hypothyroidism. It has a narrow therapeutic window. An acidic gastric pH is required to dissolve levothyroxine in order for it to be absorbed in the small intestine [42]. Many medications and supplements commonly used by patients with CKD interfere with the absorption of levothyroxine [43].

Phosphate Binders

Phosphate binders, used to treat hyperphosphatemia in ESRD, impair the absorption of levothyroxine. Both calcium-containing (e.g., calcium carbonate and calcium acetate) and noncalcium-containing phosphate binders (e.g., sevelamer and lanthanum) have this effect [44]. For example, coadministration of levothyroxine and calcium carbonate for 3 months led to an increase in mean serum TSH of 69%, with 20% of patients developing TSH levels above the normal range [45]. Thus, it is recommended to administer levothyroxine at least 4 h apart from calcium-containing products and at least several hours apart from noncalcium-containing phosphate binders to avoid impact on absorption.

Proton Pump Inhibitors

Proton pump inhibitors (PPIs) have been shown to increase TSH levels, necessitating levothyroxine dose escalations when used concomitantly for several months [46, 47]. The mechanism is thought to involve impairment of levothyroxine dissolution in higher gastric pH environments. These findings were not supported by two short-term pharmacokinetic studies, which found no difference in thyroid hormone levels after a single large dose of levothyroxine whether it was administered before or after 1 week of PPI therapy [48, 49]. A major limitation of these pharmacokinetic studies is that thyroid hormone levels were measured only up to 10 h after a single dose of levothyroxine, while thyroid hormone replacement therapy takes days to weeks to reach steady state. In practice, the impaired absorption of levothyroxine with concomitant use of PPI may be ameliorated by increasing the dose or switching to oral solution formulation [50].

Ferrous Sulfate and Fiber Supplements

Ferrous sulfate may cause impaired absorption of levothyroxine likely via formation of insoluble ferric-thyroxine complexes. Simultaneous administration of levothyroxine and ferrous sulfate for 12 weeks resulted in increased TSH from baseline, but stable free and total T4 levels [51]. Similarly, fiber supplementation can interfere with levothyroxine absorption likely from nonspecific adsorption of T4 to dietary fibers [52]. These substances should be separated from levothyroxine administration by at least 4 h.

Simvastatin

Although evidence is sparse, three case reports described increased TSH levels after simvastatin was administered to patients on replacement levothyroxine. The proposed mechanism is excess CYP3A4 formation in the liver by simvastatin resulting in accelerated levothyroxine catabolism [53, 54]. Thyroid function tests should be monitored after initiation of simvastatin, and dose increases may be necessary.

Selective Serotonin Reuptake Inhibitors

Selective serotonin reuptake inhibitors (SSRIs), such as citalopram, escitalopram, fluoxetine, and sertraline, are commonly used medications in the treatment of depression and anxiety. Through unknown mechanisms, but likely accelerated levothyroxine metabolism, SSRIs may increase TSH levels when started by patients on levothyroxine replacement. Increases in the dose of levothyroxine may be required [55].

Tricyclic Antidepressants

Tricyclic antidepressants, such as amitriptyline, nortriptyline, and imipramine, are commonly used to treat diabetic peripheral neuropathy and other types of chronic pain. Coadministration of TCAs and levothyroxine may increase the therapeutic and toxic effects of both medications. The mechanism may involve increased receptor sensitivity to catecholamines. This may increase the risk of cardiac arrhythmias and central nervous system stimulation. In addition, the onset of action of the TCA may be accelerated. Patients should be monitored clinically for toxicity. Dose adjustments of one or both of the drugs may be necessary [55]. Table 7.2 shows the impact of medications on thyroid hormone function tests.

Table 7.2 Impact of medications on thyroid hormone function tests

Medication	Effect on thyroid function tests	Mechanism	Strategies
Furosemide	Increase FT4, FT3. Stable total T4, total T3, TSH.	Displacement of thyroid hormone from thyroid hormone-binding sites in vivo and in vitro.	Measure total thyroid hormone, TBG, and TSH instead of free thyroid hormone. If measuring free thyroid hormone, do so at least 6 h after furosemide dose.
Heparin	Lab artifact: increase FT4, FT3. Stable total T4, total T3, TSH.	Displacement of thyroid hormone from thyroid hormone-binding sites in vitro.	Measure total thyroid hormone, TBG, TSH. If measuring free thyroid hormone, do so at least 10 h after heparin dose.
Aspirin	Decrease total T4, total T3, FT3, TSH. Stable FT4.	Displacement of thyroid hormone from thyroid hormone-binding sites in vitro and in vivo. This, in turn, suppresses TSH, resulting in reduction of thyroid hormone secretion.	Assays that dilute the aspirin concentration will cause less thyroid hormone displacement (less FT4 elevation) in vitro than in vivo. Direct ultrafiltration may be more accurate in measuring free thyroid hormone concentration because it does not dilute the concentration of aspirin.
Phosphate binders Calcium-containing (calcium carbonate, calcium acetate) Noncalcium-containing (sevelamer, lanthanum)	Decrease free and total thyroid hormone. Increase TSH.	Impairs absorption of levothyroxine.	Separate administration of levothyroxine and calcium, lanthanum, and sevelamer by at least 4, 2, and several hours, respectively.
Other: proton pump inhibitor, ferrous sulfate, fiber supplements	Decrease free and total thyroid hormone. Increase TSH.	Impairs absorption of levothyroxine.	Separate administration of levothyroxine and iron salts and fiber by at least 4 h. With PPI use, monitor thyroid hormone levels. May require increased dose of levothyroxine Consider switching to oral solution formula of levothyroxine.
Simvastatin	May increase TSH.	Possibly accelerated catabolism of levothyroxine from excess formation of CYP3A4 by simvastatin.	May require increased dose of levothyroxine.
Selective serotonin reuptake inhibitors	May decrease free and total thyroid hormone. Increase TSH.	Unknown.	May require increased dose of levothyroxine.
Tricyclic antidepressants	No change.	Increased therapeutic and toxic effects of both levothyroxine and tetracyclic antidepressant, possibly due to increased receptor sensitivity to catecholamines.	Monitor clinically and consider adjusting the timing or dosage of one or both of the drugs.

References

1. Rhee CM. The interaction between thyroid and kidney disease: an overview of the evidence. Curr Opin Endocrinol Diabetes Obes. 2016;23(5):407–15.
2. Brent GA. Thyroid function testing. New York: Springer; 2010. Available from: SpringerLink. Restricted to UC campuses https://doi.org/10.1007/978-1-4419-1485-9.
3. Hershman JM. Regulation of thyroid hormone production and measurement of thyrotropin. In: Brent GA, editor. Thyroid function testing. New York: Springer; 2010. p. 79–90.
4. Spencer CA. Assay of thyroid hormones and related substances. South Dartmouth: MDText.com, Inc. Updated Jan 2013.
5. Spencer CA, LoPresti JS, Patel A, Guttler RB, Eigen A, Shen D, et al. Applications of a new chemiluminometric thyrotropin assay to subnormal measurement. J Clin Endocrinol Metab. 1990;70(2):453–60.
6. Kaptein EM. Thyroid hormone metabolism and thyroid diseases in chronic renal failure. Endocr Rev. 1996;17(1):45–63.
7. Beckers C, Machiels J, Soyez C, Cornette C. Metabolic clearance rate and production rate of thyroid-stimulating hormone in man. Horm Metab Res. 1971;3(1):34–6.
8. Kaptein EM, Quion-Verde H, Chooljian CJ, Tang WW, Friedman PE, Rodriquez HJ, et al. The thyroid in end-stage renal disease. Medicine (Baltimore). 1988;67(3):187–97.
9. Lo JC, Chertow GM, Go AS, Hsu CY. Increased prevalence of subclinical and clinical hypothyroidism in persons with chronic kidney disease. Kidney Int. 2005;67(3):1047–52.
10. Asvold BO, Bjøro T, Vatten LJ. Association of thyroid function with estimated glomerular filtration rate in a population-based study: the HUNT study. Eur J Endocrinol. 2011;164(1):101–5.
11. Woodward A, McCann S, Al-Jubouri M. The relationship between estimated glomerular filtration rate and thyroid function: an observational study. Ann Clin Biochem. 2008;45(Pt 5):515–7.
12. Chaker L, Sedaghat S, Hoorn EJ, Elzen WP, Gussekloo J, Hofman A, et al. The association of thyroid function and the risk of kidney function decline: a population-based cohort study. Eur J Endocrinol. 2016;175(6):653–60.
13. Zhang Y, Chang Y, Ryu S, Cho J, Lee WY, Rhee EJ, et al. Thyroid hormone levels and incident chronic kidney disease in euthyroid individuals: the Kangbuk Samsung Health Study. Int J Epidemiol. 2014;43(5):1624–32.
14. Koulouri O, Moran C, Halsall D, Chatterjee K, Gurnell M. Pitfalls in the measurement and interpretation of thyroid function tests. Best Pract Res Clin Endocrinol Metab. 2013;27(6):745–62.
15. Kaptein EM, LoPresti JS, Kaptein MJ. Is an isolated TSH elevation in chronic nonthyroidal illness "subclinical hypothyroidism". J Clin Endocrinol Metab. 2014;99(11):4015–26.
16. Paudel K. Prevalence and clinical characteristics of hypothyroidism in a population undergoing maintenance hemodialysis. J Clin Diagn Res. 2014;8(4):MC01–4.
17. Kalk WJ, Morley JE, Gold CH, Meyers A. Thyroid function tests in patients on regular hemodialysis. Nephron. 1980;25(4):173–8.
18. Hardy MJ, Ragbeer SS, Nascimento L. Pituitary-thyroid function in chronic renal failure assessed by a highly sensitive thyrotropin assay. J Clin Endocrinol Metab. 1988;66(1):233–6.
19. Du X, Pan B, Li W, Zou Y, Hua X, Huang W, et al. Albuminuria is an independent risk factor of T4 elevation in chronic kidney disease. Sci Rep. 2017;7:41302.
20. Klee G. Laboratory techniques for recognition of endocrine disorders. In: Melmed S, Polonsky K, Larson PR, Kronenberg HM, editors. Williams textbook of endocrinology. 13th ed. Philadelphia: Elsevier; 2015. p. 83–99.
21. Midgley JE. Direct and indirect free thyroxine assay methods: theory and practice. Clin Chem. 2001;47(8):1353–63.
22. Iitaka M, Kawasaki S, Sakurai S, Hara Y, Kuriyama R, Yamanaka K, et al. Serum substances that interfere with thyroid hormone assays in patients with chronic renal failure. Clin Endocrinol. 1998;48(6):739–46.
23. d'Herbomez M, Forzy G, Gasser F, Massart C, Beaudonnet A, Sapin R. Clinical evaluation of nine free thyroxine assays: persistent problems in particular populations. Clin Chem Lab Med. 2003;41(7):942–7.
24. Nishikawa M, Ogawa Y, Yoshikawa N, Yoshimura M, Toyoda N, Shouzu A, et al. Plasma free thyroxine (FT4) concentrations during hemodialysis in patients with chronic renal failure: effects of plasma non-esterified fatty acids on FT4 measurement. Endocr J. 1996;43(5):487–93.
25. Wiederkehr MR, Kalogiros J, Krapf R. Correction of metabolic acidosis improves thyroid and growth hormone axes in haemodialysis patients. Nephrol Dial Transplant. 2004;19(5):1190–7.
26. Stevenson HP, Archbold GP, Johnston P, Young IS, Sheridan B. Misleading serum free thyroxine results during low molecular weight heparin treatment. Clin Chem. 1998;44(5):1002–7.
27. Kulkarni DP, Holley JL. Thyroid function tests in end-stage renal disease. Semin Dial. 2014;27(6):552–5.
28. Fan J, Yan P, Wang Y, Shen B, Ding F, Liu Y. Prevalence and clinical significance of low T3 syndrome in non-dialysis patients with chronic kidney disease. Med Sci Monit. 2016;22:1171–9.
29. Song SH, Kwak IS, Lee DW, Kang YH, Seong EY, Park JS. The prevalence of low triiodothyronine according to the stage of chronic kidney disease in subjects with a normal thyroid-stimulating hormone. Nephrol Dial Transplant. 2009;24(5):1534–8.
30. Malyszko J, Malyszko JS, Pawlak K, Mysliwiec M. Thyroid function, endothelium, and inflammation

in hemodialyzed patients: possible relations? J Ren Nutr. 2007;17(1):30–7.
31. Iglesias P, Díez JJ. Thyroid dysfunction and kidney disease. Eur J Endocrinol. 2009;160(4):503–15.
32. Horáček J, Dusilová Sulková S, Kubišová M, Safránek R, Malířová E, Kalousová M, et al. Thyroid hormone abnormalities in hemodialyzed patients: low triiodothyronine as well as high reverse triiodothyronine are associated with increased mortality. Physiol Res. 2012;61(5):495–501.
33. Melmed S, Polonsky KS, Larsen PR, Kronenberg H. Williams textbook of endocrinology. 13th ed. Philadelphia: Elsevier; 2016. Print
34. Kraiem Z, Lahat N, Glaser B, Baron E, Sadeh O, Sheinfeld M. Thyrotrophin receptor blocking antibodies: incidence, characterization and in-vitro synthesis. Clin Endocrinol. 1987;27:409–21.
35. Barbesino G, Tomer Y. Clinical utility of TSH receptor antibodies. J Clin Endocrinol Metab. 2013;98:2247–55.
36. Tozolli R, Bagnasco M, Giavarina D, Bizzaro N. TSH receptor autoantibody immunoassay in patients with Graves' disease: improvement of diagnostic accuracy over different generations of methods. Systematic review and meta-analysis. Autoimmun Rev. 2012;12:107–13.
37. Lukinac L, Kusic Z, Kes P. False-positive titers of thyroid autoantibodies in patients undergoing hemodialysis? Clin Chem. 1991;37:2153–4.
38. Targher G, Chonchol M, Zoppini G, Salvagno G, Pichiri I, Franchini M, Lippi G. Prevalence of thyroid autoimmunity and subclinical hypothyroidism in persons with chronic kidney disease not requiring chronic dialysis. Clin Chem Lab Med. 2009;47: 1367–71.
39. Christofides ND. Furosemide interference in newer free thyroxine assays. Clin Chem. 1999;45:1315.
40. Jaume JC, Mendel CM, Frost PH, Greenspan FS, Laughton CW. Extremely low doses of heparin release lipase activity into the plasma and can thereby cause artifactual elevations in the serum-free thyroxine concentration as measured by equilibrium. Thyroid. 1996;6:79–83.
41. Samuels MH, Pillote K, Asher D, Nelson JC. Variable effects of nonsteroidal anti-inflammatory agents on thyroid test results. J Clin Endocrinol Metab. 2003;88:5710–6.
42. Pabla D, Akhlaghi F, Zia H. A comparative pH-dissolution profile study of selected commercial levothyroxine products using induc- tively coupled plasma mass spectrometry. Eur J Pharm Biopharm. 2009;72:105–10.
43. Liwanpo L, Hershman JM. Conditions and drugs interfering with thyroxine absorption. Best Pract Res Clin Endocrinol Metab. 2009;23:781–92.
44. Diskin CJ, Stokes TJ, Dansby LM, et al. Effect of phosphate binders upon TSH and L-thyroxine dose in patients on thyroid replacement. Int Urol Nephrol. 2007;39:599–602.
45. Singh N, Singh PN, Hershman JM. Effect of calcium carbonate on the absorption of levothyroxine. JAMA. 2000;283:2822.
46. Sachmechi I, Reich DM, Aninyei M, Wibowo F, Gupta G, Kim PJ. Effect of proton pump inhibitors on serum thyroid-stimulating hormone level in euthyroid patients treated with levothyroxine for hypothyroidism. Endocr Pract. 2007;13:345–9.
47. Centanni M, Gargano L, Canettieri G, et al. Thyroxine in goiter, helicobacter pylori infection, and chronic gastritis. N Engl J Med. 2006;354:1787.
48. Dietrich JW, Gieselbrecht K, Holl RW, Boehm BO. Absorption kinetics of levothyroxine is not altered by proton-pump inhibitor therapy. Horm Metab Res. 2006;38:57–9.
49. Ananthakrishnan S, Braverman LE, Levin RM, Magnani B, Pearce EN. The effect of famotidine, esomeprazole, and ezetimibe on levothyroxine absorption. Thyroid. 2008;18:493–8.
50. Vita R, Saraceno G, Trimarchi F, Benvenga S. Switching levothyroxine from the tablet to the oral solution formulation corrects the impaired absorption of levothyroxine induced by proton-pump inhibitors. J Clin Endocrinol Metab. 2014;99:4481–6.
51. Campbell RC, Hasinoff BB, Stalts H, Rao B, Wong NC. Ferrous sulfate reduces thyroxine efficacy in patients with hypothyroidism. Ann Intern Med. 1992;117:1010–3.
52. Liel Y, Harman-Boehm I, Shany S. Evidence for a clinically important adverse effect of fiber-enriched diet on the bioavailability of levothyroxine in adult hypothyroid patients. J Clin Endocrinol Metab. 1996;81:857–9.
53. Kisch E, Segall HS. Interaction between simvastatin and L-thyroxine. Ann Intern Med. 2005;143:547.
54. Kiernan TJ. Simvastatin induced rhabdomyolysis and an important clinical link with hypothyroidism. Int J Cardiol. 2007;119(3):374–6.
55. Product Information: Synthroid(R) oral tablets, levothyroxine sodium oral tablets. Abbott Laboratories (per DailyMed), North Chicago, IL, June 2011.

8 Thyroid Status and Outcomes in Kidney Disease

Connie M. Rhee, Gregory A. Brent, and Kamyar Kalantar-Zadeh

Introduction

Thyroid dysfunction is a common yet under-recognized complication among chronic kidney disease (CKD) patients, including those with end-stage renal disease (ESRD) receiving treatment with dialysis [1, 2]. While comparatively greater focus has been placed upon other endocrine derangements in kidney disease, such as diabetes and secondary hyperparathyroidism, population-based studies have shown that advanced CKD and ESRD patients have a higher prevalence of hypothyroidism compared to the general population [3–10]. Despite this disproportionate burden, hypothyroidism may be frequently overlooked in dialysis patients, possibly due to overlap of its accompanying signs and symptoms with those of uremia (e.g., fatigue, depression, impaired cognition, impaired physical function), as well as attribution of thyroid function test changes to underlying illness rather than primary thyroid disease [1, 2].

In this chapter, we aim to review epidemiologic data on thyroid dysfunction in the CKD and ESRD populations, as well as recent studies examining the association of thyroid status and CKD-related outcomes, including incident CKD and CKD progression, mortality, and patient-centered outcomes such as health-related quality of life (HRQOL).

Definitions and Epidemiology

Primary hypothyroidism is typically identified by biochemical tests, which include an elevated serum thyrotropin (TSH) level in conjunction with a low or normal thyroxine (T4) level indicating overt (moderate-to-severe) or subclinical (mild) hypothyroidism, respectively [11]. Using these criteria, landmark data from the Third National Health and Nutrition Examination Survey (NHANES III) have shown that ~ten

C. M. Rhee (✉)
Division of Nephrology and Hypertension, Departments of Medicine and Public Health, University of California Irvine School of Medicine, Orange, CA, USA
e-mail: crhee1@uci.edu

G. A. Brent
Division of Endocrinology, Diabetes, and Hypertension, Departments of Medicine and Physiology, David Geffen School of Medicine at UCLA, Los Angeles, CA, USA

K. Kalantar-Zadeh
Division of Nephrology and Hypertension, Departments of Medicine, Pediatrics, Public Health, and Nursing Sciences, University of California Irvine School of Medicine, Orange, CA, USA

C. M. Rhee et al. (eds.), *Endocrine Disorders in Kidney Disease*,
https://doi.org/10.1007/978-3-319-97765-2_8

million adults in the United States are affected by this condition [12], and various cohorts suggest that 4–10% and 0.1–2% of the US population have subclinical and overt hypothyroidism, respectively [11].

Epidemiologic studies have shown a substantially higher prevalence of hypothyroidism in CKD. For example, in a study of 14,623 NHANES III participants stratified by kidney function, an increasingly higher prevalence of hypothyroidism was observed with incrementally impaired eGFR, such that those with moderate-to-advanced kidney dysfunction had a nearly five-fold higher prevalence compared to those with normal kidney function: 5, 11, 20, 23, and 23% among those who had estimated glomerular filtration rates (eGFRs) of ≥90, 60–89, 45–59, 30–44, and <30 ml/min/1.73m^2, respectively [4]. After accounting for differences in sociodemographic characteristics (i.e., age, sex, race/ethnicity), participants in the lower eGFR categories persisted in having a two-fold higher risk of hypothyroidism compared to those with normal eGFR, with approximately half of cases due to subclinical disease. In a large population-based study of 461,607 US Veterans with stage 3–5 CKD, it was also shown that each 10 ml/min/1.73m^2 decrement in eGFR was associated with an 18% higher risk of hypothyroidism independent of patients' case-mix characteristics [6]. Studies of thyroid status in the ESRD population have been conducted in comparatively smaller-sized cohorts, yet have shown a similarly high prevalence of hypothyroidism ranging from ~13 to 23% of hemodialysis and peritoneal dialysis patients [3, 5, 7–9, 13].

Potential Links Between Thyroid and Kidney Disease

While the mechanistic link between thyroid and kidney disease has not been fully elucidated, basic and clinical studies suggest that the relationship may be bi-directional (Fig. 8.1) [1, 2].

Thyroid Dysfunction as a Risk Factor for Kidney Disease

In animal models, hypothyroidism has been shown to adversely impact kidney size and structure in both development and adulthood. In neonatal rats, low serum thyroxine results in (1) reduced kidney-to-body weight ratio [14, 15], (2) truncated tubular mass [14, 16, 17], and (3) glomerular basement membrane (GBM) changes that include reduced volume and area,

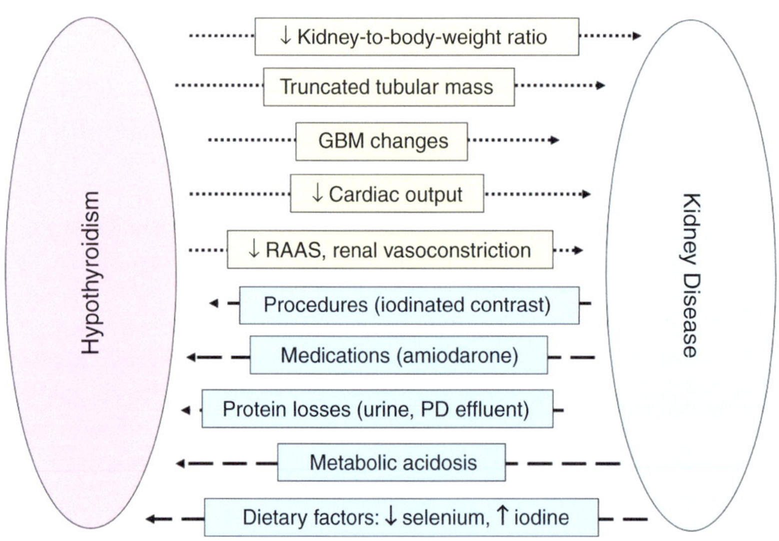

Fig. 8.1 Proposed bi-directional links between hypothyroidism and kidney disease (Abbreviations: GBM glomerular basement membrane, RAAS renin-angiotensin-aldosterone system, PD peritoneal dialysis)

GBM thickening, mesangial matrix expansion, and increased glomerular capillary permeability [18–20].

Thyroid Dysfunction as a Risk Factor for Kidney Dysfunction

Hypothyroidism may be a risk factor for kidney dysfunction via several potential mechanisms, including (1) decreased cardiac output due to systolic and diastolic dysfunction, reduced inotropy and chronotropy, and blood volume [21, 22], (2) intrarenal vasoconstriction resulting from decreased vasodilator synthesis and activity [22, 23], and (3) altered chloride channel expression leading to increased distal tubular chloride delivery and tubuloglomerular feedback [24]. In animal studies, hypothyroidism has resulted in decreased single nephron GFR, renal plasma flow, and glomerular transcapillary hydrostatic pressure [25, 26]. Human case series have also shown that hypothyroidism results in reversible serum creatinine elevations, as well as reduced renal plasma flow and eGFR as measured by creatinine-based estimating equations and gold-standard isotopic scans [22, 23, 27–29].

Many large population-based studies have corroborated a cross-sectional link between hypothyroidism and kidney dysfunction [4, 6, 30–35]. However, there have been few longitudinal studies of thyroid status and kidney function, and those reported have shown mixed findings. In a study of 104,633 participants in the Kangbuk Samsung Health Study with normal baseline kidney function who underwent annual to biennial TSH measurements, it was shown that those in the highest TSH quintile (2.85–5.00 mIU/L) had a 26% higher risk of developing incident CKD (defined as an eGFR <60 ml/min/1.73m^2) compared to those in the lowest TSH quintile (0.25–1.18 mIU/L) [36]. When TSH was examined as a continuous variable using restricted cubic spline analyses, a higher TSH was associated with a progressively higher risk of developing CKD up to a TSH threshold of ~3.0 mIU/L above which risk plateaued. However, in an investigation of 558 "oldest-old" (85-year-old) participants from the Leiden 85-Plus Study, while cross-sectional analyses showed that participants with overt and subclinical hypothyroidism had lower mean eGFRs, an association between baseline thyroid status and change in kidney function over time was not observed [33]. Yet in a longitudinal analysis of 309 participants with stage 2–4 CKD and subclinical hypothyroidism among whom 58% vs. 42% did vs. did not receive exogenous thyroid hormone supplementation at baseline, after a mean follow-up of 3 years, those who were treated had a slower decline in kidney function over time vs. those who were untreated (eGFR decline of −2 vs. −6 ml/min/1.73m^2 per year, respectively) [37]. Those in the treated group were also less likely to experience a 50% decline in eGFR or incident ESRD: HRs (95% CIs) 0.64 (0.19–00.67) and 0.85 (0.03–0.71), respectively.

Kidney Disease as a Risk Factor for Thyroid Dysfunction

It has also been suggested that CKD and its associated complications may lead to thyroid dysfunction, although further study elucidating these pathways is needed (Fig. 8.1). For example, alterations in measurements of serum TSH, triiodothyronine (T3), and T4 have been observed in metabolic acidosis, with some of the changes reversed by oral sodium citrate therapy [38]. Trace element deficiencies (e.g., selenium, zinc) are frequently observed in hemodialysis patients, and in the general population, selenium deficiency is thought to be a trigger for autoimmune thyroid disease. In addition, selenium is required for thyroid hormone metabolism [39, 40]. With respect to other dietary factors, case series have shown the excess dietary iodine consumption may also lead to thyroid dysfunction in dialysis patients, presumably due to impaired renal clearance and retention of iodine leading to hypothyroidism via the Wolff-Chaikoff effect [41, 42]. Furthermore, hemodialysis and peritoneal dialysis patients may frequently be exposed to iodine-containing agents such as iodine contrast media (i.e., in the form of contrast-enhanced CT scans, cardiac catheterizations, peripheral angiograms, fistulograms) or povidone-iodine cleansing agents that may result in iodine-induced hypothyroidism or thyrotoxicosis (via the Jod-Basedow phenomenon) [43–46]. Medications commonly administered to CKD and ESRD patients due to coexisting comorbidities (i.e., amiodarone for atrial fibrillation) may also contribute to thyroid dysfunction. Given that the vast majority of thyroid hormone is protein-bound [47], heavy protein losses in nephrotic syndrome and via the peritoneal effluent may lead to total body thyroid hormone depletion [48, 49]. Finally, non-thyroidal illness and malnutrition may contribute to some of the thyroid functional test abnormalities (i.e., low T3 levels) observed in advanced CKD and ESRD patients [50].

Thyroid Dysfunction and Outcomes

General Population: Cardiovascular Disease and Mortality

In the general population, hypothyroidism has been associated with a number of adverse cardiovascular outcomes, which include (1) systolic and diastolic dysfunction [21]; (2) endothelial dysfunction and diastolic hypertension [24, 51–53], which in conjunction with (3) dyslipidemia [51] may lead to (4) accelerated atherosclerosis [21, 54]; and (5) alterations in cardiac ion channel expression [21], which may potentially lead to prolongation of the electrophysiologic QT intervals and heightened risk of malignant arrhythmias. Emerging data suggest that thyroid hormone deficiency may lead to cardiovascular risk factors that may be particularly relevant to CKD and ESRD patients, such as (6) downregulation of matrix Gla protein and Klotho (i.e., vascular calcification inhibitors) thereby predisposing to vascular calcification [55–57]; (7) reduced erythropoietin production, iron and B12 deficiency, and blood loss from impaired hemostasis leading to anemia and erythropoietin-stimulating agent resistance [58–62]; and (8) increased platelet size and activation [63–66].

General population studies examining hard outcomes (i.e., cardiovascular events, mortality) have largely focused upon subclinical hypothyroidism, which have shown mixed findings. However, in a meta-analysis of 55,287 participants across 11 prospective cohorts from the United States, Europe, South America, Asia, and Australia conducted by the Thyroid Studies Collaboration, patients with subclinical hypothyroidism with TSH levels >10 mIU/L and >7 mIU/L had a higher risk of coronary heart disease (CHD) events and CHD death, respectively [67]. In a subsequent pooled analysis of 25,390 participants across six prospective cohorts in the United States and Europe, those with subclinical hypothyroidism and a TSH level >10 mIU/L as well as those with subclinical hyperthyroidism with a TSH level <0.1 mIU/L each had a higher risk of congestive heart failure events [68].

It has also been suggested that the impact of hypothyroidism upon cardiovascular disease and mortality may depend upon one's underlying risk, as there has been a tendency toward positive associations in studies of populations with high cardiovascular risk but not in lower-risk groups [1, 2]. Indeed, in a study of 14,879 NHANES III participants, it was shown that both hypothyroidism overall and subclinical hypothyroidism were each independently associated with higher mortality risk in those with heart failure, whereas significant associations were not observed in those without heart failure [69]. Similarly, in a study of 52,856 patients from a large university-based tertiary care center, hypothyroidism was associated with higher risk of hospitalization in those with congestive heart failure but not in those without heart failure [70]. These findings may have particular relevance among advanced CKD and ESRD patients given their high prevalence of structural heart disease [71].

Kidney Disease Population: Cardiovascular Disease and Mortality

Early investigations of hypothyroidism in kidney disease proposed that thyroid hormone deficiency may be a physiologic adaptation and/or a means to reduce metabolism in kidney disease patients who are prone to hypercatabolism, malnutrition, and dialytic protein and amino acid losses [72]. However, more recent data have suggested that thyroid hormone deficiency may be a novel risk factor for the high burden of cardiovascular disease and mortality (i.e., ~40% of deaths [71]) observed in the advanced CKD and ESRD population which are not wholly explained by traditional risk factors.

Thyroid Status Defined by Serum Triiodothyronine and Thyroxine Levels

There has been an increasing body of evidence suggesting that low T3 and T4 levels are associated with adverse cardiovascular outcomes in CKD and ESRD patients, such as decreased systolic function, endothelial dysfunction, atherosclerosis, vascular calcification, and altered ventricular conduction (Table 8.1) [56, 73–77]. A number of CKD and ESRD studies have also shown that low T3 and T4 levels are associated with higher mortality risk (Table 8.1) [56, 78–87]. In one study of 210 hemodialysis patients who underwent repeated examination of T3 and T4 levels at baseline and 3 months follow-up, it was found that those with persistently low T3 and T4 levels (defined as <66th percentile) had a three- to fourfold higher all-cause and cardiovascular death risk compared to those with persistently high levels in analyses adjusted for sociodemographic characteristics, comorbidities, and proxies of nutritional and inflammatory status [85].

However, there are limitations with respect to using T3 and T4 levels to ascertain thyroid status in studies of CKD and ESRD patients. Approximately 80% of T3 is derived from the peripheral deiodination of T4 to T3, and this process is highly sensitive to non-thyroidal illness, malnutrition, inflammation, elevated cortisol levels, and a number of medications that are commonly used in these populations [1, 2, 50, 88, 89]. In addition, given that the vast majority of T4 is protein-bound, routinely used free T4 assays that indirectly measure the minute fraction of bioavailable-free T4 are hormone-protein-binding dependent and may lead to spurious results in the presence of uremic toxins, non-thyroidal illness, and certain medications (e.g., heparin, furosemide) [47]. In contrast, serum TSH is considered to be the most sensitive and specific single biochemical metric of thyroid function, owing to its negative logarithmic association with T3 and T4 levels (i.e., small changes in T3 and T4 result in exponential changes in TSH) [11]. Although some TSH alterations have been described in kidney disease (e.g., altered clearance, blunted response to thyrotropin-releasing hormone, decreased pulsatility, increased half-life, impaired glycosylation and function [90, 91]), it is still considered a more accurate measure of thyroid status vs. T3/T4 in non-thyroidal illness.

Thyroid Status Defined by Serum Thyrotropin Levels

Given its robust characteristics, serum TSH has been increasingly used to define thyroid status in studies examining hypo- and hyperthyroidism and outcomes in the ESRD population (Table 8.2). In one of the first studies conducted to date, among 2715 dialysis patients who underwent one or more serum TSH measurements within two tertiary care centers in Boston, ~13% had hypothyroidism at baseline [5]. Compared to patients who were euthyroid, hypothyroid patients had a 35% higher risk of mortality independent of sociodemographics and comorbidity burden (e.g., diabetes status and non-cardiovascular hospitalization within the past year). Yet in a subsequent study of 1000 diabetic hemodialysis patients from the *Die Deutsche Diabetes Dialyse* (4D Trial), baseline subclinical hypothyroidism examined separately or in conjunction with overt hypothyroidism was not associated with sudden cardiac death, cardiovascular events, or all-cause death [93]. However, it bears mention that only 1.8% ($N = 18$) of the study population had hypothyroidism which may have resulted in underpowered analyses. Notably, subclinical hyperthyroidism was associated with a higher risk of short-term (i.e., 1 year) sudden cardiac death.

As interpretation of the aforementioned studies may be limited by their focus on thyroid status measured at a single-point-in-time (i.e., baseline thyroid status only), a series of studies have sought to define hypo- and hyperthyroidism using repeated measures of serum TSH over time. First, in a study of 8840 incident hemodialysis patients from a large US dialysis organization,

Table 8.1 Studies of thyroid status defined by serum triiodothyronine (T3) and thyroxine (T4) levels and outcomes in the non-dialysis-dependent chronic kidney disease (NDD-CKD) and end-stage renal disease (ESRD) populations

Study (year)	Study population (N)	Thyroid test	Outcome
Cardiovascular outcomes			
Jaroszynski et al. (2005) [73]	Hemodialysis patients (52)	↓ FT3	Delayed ventricular depolarization
Zoccali et al. (2006) [74]	Hemodialysis and peritoneal dialysis patients (234)	↓ FT3	↓ Left ventricular systolic function ↑ Left ventricular mass Estimates attenuated to the null after adjusting for inflammatory and nutritional markers
Tatar et al. (2011) [75]	Peritoneal dialysis patients (57)	↓ FT3	↑ Arterial stiffness
Tatar et al. (2011) [76]	Hemodialysis patients (137)	↓ FT3	↑ Carotid artery atherosclerosis and arterial stiffness among nondiabetic patients only
Yilmaz et al. (2011) [77]	Nondiabetic stage 3 to 4 NDD-CKD patients	↓ FT3	↓ Flow-mediated vasodilation
Meuwese et al. (2013) [56]	Peritoneal dialysis patients (84)	↓ FT3	↑ Vascular calcification
Meuwese et al. (2015) [57]	ESRD patients eligible for living donor transplantation (94)	↓ FT3 and FT4	↓ FT3 associated with ↑ coronary calcification and arterial stiffness ↓ FT4 associated with ↑ coronary calcification only
Mortality			
Zoccali et al. (2006) [78]	Hemodialysis patients (200)	↓ FT3	↑ All-cause mortality
Enia et al. (2007) [79]	Peritoneal dialysis patients (41)	↓ FT3	↑ All-cause mortality
Carrero et al. (2007) [80]	Dialysis patients (187)	↓ TT3 and ↓ FT3	↓ TT3 associated with ↑ all-cause and cardiovascular mortality No association between ↓ FT3 with mortality
Fernandez-Reyes et al. (2010) [81]	Hemodialysis patients (89)	↓ FT3	No association with all-cause mortality
Ozen et al. (2011) [82]	Hemodialysis patients (669)	↓ FT3	↑ All-cause mortality Estimates attenuated to the null after adjusting for inflammatory and nutritional markers
Horacek et al. (2012) [83]	Hemodialysis patients (167)	↓ TT3	↑ All-cause mortality
Lin et al. (2012) [84]	Peritoneal dialysis patients (46)	↓ TT3 and ↓ TT4	↓ TT3 and ↓ TT4 each associated with ↑ all-cause mortality
Meuwese et al. (2012) [85]	Hemodialysis patients (210)	↓ TT3 and ↓ TT4	Baseline and persistently ↓ TT3 and ↓ TT4 each associated with ↑ all-cause mortality
Yang et al. (2012) [86]	Proteinuric NDD-CKD patients (211)	↓ T3	↑ All-cause and cardiovascular mortality
Meuwese et al. (2013) [56]	Peritoneal dialysis patients (84)	↓ FT3	↑ All-cause mortality
Chang et al. (2015) [87]	Peritoneal dialysis patients (447)	↓ FT3	↑ All-cause, combined cardiovascular, and sudden cardiac death

Abbreviations: *FT3* free triiodothyronine, *TT3* total triiodothyronine, *TT4* total thyroxine, *NDD-CKD* non-dialysis dependent chronic kidney disease

Table 8.2 Studies of thyroid status defined by serum thyrotropin (TSH) levels and outcomes in the chronic kidney disease (CKD) and end-stage renal disease (ESRD) populations

Study (year)	Study population (N)	Thyroid test	Outcome
Cardiovascular outcomes			
Kang et al. (2008) [92]	Peritoneal dialysis patients (51)	↑ TSH and subclinical hypothyroidism (defined as ↑ TSH + normal FT4)	↑ TSH and subclinical hypothyroidism each associated with decreased left ventricular function
Meuwese et al. (2015) [57]	ESRD patients eligible for living donor transplantation (94)	↓ TSH	↓ TSH associated with ↑ coronary calcification
Rhee et al. (2018) [55]	Hemodialysis patients (104)	↑ TSH	↑ Coronary artery calcification
Mortality			
Rhee et al. (2013) [5]	Peritoneal dialysis and hemodialysis patients (2715)	↑ TSH	↑ All-cause mortality
Dreschler et al. (2014) [93]	Diabetic hemodialysis patients (1000)	Subclinical hypothyroidism (defined as ↑ TSH + normal FT4) Subclinical hyperthyroidism (defined as ↓ TSH + normal FT4)	Subclinical hypothyroidism not associated with all-cause mortality, cardiovascular events, or sudden cardiac death Subclinical hyperthyroidism associated with short-term (1 year) sudden cardiac death
Rhee et al. (2015) [7]	Hemodialysis patients (8840)	↑ TSH	↑ All-cause mortality
Rhee et al. (2015) [8]	Peritoneal dialysis patients (1484)	↑ TSH and ↓ TSH	↑ All-cause mortality
Rhee et al. (2017) [9]	Prospective hemodialysis patient cohort (541)	↑ TSH	↑ All-cause mortality
Rhee et al. (2018) [94]	Stage 3 NDD-CKD patients (227,426)	↑ TSH and ↓ TSH	↑ All-cause mortality
Rhee et al. (2018) [95]	Advanced NDD-CKD patients transitioning to ESRD (15,335)	↑ TSH	↑ All-cause mortality
Patient-centered outcomes			
Rhee et al. (2017) [96]	Prospective hemodialysis patient cohort (450)	↑ TSH	↓ HRQOL subscale scores: Role limitations due to physical health Physical function Energy/fatigue Pain

Abbreviations: *TSH* thyrotropin, *FT4* free thyroxine, *HRQOL* health-related quality of life, *ESRD* end-stage renal disease, *NDD-CKD* non-dialysis dependent chronic kidney disease

the association of thyroid status with mortality was examined using baseline and time-dependent TSH levels (i.e., repeated measures of TSH) to approximate long-term and short-term exposure—mortality associations, respectively [7]. In baseline and time-dependent analyses, it was found that hypothyroidism was associated with a 47% and 62% higher mortality risk, respectively, independent of case-mix covariates. Upon examining finer gradations of TSH, higher TSH levels even in the normal range (TSH >3 mIU/L) were associated with a 37% and 42% higher mortality risk in baseline and time-dependent analyses, respectively. Similarly, among a cohort of 1484 national peritoneal dialysis patients from a large dialysis organization, time-dependent analyses adjusted for case-mix covariates showed that both hypo- and hyperthyroidism were each associated with higher death risk [8]. As the indications for thyroid functional testing in these clinical datasets are not known, an ongoing study of prospective hemodialysis patients (*Hypothyroidism,*

Cardiovascular Disease, and Survival in Kidney Disease [HyCARDS] Study) has sought to define thyroid status using protocolized TSH measurements every 6 months [9]. In an interim analysis of 514 HyCARDS participants recruited across 17 outpatient dialysis units in Southern California, it was found that 11% had hypothyroidism at baseline. In time-dependent analyses, it was found that hemodialysis patients with TSH levels in the highest tertile (TSH >2.11 mIU/L) had a 2.5-fold higher death risk independent of case-mix characteristics (reference: lowest TSH tertile).

Recent data in the non-dialysis-dependent CKD (NDD-CKD) population have shown a similar pattern of findings (Table 8.2). In the largest study of thyroid status and mortality conducted to date, among 227,426 US Veterans with stage 3 CKD, baseline and time-dependent analyses showed that both hypo- and hyperthyroidism were independently associated with higher mortality risk [94]. Upon examining thyroid status using finer gradations of TSH, it was again found that higher TSH levels even in the normal range (TSH >3.0 mIU/L) were associated with higher death risk. Most recently, an analysis of the relationship between pre-ESRD thyroid status with post-ESRD outcomes was conducted to determine the long-term "legacy effect" of thyroid status [95]. Among 15,335 US Veterans with advanced NDD-CKD transitioning to ESRD, it was similarly found that higher pre-ESRD hypothyroid-range TSH levels (i.e., TSH >5.0 mIU/L) were associated with higher post-ESRD mortality risk.

Kidney Disease Population: Health-Related Quality of Life

Thyroid Status Defined by Serum Triiodothyronine and Thyroxine Levels

In the general population, thyroid dysfunction has been linked with reduced HRQOL [97]. Given that dialysis patients suffer from higher rates of impaired physical and mental health [98], there has been particular interest in thyroid dysfunction as a modifiable risk factor for adverse patient-centered outcomes (e.g., impaired HRQOL, decreased physical function). Indeed, in a recent prospective study of 450 patients from the HyCARDS cohort who underwent protocolized serum TSH measurements and Short Form 36 surveys every 6 months, when examined as a continuous variable it was found that higher baseline TSH levels were associated with lower HRQOL scores for the subscales of role limitations due to physical health, energy/fatigue, and pain [96]. Similarly, higher time-dependent TSH levels were associated with lower scores for role limitations due to physical health. When examined as a categorical variable, the highest baseline and time-dependent TSH tertiles were associated with lower HRQOL subscale scores for energy/fatigue and physical function, respectively. Further studies are needed to determine if thyroid-modulating therapy improves HRQOL and physical function among hemodialysis patients with thyroid dysfunction.

Treatment

Studying the impact of thyroid hormone replacement therapy may shed greater light into the causal implications of thyroid dysfunction in the CKD and ESRD populations. In fact, the US Renal Data System data show that levothyroxine is among the most commonly prescribed medications in NDD-CKD and ESRD patients who are Medicare Part D enrollees [99].

General Population

In the general population, small clinical trials have shown that exogenous thyroid hormone replacement improves adverse cardiovascular outcomes, including diastolic dysfunction, dyslipidemia, endothelial dysfunction, and atherosclerosis [100–103]. Large population-based studies examining the impact of treatment are comparatively sparse. However, in one study of 4735 patients with subclinical hypothyroidism identified from the UK General Practitioner Research Database, it was found that treatment with levothyroxine was associated with fewer ischemic heart disease events in younger individuals (i.e., 40–70 years of age; $N = 3093$), while this was not observed in older individuals (i.e., greater than 70 years of age; $N = 1642$) [104].

Kidney Disease Population

Studies examining the impact of exogenous thyroid hormone replacement among hypothyroid CKD and ESRD patients are also limited. However, in one study of 2715 dialysis patients in whom thyroid function and treatment status were ascertained at baseline, it was found that those who were euthyroid on medication (i.e., presumed to be hypothyroid treated-to-target) had similar mortality risk as those who were spontaneously euthyroid, whereas those who were hypothyroid irrespective of treatment status had higher mortality risk [5]. Similarly, in an analysis of 227,426 US Veterans with stage 3 NDD-CKD, compared to those who were spontaneously euthyroid, those who had untreated or undertreated hypothyroidism as well as untreated hyperthyroidism had higher mortality risk, whereas those who were hypothyroid treated-to-target had similar to slightly decreased mortality risk [94].

While these limited data highlight the benefits of treatment, levothyroxine is a medication with a narrow toxic-to-therapeutic window and may carry potential risk of (1) increased protein catabolism, (2) adverse cardiovascular events (e.g., atrial fibrillation, high output heart failure) among those with underlying cardiovascular disease, and (3) bone loss in postmenopausal women [1, 2, 105]. Hence, rigorous studies including clinical trials are needed to definitively determine the efficacy and safety of exogenous thyroid hormone replacement in the CKD and ESRD populations.

Future Directions and Conclusion

In summary, CKD and ESRD patients have a disproportionately higher prevalence of hypothyroidism, although many cases may remain latent and undiagnosed. While basic, clinical, and translational studies suggest a bi-directional association between thyroid and kidney disease, further studies are needed to determine the mechanistic links between these entities. A growing body of evidence suggests that hypo- and hyperthyroidism are associated with higher risk of mortality, as well as cardiovascular events and adverse patient-centered outcomes in the general and kidney disease populations. However, to better understand the causal implications of thyroid dysfunction in kidney disease, rigorous studies including randomized controlled trials are needed to determine the impact of exogenous thyroid hormone replacement, as well as optimal treatment targets, upon these CKD-related outcomes.

References

1. Rhee CM. The interaction between thyroid and kidney disease: an overview of the evidence. Curr Opin Endocrinol Diabetes Obes. 2016;23(5):407–15.
2. Rhee CM, Brent GA, Kovesdy CP, et al. Thyroid functional disease: an under-recognized cardiovascular risk factor in kidney disease patients. Nephrol Dial Transplant. 2015;30(5):724–37.
3. Kutlay S, Atli T, Koseogullari O, Nergizoglu G, Duman N, Gullu S. Thyroid disorders in hemodialysis patients in an iodine-deficient community. Artif Organs. 2005;29(4):329–32.
4. Lo JC, Chertow GM, Go AS, Hsu CY. Increased prevalence of subclinical and clinical hypothyroidism in persons with chronic kidney disease. Kidney Int. 2005;67(3):1047–52.
5. Rhee CM, Alexander EK, Bhan I, Brunelli SM. Hypothyroidism and mortality among dialysis patients. Clin J Am Soc Nephrol: CJASN. 2013;8(4):593–601.
6. Rhee CM, Kalantar-Zadeh K, Streja E, et al. The relationship between thyroid function and estimated glomerular filtration rate in patients with chronic kidney disease. Nephrol Dial Transplant. 2015;30(2):282–7.
7. Rhee CM, Kim S, Gillen DL, et al. Association of thyroid functional disease with mortality in a national cohort of incident hemodialysis patients. J Clin Endocrinol Metab. 2015;100(4):1386–95.
8. Rhee CM, Ravel VA, Streja E, et al. Thyroid functional disease and mortality in a national peritoneal dialysis cohort. J Clin Endocrinol Metab. 2016;101(11):4054–61.
9. Rhee CM, You AS, Nguyen DV, et al. Thyroid status and mortality in a prospective hemodialysis cohort. J Clin Endocrinol Metab. 2017;102(5):1568–77.

10. Shantha GP, Kumar AA, Bhise V, Khanna R, Sivagnanam K, Subramanian KK. Prevalence of subclinical hypothyroidism in patients with end-stage renal disease and the role of serum albumin: a cross-sectional study from South India. Cardiorenal Med. 2011;1(4):255–60.
11. Ladenson PW. Diagnosis of hypothyroidism. In: Braverman LE, Philadelphia CDS, editors. Werner and Ingbar's the thyroid. 10th ed. Philadelphia: Lippincott Williams and Wilkins; 2013. p. 606–11.
12. Hollowell JG, Staehling NW, Flanders WD, et al. Serum TSH, T(4), and thyroid antibodies in the United States population (1988 to 1994): National Health and Nutrition Examination Survey (NHANES III). J Clin Endocrinol Metab. 2002;87(2):489–99.
13. Lin CC, Chen TW, Ng YY, Chou YH, Yang WC. Thyroid dysfunction and nodular goiter in hemodialysis and peritoneal dialysis patients. Perit Dial Int. 1998;18(5):516–21.
14. Canavan JP, Holt J, Easton J, Smith K, Goldspink DF. Thyroid-induced changes in the growth of the liver, kidney, and diaphragm of neonatal rats. J Cell Physiol. 1994;161(1):49–54.
15. Slotkin TA, Seidler FJ, Kavlock RJ, Bartolome JV. Thyroid hormone differentially regulates cellular development in neonatal rat heart and kidney. Teratology. 1992;45(3):303–12.
16. Bentley AG, Madsen KM, Davis RG, Tisher CC. Response of the medullary thick ascending limb to hypothyroidism in the rat. Am J Pathol. 1985;120(2):215–21.
17. Salomon MI, Di Scala V, Grishman E, Brener J, Churg J. Renal lesions in hypothyroidism: a study based on kidney biopsies. Metab Clin Exp. 1967;16(9):846–52.
18. Bradley SE, Coelho JB, Sealey JE, Edwards KD, Stephan F. Changes in glomerulotubular dimensions, single nephron glomerular filtration rates and the renin-angiotensin system in hypothyroid rats. Life Sci. 1982;30(7–8):633–9.
19. Rodriguez-Gomez I, Banegas I, Wangensteen R, et al. Influence of thyroid state on cardiac and renal capillary density and glomerular morphology in rats. J Endocrinol. 2013;216(1):43–51.
20. Wheatley T, Edwards OM. Mild hypothyroidism and oedema: evidence for increased capillary permeability to protein. Clin Endocrinol. 1983;18(6):627–35.
21. Klein I, Ojamaa K. Thyroid hormone and the cardiovascular system. N Engl J Med. 2001;344(7):501–9.
22. Mariani LH, Berns JS. The renal manifestations of thyroid disease. J Am Soc Nephrol: JASN. 2012;23(1):22–6.
23. Basu G, Mohapatra A. Interactions between thyroid disorders and kidney disease. Indian J Endocrinol Metab. 2012;16(2):204–13.
24. Vargas F, Moreno JM, Rodriguez-Gomez I, et al. Vascular and renal function in experimental thyroid disorders. Eur J Endocrinol/Eur Fed Endocr Soc. 2006;154(2):197–212.
25. Bradley SE, Stephan F, Coelho JB, Reville P. The thyroid and the kidney. Kidney Int. 1974;6(5):346–65.
26. Falk SA, Buric V, Hammond WS, Conger JD. Serial glomerular and tubular dynamics in thyroidectomized rats with remnant kidneys. Am J Kidney Dis. 1991;17(2):218–27.
27. Karanikas G, Schutz M, Szabo M, et al. Isotopic renal function studies in severe hypothyroidism and after thyroid hormone replacement therapy. Am J Nephrol. 2004;24(1):41–5.
28. Kreisman SH, Hennessey JV. Consistent reversible elevations of serum creatinine levels in severe hypothyroidism. Arch Intern Med. 1999;159(1):79–82.
29. Villabona C, Sahun M, Roca M, et al. Blood volumes and renal function in overt and subclinical primary hypothyroidism. Am J Med Sci. 1999;318(4):277–80.
30. Asvold BO, Bjoro T, Vatten LJ. Association of thyroid function with estimated glomerular filtration rate in a population-based study: the HUNT study. European J Endocrinol/Eur Fed Endocr Soc. 2011;164(1):101–5.
31. Chonchol M, Lippi G, Salvagno G, Zoppini G, Muggeo M, Targher G. Prevalence of subclinical hypothyroidism in patients with chronic kidney disease. Clin J Am Soc Nephrol: CJASN. 2008;3(5):1296–300.
32. Lippi G, Montagnana M, Targher G, Salvagno GL, Guidi GC. Relationship between thyroid status and renal function in a general population of unselected outpatients. Clin Biochem. 2008;41(7–8):625–7.
33. Meuwese CL, Gussekloo J, de Craen AJ, Dekker FW, den Elzen WP. Thyroid status and renal function in older persons in the general population. J Clin Endocrinol Metab. 2014;99(8):2689–96.
34. Targher G, Chonchol M, Zoppini G, et al. Prevalence of thyroid autoimmunity and subclinical hypothyroidism in persons with chronic kidney disease not requiring chronic dialysis. Clin Chem Lab Med. 2009;47(11):1367–71.
35. Woodward A, McCann S, Al-Jubouri M. The relationship between estimated glomerular filtration rate and thyroid function: an observational study. Ann Clin Biochem. 2008;45.(Pt 5:515–7.
36. Zhang Y, Chang Y, Ryu S, et al. Thyroid hormone levels and incident chronic kidney disease in euthyroid individuals: the Kangbuk Samsung Health Study. Int J Epidemiol. 2014;43(5):1624–32.
37. Shin DH, Lee MJ, Kim SJ, et al. Preservation of renal function by thyroid hormone replacement therapy in chronic kidney disease patients with subclinical hypothyroidism. J Clin Endocrinol Metab. 2012;97(8):2732–40.
38. Wiederkehr MR, Kalogiros J, Krapf R. Correction of metabolic acidosis improves thyroid and growth hormone axes in haemodialysis patients. Nephrol Dial Transplant. 2004;19(5):1190–7.
39. Napolitano G, Bonomini M, Bomba G, et al. Thyroid function and plasma selenium in chronic uremic

patients on hemodialysis treatment. Biol Trace Elem Res. 1996;55(3):221–30.
40. Schomburg L. Selenium, selenoproteins and the thyroid gland: interactions in health and disease. Nat Rev Endocrinol. 2011;8(3):160–71.
41. Sanai T, Inoue T, Okamura K, et al. Reversible primary hypothyroidism in Japanese patients undergoing maintenance hemodialysis. Clin Nephrol. 2008;69(2):107–13.
42. Takeda S, Michigishi T, Takazakura E. Iodine-induced hypothyroidism in patients on regular dialysis treatment. Nephron. 1993;65(1):51–5.
43. Brough R, Jones C. Iatrogenic iodine as a cause of hypothyroidism in infants with end-stage renal failure. Pediatr Nephrol. 2006;21(3):400–2.
44. Lee SY, Rhee CM, Leung AM, Braverman LE, Brent GA, Pearce EN. A review: radiographic iodinated contrast media-induced thyroid dysfunction. J Clin Endocrinol Metab. 2015;100(2):376–83.
45. Moisey RS, McPherson S, Wright M, Orme SM. Thyroiditis and iodide mumps following an angioplasty. Nephrol Dial Transplant. 2007;22(4):1250–2.
46. Rhee CM, Bhan I, Alexander EK, Brunelli SM. Association between iodinated contrast media exposure and incident hyperthyroidism and hypothyroidism. Arch Intern Med. 2012;172(2):153–9.
47. Soldin OP. Measuring serum thyroid-stimulating hormone, thyroid hormones, thyroid-directed antibodies, and transport proteins. In: Braverman LE, Cooper DS, editors. Werner and Ingbar's the thyroid. 10th ed. Philadelphia: Lippincott Williams and Wilkins; 2013. p. 279–97.
48. Feinstein EI, Kaptein EM, Nicoloff JT, Massry SG. Thyroid function in patients with nephrotic syndrome and normal renal function. Am J Nephrol. 1982;2(2):70–6.
49. Gilles R, den Heijer M, Ross AH, Sweep FC, Hermus AR, Wetzels JF. Thyroid function in patients with proteinuria. Neth J Med. 2008;66(11):483–5.
50. Langton JE, Brent GA. Nonthyroidal illness syndrome: evaluation of thyroid function in sick patients. Endocrinol Metab Clin N Am. 2002;31(1):159–72.
51. Klein I. In: Bonow RO, Mann DL, Zipes DP, Libby P, editors. Braunwald's heart disease. 9th ed. Philadelphia: Elsevier Saunders; 2012. p. 1829–43.
52. Imai T, Hirata Y, Iwashina M, Marumo F. Hormonal regulation of rat adrenomedullin gene in vasculature. Endocrinology. 1995;136(4):1544–8.
53. Taddei S, Caraccio N, Virdis A, et al. Impaired endothelium-dependent vasodilatation in subclinical hypothyroidism: beneficial effect of levothyroxine therapy. J Clin Endocrinol Metab. 2003;88(8):3731–7.
54. Hak AE, Pols HA, Visser TJ, Drexhage HA, Hofman A, Witteman JC. Subclinical hypothyroidism is an independent risk factor for atherosclerosis and myocardial infarction in elderly women: the Rotterdam Study. Ann Intern Med. 2000;132(4):270–8.
55. Rhee CM, Budoff MJ, Novoa A, You AS, Nakata T, Nguyen DV, Brent GA, Kalantar-Zadeh K. Thyroid status: a novel coronary artery calcification risk factor in hemodialysis patients. Abstract submitted to the 2018 American Heart Association Scientific Session.
56. Meuwese CL, Carrero JJ, Cabezas-Rodriguez I, et al. Nonthyroidal illness: a risk factor for coronary calcification and arterial stiffness in patients undergoing peritoneal dialysis? J Intern Med. 2013;274(6):584–93.
57. Meuwese CL, Olauson H, Qureshi AR, et al. Associations between thyroid hormones, calcification inhibitor levels and vascular calcification in end-stage renal disease. PLoS One. 2015;10(7):e0132353.
58. Chadarevian R, Bruckert E, Leenhardt L, Giral P, Ankri A, Turpin G. Components of the fibrinolytic system are differently altered in moderate and severe hypothyroidism. J Clin Endocrinol Metab. 2001;86(2):732–7.
59. Donati RM, Fletcher JW, Warnecke MA, Gallagher NI. Erythropoiesis in hypothyroidism. Proc Soc Exp Biol Med. 1973;144(1):78–82.
60. Erdogan M, Kosenli A, Ganidagli S, Kulaksizoglu M. Characteristics of anemia in subclinical and overt hypothyroid patients. Endocr J. 2012;59(3):213–20.
61. Fein HG, Rivlin RS. Anemia in thyroid diseases. Med Clin North Am. 1975;59(5):1133–45.
62. Ng YY, Lin HD, Wu SC, et al. Impact of thyroid dysfunction on erythropoietin dosage in hemodialysis patients. Thyroid. 2013;23(5):552–61.
63. Coban E, Yazicioglu G, Ozdogan M. Platelet activation in subjects with subclinical hypothyroidism. Med Sci Monit. 2007;13(4):CR211–4.
64. Kim JH, Park JH, Kim SY, Bae HY. The mean platelet volume is positively correlated with serum thyrotropin concentrations in a population of healthy subjects and subjects with unsuspected subclinical hypothyroidism. Thyroid. 2013;23(1):31–7.
65. Masunaga R, Nagasaka A, Nakai A, et al. Alteration of platelet aggregation in patients with thyroid disorders. Metab Clin Exp. 1997;46(10):1128–31.
66. Yilmaz H, Ertugrul O, Ertugrul B, Ertugrul D. Mean platelet volume in patients with subclinical hypothyroidism. Platelets. 2011;22(2):143–7.
67. Rodondi N, den Elzen WP, Bauer DC, et al. Subclinical hypothyroidism and the risk of coronary heart disease and mortality. JAMA. 2010;304(12):1365–74.
68. Gencer B, Collet TH, Virgini V, et al. Subclinical thyroid dysfunction and the risk of heart failure events: an individual participant data analysis from 6 prospective cohorts. Circulation. 2012;126(9):1040–9.
69. Rhee CM, Curhan GC, Alexander EK, Bhan I, Brunelli SM. Subclinical hypothyroidism and survival: the effects of heart failure and race. J Clin Endocrinol Metab. 2013;98(6):2326–36.

70. Ro K, Yuen AD, Du L, et al. The impact of hypothyroidism and heart failure on hospitalization risk. Thyroid. 2018.
71. United States Renal Data System. USRDS 2017 Annual Data Report: Atlas of End-Stage Renal Disease in the United States. Bethesda; 2017.
72. Lim VS. Thyroid function in patients with chronic renal failure. Am J Kidney Dis. 2001;38(4 Suppl 1):S80–4.
73. Jaroszynski AJ, Glowniak A, Chrapko B, et al. Low-T3 syndrome and signal-averaged ECG in haemodialysed patients. Physiol Res/Academia Scientiarum Bohemoslovaca. 2005;54(5):521–6.
74. Zoccali C, Benedetto F, Mallamaci F, et al. Low triiodothyronine and cardiomyopathy in patients with end-stage renal disease. J Hypertens. 2006;24(10):2039–46.
75. Tatar E, Sezis Demirci M, Kircelli F, et al. The association between thyroid hormones and arterial stiffness in peritoneal dialysis patients. Int Urol Nephrol. 2012;44(2):601–6.
76. Tatar E, Kircelli F, Asci G, et al. Associations of triiodothyronine levels with carotid atherosclerosis and arterial stiffness in hemodialysis patients. Clin J Am Soc Nephrol: CJASN. 2011;6(9):2240–6.
77. Yilmaz MI, Sonmez A, Karaman M, et al. Low triiodothyronine alters flow-mediated vasodilatation in advanced nondiabetic kidney disease. Am J Nephrol. 2011;33(1):25–32.
78. Zoccali C, Mallamaci F, Tripepi G, Cutrupi S, Pizzini P. Low triiodothyronine and survival in end-stage renal disease. Kidney Int. 2006;70(3):523–8.
79. Enia G, Panuccio V, Cutrupi S, et al. Subclinical hypothyroidism is linked to micro-inflammation and predicts death in continuous ambulatory peritoneal dialysis. Nephrol Dial Transplant. 2007;22(2):538–44.
80. Carrero JJ, Qureshi AR, Axelsson J, et al. Clinical and biochemical implications of low thyroid hormone levels (total and free forms) in euthyroid patients with chronic kidney disease. J Intern Med. 2007;262(6):690–701.
81. Fernandez-Reyes MJ, Diez JJ, Collado A, et al. Are low concentrations of serum triiodothyronine a good marker for long-term mortality in hemodialysis patients? Clin Nephrol. 2010;73(3):238–40.
82. Ozen KP, Asci G, Gungor O, et al. Nutritional state alters the association between free triiodothyronine levels and mortality in hemodialysis patients. Am J Nephrol. 2011;33(4):305–12.
83. Horacek J, Dusilova Sulkova S, Kubisova M, et al. Thyroid hormone abnormalities in hemodialyzed patients: low triiodothyronine as well as high reverse triiodothyronine are associated with increased mortality. Physiol Res/Academia Scientiarum Bohemoslovaca. 2012;61(5):495–501.
84. Lin YC, Lin YC, Chen TW, Yang WC, Lin CC. Abnormal thyroid function predicts mortality in patients receiving long-term peritoneal dialysis: a case-controlled longitudinal study. J Chin Med Assoc. 2012;75(2):54–9.
85. Meuwese CL, Dekker FW, Lindholm B, et al. Baseline levels and trimestral variation of triiodothyronine and thyroxine and their association with mortality in maintenance hemodialysis patients. Clin J Am Soc Nephrol: CJASN. 2012;7(1):131–8.
86. Yang JW, Han ST, Song SH, et al. Serum T3 level can predict cardiovascular events and all-cause mortality rates in CKD patients with proteinuria. Ren Fail. 2012;34(3):364–72.
87. Chang TI, Nam JY, Shin SK, Kang EW. Low triiodothyronine syndrome and long-term cardiovascular outcome in incident peritoneal Dialysis patients. Clin J Am Soc Nephrol: CJASN. 2015;10(6):975–82.
88. Wiersinga WM, Van den Berghe G. Nonthyroidal illness syndrome. In: Braverman LE, Cooper DS, editors. Werner and Ingbar's the thyroid. 10th ed. Philadelphia: Lippincott Williams and Wilkins; 2013. p. 203–16.
89. Meuwese CL, Dekkers OM, Stenvinkel P, Dekker FW, Carrero JJ. Nonthyroidal illness and the cardiorenal syndrome. Nat Rev Nephrol. 2013;9(10):599–609.
90. Carrero JJ, Stenvinkel P, Lindholm B. Endocrine aspects of chronic kidney disease. In: Taal MW, Chertow GM, Marsden PA, Skorecki K, Yu AS, Brenner BM, editors. Taal Brenner and Rector's the kidney. 9th ed. Philadelphia: Elsevier Saunders; 2012. p. 2122–37.
91. Kaptein EM. Thyroid hormone metabolism and thyroid diseases in chronic renal failure. Endocr Rev. 1996;17(1):45–63.
92. Kang EW, Nam JY, Yoo TH, et al. Clinical implications of subclinical hypothyroidism in continuous ambulatory peritoneal dialysis patients. Am J Nephrol. 2008;28(6):908–13.
93. Drechsler C, Schneider A, Gutjahr-Lengsfeld L, et al. Thyroid function, cardiovascular events, and mortality in diabetic hemodialysis patients. Am J Kidney Dis. 2014;63(6):988–96.
94. Rhee CM, Kalantar-Zadeh K, Ravel V, et al. Thyroid status and death risk in US veterans with chronic kidney disease. Mayo Clin Proc. 2018;93(5):573–85.
95. You AS, Sim JJ, Kovesdy CP, Streja E, Nguyen DV, Brent GA, Kalantar-Zadeh K, Rhee CM. Association of thyroid status prior to transition to end-stage renal disease with early dialysis mortality. Abstract submitted to the 2018 International Congress of Nutritional and Metabolism.
96. Rhee CM, Chen Y, You AS, et al. Thyroid status, quality of life, and mental health in patients on hemodialysis. Clin J Am Soc Nephrol : CJASN. 2017;12(8):1274–83.
97. Vigario Pdos S, Vaisman F, Coeli CM, et al. Inadequate levothyroxine replacement for primary hypothyroidism is associated with poor health-related quality of life-a Brazilian multicentre study. Endocrine. 2013;44(2):434–40.

98. Kalantar-Zadeh K, Unruh M. Health related quality of life in patients with chronic kidney disease. Int Urol Nephrol. 2005;37(2):367–78.
99. United States Renal Data System. USRDS 2012 Annual Data Report: Atlas of End-Stage Renal Disease in the United States. Bethesda, MD; 2012.
100. Biondi B, Fazio S, Palmieri EA, et al. Left ventricular diastolic dysfunction in patients with subclinical hypothyroidism. J Clin Endocrinol Metab. 1999;84(6):2064–7.
101. Monzani F, Di Bello V, Caraccio N, et al. Effect of levothyroxine on cardiac function and structure in subclinical hypothyroidism: a double blind, placebo-controlled study. J Clin Endocrinol Metab. 2001;86(3):1110–5.
102. Owen PJ, Rajiv C, Vinereanu D, Mathew T, Fraser AG, Lazarus JH. Subclinical hypothyroidism, arterial stiffness, and myocardial reserve. J Clin Endocrinol Metab. 2006;91(6):2126–32.
103. Razvi S, Ingoe L, Keeka G, Oates C, McMillan C, Weaver JU. The beneficial effect of L-thyroxine on cardiovascular risk factors, endothelial function, and quality of life in subclinical hypothyroidism: randomized, crossover trial. J Clin Endocrinol Metab. 2007;92(5):1715–23.
104. Razvi S, Weaver JU, Butler TJ, Pearce SH. Levothyroxine treatment of subclinical hypothyroidism, fatal and nonfatal cardiovascular events, and mortality. Arch Intern Med. 2012;172(10):811–7.
105. Wartofsky L. Levothyroxine: therapeutic use and regulatory issues related to bioequivalence. Expert Opin Pharmacother. 2002;3(6):727–32.

Part III

Gonadal Disorders

Testosterone Deficiency and Other Testicular Disorders in Kidney Disease

9

Anna L. Goldman and Shalender Bhasin

Introduction

The kidney is an important endocrine organ; it regulates endocrine functions and also serves as a target of hormonal action. Chronic kidney disease (CKD), which encompasses a wide variety of clinical syndromes and disorders, is associated with abnormalities in the secretion, transport, metabolism, protein binding, elimination, and target tissue response of multiple, different hormones, leading to alterations in feedback loops and poor patient outcomes [1]. Testicular dysfunction is common in men with CKD, especially in those with end-stage renal disease (ESRD) who are on maintenance hemodialysis. The cause of testicular dysfunction in ESRD is often multifactorial [1–3]. Hypogonadism, in general, is manifested clinically by decreased libido, erectile dysfunction, low mood, fatigue, loss of muscle mass, decreased bone mineral density, and secondary sex characteristics. Some signs and symptoms of testosterone deficiency, such as fatigue and low mood, are non-specific and difficult to distinguish from those resulting from chronic disease or aging. Diagnosis of testosterone dysfunction is based on confirmation of signs and symptoms of testosterone deficiency along with clearly low levels of circulating testosterone on at least two occasions, using a reliable assay [4]. This chapter will provide an overview of the pathogenesis and treatment of testicular dysfunction in men with CKD.

Epidemiology

The estimates of the prevalence of hypogonadism in the general population have varied due to the heterogeneity of study populations, the clinical definition of hypogonadism used, and the assay employed to measure circulating testosterone concentrations [5–9]. Recent studies using the liquid chromatography-tandem mass spectrometry (LC-MS/MS) assay for the measurement of total testosterone concentrations in early morning samples have reported a 10–14% prevalence in healthy, community-dwelling men who are 65 years of age and older [5–9]. However, testicular dysfunction is more common in men with CKD than in the general population [10]. Changes in androgen synthesis tend to occur in early stages of renal failure [1, 11–13], and by the time men have progressed to ESRD requiring dialysis, approximately two-thirds will have testosterone levels in the hypogonadal range

A. L. Goldman (✉) · S. Bhasin
Research Program in Men's Health: Aging and Metabolism, Brigham and Women's Hospital/Harvard Medical School, Boston, MA, USA
e-mail: Algoldman1@bwh.harvard.edu

C. M. Rhee et al. (eds.), *Endocrine Disorders in Kidney Disease*,
https://doi.org/10.1007/978-3-319-97765-2_9

[1, 3, 13–19]. In one study of 260 men with ESRD, low total testosterone levels (defined as total testosterone <10 nmol/L) were present in 44% of the group [14]. Both total and free testosterone levels fall in parallel with the decline of estimated glomerular filtration rate (eGFR) [19]. In a cross-sectional analysis of 1470 men in the United States, there was no independent association between total testosterone and CKD, suggesting that low total testosterone may be a surrogate marker of disease severity and overall health rather than a causal risk factor [20].

Pathophysiology of Testicular Dysfunction in CKD

Hypogonadism in CKD results from alterations in the hypothalamic-pituitary-gonadal (HPG) axis at multiple levels (Fig. 9.1) [3, 21]. Patients frequently have damage to the seminiferous tubules and Sertoli cells with semen analysis typically showing a decreased volume of ejaculate, oligo- or azoospermia, and a low motility even at modest reductions of the GFR [13]. A reduction in 5-alpha-reductase activity is evidenced by a reduced dihydrotestosterone (DHT) to testosterone ratio. Sex hormone-binding globulin (SHBG) levels and its binding capacity are usually normal [22–24]. Overall, low testosterone levels appear to be due to a low testicular production rather than an increase in metabolic clearance [1]. Decreased testosterone levels are associated with a loss of muscle mass and strength, decreased bone mineral density (BMD) and libido, poor erectile function, anemia, and fatigue.

Secretion of inhibin, a protein produced by the Sertoli cells that exerts a negative feedback on follicle-stimulating hormone (FSH) release, tends to decrease, leading to higher FSH concentrations [13]. Uremic inhibition of luteinizing hormone (LH) signaling at the level of the Leydig cells in the testes diminishes negative feedback inhibition by testosterone, and decreased clearance is associated with an elevated plasma concentration of LH [25]. However, the acidic and bioactive forms

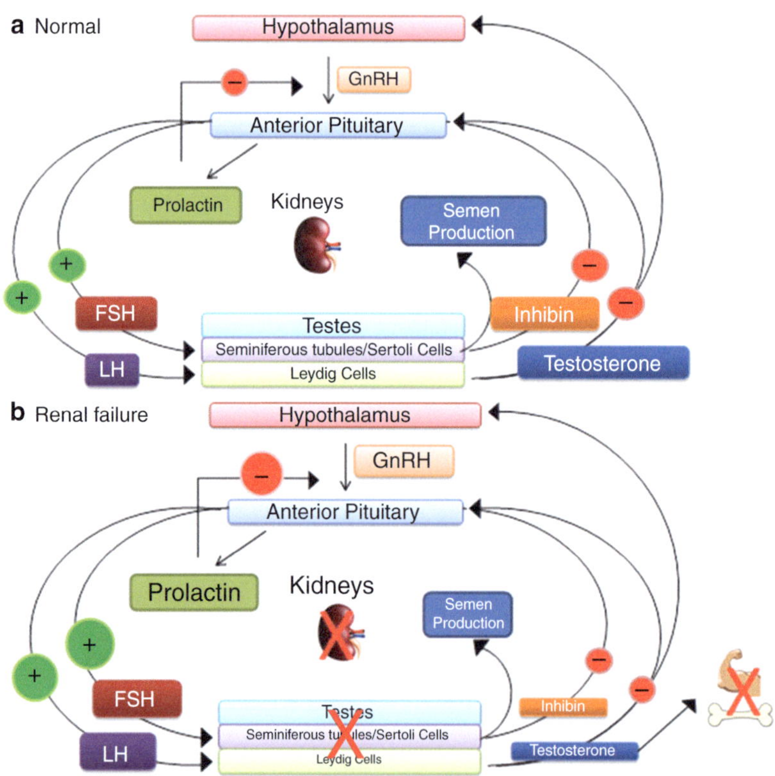

Fig. 9.1 Hypothalamic-pituitary-gonadal (HPG) axis under normal conditions and in chronic kidney disease (CKD). (**a**) The hypothalamic-pituitary-gonadal (HPG) axis in a normal, healthy man. (**b**) Hypogonadism in CKD results primarily from testicular damage and from alterations in the HPG at multiple levels

of LH are decreased in men on dialysis [26]. Hyperprolactinemia, which results from reduced clearance of prolactin in CKD [17], inhibits LH secretion and pulsatile gonadotropin-releasing hormone (GnRH) secretion at the hypothalamus and attenuates pituitary responsiveness to GnRH [27–29]. However, basal GnRH levels have been shown to be increased in ESRD and are corrected by dialysis [30]. Hyperparathyroidism, a common condition among CKD patients, also stimulates the secretion of prolactin, contributing to hyperprolactinemia [17]. Interestingly, the calcium-sensing receptor (CaSR) is expressed in the testis, and treatment of secondary hyperparathyroidism in male ESRD patients with a calcimimetic is associated with a further decrease in serum total and free testosterone concentrations [31].

Adverse Health Consequences of Testicular Dysfunction

In a cross-sectional study of 160 obese men, total testosterone and free testosterone were below normal in 57.5% and 35.6%, respectively, of the population, and decreased libido and erectile dysfunction were 7.1 and 6.7 times more common, respectively, in those with biochemical evidence of hypogonadism than in eugonadal obese men [32]. Erectile dysfunction (ED) and CKD share common risk factors, and both are associated with diseases involving endothelial impairment such as diabetes mellitus, anemia, hypertension, dyslipidemia, coronary artery disease, smoking, and obesity [33]. The bioavailability of nitrous oxide (NO), which is the primary neurotransmitter of penile erection, is reduced in CKD as a result of altered expression of NO synthase (NOS) [34]. As such, sexual dysfunction is very prevalent in men with CKD, especially in those with ESRD. A large systematic review and meta-analysis of observational studies in men with CKD reported that ED affected approximately 70% with no difference in prevalence rates among those on hemodialysis vs. peritoneal dialysis [35]. Using the validated International Index of Erectile Function (IIEF), the prevalence and severity of ED in hemodialysis patients were significantly higher than that of the controls in each age group [36]. In a cross-sectional study of 302 ESRD patients, increasing age, diabetes, and nonuse of angiotensin-converting enzyme (ACE) inhibitors were associated with higher prevalence of ED [37]. Even after renal transplantation, prevalence rates of ED still approach 50% [38].

A reduction in testosterone levels has been associated with the metabolic syndrome (MetS) and its individual components (visceral obesity, high triglycerides/low HDL cholesterol, hyperglycemia, and hypertension) regardless of age [39–43]. There seems to be a bidirectional relationship between hypogonadism and increased body fat mass, inflammation, and insulin sensitivity [44].

An independent role for sex in the progression of CKD has not been clearly established and remains controversial [45, 46]. A meta-analysis of 11,345 subjects by Neugarten et al. concluded that male sex was associated with a more rapid rate of progression and worse renal outcomes in patients with nondiabetic CKD [45]. Meta-analyses also have shown an association between progression of IgA nephropathy, polycystic kidney disease, and membranous nephropathy with male sex [47–49]. It is unclear whether the association of sex with renal disease progression is related to sex differences in other risk factors such as diet, blood pressure, or serum lipid levels or the result of complex interactions between chromosomal sex and epigenetic and activational effects of androgens and estrogens. Estrogen may have a protective effect by attenuating injury-induced superoxide production [50].

Hypertension is more widely prevalent in men than in women, although women have an increase in blood pressure after menopause, similar to measurements in men [51]. Androgen receptor expression has been found in the proximal tubule and in the cortical collecting ducts of human kidneys, suggesting that testosterone plays a local role in blood pressure regulation [52]. In an animal model of hypertension, male rats have higher blood pressures than female rats, which are reduced to female levels after castration [53–55]. Castration of spontaneously hypertensive rats (SHR) or treatment with the androgen receptor antagonist flutamide not only attenuates hypertension but also improves renal hemodynamics, decreases renin activity, and prevents age-related glomerular sclerosis [55, 56]. Baylis et al. studied glomerulosclerosis in aging rats and found that intact males developed progressive glomerular damage and proteinuria, whereas females are both intact and ovariectomized, and castrated males were protected from renal injury [57]. Exogenous administration of testosterone may exacerbate renal injury by stimulating TNF-α production and increasing pro-apoptotic and pro-fibrotic signaling [58] and increasing tubular sodium and water resorption through activation of the renin-angiotensin-aldosterone system (RAAS) and upregulation of endothelin [59–62]. Some effects of testosterone may be mediated through its aromatization to estradiol, thereby activating the estrogen receptor, thus complicating our understanding of the impact of testosterone levels on progression to CKD [63]. This rodent data is highly strain-specific.

In epidemiologic studies, low testosterone levels have been associated with all-cause mortality, especially cardiovascular mortality. Low testosterone levels have been associated with endothelial dysfunction and atherosclerosis in male ESRD patients [64]. Although low testosterone levels have been reported to be associated with an increased risk of death in patients with CKD, it remains controversial whether this association is independent of age [15, 65]. Yilmaz et al. showed that in male, non-dialysis CKD patients, the reduction in endogenous free and total testosterone levels was negatively associated with endothelial dysfunction [19]. Low testosterone levels have also been associated with increased arterial stiffness [66]. In a population-based study (n = 1822), men with both renal dysfunction and low testosterone had a more than twofold increase in all-cause mortality (HR 2.52) [67]. A low testosterone level at the time of renal transplantation was found to be independently associated with patient death (HR 2.27) and graft loss (HR 2.05) [68]. However, epidemiologic studies can only demonstrate association but not causality; in fact, reverse causality cannot be excluded. It is possible that low testosterone levels are a marker of poor health and men with increased burden of chronic conditions who are at increased risk of death may have low testosterone levels.

Testosterone deficiency is associated with low bone density, and testosterone replacement increases areal bone mineral density in the spine and volumetric bone density and bone strength in both the spine and hip in older men with unequivocally low testosterone levels [69, 70]. However, the effects of testosterone on fracture have not been studied. Reductions in BMD and elevation of biochemical markers of bone turnover progress as renal function declines [71]. Data from large, epidemiological studies have reported an increased risk of fractures among patients with CKD compared with the general population [72, 73]. This risk may be explained by a combination of factors including secondary hyperparathyroidism, osteomalacia, medications (like corticosteroids), immobilization, osteopenia, and osteoporosis [74]. Older men with reduced renal function are at increased risk of hip bone loss [75]. No randomized trials have evaluated the efficacy of testosterone therapy on fracture risk in men with CKD.

Diagnosis of Testosterone Deficiency in CKD

The Endocrine Society recommends screening for hypogonadism in symptomatic men who have conditions which are associated with a high risk of testosterone deficiency [76], which includes individuals with CKD. In men deemed to be testosterone deficient, measurement of LH and FSH concentrations can help to distinguish between primary and secondary hypogonadism. In primary hypogonadism, LH and FSH levels are elevated, while in secondary or hypogonadotropic hypogonadism, low testosterone levels are associated with low or inappropriately normal LH and FSH levels. Primary hypogonadism is the more common metabolic derangement associated with CKD [1–3]. However, men with CKD may typically have defects at all levels of the HPG axis.

The diagnosis of hypogonadism should be based upon the ascertainment of signs and symptoms of androgen deficiency along with unequivocally low fasting levels of circulating testosterone on at least two occasions, using a reliable assay (Fig. 9.2) [4]. Physical examination should be conducted with particular attention paid to hair growth, testicular volume, and the presence of gynecomastia. Testicular size should be measured using a Prader orchidometer. Damage to the seminiferous tubules may result in a decrease in the size of the testes.

Total testosterone represents the sum of free testosterone and testosterone that is bound to plasma proteins including albumin, SHBG, orosomucoid, and cortisol-binding globulin. Liquid chromatography-tandem mass spectrometry (LC-MS/MS) has emerged as the reference method with the highest accuracy and precision for measuring total testosterone levels. The reported reference ranges for total and free testosterone levels in healthy young men vary considerably among laboratories and assays [6, 77–79]. In one comparison of six different assays, the lower limit of the reported reference range for total testosterone varied from 132 to 298 ng/dL (4.6–10.3 nmol/L) [80]. A substantial amount of the variation in reference ranges is due to the lack of standardization of testosterone assays and differences in the reference populations used to generate ranges. Recently, the Endocrine Society and the Partnership for the Accurate Testing of Hormones (PATH) supported a project to develop a harmonized reference range utilizing community-dwelling men from four large cohorts in the United States and Europe, by cross-calibrating the assays used in each epidemiologic study against a higher-order method and calibrator developed by the Centers for Disease Control (CDC), and then harmonizing the local values to the CDC-standardized measurements using the Deming-Bablok regression [77]. The harmonized reference range for total testosterone in healthy, nonobese young men (aged 19–39 years) was 264–916 ng/dL (9.2–31.8 nmol/L) using harmonized 2.5th and 97.5th percentile values and 303–852 ng/dL (10.5– 29.5 nmol/L) using harmonized 5th and 95th percentile values [77]. This range can be used for CDC-certified total testosterone assays [6].

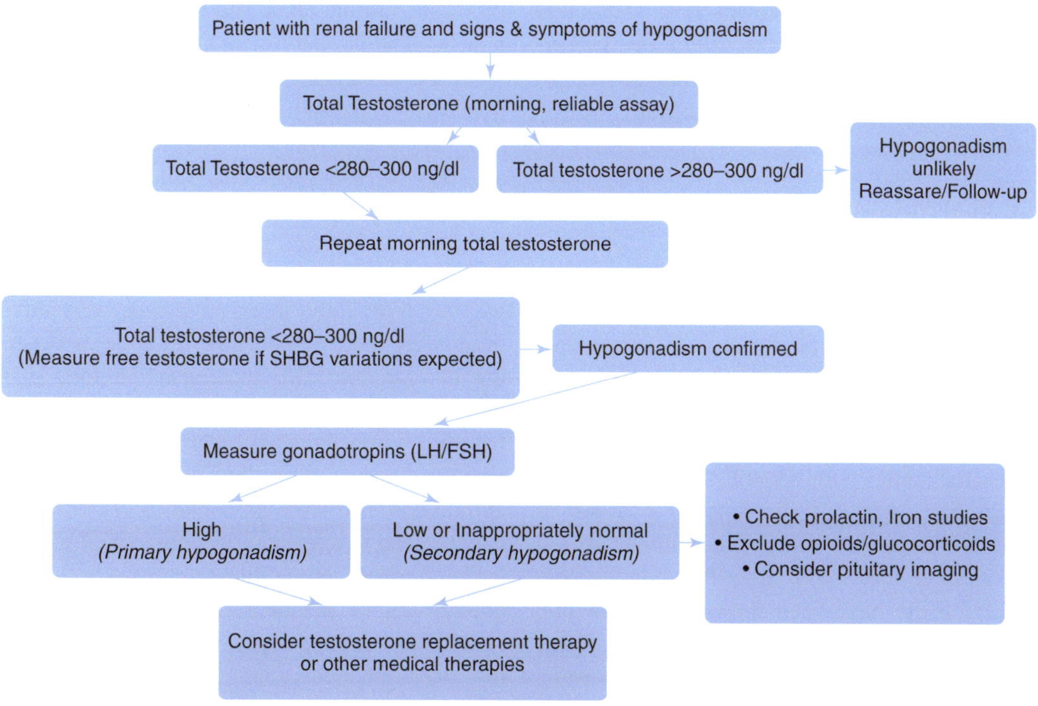

Fig. 9.2 Diagnosis of hypogonadism in patients with renal failure

As total testosterone concentrations are affected by the circulating concentrations of SHBG, measurement of free testosterone levels is important in conditions in which alterations in binding protein concentrations may occur, such as kidney disease. Free testosterone concentrations can be measured using equilibrium dialysis, ultrafiltration, or estimated from formulas that use the total testosterone, SHBG, and albumin concentrations. Free testosterone measurements by tracer analog methods are not accurate and are therefore not recommended [81]. The linear law of mass actions for estimating free testosterone concentrations is based on assumptions of linear binding of testosterone to SHBG with a single binding constant [82], and these assumptions have recently been shown to be inaccurate [83]. Zakharov and colleagues showed that the binding of testosterone to SHBG is a complex, multistep process, which involves allostery between the binding sites [83]. The estimates of free testosterone concentration using this new multistep ensemble binding model with allostery provide close approximation to those measured using equilibrium dialysis [83]. However, it is unclear how kidney failure might affect the performance of this algorithm, which was established in those with normal kidney function.

Clinical Manifestations

In the general population, hypogonadal men may present with a variety of symptoms including decreased libido, difficulty with erections, low energy, depression, fatigue, poor mood, gynecomastia, and/or infertility. In the European Male Aging Study (EMAS), only three sexual symptoms including poor morning erections, low libido, and erectile dysfunction were shown to have a syndromic association with decreased testosterone levels [9]. ED, decreased libido, and infertility have been shown to be common features of men with CKD. Up to 56% of men receiving dialysis develop ED [84]. Hypogonadal men with CKD also have a diminished quality of life [85].

Skeletal muscle atrophy and weakness (sarcopenia) are prominent features of renal disease, especially in those who are hemodialysis-dependent [86], as testosterone is thought to play an important anabolic role in muscle synthesis. Hemodialysis itself is a catabolic process and likely contributes to sarcopenia [87–90]. Cigarrán and colleagues showed that in men with moderate CKD, endogenous testosterone was independently associated with muscle strength and fat-free mass [91].

Treatment

Testosterone Therapy

Therapy for progressive CKD is initially directed at optimizing dialysis and nutritional status, correcting anemia with recombinant erythropoietin, and limiting the maladaptive metabolic consequences of secondary hyperparathyroidism with vitamin D and phosphate binders. Phosphodiesterase inhibitors have become a first-line agent in treating erectile dysfunction. In hypogonadal men with CKD who complain of decreased libido, decreased muscle mass, and fatigue, testosterone may be of additional benefit as well.

In a comparison of the pharmacokinetics of transdermal testosterone in testosterone-deficient men with ESRD on maintenance hemodialysis and men with normal renal function who had classical hypogonadism, Singh et al. reported that the time-average, steady-state total and free testosterone concentrations and minimum and maximum total and free testosterone concentrations were not significantly different between the two groups [18]. Increments in total and free testosterone concentrations above baseline, baseline-subtracted areas under the total and free testosterone curves, and half-life of testosterone elimination also were not significantly different between the two groups. The amount of testosterone removed in the dialysate (8.4 +/− 1.6 μg during 4 h of hemodialysis) was quite small compared with the daily testosterone production rates in healthy young men [18]. Therefore, testosterone replacement therapy in hypogonadal men with CKD patients who are receiving maintenance hemodialysis can be accomplished using the same dosages and regimens that the Endocrine Society has recommended for testosterone replacement of healthy hypogonadal men [92, 93]. Patients should be counseled that long-term data showing the risks and benefits of testosterone replacement therapy in men with CKD are lacking.

Because of the high burden of functional limitations and disability in CKD patients, several trials have investigated whether androgen administration can increase muscle mass, strength, and physical function in CKD. Johansen and colleagues investigated the effects of nandrolone decanoate on lean body mass (LBM), functional status, and quality of life in hypogonadal men with CKD on dialysis; nandrolone administration resulted in a significant increase in LBM with an associated improvement in measures of physical function [94]. In another trial, nandrolone decanoate also significantly improved LBM in pre-dialysis patients with CKD without altering renal function or causing serious adverse effects [95]. However, the effects of long-term androgen therapy on hard patient-important outcomes such as disability, falls, fractures, health-related quality of life, and mortality remain to be determined. Furthermore, the long-term safety of androgen administration has not been established in well-powered randomized trials.

Epidemiologic and clinical trials data support the notion that testosterone is an important regulator of erythropoiesis [96, 97]. Testosterone levels are associated with hemoglobin levels in boys and girls during the pubertal transition and in older men and women [98, 99]. Hemoglobin and hematocrit levels are higher in men than in women [100]. Androgen deficiency in hypogonadal men and in patients with prostate cancer receiving androgen deprivation therapy is associated with anemia [101]; conversely, testosterone therapy of androgen-deficient men and patients with renal disease increases hematocrit [102]. Erythrocytosis is a common adverse effect of testosterone therapy. Testosterone-induced increases in hemoglobin and hematocrit are related to testosterone dose and circulating testosterone concentrations in young and older men. Before the advent of erythropoietin, androgens were often used to treat anemia of chronic disease, and some androgens were even approved for the treatment of anemia of chronic kidney disease [103]. Although the molecular mechanisms by which testosterone increases hemoglobin and hematocrit are not fully understood [104], testosterone has been shown to stimulate iron-dependent erythropoiesis. Testosterone inhibits hepcidin transcription and increases iron availability and incorporation into the red blood cells [97]. Additionally, testosterone stimulates erythropoietin and erythropoiesis in the bone marrow [105, 106].

Although nandrolone decanoate was approved in the United States for the treatment of anemia of kidney disease, few large, adequately powered randomized trials of testosterone or other androgens have been conducted. The published trials have been limited by their small sample size, variable doses and durations, heterogeneity of patient population, and suboptimal attention to the adequacy of iron stores [107–109]. Not surprisingly, a Cochrane review found the evidence inconclusive about the efficacy of androgen therapy for the treatment of anemia of renal disease [103]. In one study of hypogonadal men on erythropoiesis-stimulating agents (ESA) undergoing hemodialysis, higher ESA doses were required in men with low testosterone levels, suggesting that hypogonadism may be an additional contributor to anemia and reduced responsiveness to ESA in men with CKD [110]. The hypothesis that testosterone treatment may restore responsiveness to erythropoietin has not been tested rigorously in randomized trials. The Clinical Guidelines from the Kidney Disease Improving Global Outcome (KDIGO) for Anemia in Chronic Kidney Disease recommend against the use of androgens as an adjuvant to ESA, citing a lack of evidence from large, randomized controlled trials and the uncertain long-term risks of androgen use [111].

Other Medical Therapies

Aside from testosterone, other medications that impact the HPG axis have been considered for treating hypogonadism in CKD patients; however, limited efficacy and safety data are available. Clomiphene citrate is a weak estrogen receptor antagonist that stimulates gonadotropin secretion and raises testosterone levels in CKD patients [112, 113]. Treatment of anemic hypogonadal patients with recombinant human erythropoietin (rhEPO) has been associated with modest improvements in circulating testosterone levels [114] and sexual function in some studies [115, 116] but not in others [117]. In patients with CKD who have hyperprolactinemia, dopaminergic agonists such as bromocriptine lower prolactin and raise testosterone levels [118, 119], but sexual function and libido are not necessarily normalized [120]. In one short-term trial, human chorionic gonadotropin (hCG) administration did not result in a satisfactory rise in testosterone as compared with controls [121]. However, during prolonged hCG administration, plasma testosterone levels were normalized [121]. For these reasons, replacement therapy using one of many approved testosterone formulations remains the best option for treating CKD patients who have confirmed hypogonadism.

Phosphodiesterase type 5 (PDE5) inhibitors are highly effective drugs for treating men with ED; however, few randomized trials have systematically evaluated their efficacy and safety in men with CKD. There is an unmet need for studying interventions for sexual dysfunction in CKD.

Renal Transplantation

The HPG axis dysfunction typically does not improve and may continue to progress with initiation of hemodialysis [1, 11, 122, 123]. In contrast, renal transplantation usually results in reductions of high levels of prolactin and elevation of circulating testosterone concentrations [124–127]. Although there is normalization of testosterone levels by 6–12 months after transplantation in many men, approximately 25% of men evaluated 1–2 years after transplantation still have biochemical evidence of testosterone deficiency [128]. Several studies suggest that ED still remains highly prevalent, affecting ~50% of patients after kidney transplantation [38, 129]. Factors associated with posttransplant ED include older age, longer time on hemodialysis prior to transplantation, pre-existing comorbid conditions including diabetes and hypertension, and the use of certain antihypertensive drugs [129, 130]. Though the elevation of FSH in CKD tends to be variable, an increased FSH level may portend a poor prognosis for return of spermatogenic function after transplantation [21]. Inhibin B levels may be helpful in predicting testicular impairment post-kidney transplant [128]. Sirolimus, an immunosuppressant widely used in renal transplantation, is associated with decreased testosterone levels and impaired spermatogenesis in recipients [131–133].

Conclusions

Testosterone deficiency and sexual dysfunction are common among patients with CKD. It remains unclear whether low, endogenous levels of circulating testosterone are adaptive or maladaptive. Dysfunction of the HPG axis can usually be detected early in the course of CKD but will often continue to progress even after hemodialysis is initiated. Kidney transplantation is the most effective treatment available for reversing uremic hypogonadism, but erectile dysfunction persists in a large percentage of patients even after renal transplantation. Posttransplant hypogonadism may even be exacerbated by certain immunosuppressants. Testosterone replacement therapy can be administered using the same dose regimens that are recommended for healthy hypogonadal men with normal kidney function. Long-term risks and benefits of testosterone replacement therapy need to be further studied in adequately powered randomized control trials.

Disclosures Dr. Goldman has no commercial or financial conflicts of interest to disclose.

Dr. Bhasin has received research grants from the National Institute on Aging, the National Institute of Nursing Research, the Foundation for the NIH, the Patient-Centered Outcomes Research Institute, AbbVie, Transition Therapeutics, and Metro International Biotechnology; he has consulted for AbbVie and Novartis and has equity interest in FPT, LLC.

References

1. Handelsman DJ. Hypothalamic-pituitary gonadal dysfunction in renal failure, dialysis and renal transplantation. Endocr Rev. 1985;6(2):151–82.
2. Foulks CJ, Cushner HM. Sexual dysfunction in the male dialysis patient: pathogenesis, evaluation, and therapy. Am J Kidney Dis. 1986;8(4):211–22.
3. Holley JL. The hypothalamic pituitary axis in men and women with chronic kidney disease. Adv Chronic Kidney Dis. 2004;11(4):337–41.
4. Traish AM, Miner MM, Morgentaler A, Zitzmann M. Testosterone deficiency. Am J Med. 2011;124(7):578–87.
5. Araujo AB, Esche GR, Kupelian V, et al. Prevalence of symptomatic androgen deficiency in men. J Clin Endocrinol Metab. 2007;92(11):4241–7.
6. Bhasin S, Pencina M, Jasuja GK, et al. Reference ranges for testosterone in men generated using liquid chromatography tandem mass spectrometry in a community-based sample of healthy nonobese young men in the Framingham Heart Study and applied to three geographically distinct cohorts. J Clin Endocrinol Metab. 2011;96(8):2430–9.
7. Hans D, Barthe N, Boutroy S, Pothuaud L, Winzenrieth R, Krieg MA. Correlations between trabecular bone score, measured using anteroposterior dual-energy X-ray absorptiometry acquisition, and 3-dimensional parameters of bone microarchitecture: an experimental study on human cadaver vertebrae. J Clin Densitom. 2011;14(3):302–12.
8. Orwoll E, Lambert LC, Marshall LM, et al. Testosterone and estradiol among older men. J Clin Endocrinol Metab. 2006;91(4):1336–44.
9. Wu FC, Tajar A, Beynon JM, et al. Identification of late-onset hypogonadism in middle-aged and elderly men. N Engl J Med. 2010;363(2):123–35.
10. Schaefer F, Mehls O, Ritz E. New insights into endocrine disturbances of chronic renal failure. Miner Electrolyte Metab. 1992;18(2–5):169–73.
11. Albaaj F, Sivalingham M, Haynes P, et al. Prevalence of hypogonadism in male patients with renal failure. Postgrad Med J. 2006;82(972):693–6.
12. Cerqueira J, Moraes M, Glina S. Erectile dysfunction: prevalence and associated variables in patients with chronic renal failure. Int J Impot Res. 2002;14(2):65–71.
13. Palmer BF. Sexual dysfunction in uremia. J Am Soc Nephrol. 1999;10(6):1381–8.
14. Carrero JJ, Qureshi AR, Nakashima A, et al. Prevalence and clinical implications of testosterone deficiency in men with end-stage renal disease. Nephrol Dial Transplant. 2010;26(1):184–90.
15. Carrero JJ, Qureshi AR, Parini P, et al. Low serum testosterone increases mortality risk among male dialysis patients. J Am Soc Nephrol. 2009;20(3):613–20.
16. Leavey SF, Weitzel WF. Endocrine abnormalities in chronic renal failure. Endocrinol Metab Clin N Am. 2002;31(1):107–19.
17. Schmidt A, Luger A, Horl WH. Sexual hormone abnormalities in male patients with renal failure. Nephrol Dial Transplant. 2002;17(3):368–71.
18. Singh AB, Norris K, Modi N, et al. Pharmacokinetics of a transdermal testosterone system in men with end stage renal disease receiving maintenance hemodialysis and healthy hypogonadal men. J Clin Endocrinol Metab. 2001;86(6):2437–45.
19. Yilmaz MI, Sonmez A, Qureshi AR, et al. Endogenous testosterone, endothelial dysfunction, and cardiovascular events in men with nondialysis chronic kidney disease. Clin J Am Soc Nephrol. 2011;6(7):1617–25.
20. Yi S, Selvin E, Rohrmann S, et al. Endogenous sex steroid hormones and measures of chronic kidney disease (CKD) in a nationally representative sample of men. Clin Endocrinol. 2009;71(2):246–52.
21. Prem AR, Punekar SV, Kalpana M, Kelkar AR, Acharya VN. Male reproductive function in uraemia: efficacy of haemodialysis and renal transplantation. Br J Urol. 1996;78(4):635–8.
22. de Vries CP, Gooren LJ, Oe PL. Haemodialysis and testicular function. Int J Androl. 1984;7(2):97–103.
23. Ramirez G, Butcher D, Brueggemeyer CD, Ganguly A. Testicular defect: the primary abnormality in gonadal dysfunction of uremia. South Med J. 1987;80(6):698–701.
24. Hylander B, Lehtihet M. Testosterone and gonadotropins but not SHBG vary with CKD stages in young and middle aged men. Basic Clin Androl. 2015;25:9.
25. Dunkel L, Raivio T, Laine J, Holmberg C. Circulating luteinizing hormone receptor inhibitor(s) in boys with chronic renal failure. Kidney Int. 1997;51(3):777–84.
26. Mitchell R, Bauerfeld C, Schaefer F, Scharer K, Robertson WR. Less acidic forms of luteinizing hormone are associated with lower testosterone secretion in men on haemodialysis treatment. Clin Endocrinol (Oxf). 1994;41(1):65–73.
27. Cheung CY. Prolactin suppresses luteinizing hormone secretion and pituitary responsiveness to luteinizing hormone-releasing hormone by a direct action at the anterior pituitary. Endocrinology. 1983;113(2):632–8.
28. Veldhuis JD, Wilkowski MJ, Zwart AD, et al. Evidence for attenuation of hypothalamic gonadotropin-releasing hormone (GnRH) impulse strength with preservation of GnRH pulse frequency in men with chronic renal failure. J Clin Endocrinol Metab. 1993;76(3):648–54.
29. Wheatley T, Clark PM, Clark JD, Raggatt PR, Evans D, Holder R. Pulsatility of luteinising hormone in men with chronic renal failure: abnormal rather than absent. Br Med J (Clin Res Ed). 1987;294(6570):482.
30. Matsubara M, Nakagawa K, Nonomura K, Hirota N. Plasma LRH levels in chronic renal failure before and during haemodialysis. Acta Endocrinol. 1983;103(2):145–50.

31. Kuczera P, Adamczak M, Wiecek A. Changes of serum total and free testosterone concentrations in male chronic hemodialysis patients with secondary hyperparathyroidism in response to cinacalcet treatment. Kidney Blood Press Res. 2016;41(1):1–8.
32. Hofstra J, Loves S, van Wageningen B, Ruinemans-Koerts J, Jansen I, de Boer H. High prevalence of hypogonadotropic hypogonadism in men referred for obesity treatment. Neth J Med. 2008;66(3):103–9.
33. Mesquita JF, Ramos TF, Mesquita FP, Bastos Netto JM, Bastos MG, Figueiredo AA. Prevalence of erectile dysfunction in chronic renal disease patients on conservative treatment. Clinics (Sao Paulo). 2012;67(2):181–3.
34. Palmer BF. Outcomes associated with hypogonadism in men with chronic kidney disease. Adv Chronic Kidney Dis. 2004;11(4):342–7.
35. Navaneethan SD, Vecchio M, Johnson DW, et al. Prevalence and correlates of self-reported sexual dysfunction in CKD: a meta-analysis of observational studies. Am J Kidney Dis. 2010;56(4):670–85.
36. Naya Y, Soh J, Ochiai A, et al. Significant decrease of the International Index of Erectile Function in male renal failure patients treated with hemodialysis. Int J Impot Res. 2002;14(3):172–7.
37. Rosas SE, Joffe M, Franklin E, et al. Prevalence and determinants of erectile dysfunction in hemodialysis patients. Kidney Int. 2001;59(6):2259–66.
38. Espinoza R, Gracida C, Cancino J, Ibarra A. Prevalence of erectile dysfunction in kidney transplant recipients. Transplant Proc. 2006;38(3):916–7.
39. Brand JS, Rovers MM, Yeap BB, et al. Testosterone, sex hormone-binding globulin and the metabolic syndrome in men: an individual participant data meta-analysis of observational studies. PLoS One. 2014;9(7):e100409.
40. Corona G, Monami M, Rastrelli G, et al. Testosterone and metabolic syndrome: a meta-analysis study. J Sex Med. 2011;8(1):272–83.
41. Garcia-Cruz E, Leibar-Tamayo A, Romero J, et al. Metabolic syndrome in men with low testosterone levels: relationship with cardiovascular risk factors and comorbidities and with erectile dysfunction. J Sex Med. 2013;10(10):2529–38.
42. Laaksonen DE, Niskanen L, Punnonen K, et al. Sex hormones, inflammation and the metabolic syndrome: a population-based study. Eur J Endocrinol. 2003;149(6):601–8.
43. Grosman H, Rosales M, Fabre B, et al. Association between testosterone levels and the metabolic syndrome in adult men. Aging Male. 2014;17(3):161–5.
44. Ebrahimi F, Christ-Crain M. Metabolic syndrome and hypogonadism - two peas in a pod. Swiss Med Wkly. 2016;146:w14283.
45. Neugarten J, Acharya A, Silbiger SR. Effect of gender on the progression of nondiabetic renal disease: a meta-analysis. J Am Soc Nephrol. 2000;11(2):319–29.
46. Jafar TH, Schmid CH, Stark PC, et al. The rate of progression of renal disease may not be slower in women compared with men: a patient-level meta-analysis. Nephrol Dial Transplant. 2003;18(10):2047–53.
47. Hall YN, Fuentes EF, Chertow GM, Olson JL. Race/ethnicity and disease severity in IgA nephropathy. BMC Nephrol. 2004;5:10.
48. Terada N, Arai Y, Kinukawa N, Yoshimura K, Terai A. Risk factors for renal cysts. BJU Int. 2004;93(9):1300–2.
49. Donadio JV Jr, Torres VE, Velosa JA, et al. Idiopathic membranous nephropathy: the natural history of untreated patients. Kidney Int. 1988;33(3):708–15.
50. Sandberg K. Mechanisms underlying sex differences in progressive renal disease. Gend Med. 2008;5(1):10–23.
51. Khoury S, Yarows SA, O'Brien TK, Sowers JR. Ambulatory blood pressure monitoring in a nonacademic setting. Effects of age and sex. Am J Hypertens. 1992;5(9):616–23.
52. Kimura N, Mizokami A, Oonuma T, Sasano H, Nagura H. Immunocytochemical localization of androgen receptor with polyclonal antibody in paraffin-embedded human tissues. J Histochem Cytochem. 1993;41(5):671–8.
53. Reckelhoff JF, Samsell L, Dey R, Racusen L, Baylis C. The effect of aging on glomerular hemodynamics in the rat. Am J Kidney Dis. 1992;20(1):70–5.
54. Reckelhoff JF, Zhang H, Granger JP. Testosterone exacerbates hypertension and reduces pressure-natriuresis in male spontaneously hypertensive rats. Hypertension. 1998;31(1 Pt 2):435–9.
55. Reckelhoff JF, Zhang H, Srivastava K, Granger JP. Gender differences in hypertension in spontaneously hypertensive rats: role of androgens and androgen receptor. Hypertension. 1999;34(4 Pt 2):920–3.
56. Fortepiani LA, Yanes L, Zhang H, Racusen LC, Reckelhoff JF. Role of androgens in mediating renal injury in aging SHR. Hypertension. 2003;42(5):952–5.
57. Baylis C. Age-dependent glomerular damage in the rat. Dissociation between glomerular injury and both glomerular hypertension and hypertrophy. Male gender as a primary risk factor. J Clin Invest. 1994;94(5):1823–9.
58. Metcalfe PD, Leslie JA, Campbell MT, Meldrum DR, Hile KL, Meldrum KK. Testosterone exacerbates obstructive renal injury by stimulating TNF-alpha production and increasing proapoptotic and profibrotic signaling. Am J Physiol Endocrinol Metab. 2008;294(2):E435–43.
59. Chen YF, Naftilan AJ, Oparil S. Androgen-dependent angiotensinogen and renin messenger RNA expression in hypertensive rats. Hypertension. 1992;19(5):456–63.
60. Ellison KE, Ingelfinger JR, Pivor M, Dzau VJ. Androgen regulation of rat renal angiotensinogen messenger RNA expression. J Clin Invest. 1989;83(6):1941–5.
61. Alexander BT, Cockrell KL, Rinewalt AN, Herrington JN, Granger JP. Enhanced renal expression of preproendothelin mRNA during chronic

angiotensin II hypertension. Am J Physiol Regul Integr Comp Physiol. 2001;280(5):R1388–92.
62. Reckelhoff JF, Yanes LL, Iliescu R, Fortepiani LA, Granger JP. Testosterone supplementation in aging men and women: possible impact on cardiovascular-renal disease. Am J Physiol Renal Physiol. 2005;289(5):F941–8.
63. Dousdampanis P, Trigka K, Fourtounas C, Bargman JM. Role of testosterone in the pathogenesis, progression, prognosis and comorbidity of men with chronic kidney disease. Ther Apher Dial. 2014;18(3):220–30.
64. Karakitsos D, Patrianakos AP, De Groot E, et al. Androgen deficiency and endothelial dysfunction in men with end-stage kidney disease receiving maintenance hemodialysis. Am J Nephrol. 2006;26(6):536–43.
65. Gungor O, Kircelli F, Carrero JJ, et al. Endogenous testosterone and mortality in male hemodialysis patients: is it the result of aging? Clin J Am Soc Nephrol. 2010;5(11):2018–23.
66. Kyriazis J, Tzanakis I, Stylianou K, et al. Low serum testosterone, arterial stiffness and mortality in male haemodialysis patients. Nephrol Dial Transplant. 2011;26(9):2971–7.
67. Haring R, Nauck M, Volzke H, et al. Low serum testosterone is associated with increased mortality in men with stage 3 or greater nephropathy. Am J Nephrol. 2011;33(3):209–17.
68. Shoskes DA, Kerr H, Askar M, Goldfarb DA, Schold J. Low testosterone at time of transplantation is independently associated with poor patient and graft survival in male renal transplant recipients. J Urol. 2014;192(4):1168–71.
69. Deb P, Gupta SK, Godbole MM. Effects of short-term testosterone replacement on areal bone mineral density and bone turnover in young hypogonadal males. Indian J Endocrinol Metab. 2012;16(6):947–51.
70. Snyder PJ, Kopperdahl DL, Stephens-Shields AJ, et al. Effect of testosterone treatment on volumetric bone density and strength in older men with low testosterone: a controlled clinical trial. JAMA Intern Med. 2017;177(4):471–9.
71. Rix M, Andreassen H, Eskildsen P, Langdahl B, Olgaard K. Bone mineral density and biochemical markers of bone turnover in patients with predialysis chronic renal failure. Kidney Int. 1999;56(3):1084–93.
72. Stehman-Breen CO, Sherrard DJ, Alem AM, et al. Risk factors for hip fracture among patients with end-stage renal disease. Kidney Int. 2000;58(5):2200–5.
73. Alem AM, Sherrard DJ, Gillen DL, et al. Increased risk of hip fracture among patients with end-stage renal disease. Kidney Int. 2000;58(1):396–9.
74. Lindberg JS, Moe SM. Osteoporosis in end-state renal disease. Semin Nephrol. 1999;19(2):115–22.
75. Ishani A, Paudel M, Taylor BC, et al. Renal function and rate of hip bone loss in older men: the Osteoporotic Fractures in Men Study. Osteoporos Int. 2008;19(11):1549–56.
76. Bhasin S, Cunningham GR, Hayes FJ, et al. Testosterone therapy in men with androgen deficiency syndromes: an Endocrine Society clinical practice guideline. J Clin Endocrinol Metab. 2010;95(6):2536–59.
77. Travison TG, Vesper HW, Orwoll E, et al. Harmonized reference ranges for circulating testosterone levels in men of four cohort studies in the United States and Europe. J Clin Endocrinol Metab. 2017;102(4):1161–73.
78. Sikaris K, McLachlan RI, Kazlauskas R, de Kretser D, Holden CA, Handelsman DJ. Reproductive hormone reference intervals for healthy fertile young men: evaluation of automated platform assays. J Clin Endocrinol Metab. 2005;90(11):5928–36.
79. Boyce MJ, Baisley KJ, Clark EV, Warrington SJ. Are published normal ranges of serum testosterone too high? Results of a cross-sectional survey of serum testosterone and luteinizing hormone in healthy men. BJU Int. 2004;94(6):881–5.
80. Wang C, Catlin DH, Demers LM, Starcevic B, Swerdloff RS. Measurement of total serum testosterone in adult men: comparison of current laboratory methods versus liquid chromatography-tandem mass spectrometry. J Clin Endocrinol Metab. 2004;89(2):534–43.
81. Rosner W, Auchus RJ, Azziz R, Sluss PM, Raff H. Position statement: utility, limitations, and pitfalls in measuring testosterone: an Endocrine Society position statement. J Clin Endocrinol Metab. 2007;92(2):405–13.
82. Vermeulen A, Verdonck L, Kaufman JM. A critical evaluation of simple methods for the estimation of free testosterone in serum. J Clin Endocrinol Metab. 1999;84(10):3666–72.
83. Zakharov MN, Bhasin S, Travison TG, et al. A multi-step, dynamic allosteric model of testosterone's binding to sex hormone binding globulin. Mol Cell Endocrinol. 2015;399:190–200.
84. Sherman FP. Impotence in patients with chronic renal failure on dialysis: its frequency and etiology. Fertil Steril. 1975;26(3):221–3.
85. Carrero JJ, Stenvinkel P. The vulnerable man: impact of testosterone deficiency on the uraemic phenotype. Nephrol Dial Transplant. 2012;27(11):4030–41.
86. Chauveau P, Moreau K, Lasseur C, Fouque D, Combe C, Aparicio M. [Sarcopenia or uremic myopathy in CKD patients]. Nephrol Ther. 2016;12(2):71–5.
87. Lim VS, Ikizler TA, Raj DS, Flanigan MJ. Does hemodialysis increase protein breakdown? Dissociation between whole-body amino acid turnover and regional muscle kinetics. J Am Soc Nephrol. 2005;16(4):862–8.
88. Ikizler TA, Pupim LB, Brouillette JR, et al. Hemodialysis stimulates muscle and whole body protein loss and alters substrate oxidation. Am J Physiol Endocrinol Metab. 2002;282(1):E107–16.
89. Raj DS, Dominic EA, Wolfe R, et al. Coordinated increase in albumin, fibrinogen, and muscle protein

synthesis during hemodialysis: role of cytokines. Am J Physiol Endocrinol Metab. 2004;286(4):E658–64.
90. Pupim LB, Majchrzak KM, Flakoll PJ, Ikizler TA. Intradialytic oral nutrition improves protein homeostasis in chronic hemodialysis patients with deranged nutritional status. J Am Soc Nephrol. 2006;17(11):3149–57.
91. Cigarran S, Pousa M, Castro MJ, et al. Endogenous testosterone, muscle strength, and fat-free mass in men with chronic kidney disease. J Ren Nutr. 2013;23(5):e89–95.
92. Johansen KL. Testosterone metabolism and replacement therapy in patients with end-stage renal disease. Semin Dial. 2004;17(3):202–8.
93. Johansen KL. Treatment of hypogonadism in men with chronic kidney disease. Adv Chronic Kidney Dis. 2004;11(4):348–56.
94. Johansen KL, Mulligan K, Schambelan M. Anabolic effects of nandrolone decanoate in patients receiving dialysis: a randomized controlled trial. JAMA. 1999;281(14):1275–81.
95. Eiam-Ong S, Buranaosot S, Wathanavaha A, Pansin P. Nutritional effect of nandrolone decanoate in predialysis patients with chronic kidney disease. J Ren Nutr. 2007;17(3):173–8.
96. Shin YS, You JH, Cha JS, Park JK. The relationship between serum total testosterone and free testosterone levels with serum hemoglobin and hematocrit levels: a study in 1221 men. Aging Male. 2016;19(4):209–14.
97. Bachman E, Travison TG, Basaria S, et al. Testosterone induces erythrocytosis via increased erythropoietin and suppressed hepcidin: evidence for a new erythropoietin/hemoglobin set point. J Gerontol A Biol Sci Med Sci. 2014;69(6):725–35.
98. Krabbe S, Christensen T, Worm J, Christiansen C, Transbol I. Relationship between haemoglobin and serum testosterone in normal children and adolescents and in boys with delayed puberty. Acta Paediatr Scand. 1978;67(5):655–8.
99. Thomsen K, Riis B, Krabbe S, Christiansen C. Testosterone regulates the haemoglobin concentration in male puberty. Acta Paediatr Scand. 1986;75(5):793–6.
100. Murphy WG. The sex difference in haemoglobin levels in adults – mechanisms, causes, and consequences. Blood Rev. 2014;28(2):41–7.
101. Grossmann M, Zajac JD. Hematological changes during androgen deprivation therapy. Asian J Androl. 2012;14(2):187–92.
102. Kraft D. Long-term treatment of renal anaemia with mesterolone (author's transl). Dtsch Med Wochenschr. 1980;105(23):830–2.
103. Yang Q, Abudou M, Xie XS, Wu T. Androgens for the anaemia of chronic kidney disease in adults. Cochrane Database Syst Rev. 2014;(10):CD006881.
104. Maggio M, Snyder PJ, Ceda GP, et al. Is the haematopoietic effect of testosterone mediated by erythropoietin? The results of a clinical trial in older men. Andrology. 2013;1(1):24–8.
105. Perretta M, Valladares L, Romero C, et al. Hormone action on the cell nucleus: effect of erythropoietin and testosterone on bone marrow. Arch Biol Med Exp (Santiago). 1976;10(1–3):35–40.
106. Ohlander SJ, Varghese B, Pastuszak AW. Erythrocytosis following testosterone therapy. Sex Med Rev. 2018;6(1):77–85.
107. Paul AK, Latif ZA, Iqbal S, Amin F, Shefin SM, Ashrafuzzaman SM. Androgen versus erythropoietin for the treatment of anaemia of pre-dialysis chronic kidney disease. Mymensingh Med J. 2012;21(1):125–8.
108. Gaughan WJ, Liss KA, Dunn SR, et al. A 6-month study of low-dose recombinant human erythropoietin alone and in combination with androgens for the treatment of anemia in chronic hemodialysis patients. Am J Kidney Dis. 1997;30(4):495–500.
109. Teruel JL, Aguilera A, Marcen R, Navarro Antolin J, Garcia Otero G, Ortuno J. Androgen therapy for anaemia of chronic renal failure. Indications in the erythropoietin era. Scand J Urol Nephrol. 1996;30(5):403–8.
110. Carrero JJ, Barany P, Yilmaz MI, et al. Testosterone deficiency is a cause of anaemia and reduced responsiveness to erythropoiesis-stimulating agents in men with chronic kidney disease. Nephrol Dial Transplant. 2012;27(2):709–15.
111. Akbari A, Clase CM, Acott P, et al. Canadian Society of Nephrology commentary on the KDIGO clinical practice guideline for CKD evaluation and management. Am J Kidney Dis. 2015;65(2):177–205.
112. Martin-Malo A, Benito P, Castillo D, et al. Effect of clomiphene citrate on hormonal profile in male hemodialysis and kidney transplant patients. Nephron. 1993;63(4):390–4.
113. Lim VS, Fang VS. Restoration of plasma testosterone levels in uremic men with clomiphene citrate. J Clin Endocrinol Metab. 1976;43(6):1370–7.
114. Tokgoz B, Utas C, Dogukan A, et al. Effects of long-term erythropoietin therapy on the hypothalamo-pituitary-testicular axis in male CAPD patients. Perit Dial Int. 2001;21(5):448–54.
115. Anantharaman P, Schmidt RJ. Sexual function in chronic kidney disease. Adv Chronic Kidney Dis. 2007;14(2):119–25.
116. Wu SC, Lin SL, Jeng FR. Influence of erythropoietin treatment on gonadotropic hormone levels and sexual function in male uremic patients. Scand J Urol Nephrol. 2001;35(2):136–40.
117. Suzuki H, Murakami M, Ichihara A, Saruta T. Alterations in sex hormones and sexual function of patients with renal failure treated with recombinant human erythropoietin. Nihon Jinzo Gakkai Shi. 1992;34(1):79–84.
118. Ramirez G, Butcher DE, Newton JL, Brueggemeyer CD, Moon J, Gomez-Sanchez C. Bromocriptine and the hypothalamic hypophyseal function in patients with chronic renal failure on chronic hemodialysis. Am J Kidney Dis. 1985;6(2):111–8.

119. Vircburger MI, Prelevic GM, Peric LA, Knezevic J, Djukanovic L. Testosterone levels after bromocriptine treatment in patients undergoing long-term hemodialysis. J Androl. 1985;6(2):113–6.
120. Stegmayr B, Skogstrom K. Hyperprolactinaemia and testosterone production. Observations in 2 men on long-term dialysis. Horm Res. 1985;21(4):224–8.
121. Bundschu HD, Rager K, Heller S, et al. Effects of long term HCG administration on testicular function in hemodialysis patients (author's transl). Klin Wochenschr. 1976;54(21):1039–46.
122. Karagiannis A, Harsoulis F. Gonadal dysfunction in systemic diseases. Eur J Endocrinol. 2005;152(4):501–13.
123. Zhang R, Alper B, Simon E, Florman S, Slakey D. Management of metabolic bone disease in kidney transplant recipients. Am J Med Sci. 2008;335(2):120–5.
124. Burgos FJ, Pascual J, Gomez V, Orofino L, Liano F, Ortuno J. Effect of kidney transplantation and cyclosporine treatment on male sexual performance and hormonal profile: a prospective study. Transplant Proc. 1997;29(1–2):227–8.
125. Chu SH, Tay SK, Chiang YJ, et al. Male sexual performance and hormonal studies in uremic patients and renal transplant recipients. Transplant Proc. 1998;30(7):3062–3.
126. Akbari F, Alavi M, Esteghamati A, et al. Effect of renal transplantation on sperm quality and sex hormone levels. BJU Int. 2003;92(3):281–3.
127. Tsujimura A, Matsumiya K, Tsuboniwa N, et al. Effect of renal transplantation on sexual function. Arch Androl. 2002;48(6):467–74.
128. Hamdi SM, Walschaerts M, Bujan L, Rostaing L, Kamar N. A prospective study in male recipients of kidney transplantation reveals divergent patterns for inhibin B and testosterone secretions. Basic Clin Androl. 2014;24:11.
129. Malavaud B, Rostaing L, Rischmann P, Sarramon JP, Durand D. High prevalence of erectile dysfunction after renal transplantation. Transplantation. 2000;69(10):2121–4.
130. Rebollo P, Ortega F, Valdes C, et al. Factors associated with erectile dysfunction in male kidney transplant recipients. Int J Impot Res. 2003;15(6):433–8.
131. Lee S, Coco M, Greenstein SM, Schechner RS, Tellis VA, Glicklich DG. The effect of sirolimus on sex hormone levels of male renal transplant recipients. Clin Transpl. 2005;19(2):162–7.
132. Huyghe E, Zairi A, Nohra J, Kamar N, Plante P, Rostaing L. Gonadal impact of target of rapamycin inhibitors (sirolimus and everolimus) in male patients: an overview. Transpl Int. 2007;20(4):305–11.
133. Zuber J, Anglicheau D, Elie C, et al. Sirolimus may reduce fertility in male renal transplant recipients. Am J Transplant. 2008;8(7):1471–9.

Amenorrhea and Estrogen Disorders in Women with Kidney Disease

10

Kavitha Vellanki and Holly Kramer

Introduction

Disorders of the reproductive system are common in women with chronic kidney disease (CKD). Women constitute approximately 42% of all adults receiving maintenance dialysis with the total number of women receiving dialysis in the United States increasing from 233,066 in 2008 to 293,936 in 2014 [1]. Health issues unique to women with CKD remain the most under-recognized and neglected patient problems in clinical practice. Data on reproductive hormonal control in women with CKD but not yet on dialysis remain limited and conflicting, with the variability of results partly attributed to the cyclical nature of hormonal control and temporal differences in the measurement of hormone levels in conjunction with the menstrual cycle. While the exact pathophysiology of the disrupted reproductive cycle in women with CKD lacks details regarding the cellular mechanisms, hormonal imbalance leading to low estrogen levels plays a key role (Table 10.1). Hence, understanding the menstrual cycle and hypothalamic-pituitary-gonadal axis of sex hormone production in normal women is crucial to differentiate the changes noted in women with kidney disease.

Menstrual Cycle and Hypothalamic-Pituitary-Gonadal Function in a Normal Woman

The menstrual cycle in a normal woman results in the release of a single mature oocyte, the process referred to as ovulation (Fig. 10.1). This generally occurs midway through the cycle and is facilitated by cyclical changes in various hormones. A menstrual cycle, which typically lasts 28 days, is normally composed of three phases: a follicular or proliferative phase beginning with the onset of menses, an ovulatory phase when ovulation occurs, and a luteal or secretory phase which ends at the onset of menses. Pulsatile hypothalamic release of gonadotropin-releasing hormone (GnRH) regulates secretion of follicle-stimulating hormone (FSH) and luteinizing hormone (LH) from the pituitary gland. During the

Table 10.1 Estrogen-related disorders in women with kidney disease

1. Menstrual disorders: amenorrhea 30–40%
2. Premature ovarian failure
3. Early menopause
4. Sexual dysfunction
5. Infertility

K. Vellanki (✉)
Department of Medicine, Loyola University Medical Center, Maywood, IL, USA
e-mail: kpotluri@lumc.edu

H. Kramer
Department of Public Health Sciences and Medicine, Loyola University Medical Center, Maywood, IL, USA
e-mail: hkramer@lumc.edu

C. M. Rhee et al. (eds.), *Endocrine Disorders in Kidney Disease*,
https://doi.org/10.1007/978-3-319-97765-2_10

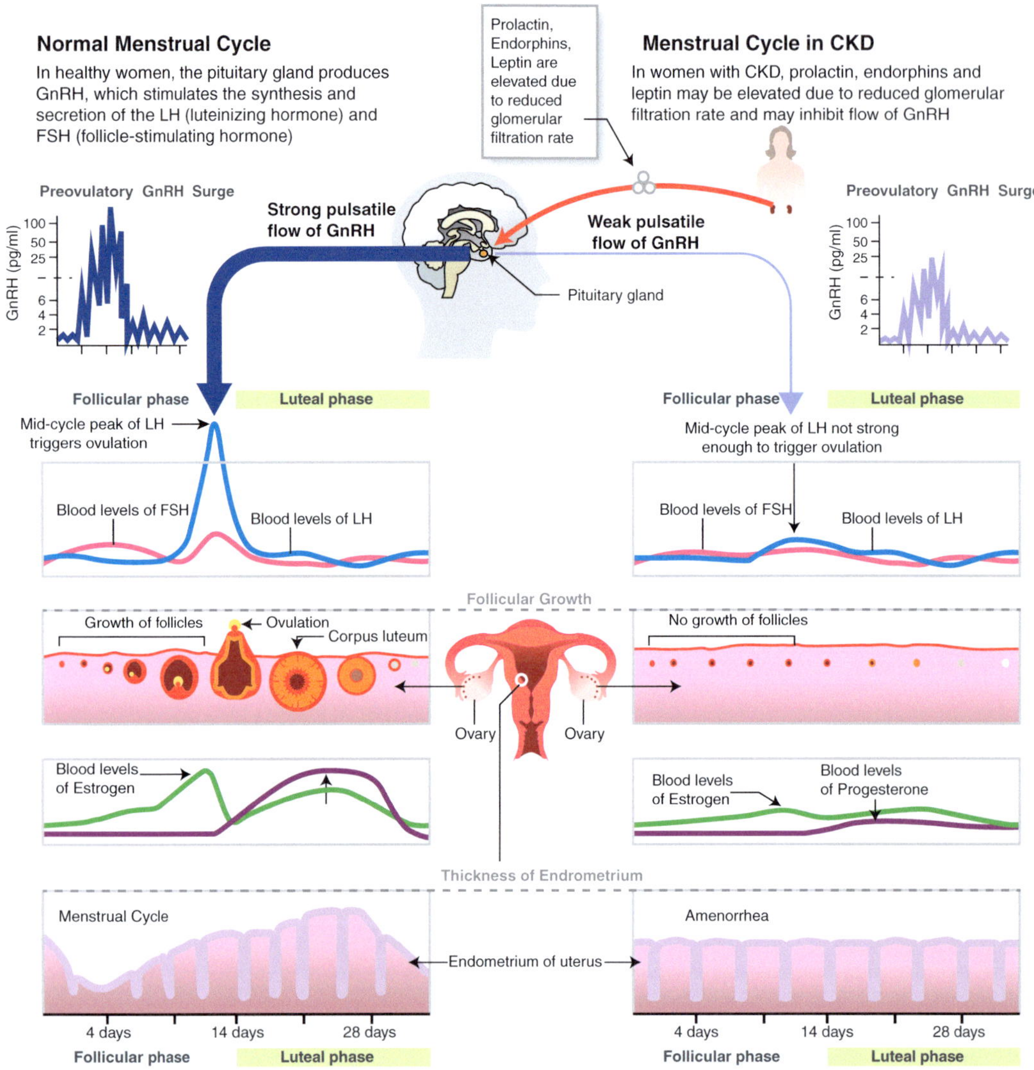

Fig. 10.1 Cartoon depicting the menstrual cycle in healthy women and in women with chronic kidney disease (CKD). Gonadotropin-releasing hormone is released by the hypothalamus, and the strength of the pulsatile frequency is reduced in CKD. This figure depicts absent ovulation and amenorrhea, but not all premenopausal women with CKD have amenorrhea

follicular phase, FSH secretion stimulates the development of follicles, which increase estradiol production. The increase in estradiol levels stimulates proliferation of the uterine endometrium in preparation for the oocyte released by the dominant follicle. Then LH increases slowly through the follicular phase with estradiol levels peaking approximately 7–8 days before the preovulatory surge of LH. During the latter part of the follicular phase, a rapid increase in the pulsatile cycling of GnRH from the hypothalamus leads to marked increases in LH and FSH release from the anterior pituitary gland. This surge in LH culminates in ovulation. Androgens and progestins also increase a few days before the LH surge, with progesterone increasing just before the LH surge. This increase in progesterone primes the endometrial surface. After release of the ovum, the follicle becomes the corpus luteum and continues to secrete progesterone and estrogen. In the absence of a fertilized oocyte, both estrogen and progesterone secretions gradually decrease toward the end of luteal phase with subsequent sloughing of the endometrium by the end of luteal phase with normal menses beginning approximately 14 days after the LH surge.

Menstrual Cycle and Hypothalamic-Pituitary-Gonadal Function in Woman with CKD

Menstrual irregularities occur frequently among premenopausal women with CKD with wide variability reported for menstrual cycle patterns. Amenorrhea (absence of menstrual cycles) that is often defined as primary (absence of menstrual cycles by 15 years of age) or secondary (absence of menstrual cycles for more than 3 months with previously regular menstrual cycles or absence of menses for more than 6 months with previously irregular menstrual cycles) occurs in 30–40% of premenopausal women with CKD. The major menstrual abnormality in women with CKD is anovulation leading to amenorrhea. Approximately one-third of premenopausal women with CKD report amenorrhea with less than 40% reporting regular menstrual cycles [2–6]. Irregular menstrual patterns ranging from occasional spotting to frequent dysfunctional uterine bleeding thus occur in up to 30% of premenopausal women with CKD.

The disruption of the hypothalamic-pituitary-gonadal axis at various levels is hypothesized to be the major factor leading to low estrogen levels and menstrual irregularities in premenopausal women with CKD. Elevated levels of hormones like prolactin, endorphins, and leptin in CKD have been implicated in the downregulation of hypothalamic secretion of GnRH in women with CKD (Fig. 10.2). The weakened pulsatile frequency of the hypothalamic secretion of GnRH abrogates the surge in LH and FSH release from the anterior pituitary gland (Fig. 10.1). While FSH and LH levels are normal to high in the early follicular phase in premenopausal women with

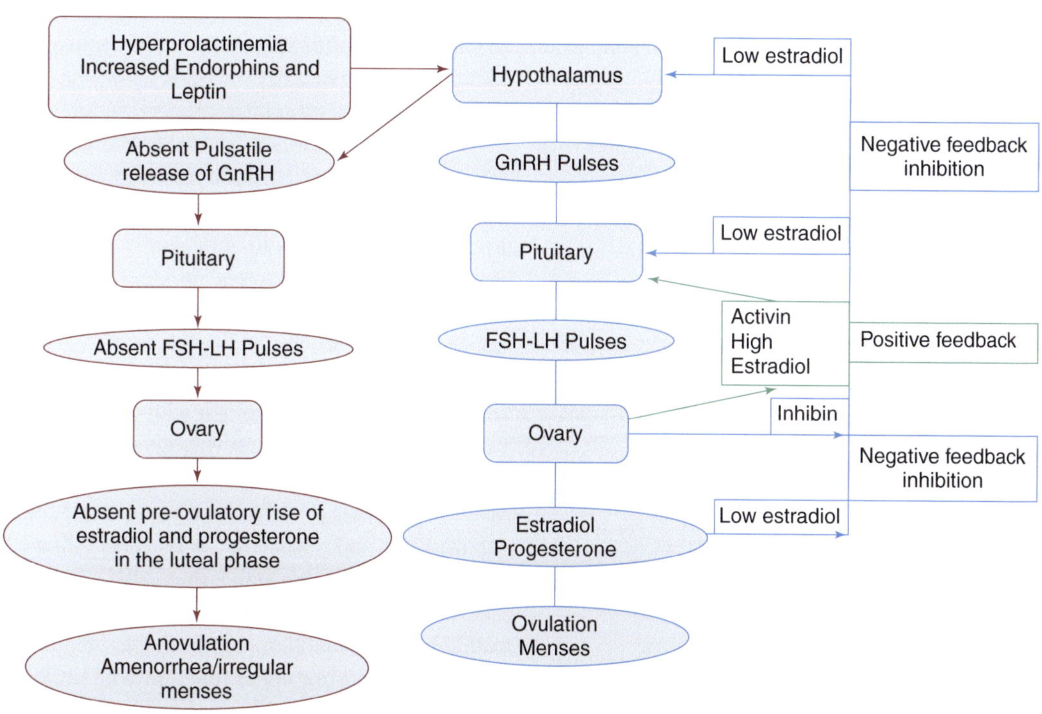

Fig. 10.2 Hypothalamic-pituitary axis in normal women and women with kidney disease. Red outline, kidney disease; blue outline, normal hormonal pattern

CKD, the lack of an FSH and LH surge leads to anovulation. In addition, progesterone, which helps prime the endometrium, does not rise normally during the latter half of the menstrual cycle. This abnormal pattern in LH, FSH, and progesterone levels throughout the menstrual cycle all contributes to menstrual irregularities in premenopausal women with CKD (Table 10.2).

The primary defect for anovulation in premenopausal women with CKD resides in the hypothalamus as demonstrated by a normal response to clomiphene administration in this population. Clomiphene citrate blocks the negative feedback of estrogen on GnRH release by the hypothalamus by competitively blocking estrogen from binding to hypothalamic receptors [7]. Clomiphene then increases the cyclical frequency and amount of GnRH release by the hypothalamus, and this surge in GnRH stimulates release of FSH and LH from the anterior pituitary. In one of the only studies to examine clomiphene for restoration of menstrual cycles in women receiving maintenance dialysis, a 5-day course of clomiphene citrate resulted in 64% fractional increase in LH, 36% fractional increase in estradiol, and 25% increase in FSH in premenopausal uremic women [8]. To date, no study has examined whether long-term clomiphene use improves sexual and reproductive function in women with CKD.

Table 10.2 Hormonal changes during menstrual cycle in normal women and women with CKD

Menstrual cycle	Normal women	Women with CKD
Pulsatile release of GnRH	Present	Absent
Estradiol secretion in luteal phase	Increased	Absent
Cyclical release of FSH	Present	Absent
LH surge prior to ovulation	Present	Absent
Increase in progesterone	Present	Absent
Ovulation	Present	Absent (especially in uremia)
Endometrial priming by progesterone	Present	Absent
Menstrual cycles	Normal	Irregular to absent

Reasons for a defect at the hypothalamus are numerous and include elevated levels of prolactin, endorphins, and leptin, which all inhibit GnRH release from the hypothalamus. Elevated prolactin levels are common in women with CKD, and the rise in prolactin levels parallels the decline in glomerular filtration rate [9–11]. Increased autonomous production of prolactin from the anterior pituitary gland and decreased metabolic clearance of prolactin are thought to be the most probable causes of elevated prolactin levels in women with CKD [12]. Elevated prolactin levels are thought to be more common in women than men with CKD, but the cause for the female predilection remains unknown. In normal women, secretion of prolactin by the pituitary gland is stimulated by thyrotropin-releasing hormone and estrogen. For example, both pregnancy and use of estrogen-based oral contraceptives are associated with elevated prolactin levels. While the kidneys play a minor role in prolactin catabolism in persons with normal kidney function, women with CKD may have a 30% reduction in prolactin clearance leading to elevated prolactin levels [12]. Because prolactin levels return toward normal after successful kidney transplantation, menses generally resumes with time after kidney transplantation [10].

Hyperprolactinemia suppresses pulsatile release of GnRH from the hypothalamus which in turn affects FSH and LH secretion by the pituitary gland. This leads to anovulatory cycles and irregular menstrual cycles in premenopausal women with CKD. Resumption of ovulation and normalization of prolactin levels have been reported with administration of bromocriptine (dopamine agonist) in women with chronic renal failure [8]. Bromocriptine was given at 2.5 mg every 12 h to three women on dialysis with elevated prolactin levels. While prolactin levels normalized in all women, only one showed restoration of normal menstrual cycles. Therapeutic use of dopamine agonists in idiopathic hyperprolactinemia is well documented in women with normal renal function with an 80% response rate reported with bromocriptine use [13]. However, data on the clinical utility of dopamine agonist use in premenopausal women with CKD and irregular menstrual cycles or amenorrhea remain limited [10].

Due to reduced clearance, plasma endorphin levels are also elevated in women with CKD. Similar to prolactin, endorphins block the pulsatile hypothalamic surge of GnRH leading to loss of the cyclic release of FSH and LH and ovulation in premenopausal women with CKD. Leptin, a small peptide hormone produced by adipose tissue, is also predominantly cleared by the kidneys. Increased circulating levels of leptin in CKD [14] may also be a contributing factor for loss of the pulsatile hypothalamic secretion of GnRH. Leptin influences the maturation of the GnRH pulse generator [15] which facilitates the rapid pulsatile release of large amounts of GnRH leading to LH surge.

As a result of the abnormal cycling of LH, estradiol, and progesterone, altered endometrial morphology is present in majority of women receiving maintenance dialysis with normal endometrial morphology seen in only 20% [5]. In a study that included 40 women aged 18–45 years receiving maintenance dialysis with endometrial biopsies, 30 out of the 40 women reported menses, but only half of the women stated the menses was normal [5]. The other ten women with CKD reported complete absence of menses, and these women with amenorrhea had substantially lower mean estradiol levels (25.6 ± 21.8 pg/ml) compared to mean estradiol levels in the entire group of 40 women (63.9 ± 42.1 pg/ml) or compared to 20 women with normal menses (95.9 ± 43.1 pg/ml). Among women with normal or abnormal menses, 36% had proliferative changes in the endometrium, while atrophic changes were noted among the ten women with amenorrhea. The reactivity of the endometrium to circulating estrogens appears to remain intact in premenopausal women with amenorrhea receiving maintenance dialysis. In a small study of 13 dialysis-dependent women aged 18–45 years with amenorrhea and serum estradiol levels <30 pg/ml, treatment with transdermal estradiol with cyclic addition of norethisterone acetate, a steroidal progestin, induced regular menses [16].

Kidney transplantation generally restores normal menstrual cycles and fertility [17–21]. Resumption of menses occurs in over 70% of premenopausal women with amenorrhea after receiving a kidney transplant, but it may take over 6 months before menses returns and cycles normally [17, 22]. The restoration of menstrual cycles after kidney transplantation varies by several factors including age at CKD onset and at kidney transplantation, hemoglobin level at the time of discharge after kidney transplantation, and dose of prednisone at 6 and 12 months posttransplant.

Premature Ovarian Failure (POF)

The diagnosis of premature ovarian failure is made when women less than age 40 years have abnormal menstrual cycles with FSH concentrations in the range of normal values for a menopausal state [23]. The risk of POF in women with CKD exposed to cyclophosphamide may be up to 14-fold higher compared to the general population. Women with glomerulonephritis (GN) are especially at risk for POF because this group can have both CKD and prior cyclophosphamide exposure. In a review of the effects of cyclophosphamide on ovarian function in women with breast cancer, the average cumulative dose among women experiencing amenorrhea was 5.2 g for women in their 40s and 9.3 g for women in their 30s [24]. Age at the time of exposure and cumulative dose of cyclophosphamide are both major determinants of POF risk. While the suggested cumulative cyclophosphamide dose for induction therapy for lupus nephritis has decreased to 3 g since publication of the 2002 Euro-Lupus clinical trial [25], the cumulative cyclophosphamide dose among women with non-lupus forms of GN continues to be high because 1.5–2 mg/kg/day of oral cyclophosphamide is generally used for several months for treatment [26, 27]. Regardless of the limited data on POF risk, premenopausal women must be counseled about the potential risks of POF before initiating cyclophosphamide treatment and the potential benefits of blocking ovulation with use of GnRH analogs [28–30]. The mechanism by which GnRH analogs prevent ovarian dysfunction remains controversial but includes the induction of a prepubertal state by shutting down the hypothalamic-pituitary axis and the reduction of ovarian blood flow with minimization of the amount of cyclophosphamide reaching the ovaries [28]. A meta-analysis on ovarian preservation by GnRH agonists during chemotherapy for cancers and autoimmune diseases reported a 68% increased rate of preserved ovarian function compared to women not receiving GnRH agonists [28]. However, GnRH agonists are not routinely used in clinical practice in premenopausal women receiving cyclophosphamide for kidney disorders.

Infertility in Women with CKD

Fertility rates decline proportionately with increasing CKD severity, but the stage of CKD at which infertility becomes irreversible has not been determined and may vary substantially by patient demographics. Estimates of the frequency of conception in patients receiving maintenance dialysis range from 0.3% to 1.8% per year [31–33]. However, the frequency of conception in women receiving nocturnal maintenance dialysis is much higher at 15.6% per year [34]. Fertility improves markedly and quickly after transplantation. In a study that looked into hormonal profile and fertility rates pre- and posttransplantation in premenopausal women, LH, FSH, and estradiol levels normalized within 3–4 months after a successful kidney transplant with conception achieved in 17 out of 21 women in a 3-year follow-up period [21].

Restoration of fertility in women with moderate to severe non-dialysis-dependent CKD should be discouraged due to risk of progression of kidney disease. Data suggest that pregnancy may incite a rapid decline in glomerular filtration rate if the prepregnancy serum creatinine exceeds >1.4 mg/dl and/or urine protein excretion exceeds 1 g/day [35, 36]. The mechanisms by which pregnancy accelerates progression in moderate to severe kidney disease have not been fully elucidated. Whatever the mechanisms, pregnancy exerts adverse effects only after a critical amount of glomerular filtration rate has been lost regardless of the cause of CKD. Once glomerular filtration rate declines during pregnancy, it cannot be predictably reversed, even by terminating the pregnancy via abortion or early delivery. Women with a pregnancy-related decline in glomerular filtration rate account for approximately 20% of women dialyzed during pregnancy [37]. Thus, women with stage 3–5 non-dialysis-dependent CKD should be encouraged to use birth control. Should a woman with CKD conceive, the complications of pregnancy are higher than the risks associated with use of oral contraceptive pills if low-dose estrogen pills are used. Studies suggest that oral contraceptives increase the risk of CKD progression [38–41], which may be related to increased blood pressure. Use of oral contraceptive drugs may also increase the risk of thromboembolic disease, and this may be heightened in patients with CKD. The venous thrombosis risks cannot be avoided with use of the transdermal patch. Intrauterine devices (IUD) may provide a useful alternative to oral contraceptives, which hold important risks for women with CKD. The infection risks associated with IUDs for contraception do not appear to differ in women with CKD or in women who have received a kidney transplant compared to healthy women [42, 43]. The efficacy for pregnancy prevention with an IUD also does not appear to be affected by CKD status.

Early Menopause and Long-Term Effects

Menopause, the permanent cessation of menstrual periods, is clinically defined as the absence of menstrual cycles for at least 12 months. The median age of menopause onset in the general population is 51–52 years, but menopause onset in women with CKD begins at younger ages. The overall median age of menopause onset in women with CKD is about 4 years earlier than healthy women and ranges from 46 to 48 years [3, 44]. Early menopause in CKD likely occurs due to disruption of the hypothalamic-pituitary axis and from accelerated aging of the ovaries from uremic toxins, oxidative stress, and persistent inflammation. In healthy women, menopause is frequently accompanied by vasomotor symptoms called "hot flashes" or brief periods of intense warmth over the upper body with sweating and often followed by a chill sensation. Hot flashes are usually transient with less than 15% of women in the general population reporting hot flashes to occur for more than 5 years after menopause onset. Women with CKD, however, are less likely to have such vasomotor symptoms than women without CKD. In the 17,891 postmenopausal women from the multiethnic Women's Health Initiative cohort, women with mild CKD (mean eGFR of 50 ml/min) had younger age of menopause onset but were also less likely to self-report hot flashes and night sweats than women without CKD (38% vs 46%, respectively). Although the frequency of severe vasomotor symptoms was not significantly different between women with and without CKD, persistent symptoms were less frequent in women with CKD [45].

In the general population, the risk of cardiovascular disease (CVD) increases after menopause, possibly due to loss of the protective effect of estrogen on lipids and vascular function. Accelerated CVD is characteristic of CKD, and the impact of earlier onset of menopause for CVD risk remains poorly explored. Menopausal women receiving dialysis have very low estradiol levels compared to the general population. Low estradiol levels are associated with Caucasian race and low body mass index but not with dialysis-related factors [46].

Bone loss during the perimenopausal period has been well documented in the general population [47–49] but not among women with CKD. The CKD state is usually accompanied by abnormal levels of calcium, phosphate, parathyroid hormone, and vitamin D, all of which may adversely impact bone health [50]. Disentangling osteoporosis due to menopause from the broad spectrum of metabolic disorders in CKD which may impact bone volume and density is extremely important as management differs vastly. The World Health Organization (WHO) classification of bone mineral density (BMD) measured by dual-energy X-ray absorptiometry (DEXA) was based upon fracture risk in healthy postmenopausal women [51]. Thus, the WHO classification system for normal and abnormal BMD for assessment of fracture risk may not be applicable to women with CKD. DEXA measures attenuation through the body tissues of low doses of X-ray, allowing the determination of both bone mineral content and bone area, from which BMD is calculated. Among patients receiving maintenance hemodialysis, DEXA of the lumbar spine often overestimates BMD as measured by bone histomorphometry [52]. Hence, existing guidelines do not recommend the routine testing of BMD in patients with CKD stages 3–5 [53]. Bone biopsy remains the gold standard for establishing the type and degree of any bone disease in patients with stage 3–5 CKD, since no single or combination of biochemical parameters accurately diagnose bone disease among this population. Due to the invasive nature and need for histologic expertise, bone biopsies in patients with CKD are rarely performed in clinical practice which markedly limits interventions for bone disease. While bisphosphonates are routinely used for management of osteoporosis in adults without CKD, their use is generally contraindicated when eGFR is below 30 mL/min/1.73 m^2. Pooled data from post hoc and retrospective analyses report increased BMD and decreased vertebral fracture risk with alendronate and risedronate in women with non-dialysis-dependent CKD compared to a placebo [54, 55]. However, to date, no clinical trial has examined bisphosphonate therapy and bone fractures risk specifically in postmenopausal women with CKD.

The effect of the selective estrogen receptor mediator raloxifene on BMD has been reported in women with CKD in several studies. In a post hoc analysis of a randomized placebo controlled trial of raloxifene in 7705 postmenopausal women with osteoporosis, the effects of raloxifene on the rate of BMD loss, fracture incidence, and adverse events by CKD stage were examined over a 3-year follow-up period [56]. Women were randomly assigned to receive one of the three treatments: placebo or 60 and 120 mg/day of oral raloxifene. All women were also given daily supplements of 500 mg of calcium and 400 to 600 IU of vitamin

D. The study population was divided into three groups based on creatinine clearance (CrCl) using the Cockcroft-Gault formula (CrCl <45, 45 to 59, and ≥60 ml/min). Raloxifene increased BMD at both the hip and the spine and reduced the risk for vertebral fractures among individuals with and without CKD. Hip BMD showed the greatest increase with raloxifene use among women with mild to moderate CKD. However, only 55 women in the study had CKD stage 4 or higher. In addition, women with elevated parathyroid levels and low vitamin D levels, common among adults with CKD, were excluded from the study. A significant improvement in BMD at the lumbosacral spine with 1-year use of raloxifene has been reported in postmenopausal women receiving maintenance hemodialysis [57]. Raloxifene is not generally used in women with CKD. Long-term clinical studies are needed to accurately characterize the benefits vs. risks in postmenopausal women with CKD.

Hormone Replacement Therapy in CKD

The use of hormone replacement therapy in postmenopausal women in the general population has become increasingly controversial. The Women's Health Initiative clinical trial of estrogen with progestin was stopped early after a mean of 5.6 years of follow-up. While use of estrogen plus progestin was associated with significantly lower rates of hip fracture and colorectal cancer, incidence of venous thromboembolic events, stroke, and breast cancer were all higher in the estrogen plus progestin group vs. placebo [58]. The Heart and Estrogen/Progestin Replacement Study (HERS), a large randomized trial that included menopausal women with established cardiovascular disease, excluded women receiving maintenance dialysis, but 40% of the study population had non-dialysis-dependent CKD [59]. No significant difference in cardiovascular outcomes or mortality was noted between the treatment and placebo arms regardless of baseline CKD status [60]. In 1 small study of 11 postmenopausal women on dialysis, treatment with estradiol for 5 weeks increased high-density lipoprotein cholesterol and ApoA-I levels with no change in total cholesterol, low-density lipoprotein cholesterol levels, lipoprotein A, or triglycerides [61] levels. Currently, given the imbalance between risks and benefits of estrogen replacement therapy, hormone replacement therapy (HRT) with estrogen is recommended for treatment of menopausal symptoms alone and not for primary or secondary prevention of cardiovascular events as per the North American Menopause Society guidelines [62, 63]. Treatment for menopausal symptoms should also be brief and individualized to patient symptoms.

Sexual Dysfunction in Women with CKD

Sexual dysfunction is highly prevalent in women with advanced CKD, especially among women receiving maintenance dialysis. Vaginal symptoms such as dryness and itching and dyspareunia may occur in one out of every three women during the menopause transition alone. However, after several years of menopause, vaginal symptoms will occur in one out of every two women [64]. Vaginal symptoms appear to be more common in menopausal women with CKD compared to the general population, but studies are very limited [65]. The low estrogen levels in women with CKD lead to low libido, vaginal dryness, dyspareunia, and overall reduced sexual function. In a multinational cross-sectional study on women receiving maintenance hemodialysis, 84% of 659 women reported sexual dysfunction [66]. Sexual dysfunction was independently associated with age, depressive symptoms, less education, menopause, diabetes, and diuretic therapy. While sexual dysfunction is common among women with CKD, most affected women will never discuss this problem with health-care providers [67]. The prevalence of sexual problems is lower among adults with a successful kidney transplant but higher compared to the general population [19, 68].

Currently, there are no tested treatment options for sexual dysfunction in women with

CKD. Estrogen supplementation may improve sexual function in those patients with low circulating estradiol levels, but studies addressing the safety and efficacy of estrogen supplementation in women with CKD are lacking. Prior to the Women's Health Initiative trial, HRT use was 20% among women receiving maintenance dialysis [44] but is likely lower now given the results of the Women's Health Initiative [58].

Because CKD alters the pharmacokinetics of estrogen metabolism, the dose of estrogen replacement should be reduced by 50–70% in patients with CKD as renal failure alters the pharmacokinetics of estrogen [69]. Estrone sulfate, an estrogen conjugate derived from the liver, is the primary circulating form of estrogen in humans. Plasma concentrations of estradiol, estrone, and estrone sulfate are dependent on the menopausal state [11]. Levels of estradiol and estrone are lower in postmenopausal than premenopausal women with the ratio of estradiol to estrone being lower as well. The concentrations of estrone exceed estradiol concentrations when estrogen is administered orally, whereas the opposite occurs with the transdermal administration of estrogen. Both estrone and estradiol, being highly protein bound, are not removed by hemodialysis [70]. Free and total estradiol plasma concentrations are overall low in women with ESRD [46], but levels of both free and total estradiol levels will be higher after an oral estradiol dose in this population compared to healthy women. Measuring estradiol levels in women with CKD receiving HRT may be of value as their side effects could be related to high blood concentrations of estradiol and not the actual dose.

In conclusion, kidney disease is associated with a disruption of the hypothalamic-pituitary axis leading to irregular menses, low estrogen levels, and reduced fertility. Due to the cardiovascular and thrombosis risks associated with oral contraceptives, intrauterine devices may be a safe alternative for contraception in premenopausal women with CKD. Menopause onset is usually 5 years earlier in women with CKD, but vasomotor symptoms accompanying the menopausal transition appear to be less severe in this population. Counseling women on reasons for menstrual irregularities, infertility, sexual dysfunction, and early menopause may help women with CKD cope with these symptoms which greatly impact their overall quality of life [71].

References

1. U S Renal Data System. USRDS 2013 annual data report: Atlas of chronic kidney disease and end-stage renal disease in the United States. Bethesda: National Institutes of Health, National Institute of Diabetes and Digestive and Kidney Diseases
2. Anantharaman P, Schmidt RJ. Sexual function in chronic kidney disease. Adv Chronic Kidney Dis. 2007;14(2):119–25.
3. Holley JL, Schmidt RJ, Bender FH, Dumler F, Schiff M. Gynecologic and reproductive issues in women on dialysis. Am J Kidney Dis. 1997;29(5):685–90.
4. Lim VS. Reproductive function in patients with renal insufficiency. Am J Kidney Dis. 1987;9(4):363–7.
5. Matuszkiewicz-Rowinska J, Skorzewska K, Radowicki S, Niemczyk S, Sokalski A, Przedlacki J, Puka J, Switalski M, Wardyn K, Grochowski J, et al. Endometrial morphology and pituitary-gonadal axis dysfunction in women of reproductive age undergoing chronic haemodialysis – a multicentre study. Nephrol Dial Transplant. 2004;19(8):2074–7.
6. Morley JE, Distiller LA, Epstein S, Katz M, Gold C, Sagel J, Kaye G, Pokroy M, Kalk J. Menstrual disturbances in chronic renal failure. Horm Metab Res. 1979;11(1):68–72.
7. Holley JL. The hypothalamic-pituitary axis in men and women with chronic kidney disease. Adv Chronic Kidney Dis. 2004;11(4):337–41.
8. Lim VS, Henriquez C, Sievertsen G, Frohman LA. Ovarian function in chronic renal failure: evidence suggesting hypothalamic anovulation. Ann Intern Med. 1980;93(1):21–7.
9. Ginsburg ES, Owen WF. Reproductive endocrinology and pregnancy in women on hemodialysis. Semin Dial. 1993;6:105–16.
10. Lim VS, Kathpalia SC, Frohman LA. Hyperprolactinemia and impaired pituitary response to suppression and stimulation in chronic renal failure: reversal after transplantation. J Clin Endocrinol Metab. 1979;48(1):101–7.
11. Holley JL, Schmidt RJ. Changes in fertility and hormone replacement therapy in kidney disease. Adv Chronic Kidney Dis. 2013;20(3):240–5.
12. Sievertsen GD, Lim VS, Nakawatase C, Frohman LA. Metabolic clearance and secretion rates of human prolactin in normal subjects and in patients with chronic renal failure. J Clin Endocrinol Metab. 1980;50(5):846–52.
13. Vance ML, Evans WS, Thorner MO. Drugs five years later. Bromocriptine. Ann Intern Med. 1984;100(1):78–91.

14. Wolf G, Chen S, Han DC, Ziyadeh FN. Leptin and renal disease. Am J Kidney Dis. 2002;39(1):1–11.
15. Singh AK, Raed A, Kari J. Endocrine complications of chronic kidney disease. In: Kimmel PL, Rosenberg ME, editors. Chronic kidney diseases. 1st ed. New York: Academic; 2014. p. 310–9.
16. Matuszkiewicz-Rowinska J, Skorzewska K, Radowicki S, Sokalski A, Przedlacki J, Niemczyk S, Wlodarczyk D, Puka J, Switalski M. The benefits of hormone replacement therapy in pre-menopausal women with oestrogen deficiency on haemodialysis. Nephrol Dial Transplant. 1999;14(5):1238–43.
17. Filocamo MT, Zanazzi M, Li Marzi V, Lombardi G, Del Popolo G, Mancini G, Salvadori M, Nicita G. Sexual dysfunction in women during dialysis and after renal transplantation. J Sex Med. 2009;6(11):3125–31.
18. Ghazizadeh S, Lessan-Pezeshki M, Mahdavi M, Razeghi E, Seifi S. Menstrual problems among kidney transplant recipients. Transplant Proc. 2003;35(7):2720–1.
19. Noohi S, Azar M, Behzadi AH, Barbati ME, Haghshenas A, Amoozgar B, Karami M. Comparison of sexual function in females receiving haemodialysis and after renal transplantation. J Ren Care. 2010;36(4):212–7.
20. Pertuz W, Castaneda DA, Rincon O, Lozano E. Sexual dysfunction in patients with chronic renal disease: does it improve with renal transplantation? Transplant Proc. 2014;46(9):3021–6.
21. Wang GC, Zheng JH, Xu LG, Min ZL, Zhu YH, Qi J, Duan QL. Measurements of serum pituitary-gonadal hormones and investigation of sexual and reproductive functions in kidney transplant recipients. Int J Nephrol. 2010;2010:612126.
22. Kim JH, Chun CJ, Kang CM, Kwak JY. Kidney transplantation and menstrual changes. Transplant Proc. 1998;30(7):3057–9.
23. Taylor AE, Adams JM, Mulder JE, Martin KA, Sluss PM, Crowley WF Jr. A randomized, controlled trial of estradiol replacement therapy in women with hypergonadotropic amenorrhea. J Clin Endocrinol Metab. 1996;81(10):3615–21.
24. Koyama H, Wada T, Nishizawa Y, Iwanaga T, Aoki Y. Cyclophosphamide-induced ovarian failure and its therapeutic significance in patients with breast cancer. Cancer. 1977;39(4):1403–9.
25. Houssiau FA, Vasconcelos C, D'Cruz D, Sebastiani GD, Garrido Ed Ede R, Danieli MG, Abramovicz D, Blockmans D, Mathieu A, Direskeneli H, et al. Immunosuppressive therapy in lupus nephritis: the euro-lupus nephritis trial, a randomized trial of low-dose versus high-dose intravenous cyclophosphamide. Arthritis Rheum. 2002;46(8):2121–31.
26. Jayne D, Rasmussen N, Andrassy K, Bacon P, Tervaert JW, Dadoniene J, Ekstrand A, Gaskin G, Gregorini G, de Groot K, et al. A randomized trial of maintenance therapy for vasculitis associated with antineutrophil cytoplasmic autoantibodies. N Engl J Med. 2003;349(1):36–44.
27. Rauen T, Eitner F, Fitzner C, Sommerer C, Zeier M, Otte B, Panzer U, Peters H, Benck U, Mertens PR, et al. Intensive supportive care plus immunosuppression in IgA nephropathy. N Engl J Med. 2015;373(23):2225–36.
28. Clowse ME, Behera MA, Anders CK, Copland S, Coffman CJ, Leppert PC, Bastian LA. Ovarian preservation by GnRH agonists during chemotherapy: a meta-analysis. J Womens Health (Larchmt). 2009;18(3):311–9.
29. Munhoz RR, Pereira AA, Sasse AD, Hoff PM, Traina TA, Hudis CA, Marques RJ. Gonadotropin-releasing hormone agonists for ovarian function preservation in premenopausal women undergoing chemotherapy for early-stage breast cancer: a systematic review and meta-analysis. JAMA Oncol. 2016;2(1):65–73.
30. Somers EC, Marder W, Christman GM, Ognenovski V, McCune WJ. Use of a gonadotropin-releasing hormone analog for protection against premature ovarian failure during cyclophosphamide therapy in women with severe lupus. Arthritis Rheum. 2005;52(9):2761–7.
31. Hou S. Daily dialysis in pregnancy. Hemodial Int. 2004;8(2):167–71.
32. Souqiyyeh MZ, Huraib SO, Saleh AG, Aswad S. Pregnancy in chronic hemodialysis patients in the Kingdom of Saudi Arabia. Am J Kidney Dis. 1992;19(3):235–8.
33. Toma H, Tanabe K, Tokumoto T, Kobayashi C, Yagisawa T. Pregnancy in women receiving renal dialysis or transplantation in Japan: a nationwide survey. Nephrol Dial Transplant. 1999;14(6):1511–6.
34. Barua M, Hladunewich M, Keunen J, Pierratos A, McFarlane P, Sood M, Chan CT. Successful pregnancies on nocturnal home hemodialysis. Clin J Am Soc Nephrol. 2008;3(2):392–6.
35. Imbasciati E, Gregorini G, Cabiddu G, Gammaro L, Ambroso G, Del Giudice A, Ravani P. Pregnancy in CKD stages 3 to 5: fetal and maternal outcomes. Am J Kidney Dis. 2007;49(6):753–62.
36. Jones DC, Hayslett JP. Outcome of pregnancy in women with moderate or severe renal insufficiency. N Engl J Med. 1996;335(4):226–32.
37. Okundaye I, Abrinko P, Hou S. Registry of pregnancy in dialysis patients. Am J Kidney Dis. 1998;31(5):766–73.
38. Ahmed SB, Hovind P, Parving HH, Rossing P, Price DA, Laffel LM, Lansang MC, Stevanovic R, Fisher ND, Hollenberg NK. Oral contraceptives, angiotensin-dependent renal vasoconstriction, and risk of diabetic nephropathy. Diabetes Care. 2005;28(8):1988–94.
39. Baillargeon JP, McClish DK, Essah PA, Nestler JE. Association between the current use of low-dose oral contraceptives and cardiovascular arterial disease: a meta-analysis. J Clin Endocrinol Metab. 2005;90(7):3863–70.
40. Fung MM, Poddar S, Bettencourt R, Jassal SK, Barrett-Connor E. A cross-sectional and 10-year prospective study of postmenopausal estrogen therapy and blood pressure, renal function, and albuminuria: the Rancho Bernardo Study. Menopause. 2011;18(6):629–37.
41. Monster TB, Janssen WM, de Jong PE, de Jong-van den Berg LT, Prevention of Renal and Vascular End Stage Disease Study Group. Oral contraceptive use and hormone replacement therapy are asso-

ciated with microalbuminuria. Arch Intern Med. 2001;161(16):2000–5.
42. Krajewski CM, Geetha D, Gomez-Lobo V. Contraceptive options for women with a history of solid-organ transplantation. Transplantation. 2013;95(10):1183–6.
43. Ramhendar T, Byrne P. Use of the levonorgestrel-releasing intrauterine system in renal transplant recipients: a retrospective case review. Contraception. 2012;86(3):288–9.
44. Kramer HM, Curhan GC, Singh A, Hemodialysis and Estrogen Levels in Postmenopausal Patients Study Group. Permanent cessation of menses and postmenopausal hormone use in dialysis-dependent women: the HELP study. Am J Kidney Dis. 2003;41(3):643–50.
45. Cheung KL, Stefanick ML, Allison MA, LeBlanc ES, Vitolins MZ, Shara N, Chertow GM, Winkelmayer WC, Kurella Tamura M. Menopausal symptoms in women with chronic kidney disease. Menopause. 2015;22(9):1006–11.
46. Kramer HM, Curhan G, Singh A, HELP Study Group. Hemodialysis and estrogen levels in postmenopausal (HELP) patients: the multicenter HELP study. Am J Kidney Dis. 2003;41(6):1240–6.
47. Greendale GA, Sowers M, Han W, Huang MH, Finkelstein JS, Crandall CJ, Lee JS, Karlamangla AS. Bone mineral density loss in relation to the final menstrual period in a multiethnic cohort: results from the study of women's health across the nation (SWAN). J Bone Miner Res. 2012;27(1):111–8.
48. Slemenda C, Longcope C, Peacock M, Hui S, Johnston CC. Sex steroids, bone mass, and bone loss. A prospective study of pre-, peri-, and postmenopausal women. J Clin Invest. 1996;97(1):14–21.
49. Sowers M, Crutchfield M, Bandekar R, Randolph JF, Shapiro B, Schork MA, Jannausch M. Bone mineral density and its change in pre-and perimenopausal white women: the Michigan Bone Health Study. J Bone Miner Res. 1998;13(7):1134–40.
50. Moe S, Drueke T, Cunningham J, Goodman W, Martin K, Olgaard K, Ott S, Sprague S, Lameire N, Eknoyan G, et al. Definition, evaluation, and classification of renal osteodystrophy: a position statement from Kidney Disease: Improving Global Outcomes (KDIGO). Kidney Int. 2006;69(11):1945–53.
51. Cummings SR, Bates D, Black DM. Clinical use of bone densitometry: scientific review. JAMA. 2002;288(15):1889–97.
52. Sherman ME, Shepherd J, Frassetto L, Genant HK. Discrepancy in results between spine and hip scans of a woman with end stage renal disease. J Clin Densitom. 2002;5(1):95–8.
53. Kidney Disease: Improving Global Outcomes (KDIGO) CKD-MBD Work Group. KDIGO clinical practice guideline for the diagnosis, evaluation, prevention, and treatment of chronic kidney disease-mineral and bone disorder (CKD-MBD). Kidney Int. 2009;113:S1–S130.
54. Jamal SA, Bauer DC, Ensrud KE, Cauley JA, Hochberg M, Ishani A, Cummings SR. Alendronate treatment in women with normal to severely impaired renal function: an analysis of the fracture intervention trial. J Bone Miner Res. 2007;22(4):503–8.
55. Miller PD, Roux C, Boonen S, Barton IP, Dunlap LE, Burgio DE. Safety and efficacy of risedronate in patients with age-related reduced renal function as estimated by the Cockcroft and Gault method: a pooled analysis of nine clinical trials. J Bone Miner Res. 2005;20(12):2105–15.
56. Ishani A, Blackwell T, Jamal SA, Cummings SR, Ensrud KE, MORE Investigators. The effect of raloxifene treatment in postmenopausal women with CKD. J Am Soc Nephrol. 2008;19(7):1430–8.
57. Hernandez E, Valera R, Alonzo E, Bajares-Lilue M, Carlini R, Capriles F, Martinis R, Bellorin-Font E, Weisinger JR. Effects of raloxifene on bone metabolism and serum lipids in postmenopausal women on chronic hemodialysis. Kidney Int. 2003;63(6):2269–74.
58. Rossouw JE, Anderson GL, Prentice RL, LaCroix AZ, Kooperberg C, Stefanick ML, Jackson RD, Beresford SA, Howard BV, Johnson KC, et al. Risks and benefits of estrogen plus progestin in healthy postmenopausal women: principal results from the women's health initiative randomized controlled trial. JAMA. 2002;288(3):321–33.
59. Grady D, Applegate W, Bush T, Furberg C, Riggs B, Hulley SB. Heart and estrogen/progestin replacement study (HERS): design, methods, and baseline characteristics. Control Clin Trials. 1998;19(4):314–35.
60. Shlipak MG, Simon JA, Grady D, Lin F, Wenger NK, Furberg CD, Heart and Estrogen/Progestin Replacement Study (HERS) Investigators. Renal insufficiency and cardiovascular events in postmenopausal women with coronary heart disease. J Am Coll Cardiol. 2001;38(3):705–11.
61. Ginsburg ES, Walsh B, Greenberg L, Price D, Chertow GM, Owen WF Jr. Effects of estrogen replacement therapy on the lipoprotein profile in postmenopausal women with ESRD. Kidney Int. 1998;54(4):1344–50.
62. North American Menopause Society. The 2012 hormone therapy position statement of: the North American Menopause Society. Menopause. 2012;19(3):257–71.
63. Stuenkel CA, Davis SR, Gompel A, Lumsden MA, Murad MH, Pinkerton JV, Santen RJ. Treatment of symptoms of the menopause: an endocrine society clinical practice guideline. J Clin Endocrinol Metab. 2015;100(11):3975–4011.
64. Grady D. Clinical practice. Management of menopausal symptoms. N Engl J Med. 2006;355(22):2338–47.
65. Navaneethan SD, Vecchio M, Johnson DW, Saglimbene V, Graziano G, Pellegrini F, Lucisano G, Craig JC, Ruospo M, Gentile G, et al. Prevalence and correlates of self-reported sexual dysfunction in CKD: a meta-analysis of observational studies. Am J Kidney Dis. 2010;56(4):670–85.
66. Strippoli GF, Collaborative Depression and Sexual Dysfunction (CDS) in Hemodialysis Working Group, Vecchio M, Palmer S, De Berardis G, Craig J, Lucisano

G, Johnson D, Pellegrini F, Nicolucci A, et al. Sexual dysfunction in women with ESRD requiring hemodialysis. Clin J Am Soc Nephrol. 2012;7(6):974–81.
67. Seethala S, Hess R, Bossola M, Unruh ML, Weisbord SD. Sexual function in women receiving maintenance dialysis. Hemodial Int. 2010;14(1):55–60.
68. Diemont WL, Vruggink PA, Meuleman EJ, Doesburg WH, Lemmens WA, Berden JH. Sexual dysfunction after renal replacement therapy. Am J Kidney Dis. 2000;35(5):845–51.
69. Ginsburg ES, Owen WF, Jr GLM, Shea BF, Lazarus JM, Walsh BW. Estrogen absorption and metabolism in postmenopausal women with end-stage renal disease. J Clin Endocrinol Metab. 1996;81(12):4414–7.
70. Anderson GD, Odegard PS. Pharmacokinetics of estrogen and progesterone in chronic kidney disease. Adv Chronic Kidney Dis. 2004;11(4):357–60.
71. Holley JL, Reddy SS. Pregnancy and CKD: lessons on communication from patients. Am J Kidney Dis. 2015;66(6):936–8.

11 Pregnancy in Kidney Disease

Madeleine V. Pahl

Introduction

Chronic kidney disease (CKD) has become a healthcare epidemic with increasing incidence and prevalence rates reported internationally. It is estimated that approximately 3% of childbearing age women have CKD stages 1–2 [1] and 0.7% have CKD stages 3–5 [2]. Although clear substantiating data is not available, it is the perception of the renal community that pregnancy rates in CKD, particularly in the later stages of CKD, are less frequent when compared to the rates seen in women with normal renal function, and when pregnancies occur, they are considered to be high risk. The magnitude of this risk, however, is unclear. This is because most studies are small, do not report important outcomes such as maternal death, and include pregnancies in women with varying degrees of CKD caused by different underlying disorders with different comorbidities. This chapter will review the maternal and fetal outcomes in varying stages of CKD including end-stage kidney disease (ESKD) and discuss management recommendations.

M. V. Pahl
Division of Nephrology and Hypertension, University of California Irvine School of Medicine, Orange, CA, USA
e-mail: mpahl@uci.edu

Fertility in CKD

Fertility is reduced in women with CKD. This is likely the result of altered complex pathophysiologic changes compounded by the effects of medications, depression, fatigue, anemia, and the overall burden of chronic illness on libido. Gonadal abnormalities that result in menstrual irregularities and anovulatory cycles are common, occur early in the course of CKD, and tend to progress after the initiation of renal replacement therapy. Menstrual cycle irregularities begin in women with CKD stages 4–5 and progress to amenorrhea at glomerular filtration rates (GFR) below 5 ml/min [3–5]. In fact, 42–75% of pre-menopausal women maintained on hemodialysis report menstrual irregularities [6]. Although the pathogenesis of these abnormalities has not been extensively studied, altered hypothalamic-pituitary-ovarian hormonal patterns have been reported in women with CKD. In pre-menopausal, normal women, a sustained midcycle increase in estradiol causes an increase in hypothalamic secretion of gonadotropin-releasing hormone (GnRH). This hormone then stimulates the pituitary gland to increase luteinizing hormone (LH) secretion, and, with an increase in progesterone and estradiol, follicle-stimulating hormone (FSH) levels increase. This hormonal pattern leads to normal ovulation and menstruation. In the majority of pre-menopausal women with CKD, the positive feedback mechanism of

C. M. Rhee et al. (eds.), *Endocrine Disorders in Kidney Disease*,
https://doi.org/10.1007/978-3-319-97765-2_11

estradiol on the hypothalamus is blunted. The midcycle surge of LH and FSH is impaired, and reduction levels of progesterone are observed [7–9]. Estradiol levels may be normal in women with earlier stages of CKD in the follicular phase, but reduced midcycle peaks are observed [8]. By the late stages of CKD stage 5, women maintained on hemodialysis demonstrate extremely low estradiol levels [10]. Additionally, hyperprolactinemia is present in approximately 70% of women with CKD adding to the hormonal imbalances that can contribute to menstrual irregularities. This common abnormality is likely due to a combination of factors including reduced renal clearance, increased secretion by the anterior pituitary, and anterior pituitary resistance due to the downregulatory effects of dopamine [11, 12]. In addition to the menstrual abnormalities that result in infertility, menopause occurs at a younger age among women with CKD. The median age of menopause is 50–51 years in normal women but 47 years among women with CKD [13].

Anti-mullerian hormone (AMH) levels are currently used by infertility experts to determine ovarian reserve. AMH is a member of the transforming growth factor (TGF)-beta family that is expressed by the small preantral and early antral follicles of the ovary. AMH levels reflect the size of the follicle pool and are considered biomarkers of ovarian function. They gradually decline with age and are undetectable at menopause. In women with normal renal function, very low levels are associated with reduced ovarian reserve. A recent study of women with CKD revealed significantly lower serum AMH concentrations in regularly menstruating CKD women on hemodialysis when compared to healthy controls [14]. Interestingly, serum AMH concentration was higher in hemodialysis women with irregular menstrual cycles, similar to reports in the general population that identified increased serum AMH concentrations in women with irregular menses and polycystic ovaries syndrome or hyperandrogenism [15].

These abnormalities in the pituitary-gonadal hormones have been documented to improve 3–6 months after kidney transplantation [16] and after the conversion to intense, daily hemodialysis [17], suggesting they are reversible with improved management of CKD.

Pregnancy in CKD

Epidemiology

Rates of pregnancy in CKD are difficult to determine. There are no available studies that have systematically investigated this issue. However, most experts consider CKD a disorder that reduces fertility which results in reduced pregnancy rates. Additionally, given the maternal and fetal risks associated with CKD, many women may choose to avoid pregnancy. In spite of these observations, pregnancy is becoming more common in women with CKD [18]. Earlier studies reported prevalent rates of pregnancies from 0.1% to 1% [19], but recently, it has been estimated to be closer to 3% [1].

Maternal Outcomes

In women with CKD, pregnancy can result in a variety of maternal and fetal complications. This section will address the effects of pregnancy on the mother's underlying kidney disease and possible effects on morbidity and mortality.

The effect of pregnancy on renal function has been debated for decades, and several series have tried to address this issue. Most studies have noted that while renal function may decline as a result of the gestation in those with advanced CKD, in women with preserved renal function, pregnancy may have little effect on the course of the renal disease. When renal progression does occur, it is unclear whether these changes reflect the natural history of the underlying renal disease or the effects of the pregnancy. However, whether the clinical findings of increasing proteinuria and reduced GFR represent worsening of the underlying renal disorder or the development of pregnancy-associated complications, these risk factors need to be understood and addressed.

In women with CKD stages 1–2, pregnancy has been reported to result in progression of CKD in 0–10% of cases. Jungers et al. reported the effect of pregnancy in a group of 360 women with CKD and compared the outcomes of the 171 who became pregnant to those who did not conceive. An actuarial analyses of the data after a follow up period of up to 30 years revealed no differences in renal survival in those who became pregnant compared to those who did not. While pregnancy was not identified as a risk factor for progression to ESKD, the presence of hypertension was a major determinant [20]. Similarly, others have reported low rates of permanent decline in renal function in women with serum creatinine (Cr) < 1.4 mg/dl [21, 22]. Katz et al. reported increased hypertension in 23% and progression of proteinuria in 68% of 121 pregnancies in 89 women. Increases in serum Cr were seen in 16% but resolved postpartum in most cases. Follow-up of 3 months up to 23 years identified a permanent but minimal reduction of renal function in five women and progression to ESKD in five [22]. A recent meta-analysis of 8 cohort studies and 1268 combined cases of pregnant women with early stages of CKD further revealed little risk for progression of renal disease [23]. However, since most reported cases had preserved GFR complicated only with albuminuria, the findings appear applicable only to those women with normal baseline renal function, consistent with the previous reports.

The outcome appears to be different in women with moderate CKD. Jones et al. [24] reviewed the outcomes of 82 pregnancies in 67 women and noted that the mean serum Cr increased from 1.9 mg/dl in early pregnancy to 2.5 mg/dl in the third trimester. They observed pregnancy-related loss of renal function in 43%. In 10% of these cases, the pregnancy was associated with progression to ESKD 12 months postpartum with the highest risk among those with initial serum Cr of >2.0 mg/dl. In women with a serum Cr of >1.6 mg/dl, Bear et al. [25] reported a higher frequency in the decline of renal function when compared to those with serum Cr < 1.6 mg/dl. Hou et al. [26] noted increases in serum Cr of >1 mg/dl in 8 out of 23 pregnant women with moderate renal insufficiency during gestation and 6 months postpartum. Imbasciati et al. noted that 5 out of 18 pregnant women with creatinine clearance of <40 ml/min developed more rapid progression of their disease than expected during gestation or immediately postpartum [27]. More recently, these same authors reported their findings on a larger cohort of 49 women with preconception mean serum Cr 2.1 mg/dl and GFR of 35 ml/min. While the mean GFR dropped to 30 ml/min after delivery, the rate of GFR decrease did not change significantly from prepartum values. Factors that were associated with faster GFR loss and shorter time to dialysis therapy included the combination of a baseline GFR < 40 ml/min and proteinuria >1 g/day [2]. Piccoli et al. reported progression of CKD in 9.3% of her large cohort of pregnant women. Progression to a higher CKD stage and/or initiation of renal replacement therapy occurred in 7.6% of the cases with CKD stage 1 (28 out of 370 pregnancies), 12.6% of those with CKD stage 2 (33/87 pregnancies), 16.2% of those with CKD stage 3 (6/37 pregnancies), and 20% in those with CKD stages 4–5 (2/10 pregnancies). They reported one patient with pre-existing CKD stage 5 who went on to require dialysis during pregnancy [1]. Most recently, the same group compared pregnancy outcomes in 504 pregnancies in women with CKD to 836 low-risk pregnancies in women with normal renal function [28]. The authors reported risks of adverse outcomes increased across all stages of CKD. New-onset hypertension (HTN) was seen in increasing percentage of cases with progressive CKD (7.9% in CKD stage 1, 17.6% in CKD stage 2, 47.1% in CKD stage 3, 50% in CKD stages 4–5), and new-onset or doubling of proteinuria was noted in 20.5% of those with CKD stage 1, 37.9% in CKD stage 2, 86.5% in CKD stage 3, and in 70% of those with CKD stages 4–5. The median for follow-up time for renal events was 5 years (interquartile range, 5–14.7 years). There was an increasing trend that did not reach statistical significance in the occurrence of renal events between CKD pregnant women and those without pregnancy (OR, 0.96; 95% CI, 0.69–1.35). Subgroup analysis showed that publication year, sample size, follow-up years, type of primary disease, CKD classification, level of serum Cr at baseline, proteinuria, and level of systolic blood pressure did not modify the renal outcomes. In summary, most reports confirm that in women with CKD stages 1–2, pregnancy may have little effect on the progression of CKD, but with more advanced CKD, pregnancy carries a risk of reduction of renal function that can be irreversible.

The effects of CKD on pregnancy-related complications of HTN, proteinuria, and preeclampsia are more consistently reported. Most reports note that HTN and proteinuria are increased during pregnancy. However, whether this reflects progression of renal disease, the effect of the gestation, or the presence of superimposed preeclampsia is unclear. Preeclampsia rates are likely increased, particularly in women with advanced stages of CKD. However, a definitive diagnosis of preeclampsia can be difficult in this population, and thus rates may be subject to significant variability. The classic features of HTN and increasing proteinuria may reflect progression of renal disease and/or the effects of the gestation on renal parameters rather than the presence of superimposed preeclampsia. Thrombocytopenia and abnormal liver function tests may facilitate the diagnosis but are not always present in established cases. Some large observational studies have reported changes in blood pressures or progression of proteinuria rather than rates of preeclampsia. These complications are relatively common with increases in proteinuria being reported in approximately half of the cases and development of HTN in about one-quarter.

In a meta-analysis of 13 cohort studies, women with CKD were more likely to develop HTN, preeclampsia, eclampsia, or death [29]. The authors identified 312 adverse maternal events in 2682 pregnancies (weighted average of 11.5%) compared with 500 events in 26,149 pregnancies in normal healthy women (weighted average of 2%). Similarly, in a larger systematic review of 23 studies (14 with data for adverse pregnancy outcomes and 9 for renal outcomes) with 506,340 pregnancies, the authors confirmed that CKD had greater odds of preeclampsia (odds ratio of 10.36) particularly in those with nondiabetic nephropathy and proteinuria [23]. Interestingly, in a study that included renal biopsy data, only 7 out of 13 women with CKD that were clinically diagnosed with superimposed preeclampsia (including one diagnosed with eclampsia) had the characteristic glomerular lesions of preeclampsia, thus confirming the suspicion that the diagnosis of preeclampsia cannot be made with certainty in the face of CKD [22].

Cesarean section rates are not frequently reported but appear to be increased in women with CKD. Kendrick [30] noted a 33% increased odds of delivery by Cesarean section in a large American cohort of women with CKD when compared to those with normal renal function. An Italian group reported Cesarean sections in 54.8% of the women with CKD compared with a rate of 27.2% in normal women [28].

Although previous data suggested rates of maternal deaths may have been increased in pregnant women with CKD, a recent retrospective review of a large electronic health data system failed to confirm these findings [30]. The authors reviewed the outcomes of 778 pregnancies from women with CKD and compared them to 778 pregnancies in women without CKD. They noted no increases in hospital stays or maternal mortality.

Obstetrical and Fetal Outcomes

Many observational reports have reported adverse obstetric and fetal outcomes in pregnant women with varying stages of pre-dialysis CKD. Katz et al. reported on the outcomes of 121 pregnancies in women with CKD and noted that preterm delivery occurred in 20% and intrauterine growth retardation in 24%. Infant survival was reported to be 89% [22]. Most recently, Nevis et al. conducted a systematic review of 13 reports that included at least 5 pregnant women with CKD. Only five studies reported serum Cr levels which ranged from 0.8 to 4.61 mg/dl. There were 312 adverse maternal events among 2682 pregnancies in women with CKD (weighted average of 11.5%) compared with 500 events in 26,149 pregnancies in normal healthy women (weighted average of 2%). The risks for adverse fetal outcomes, such as premature births, intrauterine growth restriction, small for gestational age, neonatal mortality, stillbirths, and low birth weight were at least two times higher among the women with CKD. The frequency of preterm delivery was significantly higher among women with CKD (13 vs. 6%) with an odds ratio of 5.72. Intrauterine growth restriction was seen in 5% of those with CKD compared with none of the women with normal renal function, and small for gestational age babies were reported in 14% of women with CKD vs. 8% of normal women. The authors calculated an odds ratio for small for gestational age/low birth weight in CKD of 4.85. Stillbirths were also increased in women with CKD and reported in 5% of the pregnancies compared with 2% in those with normal renal function [29].

Using data from an integrated healthcare delivery system, Kendrick et al. identified 778 women with ICD-9 codes or National Kidney Foundation Kidney Disease Outcomes Quality Initiative definition for CKD (serum Cr > 1.2 mg/dl or proteinuria in the first trimester) and matched controls from a pool of 74,105 women. Compared with women without kidney disease, those with CKD had a 52% increased odds of preterm delivery with a twofold increase in infants with low birth weights. These infants had a 71% increased odds of admission to neonatal intensive care units or death [30].

General Management and Blood Pressure Control

Management of pregnant women with CKD requires a multidisciplinary approach that includes nephrologists and obstetricians experienced in high-risk pregnancies. Initial evaluation must include thorough review and discontinuation of prescribed medications that are known to affect the fetus such as inhibitors of the renin-angiotensin system, statins, and some immunosuppressive drugs such as cyclophosphamide and mycophenolate mofetil. Management should include increased frequency of prenatal visits, screening and treatment of asymptomatic bacteriuria, serial monitoring of renal function, fetal surveillance with ultrasound and fetal heart rate monitoring, and appropriate treatment of HTN. Management of blood pressure is critical as fetal survival is lower when HTN is uncontrolled [31] and is often directed by the nephrologist.

Antihypertensive regimens and blood pressure targets in pregnancy are much debated, and little information is available on women with CKD. Pharmacologic therapy needs include a consideration of the risk-benefit ratio of treatment with the potential effects of drug exposure on the fetus. While most antihypertensive agents cross the placenta, clinical experience with several agents has led to their common use in pregnancy. Alpha-methyldopa has been shown to be safe in pregnancy [32]. However, in women with CKD, this agent is often inadequate to control blood pressure at doses that are not associated with significant side effects. Labetalol, the dual alpha, beta-adrenergic blocker, is frequently used because of its rapid onset of action and tolerability. It has been shown to be safe in pregnancy [33] and has not been reported to cause neonatal bradycardia, intrauterine growth restriction, hypoglycemia, and the respiratory depression associated with beta-blockers. Among the calcium channel blockers, long-acting nifedipine has the widest use due to its minimal effect on uteroplacental flow, but non-dihydropyridine agents and amlodipine have also been used with limited data on their safety [34]. Oral hydralazine use as a single agent to control blood pressure has long been known to be poorly effective. It results in reflex tachycardia and fluid retention and thus should be added on to existing regimens. In a recent meta-analysis, hydralazine was shown to be associated with slightly higher adverse outcomes when compared with labetalol, yet it remains a commonly used agent [35]. Diuretic use is controversial, and most clinicians avoid their inclusion in blood pressure regimens because of concerns for intravascular volume depletion. In patients with CKD and volume overload however, judicious use of loop diuretics appears to be reasonable. Clonidine is not frequently used but has been successfully added to those who cannot achieve blood pressure control. Renin-angiotensin system inhibitors such as angiotensin-converting enzyme inhibitors and angiotensin receptor blockers are avoided during pregnancy because they can result in oligohydramnios, fetal kidney dysplasia, and pulmonary hypoplasia in the second and third trimester. First trimester use was thought to increase the risk of cardiovascular and neurologic abnormalities, but recent studies have questioned this association and suggest the anomalies are associated with the hypertension itself [36]. Some experts have suggested that the use of these renal protective agents be continued up to the first 8 weeks of pregnancy, but given the possible risks for fetal adverse events, it seems most reasonable at this time to transition to anti-HTN medications with safer safety profile pre-pregnancy during the planning stage or as soon as an unexpected pregnancy is detected.

There are no specific guidelines for blood pressure target levels in pregnant women with CKD. Earlier data suggested that in women with HTN, birth weight was slightly but significantly lowered in association with lowering of the mean arterial pressure with anti-HTN medications [37]. However, a recent meta-analysis of randomized studies of pregnant women with mild-moderate HTN and the results of the 2015 Control of Hypertension in Pregnancy Study (CHIPS) clinical trial that assigned pregnant women with HTN to diastolic blood pressures of 85 vs. 100 mmHg revealed that there were no adverse fetal effects in those with lower blood pressures and episodes of severe HTN were avoided in women that were targeted to have lower blood pressures [38, 39]. Additionally, in the CHIPS post hoc analysis, severe maternal HTN was shown to be associated with lower infant birth weight, more preterm delivery, preeclampsia, and features of HELLP [40]. Thus, while there is no data in women with CKD, given these recent findings, it seems reasonable to target blood pressure control in women with pre-dialysis CKD to similar levels.

Pregnancy in ESKD

Epidemiology

ESKD has been previously described as a very effective means of contraception. However, emerging data confirm the clinical impression that pregnancy rates are increasing. Since the first report of pregnancy in dialysis patients in 1965 [41], several series have reported rates that range from 1% to 7% of childbearing age women maintained of dialysis. The US Registry of Pregnancy in Dialysis Patients [42] reported rates of conception of 2.2% or 0.5% per year, and Souquiyyeh et al. noted rates as high as 7% in Saudi women [43]. The Australian-New Zealand Registry reported overall pregnancy rates of 2.0 per 1000 patient-years (PY) from 1966 to 2008 but confirmed increases in the 1996 to 2008 period (3.3/1000 PY vs. 0.54 and 0.67 in 1976–1985 and 1986–1995) [44]. It has been suggested that improved dialysis management that includes maximization of dialysis prescription and anemia, blood pressure, and volume control may be responsible for this observed increase. Dialysis modality may play a role in pregnancy rates. American women maintained on hemodialysis (HD) were noted to have rates of 2.2%, while those maintained on peritoneal dialysis (PD) had rates of 1.1% [42]. The reasons for these differences are unclear, but some have hypothesized that dialysate in the peritoneum may interfere with transport of the ovum to the fallopian tube and that episodes of peritonitis may result in adhesions that interfere with implantation.

Maternal Outcomes

Maternal outcomes in pregnant women maintained on dialysis appear to be relatively good. No clear evidence of increased maternal mortality has been noted, including in a recent survey of US experiences over the last 5 years [45]. Preeclampsia appears to be a very common complication but as previously discussed a particularly difficult challenge to diagnose. Shahir et al. [44] reported preeclampsia rates of 19.4% in Australian/New Zealand women, and Luders et al. noted similar rates (19.2%) in their Brazilian population [46]. Sachveda et al. reported rates of 44% obtained from the survey of 196 US nephrologists that cared for >187 pregnant women maintained on HD [45]. Given these alarming rates, clinicians must maintain a high level of suspicion and carefully monitor patients for the presence of symptoms and signs of preeclampsia including visual changes, blood pressure increases, presence of fetal growth restriction, altered placental Doppler blood flows, and laboratory changes suggestive of HELLP.

Cesarean section rates are not readily available in many of the large series reporting outcomes in pregnant dialysis patients, but many caring for these patients note increased rates when compared with normal women. Luders et al. reported an overall rate of 65% caesarian sections in their Brazilian population [46].

Obstetric and Fetal Outcomes

Initial reports of fetal outcomes in women maintained on HD were very poor. The registry report from the European Dialysis and Transplant Association noted a 23% live birth rate [47], and subsequent US and Saudi data was only minimally better with a live birth rates of 37% [43, 48]. More recently, live birth rates have significantly improved to levels of 87% [46]. From the earlier reports, it became clear that live birth rates were greater in those women who conceived with CKD stage 5 and then required dialysis when compared with those already maintained on dialysis when the pregnancy occurred, suggesting a beneficial role of residual renal function and enhanced clearance [42, 46]. A summary of fetal outcomes from series with >20 patients is shown in Table 11.1.

Additional obstetric complications common in this population include polyhydramnios, intrauterine growth retardation, preterm labor, and delivery of low birth weight infants. Polyhydramnios has been reported between 30 and 70% of cases and may respond to increased dialysis prescription [50]. Intrauterine growth retardation is commonly reported, and premature labor and small for gestational age babies are commonplace. Until recently, most babies born to women on dialysis had an average gestational age of 32 weeks and weights of <2000 g [51]. Similar findings of high rates of preterm deliveries were noted in large series reviews. The Australian/New Zealand data revealed 53.4% babies were born preterm, 65% had low birth weight (<2500 g), and 35% had very low birth weight (<1500 g) [44]. Although the cause of these complications is unclear, it appears that the biggest risk factor for these adverse outcomes appears to be preeclampsia and uncontrolled HTN. In the large Brazilian series, severely premature babies were almost entirely confined to women with preeclampsia, with only 3 of the 42 pregnancies without preeclampsia resulting in births before 30 weeks of gestation [46]. Most recently, a report from Toronto utilizing long, daily dialysis regimens describes six successful pregnancies with a mean gestational age of 36.2 weeks and a mean birth weight of 2417 g, suggesting dialysis prescription plays an important role in favorable outcomes [52].

Dialysis Management

Pregnant women maintained on dialysis require close, careful follow-up by a dedicated multispecialty team that includes nephrologists, high-risk obstetricians, experienced dialysis and obstetric nurses, and dietitians. Dialysis management includes close attention and appropriate adjust-

Table 11.1 Pregnancy rates and outcomes in hemodialysis and peritoneal dialysis in series with >20 cases

Site [reference]	Pregnancy rate (%)	Termination (%)	Losses (%)	Live births (%)
Europe 1980 [47]	–	39	38	23
Saudi Arabia 1992 [43]	7	0	63	37
USA 1994 [48]	1.5	8	52	37
USA 1998 [42]	2.2	11	46	42
Japan 1999 [49]	3.4	19	24	49
Australia/New Zealand 1996–2008 [44]		15	30	55
Brazil 2010 [46]	–	–	13	87

ment of the dialysis prescription including dose, type of dialyzers used, and adjustments of the dialysate composition. In addition, nephrologists must carefully adjust volume management, dry weight, blood pressure control, anemia management, mineral-bone metabolism parameters, nutrition requirements, and appropriate vitamin supplementation.

Increased duration and intensity of dialysis in pregnant women with ESKD has emerged as an important factor associated with improved fetal outcomes. Most experts suggest that after 16–20 weeks of gestation, HD sessions should be increased to daily or six times a week. Initial reports from the US Registry data noted that in women dialyzed >20 h/week, 83% of the pregnancies were successful vs. 46% in those dialyzed <14 h/week, and these findings were confirmed in more recent updates [42, 53]. Others have reported similar findings with intensified HD prescriptions. Haase et al. reported that in five pregnant women dialyzed with a mean weekly Kt/Vdp of 9.6 ± 1.4 and urea reduction rate 54.8% ± 29.4%, there were no fetal losses, and a mean gestational age is 32.8 ± 3.3 weeks with birth weights of 1765 ± 554 g [54]. Hladunewich et al. reported improved outcomes in Canadian women dialyzed for >36 h/week when compared to those reported in the US Registry and treated for <20 h ($p = 0.02$). Birth rates were greater (86.4% vs. 61.4%), and mean duration of pregnancy in the intensely dialyzed Toronto group was 36 weeks vs. 27 weeks in the US group [55]. This Canadian group had previously published their experience with a group of seven women managed with an average of 36 ± 10 h/week nocturnal HD. They increased treatment times during the pregnancy to a mean of 48 ± 5 h/week and reported excellent outcomes with minimal complications. There were six live births, two babies were small for gestational age, and one was a preterm birth. The mean gestational age was 36.2 + 3 weeks, and the mean birth weight was 2417.5 + 657 g. One pregnancy was terminated because it was thought to be a molar pregnancy [52]. Blood urea nitrogen (BUN) levels of 50 mg/dl have also been identified as important targets to achieve favorable results. Asamiya et al. reported a negative relationship with blood urea nitrogen (BUN) levels and birth weights and gestational age. Improved outcomes were observed with BUN levels of 48–49 mg/dl or less [56]. These observations have been largely translated into clinical practice; a recent survey of US experiences noted that most nephrologists prescribe 4–4.5 h of HD 6 days a week to their pregnant HD patients and that 66% target a BUN <50 mg/dl and 21% aim for a pre-dialysis BUN of <20 mg/dl [45].

Determination of dry weight during pregnancy can be a challenge and requires careful ongoing evaluation. During the first trimester, the weight gain is minimal and may only increase by 1–1.5 kg. However, during the second and third trimesters, weights are expected to increase by an average of 0.5 kg/week and should be adjusted accordingly. It is critical however that careful clinical assessments with a focus on volume status and blood pressure control be incorporated in the determination of the dry weight and ultrafiltration rates.

HTN is an extremely common problem in pregnant dialysis patients and in early series as many as 40% had BP > 170/110. The mainstay of treatment is judicious volume control targeted to an accurate dry weight. It is important to avoid aggressive ultrafiltration and maternal hypotension as it can result in fetal distress [57]. The use of antihypertensive agents follows the same approach as that outlined for women with CKD.

Anemia is a common problem among pregnant dialysis patients. In addition to the factors associated with anemia of CKD, one must account for the increased demands for red cell production during pregnancy required to support placental and fetal growth. As a result, erythropoietin (EPO) and iron requirements increase during pregnancy. To maintain targets of hemoglobin of 10–11 g/dl, EPO doses are commonly increased by >50%. Although the safety of EPO and intravenous iron has not been established, these agents have commonly been used. EPO (molecular weight 30,400 daltons) is not expected to cross the placenta, and a small study in humans noted normal EPO levels and hematocrits in neonates exposed to intrauterine exogenous EPO [58]. As in all treated patients, careful follow-up of complete blood counts and iron parameters is required to guide therapy.

Measures of mineral-bone disease should be maintained as per Kidney Disease Outcomes and Qualities Initiative guidelines. Serum phosphorus levels may be easier to control given its incorporation into fetal skeleton and the increased dialysis times, and binder use should be adjusted accordingly. In those with very long dialysis times with evidence of hypophosphatemia, supplements or addition of phosphorous to the dialysate may be required. Calcium requirements are increased in pregnancy, particularly in the third trimester. There appears to be no consensus regarding calcium concentration in the dialysate. Some have advocated increasing the concentration to 3.0 or 3.25 mEq/l [48, 52], while others have noted good outcomes with those dialyzed against a 2.5 mEq/l bath [54]. Monitoring of calcium and avoiding hypo- and or hypercalcemia should be used to individualize treatment.

Active vitamin D preparations are usually continued. As the placenta can convert 25(OH) vitamin D to 1–25 (OH) vitamin D, dose adjustments may be required. Cinacalcet safety is unclear, but in pregnant animals, it has been shown to be safe with no adverse fetal effects. Three pregnancies in two women with hypercalcemia from primary hyperparathyroidism and parathyroid malignancy treated with cinacalcet have been reported with no fetal or maternal adverse events attributed to the therapy [59, 60]. However, little to no information regarding the use of this agent in the dialysis population is available. In cases where hypercalcemia is not present, it seems reasonable to hold the agent and manage mineral-bone disease with the use of binders and active vitamin D preparations until more information is available.

There is little information available regarding nutritional requirements in pregnant dialysis patients. Some have suggested that in addition to the routine protein requirements of dialysis patients, an additional 20 g/day are required for fetal development. This has led to the suggestion that 1.8 g/kg/day of protein intake (with 3000 kcal/day) is optimal for this population [61]. As water-soluble vitamins and minerals can be removed by the intensified dialysis, prenatal vitamin supplementation is an important part of the management. Folate supplementation is an important requirement, particularly early in fetal development, and doses of folate between 2 and 5 mg/day have been described. Following folate and vitamin B-12 levels and careful attention to mean corpuscular volume measures can provide some guidance. Some provide additional B-complex and trace mineral supplements [54, 62].

Additional management issues surrounding the HD treatment include the recommendations to use only biocompatible, non-reuse dialyzers and to avoid formaldehyde or ethylene oxide exposure to avoid potential fetal malformations. Anticoagulation is continued with unfractionated heparin as required. As pregnancy normally results in respiratory alkalosis with compensatory metabolic acidosis, dialysate bicarbonate concentrations are often reduced to 25 mEq/l to avoid alkalosis [61]. With the intensified hemodialysis prescription, most women require a potassium dialysate bath of 3 mEq/l.

Peritoneal dialysis (PD), previously thought to be less stressful to the pregnancy as a result of gentle daily ultrafiltration, fewer electrolyte fluctuations, and the lack of anticoagulation, is not commonly used at this time. Early reports concluded that peritoneal dialysis was superior to hemodialysis and recommended it as the modality of choice [63]. However, early registry data from the USA could not find a statistically significant difference between PD and HD in the rate of live births [42], and a single center reported worse outcomes with PD. [64] Concerns for maternal complications unique to PD, including abdominal fullness, catheter drainage problems, and acute peritonitis have resulted in reduced utilization of this modality. Thus, while a successful pregnancy is possible on PD, particularly in those with residual renal function, there are fewer cases reported, and the greatest clinical experience is with intensified HD. An outline of HD management recommendations is provided in Table 11.2.

In summary, pregnancy in women with ESKD maintained on HD is now becoming more common. Intensified dialysis therapy and close follow-up conducted by an experienced multidisciplinary team have resulted in substantially improved outcomes.

Table 11.2 Hemodialysis management in pregnancy

Dialysis prescription	High-flux membranes No reuse of dialyzers Avoid formaldehyde- or ethylene oxide-treated dialyzers
Dialysate	3 mEq/l potassium bath 25 mEq/l bicarbonate bath 2.5–3.5 mEq/l calcium bath
Dialysis dose	>20 h/week 6 HD treatments a week Target BUN <50 mg/dl
Dry weight	Increase 1–1.5 kg in the first 12 weeks Increase 0.5 kg weekly thereafter
Anemia	Target hg 10–11 g/dl Continue erythropoietin, expect increase in dose Continue parenteral iron as required
MBD	Continue vitamin D preparations No clear data on the use of cinacalcet
Nutrition	1.8 g protein/kg/day Multivitamin use Folate 2–5 mg/day

Abbreviations: *HD* hemodialysis, *BUN* blood urea nitrogen, *Hg* hemoglobin

References

1. Piccoli GB, Attini R, Vasario E, Conijn A, Biolcati M, D'Amico F, et al. Pregnancy and chronic kidney disease: a challenge in all CKD stages. Clin J Am Soc Nephrol. 2010;5:844–55.
2. Imbasciati E, Gregorinin G, Cabiddu G, Gammaro L, Ambroso G, Del Giudice A, et al. Pregnancy in CKD stages 3 to 5: fetal and maternal outcomes. Am J Kidney Dis. 2007;49:753–62.
3. Holley JL, Schmidt RJ, Bender FH, Dumler F, Schiff M. Gynecologic and reproductive issues in woman on dialysis. Am J Kidney Dis. 1997;29:685–90.
4. Phocas I, Sarandakou A, Kassanos D, Rizos D, Tserkezis G, Koutsikos D. Hormonal and ultrasound characteristics of menstrual function during chronic dialysis and after successful renal transplantation. Int J Gynecol Obstet. 1992;37:19–28.
5. Sievertsen GD, Lim VS, Nakawatase C, Frohman LA. Metabolic clearance and secretion rates of human prolactin in normal subjects and in patients with chronic renal failure. J Clin Endocrinol Metab. 1980;50:846–52.
6. Filocamo MT, Zanazzi M, Li Marzi V, Lombardi G, Del Popolo G, Mancini G, et al. Sexual dysfunction in women during dialysis and after renal transplantation. J Sex Med. 2009;6:3125–311.
7. Lim VS. Reproductive function in patients with renal insufficiency. Am J Kidney Dis. 1987;9:363–7.
8. Lim VS, Henriquez C, Sievertsen G, Frohman LA. Ovarian function in chronic renal failure: evidence suggesting hypothalamic anovulation. Ann Intern Med. 1980;93:21–7.
9. Zingraff J, Jungers P, Pelissier C, Nahoul K, Feinstein MC, Scholler R. Pituitary and ovarian dysfunctions in women on haemodialysis. Nephron. 1982;30:149–53.
10. Mantouvalos H, Metallinos C, Makrygiannakis A, Gouskos A. Sex hormones in women on hemodialysis. Int J Gynecol Obstet. 1984;22:367–70.
11. Gomez F, de la Cueva R, Wauters JP, Lemarchand-Beraud T. Endocrine abnormalities in patients undergoing long-term hemodialysis. The role of prolactin. Am J Med. 1980;68:522–30.
12. Hou SH, Grossman S, Molitch ME. Hyperprolactinemia in patients with renal insufficiency and chronic renal failure requiring hemodialysis or chronic ambulatory peritoneal dialysis. Am J Kidney Dis. 1985;6:245–9.
13. Holley JL, Schmidt RJ, Bender FH, Dumler F, Schiff M. Gynecologic and reproductive issues in women on dialysis. Am J Kidney Dis. 1997;29:685–90.
14. Sikora-Grabkaa E, Adamczaka M, Kuczeraa P, Szotowskaa M, Madejb P, Wieceka A. Serum anti-Müllerian hormone concentration in young women with chronic kidney disease on hemodialysis, and after successful kidney transplantation. Kidney Blood Press Res. 2016;41:552–60.
15. Tal R, Seifer DB, Khanimov M, Malter HE, Grazi RV, Leader B. Characterization of women with elevated antimüllerian hormone levels (AMH): correlation of AMH with polycystic ovarian syndrome phenotypes and assisted reproductive technology outcomes. Am J Obstet Gynecol. 2014;211:1–8.
16. Wang GC, Zheng JH, Xu LG, Min ZL, Zhu YH, Qi J, Duan QL. Measurement of serum pituitary-gonadal hormones and investigation of sexual and reproductive functions in kidney transplant recipients. Int J Nephrol. 2010;2010:612126. https://doi.org/10.4061/2010/612126.
17. Pinciaroli AR. Hormonal changes in daily hemodialysis. Semin Dial. 1999;12:455–61.
18. Hou S. Historical perspective of pregnancy in chronic kidney disease. Adv Chronic Kidney Dis. 2007;14:116–8.
19. Williams D, Davison J. Chronic kidney disease in pregnancy. BMJ. 2008;336(7637):211–5.
20. Jungers P, Houillier P, Forget D, Labrunie M, Skhiri H, Giatras I, et al. Influence of pregnancy on the course of primary chronic glomerulonephritis. Lancet. 1995;346(8986):1122–4.
21. Surian M, Imbasciati E, Cosci P, Banfi G, Barbiano di Belgiojoso G, Brancaccio D, et al. Glomerular disease and pregnancy. A study of 123 pregnancies in patients with primary and secondary glomerular diseases. Nephron. 1984;36(2):101–5.
22. Katz AI, Davison JM, Hayslett JP, Singson E, Lindheimer MD. Pregnancy in women with kidney disease. Kidney Int. 1980;18:192–206.
23. Zhang JJ, Ma XX, Hao L, Liu LJ, Lv JC, Zhang H. A systematic review and meta-analysis of outcomes of

pregnancy in CKD and CKD outcomes in pregnancy. Clin J Am Soc Nephrol. 2015;10(11):1964–78.
24. Jones DC, Hayslett JP. Outcome of pregnancy in women with moderate or severe renal insufficiency. N Engl J Med. 1996;335(4):226–32.
25. Bear RA. Pregnancy in patients with renal disease: a study of 44 cases. Obstet Gynecol. 1976;48:13–8.
26. Hou SH, Grossman SD, Madias NE. Pregnancy in women with renal disease and moderate renal insufficiency. Am J Med. 1985;78:185–94.
27. Imbasciati E, Pardi G, Capetta P, Ambroso G, Bozzetti P, Pagliari B, et al. Pregnancy in women with chronic renal failure. Am J Nephrol. 1986;6(3):193–8.
28. Piccoli GB, Cabiddu G, Attini R, Vigotti FN, Maxia S, Lepori N, et al. Risk of adverse pregnancy outcomes in women with CKD. J Am Soc Nephrol. 2015;26(8):2011–22.
29. Nevis IF, Reitsma A, Dominic A, McDonald S, Thabane L, Akl EA, et al. Pregnancy outcomes in women with chronic kidney disease: a systematic review. Clin J Am Soc Nephrol. 2011;6:2587–98.
30. Kendrick J, Sharma S, Holmen J, Palit S, Nuccio E, Chonchol M. Kidney disease and maternal and fetal outcomes in pregnancy. Am J Kidney Dis. 2015;66(1):55–9.
31. Jungers P, Chauveau D. Pregnancy in renal disease. Kidney Int. 1997;52:871–85.
32. Cockburn J, Moar VA, Ounsted M, Redman CW. Final report of study on hypertension during pregnancy: the effects of specific treatment on the growth and development of the children. Lancet. 1982;1(8273):647–9.
33. Molvi SN, Mir S, Rana VS, Jabeen F, Malik AR. Role of antihypertensive therapy in mild to moderate pregnancy-induced hypertension: a prospective randomized study comparing labetalol with alpha methyldopa. Arch Gynecol Obstet. 2012;285(6):1553–62.
34. Hussain A, Karovitch A, Carson M. Blood pressure goals and treatment in patients with chronic kidney disease. Adv Chronic Kidney Dis. 2015;22(2):165–9.
35. American College of Obstetricians and Gynecologists. ACOG practice bulletin number 33. Diagnosis and management of preeclampsia and eclampsia. Obstet Gynecol. 2002;99(1):159–67.
36. Li DK, Yang C, Andrade S, Tavares V, Ferber JR. Maternal exposure to angiotensin converting enzyme inhibitors in the first trimester and risk of malformations in offspring: a retrospective cohort study. BMJ. 2011;343:d5931. https://doi.org/10.1136/bmj.d5931.
37. von Dadelszen P, Magee LA. Fall in mean arterial pressure and fetal growth restriction in pregnancy hypertension: an updated metaregression analysis. J Obstet Gynaecol Can. 2002;24(12):941–5.
38. Abalos E, Duley L, Steyn DW. Antihypertensive drug therapy for mild to moderate hypertension during pregnancy. Cochrane Database Syst Rev. 2014; https://doi.org/10.1002/14651858.CD002252.pub3.
39. Magee LA, von Dadelszen P, Rey E, Ross S, Asztalos E, Murphy KE, et al. Less-tight versus tight control of hypertension in pregnancy. N Engl J Med. 2015;372:407–17.
40. Magee LA, von Dadelszen P, Singer J, Lee T, Rey E, Ross S, et al. The CHIPS randomized, controlled trial (Control of Hypertension in Pregnancy Study): is severe hypertension just an elevated blood pressure? Hypertension. 2016;68(5):1153–9.
41. Herwig KR, Merill JP, Jackson RL, et al. Chronic renal diseases and pregnancy. Am J Obstet Gynecol. 1965;92:1117–21.
42. Okundaye I, Abrinko P, Hou S. Registry of pregnancy in dialysis patients. Am J Kidney Dis. 1998;31(5):766–73.
43. Souquiyyeh MZ, Huraib SO, Saleh AGM, et al. Pregnancy in chronic hemodialysis patients in the Kingdom of Saudi Arabia. Am J Kidney Dis. 1992;19:235–8.
44. Shahir AK, Briggs N, Katsoulis J, Levidiotis V. An observational outcomes study from 1966–2008, examining pregnancy and neonatal outcomes from dialyzed women using data from the ANZDATA Registry. Nephrology. 2013;18:276–84.
45. Sachdeva M, Barta V, Thakkar J, Sakhiya V, Miller I. Pregnancy outcomes in women on hemodialysis: a national survey. Clin Kidney J. 2017;10(2):276–81.
46. Luders C, Castro MC, Titan SM, De Castro I, Elias RM, Abensur H, Romão JE Jr. Obstetric outcome in pregnant women on long-term dialysis: a case series. Am J Kidney Dis. 2010;56(1):77–85.
47. Registration Committee of the European Dialysis and Transplant Association. Successful pregnancies in women treated by dialysis and kidney transplantation. Br J Obstet Gynecol. 1980;87:839–45.
48. Hou SH. Frequency and outcome of pregnancy in women on dialysis. Am J Kidney Dis. 1994;23:60–3.
49. Toma H, Tanabe K, Tokumoto T, Kobayashi C, Yagisawa T. Pregnancy in women receiving renal dialysis or transplantation in Japan: a nationwide survey. Nephrol Dial Transplant. 1999;14(6):1511–6.
50. Manisco G, Poti M, Maggiulli G, Di Tullio M, Losappio V, Vernaglione L. Pregnancy in end-stage renal disease on dialysis: how to achieve a successful delivery. Clin Kidney J. 2015;8:293–9.
51. Holley JL, Reddy SS. Pregnancy in dialysis patients: a review of outcomes, complications and management. Semin Dial. 2003;16(5):384–7.
52. Barua M, Hladunewich MA, Keunen J, Pierratos A, McFarlane P, Sood M, Chan C. Successful pregnancies on nocturnal home hemodialysis. Clin J Am Soc Nephrol. 2008;3:392–6.
53. Hou S. Modification of dialysis regimens for pregnancy. Int J Artif Organs. 2002;25(9):823–6.
54. Haase M, Morgera S, Bamber C, Halle H, Martini S, Hocher B, et al. A systematic approach to managing pregnant dialysis patients – the importance of an intensified haemodiafiltration protocol. Nephrol Dial Transplant. 2005;20:2537–42.
55. Hladunewich MA, Hou S, Odutayo A, Cornelis T, Pierratos A, Goldstein M, et al. Intensive hemodialysis with improved pregnancy outcomes: a Canadian

and United States Cohort Comparison. J Am Soc Nephrol. 2014;25:1103–9.
56. Asamiya Y, Otsubo S, Matsuda Y, Kimata N, Kikuchi K, Miwa N, et al. The importance of low blood urea nitrogen levels in pregnant patients undergoing hemodialysis to optimize birth weight and gestational age. Kidney Int. 2009;75:1217–22.
57. Unzelman RF, Alderfer GR, Chojnacki RE. Pregnancy and chronic hemodialysis. Trans Am Soc Artif Intern Organs. 1973;19:144–9.
58. J B, Marques R, Branco A, Gonçalves J, Lobato L, Pimentel JP, et al. Maternal and perinatal implications of the use of human recombinant erythropoietin. Acta Obstet Gynecol Scand. 1996;75(5):449–3.
59. Horjus C, Groot I, Telting D, van Setten P, van Sorge A, Kovacs CS, et al. Cinacalcet for hyperparathyroidism in pregnancy and puerperium. J Pediatr Endocrinol Metab. 2009;22(8):741–9.
60. Nadarasa K, Bailey M, Chahal H, Raja O, Bhat R, Gayle C, et al. The use of cinacalcet in pregnancy to treat a complex case of parathyroid carcinoma. Endocrinol Diabetes Metab Case Rep. 2014;2014:140056. https://doi.org/10.1530/EDM-14-0056.
61. Giatras I, Levy DP, Malone FD, Carslon JA, Jungers P. Pregnancy during dialysis: case report and management guidelines. Nephrol Dial Transplant. 1998;13:3266–72.
62. Hladunewich MA, Hercz AE, Keunen J, Chan C, Pierratos A. Pregnancy in end-stage renal disease. Semin Dial. 2011;24(6):634–9.
63. Redrow M, Cherem L, Elliott J, Mangalat J, Mishler RE, Bennett WM, et al. Dialysis in the management of pregnant patients with renal insufficiency. Medicine (Baltimore). 1988;67:199–208.
64. Chou CY, Ting IW, Lin TH, Lee CN. Pregnancy in patients on chronic dialysis: a single center experience and combined analysis of reported results. Eur J Obstet Gynecol Reprod Biol. 2008;136:165–70.

Part IV

Dyslipidemia

12 Lipid Disorders Associated with Chronic Kidney Disease and Nephrotic Syndrome

Hamid Moradi and Nosratola D. Vaziri

Introduction

Based on data from the United States Renal Data System (USRDS), there are approximately 25 million patients with chronic kidney disease (CKD) in the United States [1]. From this astonishing number, roughly 450,000 patients have end-stage renal disease (ESRD) requiring weekly/daily renal replacement therapy [1]. Furthermore, given the prevalence of the causes of CKD, it is expected that the number of patients with ESRD will increase to more than 750,000 by 2020 [1]. Treatment of CKD-/ESRD-related complications is associated with significant economic, healthcare, and societal costs, the ramification of which is becoming more and more recognized. Therefore understanding the pathophysiology of CKD and its complications has significant preventive and therapeutic value. It is well known that CKD and proteinuria are associated with significant alterations in lipid metabolism and plasma lipid and lipoprotein profiles. These abnormalities can play a substantial role in the pathogenesis and progression of renal and cardiovascular disease in this population [2–4]. There are many different factors which can impact lipid metabolism and contribute to the nature of lipid abnormalities observed in patients with kidney disease. These include preexisting genetic disorders, severity of kidney disease, presence and degree of proteinuria, dietary restrictions, features unique to each type of renal replacement therapy (hemodialysis, peritoneal dialysis), renal transplantation, and pharmacologic therapies commonly utilized in this patient population. In this chapter, we will outline the features of dyslipidemia observed in kidney disease, their underlying mechanisms, and potential significance of these observations.

H. Moradi (✉)
Division of Nephrology and Hypertension, University of California Irvine School of Medicine, Orange, CA, USA

Tibor Rubin Veterans Affairs Medical Center, Long Beach, CA, USA
e-mail: hmoradi@uci.edu

N. D. Vaziri
Division of Nephrology and Hypertension, University of California Irvine School of Medicine, Orange, CA, USA

Part I: Dyslipidemia of Chronic Kidney Disease

The lipid profile pattern of patients with advanced CKD and ESRD is marked by elevation of triglycerides and very low-density lipoprotein (VLDL) levels, and this is most likely due to impaired clearance of VLDL, chylomicrons, intermediate-density lipoprotein (IDL), and chylomicron remnants. In addition, there is increased serum concentration of small dense low-density lipoprotein (LDL), IDL, chylomicron remnants, and oxidized LDL [5–8]. Interestingly, serum total cholesterol and LDL content are not necessarily elevated and change

C. M. Rhee et al. (eds.), *Endocrine Disorders in Kidney Disease*,
https://doi.org/10.1007/978-3-319-97765-2_12

through the different stages of CKD. For instance, lipid profiles of patients with CKD and nephrotic range proteinuria frequently exhibit hypercholesterolemia and elevated LDL levels [5]. Meanwhile patients with advanced CKD and negligible proteinuria or those with ESRD on maintenance hemodialysis exhibit reduced or normal serum total and LDL cholesterol levels. Another common feature of CKD-associated dyslipidemia is reduced serum apolipoprotein AI (apoAI) and high-density lipoprotein (HDL) cholesterol levels. Moreover, there are impaired HDL-mediated reverse cholesterol transport, reduced HDL maturation and abnormal HDL antioxidant, and anti-inflammatory properties in patients with CKD [9–13].

In patients with ESRD, the renal replacement therapy modality plays a major role in the pathogenesis and clinical presentation of dyslipidemia. Much like the patients with nephrotic syndrome, the serum lipid profile of patients on chronic peritoneal dialysis frequently exhibits elevated total and LDL cholesterol levels [5, 8]. This is in contrast to patients on maintenance hemodialysis who frequently have normal or reduced serum total and LDL cholesterol levels. Other factors which complicate the dyslipidemia of kidney disease are presence of coexisting genetic disorders, pharmacologic lipid lowering therapy, and malnutrition, all of which can alter the lipid profile observed in each individual patient. Furthermore, oxidative stress and inflammation, which are common denominators in all forms of kidney disease, can lead to decreased serum cholesterol levels while increasing the risk of atherogenesis and cardiovascular disease by promoting lipid peroxidation (i.e., oxidation of LDL) [14–17]. Hence, even in patients with ESRD on hemodialysis who may have "normal" levels of LDL cholesterol, LDL particles may be significantly modified by the prooxidant and pro-inflammatory milieu such that small amounts of LDL may play a major causative role in the cardiovascular disease burden observed in this patient population. It should be noted that patients with ESRD who have undergone renal transplantation will also experience dyslipidemia due to several additional factors including residual kidney disease and immunosuppressive therapy. For instance, medications such as rapamycin, glucocorticoids, and calcineurin inhibitors adversely and significantly impact serum lipid profile independently of a patient's degree of renal disease. Therefore to gain a clear understanding of the complex processes which may impact a CKD patient's lipid profile, we first need to describe the underlying mechanisms responsible for CKD-associated abnormal lipid metabolism.

Impact of CKD on Cholesterol and LDL Metabolism

While advanced CKD is not commonly associated with elevated serum total or LDL cholesterol concentrations, there is still abnormal LDL metabolism as advanced CKD is associated with lipoprotein lipase (LPL) and hepatic lipase deficiency [18, 19]. The latter enzymes normally hydrolyze the triglyceride content of lipoproteins allowing for release of fatty acids for uptake into tissues such as the liver or muscle. LPL activity leads to conversion of VLDL to IDL and subsequently to LDL, a process vital to normal transport and metabolism of lipoproteins and their contents. Therefore, the constellation of LPL and hepatic lipase deficiency leads to impaired conversion of intermediate-density lipoprotein (IDL) to triglyceride-depleted cholesterol-rich LDL and accumulation of oxidation-prone LDL particles. Given the prooxidant environment which is characteristic of CKD, LDL oxidation leads to formation of an atherogenic moiety of this lipoprotein. Therefore it is not surprising that patients with advanced CKD and ESRD can have significantly increased risk of cardiovascular disease despite lacking a lipid profile which traditionally is considered a major risk factor for poor cardiovascular outcomes [20]. In addition, the mechanisms described help at least partly explain the recent clinical trials which have shown that HMGCoA reductase inhibitors (statins) are not effective in lowering the incidence of cardiovascular disease in patients with ESRD on maintenance hemodialysis [21, 22]. While statin therapy may reduce serum LDL cholesterol concentrations, it does not address the nature of LDL particles present in the serum. It is conceivable that accumulation of even small amounts of oxidized LDL which is a result of and contributes to the oxidative stress and inflammation of CKD makes a significant contribution to the atherogenic diathesis in this patient population. Other factors which complicate the serum LDL profile of patients with CKD and ESRD are presence of proteinuria and modality of renal replacement therapy. Patients with CKD and concomitant proteinuria can have significant elevation of their serum total and LDL cholesterol concentrations [23, 24]. In addition, patients on peritoneal dialysis experience significant protein losses in the peritoneal dialysate effluent which creates a clinical picture similar to nephrotic syndrome with elevated serum total cholesterol and LDL cholesterol levels. Interestingly, despite the increased levels of LDL cholesterol, patients on peritoneal dialysis do not experience a significantly increased risk of cardiovascular disease when compared with patients on hemodialysis. This may be due to the reduced burden of oxidative stress and inflammation in this patient population as inflammation-related issues of biocompatibility and shear stress which are unique to hemodialysis do not apply to peritoneal dialysis.

Impact of CKD on Lp(a)

Lipoprotein (a) (Lp(a)) is a low-density lipoprotein (LDL)-like particle which typically contains roughly 45% cholesterol. The serum concentrations of free and LDL-bound (Lp(a) are elevated in patients with ESRD. Using stable isotope techniques, it has been shown that the plasma residence time of these particles is more than twice as long in hemodialysis patients when compared to non-CKD controls. Therefore, increased serum Lp(a) levels are at least partly due to the lack of renal catabolism of this lipoprotein in the CKD patient population [25]. The production rate of Lp(a) in hemodialysis patients is similar to that in controls, and therefore increased synthesis is less likely to contribute to elevated Lp(a) levels [26].

Decreased catabolism of atherogenic lipoproteins such as Lp(a) which leads to its increased serum half-life can increase the risk of their further modification by oxidation, carbamylation, and glycation given the preponderance of oxidative stress and inflammation in patients with CKD. The latter will establish a vicious cycle where oxidative stress will lead to lipoprotein modification and vice versa. Therefore, it is imperative that the dyslipidemia of CKD be addressed not only based on the plasma concentrations of these lipoproteins but also in the context of their metabolic and structural qualities. In addition, the usual methods used to measure LDL cholesterol levels do not differentiate between cholesterol derived from LDL and Lp(a) and are thus the net result of cholesterol levels from both lipoproteins. Therefore, it is possible that elevated Lp(a) levels in CKD make up a significant portion of LDL cholesterol levels. Given that statin therapy typically does not impact Lp(a) concentrations, the lack of efficacy of statin trials in ESRD can be partially explained if the patients studied had markedly increased serum Lp(a) levels comprising most of their measured LDL cholesterol concentrations [27].

Impact of CKD on Triglyceride-Rich Lipoprotein Metabolism

CKD is associated with a significant increase in the level of serum triglyceride-rich lipoproteins [28]. This abnormality is mainly due to impaired clearance of VLDLs, chylomicrons, and their remnants. The major underlying mechanisms for these findings are the CKD-associated reduction of tissue LPL and VLDL receptor in organs such as skeletal muscle, adipose tissue, and myocardium [18, 29, 30]. In animals with experimental CKD, there is evidence that cardiac and skeletal muscle mRNA expression and protein abundance of VLDL receptors are significantly reduced [29]. VLDL receptors are responsible for binding and removal of VLDL particles and thereby play a key role in extrahepatic triglyceride metabolism. Hence VLDL receptor deficiency can result in hypertriglyceridemia and impaired fatty acid-related energy utilization. Another important component of impaired energy metabolism and hypertriglyceridemia of CKD is significantly reduced LPL level and activity [31, 32]. There are several mechanisms by which LPL deficiency and dysfunction is mediated in CKD. The ratio of apolipoprotein CIII (apoCIII) to apolipoprotein CII (apoCII) is significantly increased in patients with CKD [9, 33]. Given that apoC-III inhibits LPL and hepatic lipase activity while apoCII activates LPL, the increase in the ratio of these apoproteins can lead to their enzymatic inhibition result in abnormal triglyceride-rich lipoprotein metabolism in CKD. Additionally, LPL expression is downregulated, and its activity is reduced by other factors such as insulin resistance, reduced physical activity, and diminished thyroxine (T4)-to-triiodothyronine (T3) conversion all of which commonly complicate advanced CKD [34–37]. Moreover, several studies have demonstrated marked reduction of plasma post-heparin lipolytic activity in patients with CKD on maintenance hemodialysis [38–40]. This is most likely due to the release and degradation of the endothelium-bound LPL mediated via heparin anticoagulation which is commonly used in hemodialysis to avoid excess clotting [41]. Another potential side effect of heparinization is the release of angiopoietin-like proteins (ANGPTL) 3 and 4. The latter proteins have been shown to inactivate LPL, and their concentrations were found to be increased in patients on hemodialysis with heparin as their anticoagulant [42]. In addition, LPL is anchored to the endothelium by glycosylphosphatidylinositol-anchored binding protein 1 (GPIHBP1). This molecule plays an important role in LPL metabolism and function as GPIHBP1 deficiency has been shown to cause severe hypertriglyceridemia. Animals with CKD have reduced mRNA expression and protein abundance of GPIHBP1 in adipose, skeletal muscle, and myocardial tissues when compared with normal controls [43]. Furthermore, hepatic and LPL deficiency of CKD is also mediated by secondary hyperparathyroidism which has been shown to be associated with marked reductions of LPL mRNA expression and protein abundance in animals with CKD [44–48]. In fact, studies have shown that post-heparin plasma lipolytic activity is significantly improved in animals with CKD who underwent parathyroidectomy [49].

Another important mechanism responsible for abnormal triglyceride metabolism of CKD which should be mentioned are significant decreases in LDL receptor-related protein (LRP). LRP is mainly expressed in the liver and is involved in clearance of many different lipoproteins including VLDL, chylomicrons, and IDL. There is evidence that hepatic LRP gene expression and protein abundance is reduced in animal models of CKD [50]. Therefore, LRP deficiency will further exacerbate the abnormalities caused by LPL and VLDL receptor deficiency.

Consequences of Abnormal LDL, Lp(a), and Triglyceride-Rich Lipoprotein Metabolism

Impaired clearance of LDL, Lp(a), and triglyceride-rich lipoproteins and accumulation of their remnants leads to several adverse effects [51, 52]. There is evidence that elevated serum Lp(a) levels are associated with an increased risk of atherosclerosis and cardiovascular disease in patients with ESRD [53, 54]. Due to the delayed clearance of triglyceride-containing small dense LDL, chylomicron remnants, and oxidation-prone IDL, there is accumulation of the latter lipoproteins in patients with CKD [7]. In light of the increased burden of oxidative stress and inflammation in these patients, retention of these lipoproteins can result in their oxidative modification and increased concentrations of oxidized lipids. These circulating oxidized lipoproteins and their remnants play a key role in the dispersal and propagation of oxidative stress throughout the body via various mechanisms including the initiation of lipid peroxidation chain reaction (which as the name suggests leads to further dissemination of oxidation in other lipids/phospholipids). In addition, binding of these oxidized lipoproteins and their phospholipid components to receptors on immune cells such as macrophages leads to activation and release of pro-inflammatory cytokines resulting in the pathogenesis and amplification of inflammation and oxidative stress in patients with CKD [55].

Impact of CKD on HDL Function and Metabolism (Fig. 12.1)

CKD is associated with marked abnormalities in high-density lipoprotein (HDL) size, content, function, and metabolism [10]. Patients with advanced CKD often have decreased serum HDL cholesterol levels. In addition, the maturation of HDL (a key component of reverse cholesterol transport) from cholesterol ester-poor pre-beta-migrating HDL (HDL3) to cholesterol ester-enriched alpha-migrating HDL (HDL2) is significantly reduced in patients with advanced CKD and ESRD [5, 6, 56, 57]. Moreover, the triglyceride content of HDL is increased in ESRD patients on hemodialysis most likely due to reduced hepatic lipase activity given that serum cholesteryl ester transfer protein (CETP) levels and activity have been shown to be normal [48, 58, 59].

It is important to note that while serum HDL level, size, and content are valuable indices in evaluation of HDL as an antiatherogenic lipoprotein, there is accumulating evidence which points to HDL function as a key component of its cardioprotective properties [10, 60]. HDL has many different functions and properties, but in the context of this chapter, we will only discuss impact of CKD on HDL antioxidant, anti-inflammatory properties, and reverse cholesterol transport. In this regard, CKD is associated with impaired HDL antioxidant and anti-inflammatory properties when compared with healthy controls. We have shown that HDL from patients with ESRD exhibits markedly reduced antioxidant activity, and these findings were accompanied by and were most likely in part due to significant reductions in the activity of HDL-associated antioxidant enzymes paraoxonase1 and glutathione peroxidase [11, 61]. Furthermore, we demonstrated that ESRD was not only associated with reduced HDL anti-inflammatory activity, but in a subset of patients, HDL exhibited pro-inflammatory characteristics [12, 62]. Our findings have also been confirmed by several other investigators who reported that in contrast to the HDL from healthy

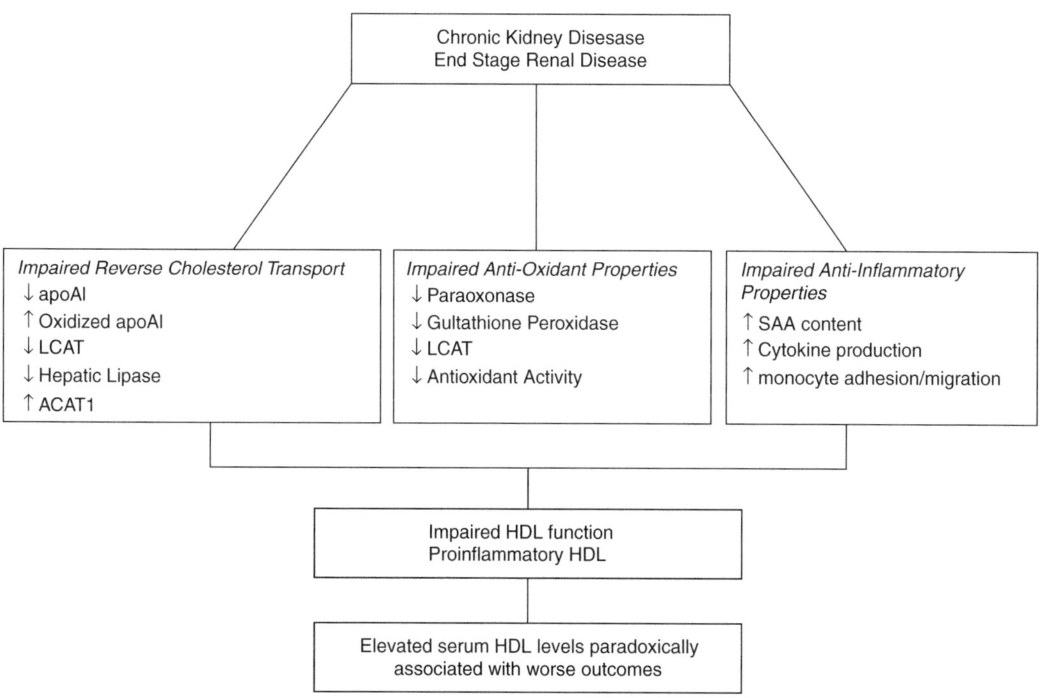

Fig. 12.1 Impact of kidney disease on HDL metabolism and potential consequences of HDL dysfunction in chronic kidney disease and end-stage renal disease

controls, HDL from hemodialysis patients promoted inflammatory cytokine production by immune cells and this was accompanied with significant reductions of the HDL antichemotactic activity [63, 64]. Using proteomics, investigators have shown that the pro-inflammatory activity of HDL is most likely due to the enrichment of this molecule with serum amyloid A whose pro-inflammatory nature was confirmed in vitro [65]. Furthermore, reduced HDL anti-oxidant and anti-inflammatory properties have been demonstrated in pediatric patients with CKD who do not have multiple comorbidities such as diabetes and hypertension and patients with functioning renal allografts [64, 66, 67]. Moreover, HDL dysfunction has been confirmed in patients with ESRD who are on peritoneal dialysis as well as hemodialysis, and hence the modality of renal replacement therapy does not seem to make a significant impact on HDL antioxidant and anti-inflammatory properties [68]. Reduced anti-inflammatory functions of HDL in patients with ESRD are most likely due to oxidative modification of this molecule by the prevailing oxidative stress. This phenomenon is not unique to ESRD and can be seen in other chronic inflammatory conditions [69, 70]. However, pro-inflammatory HDL can intensify the inciting oxidative stress and inflammation in ESRD. In fact, oxidative modification of HDL as measured by oxidized apoAI levels can be associated with a higher risk of cardiovascular mortality [71]. The significance of the latter abnormalities are highlighted in a study by our group where a sizeable minority of patients on hemodialysis had elevated serum HDL cholesterol levels that were paradoxically associated with increased cardiovascular and overall mortality [72]. In addition, recent studies have noted that the association of elevated serum HDL cholesterol levels with improved cardiovascular mortality is significantly attenuated by patients' estimated glomerular filtration rate [73]. Hence, elevated serum HDL cholesterol concentrations are not necessarily associated with improved cardiovascular outcomes in patients with CKD stage III or worse [73]. Furthermore, a recent study in a large Veterans Affairs (VA) cohort found that low and high (lowest and highest deciles) serum HDL cholesterol levels are associated with significantly increased risks of incident CKD and progression of CKD [74]. The authors noted that while it is expected that low serum HDL levels are associated with poor renal outcomes, the observation that increased serum HDL cholesterol levels can also be associated with adverse renal outcomes was surprising. However, given the mechanisms provided so far in this section, these findings can be explained by the notion that HDL particles in a subset of patients with CKD are highly oxidized and pro-inflammatory due to their enrichment in acute phase proteins such as serum amyloid A. This combined with the fact that HDL particles from patients with CKD/ESRD on maintenance hemodialysis have been shown to have impaired reverse cholesterol transport capabilities can lead to HDL dysfunction and explain the paradoxical associations of serum HDL level with outcomes noted in epidemiologic studies [75, 76].

Another important component of abnormal HDL metabolism in CKD is impaired HDL maturation and reverse cholesterol transport. Impaired maturation of HDL in CKD is mainly driven by the lower serum concentrations of enzyme lecithin-cholesterol acyltransferase (LCAT) and reduced enzymatic activity [77–81]. Under normal conditions, LCAT catalyzes the conversion of free cholesterol to cholesterol ester allowing for incorporation of hydrophobic lipids into the HDL core and loading of this lipoprotein. Therefore LCAT plays a major role in HDL maturation, and by loading the cholesterol cargo of HDL, it mediates a critical step in reverse cholesterol transport. We and other investigators have shown reduced serum LCAT concentrations and activity in patients and downregulation of LCAT mRNA expression in the liver of animals with CKD [11]. Another important step in reverse cholesterol transport which is impaired in CKD is the conversion of intracellular cholesterol esters to free cholesterol for removal from the cell. Since acetyl-CoA acetyltransferase, cytosolic 1 (ACAT)1 normally esterifies cholesterol for intracellular storage, its upregulation can lead to accumulation of lipids and reduced mobilization of free cholesterol from within the cells for transport to the liver via HDL. There is evidence that

CKD is associated with marked upregulation of renal and arterial ACAT1, and this can lead to further impairment of reverse cholesterol transport [82–84].

Additionally, an important cause of HDL deficiency and dysfunction in CKD is reduced apoAI and apoAII levels. ApoAI is the major protein constituent of HDL and plays a critical role in reverse cholesterol transport and HDL antioxidant and anti-inflammatory properties. We have shown that apoAI hepatic biosynthesis is significantly decreased in animals with CKD and in a series of in vitro studies found that the downregulation of apoAI gene expression by uremic toxins was mediated via mRNA instability [85, 86]. In addition, increased catabolism of apoAI has been demonstrated in patients with CKD and ESRD on maintenance hemodialysis [87, 88]. Moreover, a higher prevalence of anti-apoAI autoantibodies have been reported in patients with ESRD, and this can lead to reduction and dysfunction of the apoAI protein [89]. Finally, since presence of normal apoAI is crucial to HDL function, its deficiency and oxidation can make a major adverse impact on HDL properties [13]. For instance, HDL's affinity and binding to ATP-binding cassette transporter A1 (ABCA-1) transporter, the protein which normally transports free cholesterol from the intracellular space for loading into HDL, can be reduced with apoAI deficiency and oxidative modification [90]. Therefore, it is not surprising that in vitro studies have shown impaired reverse cholesterol transport and decreased HDL ability to remove cholesterol from lipid-laden macrophages in patients with CKD, ESRD, and those with renal transplant allografts [91].

Therefore, CKD-associated abnormalities of HDL metabolism are threefold. One is apoAI and HDL deficiency which on their own can be associated with adverse outcomes. There is also the defective HDL maturation and impaired reverse cholesterol transport which is mainly driven by LCAT deficiency and ACAT1 overexpression in addition to impaired apoAI-mediated free cholesterol efflux. Finally, CKD is associated with reduced HDL antioxidant and anti-inflammatory activity which can be a result of and lead to oxidative modification of HDL as demonstrated in patients with ESRD [92]. HDL deficiency and dysfunction can in turn lead to further oxidative stress, inflammation, and accumulation of oxidized LDL and phospholipids providing the ingredients needed for cardiovascular disease [93]. When combined with severely limited reverse cholesterol transport, these abnormalities can lead to a significantly increased risk of cardiovascular complications and mortality.

Impact of CKD Treated with Peritoneal Dialysis Therapy on Lipid Metabolism

Peritoneal dialysis therapy can result in substantial losses of proteins in the dialysate effluent with an average protein loss of 10 g/day. Therefore, dyslipidemia of this modality of renal replacement therapy shares some of the features of the dyslipidemia associated with proteinuria. Therefore it is not surprising that compared to patients on maintenance hemodialysis, peritoneal dialysis patients have increased LDL cholesterol, triglyceride, and Lp(a) concentrations [8, 94–98]. The mechanism of dyslipidemia unique to peritoneal dialysis which needs to be mentioned in this section is the role of dextrose-based dialysate. Dwelling of the large amounts of dextrose-containing dialysate in the peritoneum which is used to facilitate ultrafiltration can result in the absorption of significant quantities of glucose via the peritoneal membrane and hyperglycemia. This can in turn lead to the activation of carbohydrate-responsive element-binding protein (chREBP), lipogenesis, and de novo fatty acid synthesis with the end result of hyperlipidemia and hypertriglyceridemia in these patients [99]. Direct evidence for the deleterious role of dialysate glucose in peritoneal dialysis-related dyslipidemia was provided by Babazono et al. who showed significant reduction of serum LDL cholesterol, triglycerides, and small dense LDL particles in patients using icodextrin-containing dialysate instead of the glucose-based peritoneal dialysis solutions [100].

Impact of Renal Transplantation on Lipid Metabolism

The dyslipidemia observed in patients with functioning renal allografts is multifactorial with contribution from CKD, chronic allograft nephropathy, inflammation, and most importantly use of immunosuppressive agents, particularly prednisone, cyclosporine, and sirolimus. As a result of the interplay between the mentioned factors, kidney transplant recipients frequently exhibit hyperlipidemia (increased total and LDL cholesterol), hypertriglyceridemia, and normal or reduced HDL concentrations accompanied by HDL dysfunction [66, 101–103]. It is known that the major cause of mortality in patients with functioning renal allografts is cardiovascular disease, and given this highly atherogenic lipid profile, dyslipidemia most likely plays a major role in the pathogenesis of cardiovascular disease and its complications in this population [104].

Since we have so far discussed the mechanisms responsible for the pathogenesis of dyslipidemia in CKD, in this section we will focus on the impact of immunosuppressive therapy on lipid metabolism and abnormal lipid profiles in patients with renal transplantation. While not commonly used, sirolimus can cause hypertriglyceridemia and hypercholesterolemia (increased LDL and HDL cholesterol). It was recently reported that downregulation of hepatic LDL receptor expression is mediated via mTOR complex 1 pathway and leads to increased LDL cholesterol levels in mice. In addition, rapamycin therapy has been shown to cause scavenger receptor class B type 1 downregulation in human umbilical vein endothelial cells (HUVECs), hence interfering with reverse cholesterol transport and leading to increased serum HDL cholesterol levels [105, 106].

Glucocorticosteroids, which are a common feature of immunosuppressive therapy in transplantation, cause insulin resistance, increased glucose production, and hyperglycemia. Steroid therapy also leads to increased fatty acid synthesis and generation of triglycerides in addition to decreased HDL cholesterol levels [107]. Another commonly used immunosuppressive agent is cyclosporine which causes hypertriglyceridemia and elevated serum cholesterol and Lp(a) levels. The direct impact of cyclosporine on lipid metabolism was shown by Artz et al. who found that replacement of cyclosporine by alternate immunosuppressive therapy can lead to substantial reductions in LDL, total cholesterol, and triglyceride levels in transplant patients [108]. There are several mechanisms by which cyclosporine causes dyslipidemia. We have found downregulation of hepatic cholesterol 7-alpha-hydroxylase enzyme in animal treated with cyclosporine [109]. Given that 7-alpha-hydroxylase normally converts cholesterol to bile acid for its excretion in the bowel, decreased levels of this enzyme can limit this process and lead to hyperlipidemia. In addition, cyclosporine has been shown to cause downregulation of LPL in the skeletal muscle and adipose tissue of animals [109]. Cyclosporine also increases CETP activity, reduces bile acid synthesis, reduces expression of the LDL receptor, inhibits ABCA-1 mediated reverse cholesterol transport, and reduces apolipoprotein E secretion [110–112].

Part II: Dyslipidemia of Nephrotic Syndrome

Proteinuria is caused by various primary and secondary processes which ultimately damage and impair glomerular function and lead to a range of complications including CKD and dyslipidemia. Nephrotic syndrome is typically defined as proteinuria exceeding 3.5 g/day together with hypertension, sodium retention, hypoalbuminemia, edema, significant hyperlipidemia, and lipiduria. The degree of proteinuria usually corresponds with the severity of dyslipidemia and abnormal lipoprotein metabolism in patients with nephrotic syndrome. There are major structural and quantitative changes of lipoproteins in patients with nephrotic syndrome. The structural makeup of lipoproteins can be altered to a major extent as cholesterol-to-triglyceride, free cholesterol-to-cholesterol ester, and phospholipid-to-protein ratios are significantly increased in nephrotic syndrome [23, 113]. Furthermore, apolipoproteins—AI, AIV, B, C, and

E levels and the apoCIII/apoCII ratio—are markedly increased. There are also quantitative changes in the serum lipid profile of patients with nephrotic syndrome. There is a significant increase in serum content of triglycerides, apoB-containing lipoproteins (such as VLDL, IDL, and LDL), Lp(a), and total cholesterol [113, 114].

Impact of Nephrotic Syndrome on LDL, Lp(a), and Cholesterol Metabolism

Nephrotic syndrome is associated with a significant increase in serum total and LDL cholesterol. The mechanisms responsible for these findings are twofold. First, there is increased cholesterol synthesis and LDL production in nephrotic syndrome. The latter is caused by an upregulation of 3-hydroxy-3-methylglutaryl-coenzyme (HMG-CoA) reductase and ACAT2 enzyme expression and increased activity (all of which increase cholesterol production) and increased apoB-100 production [114–118]. Secondly, there is diminished catabolism and impaired clearance of apoB-containing lipoproteins such as LDL mainly due to reduced LDL receptor (LDLR) protein abundance [115, 119–122]. Under normal conditions, LDL binds to LDLR on the surface of hepatocytes thereby forming a complex which subsequently undergoes endocytosis. LDL then undergoes lysosomal degradation and LDLR is released to repeat this cycle. Proprotein convertase subtilisin/kexin type 9 (PCSK9), which is primarily produced and released by the liver, regulates this process and hence plays an important part in regulation of LDLR and cholesterol metabolism [123–125]. PCSK9 binds to the LDLR on the surface of hepatocytes and forms a complex which is internalized and leads to intracellular degradation of the LDLR [124]. Therefore, PCSK9 prevents recycling of LDLR by promoting its degradation and causes the posttranslational downregulation of this protein. In this regard, individuals with loss-of-function mutations of PCSK9 have been shown to have low plasma LDL cholesterol levels and a decreased risk of cardiovascular disease. Given the decreased abundance of LDLR in nephrotic syndrome, our group studied and found that hepatic expression of PCSK9 and inducible degrader of the LDL receptor (IDOL) is significantly increased in animals with nephrotic syndrome. In addition, plasma concentrations of PCSK9 were markedly elevated in patients with nephrotic syndrome and peritoneal dialysis. These findings explain the LDLR deficiency of nephrotic syndrome and further point toward a posttranslational mechanism [126, 127]. Furthermore, due to increased hepatic production, serum Lp(a) levels are significantly elevated in patients with nephrotic syndrome [23, 128, 129]. The direct impact of proteinuria on serum Lp(a) level has been confirmed since antiproteinuric therapy or spontaneous disease remission leads to a significant reduction in Lp(a) levels in patients with nephrotic syndrome.

Potential Consequences of Elevated LDL and Lp(a) Levels on Renal Disease

The significant elevation of serum LDL cholesterol and Lp(a) levels are not only major contributors to atherogenesis but also can adversely impact renal outcomes in patients with nephrotic syndrome. There is accumulating evidence that lipids and modified lipoproteins can play a role in pathogenesis and progression of renal disease. While there is an abundance of in vitro and animal studies which support lipid-induced renal injury [130–133], the most direct clinical evidence linking LDL cholesterol and kidney injury are from studies in patients with minimal change disease and focal segmental glomerulosclerosis. Several studies have shown that in a subset of patients with nephrotic syndrome who are resistant to immunosuppressive therapy, lowering of LDL via LDL apheresis resulted in complete or partial remission of proteinuria [134, 135]. These intriguing results are not only indicative of the causative role of hyperlipidemia in the pathogenesis and progression of renal disease but also provide support for the notion of using LDL apheresis and other lipid-reducing mechanisms as potential new strategies in treatment of patients with nephrotic syndrome. In this regard, novel pharmacologic tools are now in clinical use which inhibit PCSK9 protein and can correct the LDL receptor deficiency of nephrotic syndrome [136]. It will be intriguing to see whether such therapies can be part of the treatment of renal injury in nephrotic syndrome in addition to their current role in prevention of atherosclerosis.

Impact of Nephrotic Syndrome on HDL Metabolism

Nephrotic syndrome is associated with impaired maturation of HDL from the discoid cholesterol-poor moiety (HDL-3) to the spherical cholesterol-loaded form (HDL-2). The mechanisms responsible for this undesired morphological change are several. First, it is well known that albumin can serve as a carrier for free cholesterol, and HDL can obtain a major portion of its cholesterol content from albumin. Therefore, the amount of free cholesterol that is normally transported from the peripheral tissues to lipid-poor HDL-3 by albumin is significantly reduced in nephrotic syndrome due to hypoalbuminemia [137]. In addition, given the similar molecular weight of LCAT to albumin (63kD), there are substantial urinary losses of LCAT in patients with heavy proteinuria which leads to LCAT deficiency [138]. Since LCAT is responsible for the packing of HDL with cholesterol esters, it is not surprising that LCAT deficiency contributes to impaired cholesterol loading of HDL and reduced HDL maturation. Finally, human serum CETP normally transfers cholesterol esters from HDL and triglycerides to HDL hence increasing the triglyceride and lowering the cholesterol content of HDL. Several studies have demonstrated that nephrotic syndrome is associated with significant elevation of CETP, and this can lead to abnormal HDL content of triglycerides and impair reverse cholesterol transport [139–141]. In addition, since mature cholesterol-enriched HDL2 particles can act as apoE and apoC donors to the chylomicrons and nascent VLDL, interference in HDL maturation and reduced HDL apoE levels can also lead to impaired triglyceride metabolism in patients with nephrotic syndrome [142]. Moreover, our group has shown a significant decrease in hepatic protein abundance of scavenger receptor class B type 1 (SR-B1) accompanied by downregulation of PDZ containing domain 1 (PDZK1) (protein companion of SR-B1 in cell membrane) expression and reduced protein abundance in animals with nephrotic syndrome [143, 144]. In light of the fact that SR-B1 acts as the docking receptor for HDL in the liver and allows for unloading of HDL cholesterol cargo, its deficiency further indicates dysregulation of HDL metabolism and impaired reverse cholesterol transport in patients with nephrotic syndrome.

Altered handling of serum HDL and impaired reverse cholesterol transport in nephrotic syndrome is associated with increased oxidative modification of HDL which can alter its function. Newman et al. have demonstrated that proteinuria is associated with increased total oxylipid amounts in the HDL and VLDL fractions. Lipoprotein content of epoxides and diols increased twofold in HDL and fivefold in VLDL particles, while hydroxyeicosatetraenoic acids and hydroxyoctadecadienoic acids increased more than fourfold in HDL and more than 20-fold in VLDL [145]. Given the deleterious role of lipid peroxidation on oxidative stress and atherogenesis, these abnormalities further explain the increased risk of cardiovascular disease in patients with nephrotic syndrome.

Impact of Nephrotic Syndrome on Triglyceride-Rich Lipoprotein Metabolism (Fig. 12.2)

Heavy proteinuria and nephrotic syndrome are associated with significantly increased fasting serum levels of triglycerides, IDL, and VLDL. In addition, there is delayed resolution of postprandial lipemia and increased triglyceride loading of apoB-containing lipoproteins in nephrotic syndrome [121, 146–149]. These abnormalities are mediated via several different mechanisms. First, nephrotic syndrome is associated with VLDL deficiency and alteration of lipoprotein structure and composition, and this disrupts the interaction and binding of the triglyceride-rich lipoproteins such as VLDL and chylomicrons to their receptors and impairs their clearance [148, 150, 151].

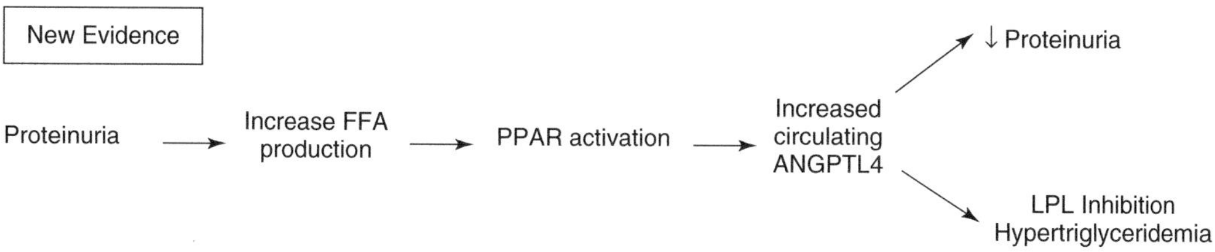

Fig. 12.2 The potential role of ANGPLT4 as the link between proteinuria and hypertriglyceridemia in nephrotic syndrome

The second mechanism responsible for abnormal triglyceride metabolism in nephrotic syndrome is LPL and hepatic lipase deficiency which together lead to impaired mobilization and metabolism of triglyceride-rich lipoproteins. Hepatic lipase inhibition was demonstrated in in vitro studies which showed a 50% decrease in heparin-releasable lipase activity in the liver of animals with nephrotic syndrome when compared to controls [149]. Furthermore, marked downregulation of hepatic lipase expression and activity and of VLDL receptor mRNA and protein abundance in the skeletal muscle and myocardium of animals with nephrotic syndrome has been reported [18, 152–154].

In regard to LPL deficiency, we have found a significant reduction of LPL protein concentration despite normal LPL messenger RNA (mRNA) expression in the adipose tissue, skeletal muscle, and myocardium of two animal models of nephrotic syndrome (Imai rats with spontaneous focal glomerulosclerosis and puromycin-induced podocyte injury resulting in nephrotic syndrome) [155]. This was associated with pronounced reductions of heparin-releasable and intracellular LPL [153]. Furthermore, other investigators have also found significant reduction of post-heparin lipolytic activity in humans and animals with nephrotic syndrome further indicating depletion of endothelium-bound LPL reserves [113, 146, 147, 156, 157]. In addition, nephrotic syndrome is associated with increased apoC-III to apoC-II ratio and reduced apoC-II and apoE content in VLDL and chylomicrons which can lead to impaired LPL function and reduced lipolysis of triglyceride-rich lipoproteins [158, 159]. Another potential cause of LPL dysfunction is nephrotic syndrome-associated impaired HDL metabolism [142, 160]. There is evidence that in rat aortic endothelial cells from nephrotic animals, there is impaired binding and LPL-induced lipolysis of VLDL and chylomicrons which can be reversed by the introduction of HDL from normal animals [160]. In addition, rats with nephrotic syndrome have impaired VLDL endothelial binding and LPL-mediated lipolysis which can be corrected using HDL from normal animals. Moreover, the ability of triglyceride-rich lipoproteins to activate lipolytic enzymes and participate in effective lipid and apoprotein exchange with other lipoproteins such as HDL is significantly reduced in nephrotic syndrome [56].

There is mounting evidence that abnormal triglyceride and fatty acid metabolism in nephrotic syndrome are not only a consequence of this disorder, but they may also be linked to its pathogenesis. The mechanisms responsible for abnormal fatty acid production and reduced catabolism in nephrotic syndrome have been studied in detail. There is evidence that nephrotic syndrome is associated with downregulation of hepatic genes involved in fatty acid catabolism, while expression of the key enzymes involved in fatty acid, phospholipid, and triglyceride production is upregulated [161–163]. However, recently Clement et al. demonstrated that circulating angiopoietin-like 4 (ANGPTL4) plays a vital role in the pathogenesis of hypertriglyceridemia and proteinuria in nephrotic syndrome thereby directly linking proteinuria to the abnormal triglyceride metabolism. There is evidence circulating ANGPTL4 causes inactivation and inhibition of LPL activity. In this regard, it was found that increasing plasma levels of ANGPTL4 was associated with elevated triglyceride levels, and patients with untreated nephrotic syndrome had a considerably higher plasma level of ANGPTL4 when compared to healthy controls [164, 165]. It was also shown that ANGPTL4 is expressed in podocytes and that circulating ANGPTL4 reduces proteinuria in nephrotic syndrome [166]. Therefore, while elevated circulating ANGPTL4 ameliorates proteinuria via its interaction with αvβ5 integrin, it also leads to hypertriglyceridemia. These findings are not unique to primary causes of nephrotic syndrome given recent studies by Herman-Edelstein et al. who found down-regulation of kidney LPL and increased expression of ANGPTL4 was associated with increased lipid deposition in renal biopsy specimens from patients with diabetic nephropathy and proteinuria [167]. Hence, it appears that elevated circulating levels of ANGPTL4 are triggered by increased free fatty acids (FFA) and are a physiologic response to proteinuria which as a side effect also interfere with triglyceride metabolism [164]. The mechanisms by which FFAs regulate ANGPTL4 have not been fully elucidated, but it is known that this molecule is a peroxisome proliferator-activated receptor (PPAR) target gene and that free fatty acids (FFAs) mediate upregulation of ANGPTL4 via members of the PPAR family [168]. Our group has shown increased hepatic PPAR alpha expression and nuclear translocation which was associated with increased tissue and plasma FFA concentration in animals with puromycin-induced minimal change disease [161]. Furthermore, these findings were not unique to the mechanism of heavy proteinuria as we have demonstrated hypertriglyceridemia, increased renal and hepatic PPAR alpha nuclear translocation, and increased plasma FFA content in a CKD model (via a 5/6 nephrectomy model) which is also associated with proteinuria [169, 170]. Therefore, it is possible that increased FFA in proteinuria activate PPARs which then leads to increase in ANGPTL4 thereby decreasing proteinuria and increasing triglycerides.

References

1. USRDS., U.S.R.D.S. and Annual Data Report: Atlas of end-stage renal disease in the United States. National Institutes of Health NIDDK; 2011.
2. Segura R, Gotto AM Jr. Lipid and lipoprotein abnormalities in renal disease. Perspect Nephrol Hypertens. 1976;3:159–200.
3. Attman PO, Alaupovic P. Pathogenesis of hyperlipidemia in the nephrotic syndrome. Am J Nephrol. 1990;10(Suppl 1):69–75.
4. Baxter JH, Goodman HC, Havel RJ. Serum lipid and lipoprotein alterations in nephrosis. J Clin Invest. 1960;39:455–65.
5. Vaziri ND. Dyslipidemia of chronic renal failure: the nature, mechanisms, and potential consequences. Am J Physiol Renal Physiol. 2006;290(2): F262–72.
6. Vaziri ND. Lipotoxicity and impaired high density lipoprotein-mediated reverse cholesterol transport in chronic kidney disease. J Ren Nutr. 2010;20(5 Suppl):S35–43.
7. Deighan CJ, et al. Atherogenic lipoprotein phenotype in end-stage renal failure: origin and extent of small dense low-density lipoprotein formation. Am J Kidney Dis. 2000;35(5):852–62.
8. Attman PO, et al. Dialysis modalities and dyslipidemia. Kidney Int Suppl. 2003;84:S110–2.
9. Vaziri ND, Moradi H. Mechanisms of dyslipidemia of chronic renal failure. Hemodial Int. 2006;10(1):1–7.
10. Moradi H, et al. Role of HDL dysfunction in end-stage renal disease: a double-edged sword. J Ren Nutr. 2013;23(3):203–6.
11. Moradi H, et al. Impaired antioxidant activity of high-density lipoprotein in chronic kidney disease. Transl Res. 2009;153(2):77–85.
12. Vaziri ND, et al. In vitro stimulation of HDL anti-inflammatory activity and inhibition of LDL pro-inflammatory activity in the plasma of patients with end-stage renal disease by an apoA-1 mimetic peptide. Kidney Int. 2009;76(4):437–44.
13. Vaziri ND, Navab M, Fogelman AM. HDL metabolism and activity in chronic kidney disease. Nat Rev Nephrol. 2010;6(5):287–96.
14. Himmelfarb J. Oxidative stress in hemodialysis. Contrib Nephrol. 2008;161:132–7.
15. Vaziri ND. Oxidative stress in uremia: nature, mechanisms, and potential consequences. Semin Nephrol. 2004;24(5):469–73.
16. Kaysen GA, Eiserich JP. The role of oxidative stress-altered lipoprotein structure and function and microinflammation on cardiovascular risk in patients with minor renal dysfunction. J Am Soc Nephrol. 2004;15(3):538–48.
17. Navab KD, et al. Chronic inflammatory disorders and accelerated atherosclerosis: chronic kidney disease. Curr Pharm Des. 2011;17(1):17–20.
18. Vaziri ND, Liang K. Down-regulation of tissue lipoprotein lipase expression in experimental chronic renal failure. Kidney Int. 1996;50(6):1928–35.
19. Bolzano K, Krempler F, Sandhofer F. Hepatic and extrahepatic triglyceride lipase activity in uraemic patients on chronic haemodialysis. Eur J Clin Investig. 1978;8(5):289–93.

20. Kalantar-Zadeh K, Balakrishnan VS. The kidney disease wasting: inflammation, oxidative stress, and diet-gene interaction. Hemodial Int. 2006;10(4):315–25.
21. Epstein M, Vaziri ND. Statins in the management of dyslipidemia associated with chronic kidney disease. Nat Rev Nephrol. 2012;8(4):214–23.
22. Vaziri ND, Norris KC. Reasons for the lack of salutary effects of cholesterol-lowering interventions in end-stage renal disease populations. Blood Purif. 2013;35(1–3):31–6.
23. Kronenberg F. Dyslipidemia and nephrotic syndrome: recent advances. J Ren Nutr. 2005;15(2):195–203.
24. Vaziri ND, Sato T, Liang K. Molecular mechanisms of altered cholesterol metabolism in rats with spontaneous focal glomerulosclerosis. Kidney Int. 2003;63(5):1756–63.
25. Trenkwalder E, et al. Increased plasma concentrations of LDL-unbound apo(a) in patients with end-stage renal disease. Kidney Int. 1997;52(6):1685–92.
26. Kronenberg F, et al. Kinetic studies of atherogenic lipoproteins in hemodialysis patients: do they tell us more about their pathology? Semin Dial. 2007;20(6):554–60.
27. Kronenberg F, et al. Lipoprotein(a)- and low-density lipoprotein-derived cholesterol in nephrotic syndrome: impact on lipid-lowering therapy? Kidney Int. 2004;66(1):348–54.
28. Wanner C, Frommherz K, Horl WH. Hyperlipoproteinemia in chronic renal failure: pathophysiological and therapeutic aspects. Cardiology. 1991;78(3):202–17.
29. Vaziri ND, Liang K. Down-regulation of VLDL receptor expression in chronic experimental renal failure. Kidney Int. 1997;51(3):913–9.
30. Goldberg IJ. Lipoprotein metabolism in normal and uremic patients. Am J Kidney Dis. 1993;21(1):87–90.
31. Stegmayr B, Olivecrona T, Olivecrona G. Lipoprotein lipase disturbances induced by uremia and hemodialysis. Semin Dial. 2009;22(4):442–4.
32. Vaziri ND. Causes of dysregulation of lipid metabolism in chronic renal failure. Semin Dial. 2009;22(6):644–51.
33. Nishizawa Y, et al. Hypertriglyceridemia and lowered apolipoprotein C-II/C-III ratio in uremia: effect of a fibric acid, clinofibrate. Kidney Int. 1993;44(6):1352–9.
34. Roullet JB, et al. Correction by insulin of disturbed TG-rich LP metabolism in rats with chronic renal failure. Am J Phys. 1986;250(4 Pt 1):E373–6.
35. Roullet JB, Lacour B, Drueke T. Partial correction of lipid disturbances by insulin in experimental renal failure. Contrib Nephrol. 1986;50:203–10.
36. Saffari B, Ong JM, Kern PA. Regulation of adipose tissue lipoprotein lipase gene expression by thyroid hormone in rats. J Lipid Res. 1992;33(2):241–9.
37. Fagher B, et al. Reduced thermogenesis in muscle and disturbed lipoprotein metabolism in relation to thyroid function in haemodialysis patients. Scand J Clin Lab Invest. 1987;47(1):91–7.
38. Nasstrom B, et al. Lipoprotein lipase during heparin infusion: lower activity in hemodialysis patients. Scand J Clin Lab Invest. 2003;63(1):45–53.
39. Chan MK, et al. Pathogenic roles of post-heparin lipases in lipid abnormalities in hemodialysis patients. Kidney Int. 1984;25(5):812–8.
40. Nasstrom B, et al. Lower plasma levels of lipoprotein lipase after infusion of low molecular weight heparin than after administration of conventional heparin indicate more rapid catabolism of the enzyme. J Lab Clin Med. 2003;142(2):90–9.
41. Mahmood D, et al. Lipoprotein lipase activity is favoured by peritoneal dialysis compared to hemodialysis. Scand J Clin Lab Invest. 2014;74(4):296–300.
42. Mahmood D, et al. Response of angiopoietin-like proteins 3 and 4 to hemodialysis. Int J Artif Organs. 2014;37(1):13–20.
43. Vaziri ND, et al. Lipoprotein lipase deficiency in chronic kidney disease is accompanied by down-regulation of endothelial GPIHBP1 expression. Clin Exp Nephrol. 2012;16(2):238–43.
44. Liang K, Oveisi F, Vaziri ND. Role of secondary hyperparathyroidism in the genesis of hypertriglyceridemia and VLDL receptor deficiency in chronic renal failure. Kidney Int. 1998;53(3):626–30.
45. Vaziri ND, Wang XQ, Liang K. Secondary hyperparathyroidism downregulates lipoprotein lipase expression in chronic renal failure. Am J Phys. 1997;273(6 Pt 2):F925–30.
46. Nishizawa Y, et al. Atherosclerosis in uremia: possible roles of hyperparathyroidism and intermediate density lipoprotein accumulation. Kidney Int Suppl. 1997;62:S90–2.
47. Massry SG, Akmal M. Lipid abnormalities, renal failure, and parathyroid hormone. Am J Med. 1989;87(5N):42N–4N.
48. Klin M, et al. Abnormalities in hepatic lipase in chronic renal failure: role of excess parathyroid hormone. J Clin Invest. 1996;97(10):2167–73.
49. Akmal M, et al. Excess parathyroid hormone adversely affects lipid metabolism in chronic renal failure. Kidney Int. 1990;37(3):854–8.
50. Kim C, Vaziri ND. Down-regulation of hepatic LDL receptor-related protein (LRP) in chronic renal failure. Kidney Int. 2005;67(3):1028–32.
51. Ikewaki K, et al. Delayed in vivo catabolism of intermediate-density lipoprotein and low-density lipoprotein in hemodialysis patients as potential cause of premature atherosclerosis. Arterioscler Thromb Vasc Biol. 2005;25(12):2615–22.
52. Vaziri ND, Norris K. Lipid disorders and their relevance to outcomes in chronic kidney disease. Blood Purif. 2011;31(1–3):189–96.
53. Kronenberg F, et al. LDL-unbound apolipoprotein(a) and carotid atherosclerosis in hemodialysis patients. Clin Genet. 1997;52(5):377–86.
54. Kronenberg F, et al. The low molecular weight apo(a) phenotype is an independent predictor for coronary

artery disease in hemodialysis patients: a prospective follow-up. J Am Soc Nephrol. 1999;10(5):1027–36.
55. Vaziri ND. Role of dyslipidemia in impairment of energy metabolism, oxidative stress, inflammation and cardiovascular disease in chronic kidney disease. Clin Exp Nephrol. 2014;18(2):265–8.
56. Vaziri ND. HDL abnormalities in nephrotic syndrome and chronic kidney disease. Nat Rev Nephrol. 2016;12(1):37–47.
57. Speer T, Zewinger S, Fliser D. Uraemic dyslipidaemia revisited: role of high-density lipoprotein. Nephrol Dial Transplant. 2013;28(10):2456–63.
58. Pahl MV, et al. Plasma phospholipid transfer protein, cholesteryl ester transfer protein and lecithin:cholesterol acyltransferase in end-stage renal disease (ESRD). Nephrol Dial Transplant. 2009;24(8):2541–6.
59. Kimura H, et al. Cholesteryl ester transfer protein as a protective factor against vascular disease in hemodialysis patients. Am J Kidney Dis. 2001;38(1):70–6.
60. Yamamoto S, Kon V. Chronic kidney disease induced dysfunction of high density lipoprotein. Clin Exp Nephrol. 2014;18(2):251–4.
61. Dantoine TF, et al. Decrease of serum paraoxonase activity in chronic renal failure. J Am Soc Nephrol. 1998;9(11):2082–8.
62. Vaziri ND, et al. Salutary effects of hemodialysis on low-density lipoprotein proinflammatory and high-density lipoprotein anti-inflammatory properties in patient with end-stage renal disease. J Natl Med Assoc. 2011;103(6):524–33.
63. Yamamoto S, et al. Dysfunctional high-density lipoprotein in patients on chronic hemodialysis. J Am Coll Cardiol. 2012;60(23):2372–9.
64. Kaseda R, et al. Dysfunctional high-density lipoproteins in children with chronic kidney disease. Metabolism. 2015;64(2):263–73.
65. Weichhart T, et al. Serum amyloid A in uremic HDL promotes inflammation. J Am Soc Nephrol. 2012;23(5):934–47.
66. Kopecky C, et al. Restoration of renal function does not correct impairment of uremic HDL properties. J Am Soc Nephrol. 2015;26(3):565–75.
67. Shroff R, et al. HDL in children with CKD promotes endothelial dysfunction and an abnormal vascular phenotype. J Am Soc Nephrol. 2014;25(11):2658–68.
68. Holzer M, et al. Dialysis modalities and HDL composition and function. J Am Soc Nephrol. 2015;26(9):2267–76.
69. Ansell BJ, Fonarow GC, Fogelman AM. The paradox of dysfunctional high-density lipoprotein. Curr Opin Lipidol. 2007;18(4):427–34.
70. McMahon M, et al. Proinflammatory high-density lipoprotein as a biomarker for atherosclerosis in patients with systemic lupus erythematosus and rheumatoid arthritis. Arthritis Rheum. 2006;54(8):2541–9.
71. Honda H, et al. Oxidized high-density lipoprotein as a risk factor for cardiovascular events in prevalent hemodialysis patients. Atherosclerosis. 2012;220(2):493–501.
72. Moradi H, et al. Elevated high-density lipoprotein cholesterol and cardiovascular mortality in maintenance hemodialysis patients. Nephrol Dial Transplant. 2014;29(8):1554–62.
73. Zewinger S, et al. HDL cholesterol is not associated with lower mortality in patients with kidney dysfunction. J Am Soc Nephrol. 2014;25(5):1073–82.
74. Bowe B, et al. Low levels of high-density lipoprotein cholesterol increase the risk of incident kidney disease and its progression. Kidney Int. 2016;89:886.
75. Kopecky C, et al. Quantification of HDL proteins, cardiac events, and mortality in patients with type 2 diabetes on hemodialysis. Clin J Am Soc Nephrol. 2015;10(2):224–31.
76. Holzer M, et al. Uremia alters HDL composition and function. J Am Soc Nephrol. 2011;22(9):1631–41.
77. Vaziri ND, Liang K, Parks JS. Down-regulation of hepatic lecithin:cholesterol acyltransferase gene expression in chronic renal failure. Kidney Int. 2001;59(6):2192–6.
78. Liang K, Kim CH, Vaziri ND. HMG-CoA reductase inhibition reverses LCAT and LDL receptor deficiencies and improves HDL in rats with chronic renal failure. Am J Physiol Renal Physiol. 2005;288(3):F539–44.
79. Moradi H, et al. Increased monocyte adhesion-promoting capacity of plasma in end-stage renal disease – response to antioxidant therapy. Clin Nephrol. 2010;74(4):273–81.
80. Miida T, et al. LCAT-dependent conversion of prebeta1-HDL into alpha-migrating HDL is severely delayed in hemodialysis patients. J Am Soc Nephrol. 2003;14(3):732–8.
81. Guarnieri GF, et al. Lecithin-cholesterol acyltransferase (LCAT) activity in chronic uremia. Kidney Int Suppl. 1978;8:S26–30.
82. Liang K, Vaziri ND. Upregulation of acyl-CoA: cholesterol acyltransferase in chronic renal failure. Am J Physiol Endocrinol Metab. 2002;283(4):E676–81.
83. Moradi H, et al. Reverse cholesterol transport pathway in experimental chronic renal failure. Am J Nephrol. 2009;30(2):147–54.
84. Vaziri ND, Liang K. ACAT inhibition reverses LCAT deficiency and improves plasma HDL in chronic renal failure. Am J Physiol Renal Physiol. 2004;287(5):F1038–43.
85. Moradi H, Said HM, Vaziri ND. Post-transcriptional nature of uremia-induced downregulation of hepatic apolipoprotein A-I production. Transl Res. 2013;161(6):477–85.
86. Vaziri ND, Deng G, Liang K. Hepatic HDL receptor, SR-B1 and Apo A-I expression in chronic renal failure. Nephrol Dial Transplant. 1999;14(6):1462–6.
87. Batista MC, et al. Apolipoprotein A-I, B-100, and B-48 metabolism in subjects with chronic kidney disease, obesity, and the metabolic syndrome. Metabolism. 2004;53(10):1255–61.
88. Okubo K, et al. Abnormal HDL apolipoprotein A-I and A-II kinetics in hemodialysis patients: a stable isotope study. J Am Soc Nephrol. 2004;15(4):1008–15.

89. Pruijm M, et al. High prevalence of anti-apolipoprotein/A-1 autoantibodies in maintenance hemodialysis and association with dialysis vintage. Ther Apher Dial. 2012;16(6):588–94.
90. Shao B. Site-specific oxidation of apolipoprotein A-I impairs cholesterol export by ABCA1, a key cardio-protective function of HDL. Biochim Biophys Acta. 2012;1821(3):490–501.
91. Kon V, Yang H, Fazio S. Residual cardiovascular risk in chronic kidney disease: role of high-density lipoprotein. Arch Med Res. 2015;46(5):379–91.
92. Kalantar-Zadeh K, Brennan ML, Hazen SL. Serum myeloperoxidase and mortality in maintenance hemodialysis patients. Am J Kidney Dis. 2006;48(1):59–68.
93. Kalantar-Zadeh K, et al. HDL-inflammatory index correlates with poor outcome in hemodialysis patients. Kidney Int. 2007;72(9):1149–56.
94. Garcia-Lopez E, et al. Risk factors for cardiovascular disease in patients undergoing peritoneal dialysis. Perit Dial Int. 2007;27(Suppl 2):S205–9.
95. Attman PO, et al. Apolipoprotein B-containing lipoproteins in renal failure: the relation to mode of dialysis. Kidney Int. 1999;55(4):1536–42.
96. Shoji T, et al. Roles of hypoalbuminemia and lipoprotein lipase on hyperlipoproteinemia in continuous ambulatory peritoneal dialysis. Metabolism. 1991;40(10):1002–8.
97. Siamopoulos KC, et al. Lipid parameters including lipoprotein (a) in patients undergoing CAPD and hemodialysis. Perit Dial Int. 1995;15(8):342–7.
98. Moberly JB, et al. Alterations in lipoprotein composition in peritoneal dialysis patients. Perit Dial Int. 2002;22(2):220–8.
99. Xu X, et al. Transcriptional control of hepatic lipid metabolism by SREBP and ChREBP. Semin Liver Dis. 2013;33(4):301–11.
100. Babazono T, et al. Effects of icodextrin on glycemic and lipid profiles in diabetic patients undergoing peritoneal dialysis. Am J Nephrol. 2007;27(4):409–15.
101. Phillips S, Heuberger R. Metabolic disorders following kidney transplantation. J Ren Nutr. 2012;22(5):451–60. e1
102. Kobashigawa JA, Kasiske BL. Hyperlipidemia in solid organ transplantation. Transplantation. 1997;63(3):331–8.
103. Tse KC, et al. A long-term study on hyperlipidemia in stable renal transplant recipients. Clin Transpl. 2004;18(3):274–80.
104. Riella LV, Gabardi S, Chandraker A. Dyslipidemia and its therapeutic challenges in renal transplantation. Am J Transplant. 2012;12(8):1975–82.
105. Fruhwurth S, et al. Inhibition of mTOR down-regulates scavenger receptor, class B, type I (SR-BI) expression, reduces endothelial cell migration and impairs nitric oxide production. Biochim Biophys Acta. 2014;1841(7):944–53.
106. Morrisett JD, et al. Effects of sirolimus on plasma lipids, lipoprotein levels, and fatty acid metabolism in renal transplant patients. J Lipid Res. 2002;43(8):1170–80.
107. Fardet L, Feve B. Systemic glucocorticoid therapy: a review of its metabolic and cardiovascular adverse events. Drugs. 2014;74(15):1731–45.
108. Artz MA, et al. Improved cardiovascular risk profile and renal function in renal transplant patients after randomized conversion from cyclosporine to tacrolimus. J Am Soc Nephrol. 2003;14(7):1880–8.
109. Vaziri ND, Liang K, Azad H. Effect of cyclosporine on HMG-CoA reductase, cholesterol 7alpha-hydroxylase, LDL receptor, HDL receptor, VLDL receptor, and lipoprotein lipase expressions. J Pharmacol Exp Ther. 2000;294(2):778–83.
110. Le Goff W, et al. Cyclosporin A traps ABCA1 at the plasma membrane and inhibits ABCA1-mediated lipid efflux to apolipoprotein A-I. Arterioscler Thromb Vasc Biol. 2004;24(11):2155–61.
111. Kockx M, et al. Cyclosporin A decreases apolipoprotein E secretion from human macrophages via a protein phosphatase 2B-dependent and ATP-binding cassette transporter A1 (ABCA1)-independent pathway. J Biol Chem. 2009;284(36):24144–54.
112. Tory R, et al. Cyclosporine A and rapamycin induce in vitro cholesteryl ester transfer protein activity, and suppress lipoprotein lipase activity in human plasma. Int J Pharm. 2008;358(1–2):219–23.
113. Vaziri ND. Molecular mechanisms of lipid disorders in nephrotic syndrome. Kidney Int. 2003;63(5):1964–76.
114. Kaysen GA, de Sain-van der Velden MG. New insights into lipid metabolism in the nephrotic syndrome. Kidney Int Suppl. 1999;71:S18–21.
115. Kim CH, et al. Hepatic tissue sterol regulatory element binding protein 2 and low-density lipoprotein receptor in nephrotic syndrome. Metabolism. 2007;56(10):1377–82.
116. Vaziri ND, Liang KH. Acyl-coenzyme A: cholesterol acyltransferase inhibition ameliorates proteinuria, hyperlipidemia, lecithin-cholesterol acyltransferase, SRB-1, and low-density lipoprotein receptor deficiencies in nephrotic syndrome. Circulation. 2004;110(4):419–25.
117. Vaziri ND, Liang K. Up-regulation of acyl-coenzyme A: cholesterol acyltransferase (ACAT) in nephrotic syndrome. Kidney Int. 2002;61(5):1769–75.
118. Vaziri ND, Liang KH. Hepatic HMG-CoA reductase gene expression during the course of puromycin-induced nephrosis. Kidney Int. 1995;48(6):1979–85.
119. Kim S, Kim CH, Vaziri ND. Upregulation of hepatic LDL receptor-related protein in nephrotic syndrome: response to statin therapy. Am J Physiol Endocrinol Metab. 2005;288(4):E813–7.
120. Vaziri ND, Liang KH. Down-regulation of hepatic LDL receptor expression in experimental nephrosis. Kidney Int. 1996;50(3):887–93.
121. Warwick GL, et al. Metabolism of apolipoprotein B-containing lipoproteins in subjects with nephrotic-range proteinuria. Kidney Int. 1991;40(1):129–38.
122. Warwick GL, et al. Low-density lipoprotein metabolism in the nephrotic syndrome. Metabolism. 1990;39(2):187–92.

123. Li J, et al. Secreted PCSK9 promotes LDL receptor degradation independently of proteolytic activity. Biochem J. 2007;406(2):203–7.
124. Lagace TA, et al. Secreted PCSK9 decreases the number of LDL receptors in hepatocytes and in livers of parabiotic mice. J Clin Invest. 2006;116(11):2995–3005.
125. Maxwell KN, Breslow JL. Adenoviral-mediated expression of Pcsk9 in mice results in a low-density lipoprotein receptor knockout phenotype. Proc Natl Acad Sci U S A. 2004;101(18):7100–5.
126. Jin K, et al. Plasma PCSK9 in nephrotic syndrome and in peritoneal dialysis: a cross-sectional study. Am J Kidney Dis. 2014;63(4):584–9.
127. Liu S, Vaziri ND. Role of PCSK9 and IDOL in the pathogenesis of acquired LDL receptor deficiency and hypercholesterolemia in nephrotic syndrome. Nephrol Dial Transplant. 2014;29(3):538–43.
128. Kronenberg F, Utermann G, Dieplinger H. Lipoprotein(a) in renal disease. Am J Kidney Dis. 1996;27(1):1–25.
129. Wanner C, et al. Elevated plasma lipoprotein(a) in patients with the nephrotic syndrome. Ann Intern Med. 1993;119(4):263–9.
130. Wahl P, Ducasa GM, Fornoni A. Systemic and renal lipids in kidney disease development and progression. Am J Physiol Renal Physiol. 2016;310(6):F433–45.
131. Kamanna VS, et al. Oxidative modification of low-density lipoprotein enhances the murine mesangial cell cytokines associated with monocyte migration, differentiation, and proliferation. Lab Investig. 1996;74(6):1067–79.
132. Kume S, et al. Role of altered renal lipid metabolism in the development of renal injury induced by a high-fat diet. J Am Soc Nephrol. 2007;18(10):2715–23.
133. Rodriguez-Iturbe B, et al. Mycophenolate mofetil ameliorates nephropathy in the obese Zucker rat. Kidney Int. 2005;68(3):1041–7.
134. Muso E, et al. Immediate therapeutic efficacy of low-density lipoprotein apheresis for drug-resistant nephrotic syndrome: evidence from the short-term results from the POLARIS study. Clin Exp Nephrol. 2015;19(3):379–86.
135. Shiraishi N, et al. Low-density lipoprotein apheresis for proteinuria in lupus nephritis with intraglomerular foam cells containing cholesterol crystals. Am J Kidney Dis. 2015;65(3):490–3.
136. Rader DJ. New therapeutic approaches to the treatment of dyslipidemia. Cell Metab. 2016;23(3):405–12.
137. Zhao Y, Marcel YL. Serum albumin is a significant intermediate in cholesterol transfer between cells and lipoproteins. Biochemistry. 1996;35(22):7174–80.
138. Vaziri ND, Liang K, Parks JS. Acquired lecithin-cholesterol acyltransferase deficiency in nephrotic syndrome. Am J Physiol Renal Physiol. 2001;280(5):F823–8.
139. Zhang C, et al. Effect of hypoalbuminemia on the increased serum cholesteryl ester transfer protein concentration in children with idiopathic nephrotic syndrome. Clin Biochem. 2007;40(12):869–75.
140. Moulin P, et al. Increased concentration of plasma cholesteryl ester transfer protein in nephrotic syndrome: role in dyslipidemia. J Lipid Res. 1992;33(12):1817–22.
141. Braschi S, et al. Role of lipoprotein-bound NEFAs in enhancing the specific activity of plasma CETP in the nephrotic syndrome. Arterioscler Thromb Vasc Biol. 1997;17(11):2559–67.
142. Shearer GC, Couser WG, Kaysen GA. Nephrotic livers secrete normal VLDL that acquire structural and functional defects following interaction with HDL. Kidney Int. 2004;65(1):228–37.
143. Vaziri ND, et al. Nephrotic syndrome causes upregulation of HDL endocytic receptor and PDZK-1-dependent downregulation of HDL docking receptor. Nephrol Dial Transplant. 2011;26(10):3118–23.
144. Liang K, Vaziri ND. Down-regulation of hepatic high-density lipoprotein receptor, SR-B1, in nephrotic syndrome. Kidney Int. 1999;56(2):621–6.
145. Newman JW, et al. Proteinuria increases oxylipid concentrations in VLDL and HDL but not LDL particles in the rat. J Lipid Res. 2007;48(8):1792–800.
146. Kaysen GA, et al. Both peripheral chylomicron catabolism and hepatic uptake of remnants are defective in nephrosis. Am J Phys. 1992;263(2 Pt 2):F335–41.
147. de Sain-van der Velden MG, et al. Increased VLDL in nephrotic patients results from a decreased catabolism while increased LDL results from increased synthesis. Kidney Int. 1998;53(4):994–1001.
148. Kaysen GA. Nephrotic hyperlipidemia: primary abnormalities in both lipoprotein catabolism and synthesis. Miner Electrolyte Metab. 1992;18(2–5):212–6.
149. Garber DW, et al. Catabolism of very low density lipoproteins in experimental nephrosis. J Clin Invest. 1984;74(4):1375–83.
150. Shearer GC, et al. Hypoalbuminemia and proteinuria contribute separately to reduced lipoprotein catabolism in the nephrotic syndrome. Kidney Int. 2001;59(1):179–89.
151. Davies RW, et al. Proteinuria, not altered albumin metabolism, affects hyperlipidemia in the nephrotic rat. J Clin Invest. 1990;86(2):600–5.
152. Sato T, Liang K, Vaziri ND. Protein restriction and AST-120 improve lipoprotein lipase and VLDL receptor in focal glomerulosclerosis. Kidney Int. 2003;64(5):1780–6.
153. Liang K, Vaziri ND. Gene expression of lipoprotein lipase in experimental nephrosis. J Lab Clin Med. 1997;130(4):387–94.

154. Liang K, Vaziri ND. Down-regulation of hepatic lipase expression in experimental nephrotic syndrome. Kidney Int. 1997;51(6):1933–7.
155. Sato T, Liang K, Vaziri ND. Down-regulation of lipoprotein lipase and VLDL receptor in rats with focal glomerulosclerosis. Kidney Int. 2002;61(1):157–62.
156. Joven J, et al. Abnormalities of lipoprotein metabolism in patients with the nephrotic syndrome. N Engl J Med. 1990;323(9):579–84.
157. Levy E, et al. Experimental nephrotic syndrome: removal and tissue distribution of chylomicrons and very-low-density lipoproteins of normal and nephrotic origin. Biochim Biophys Acta. 1990;1043(3):259–66.
158. Wang L, et al. Proteinuria decreases tissue lipoprotein receptor levels resulting in altered lipoprotein structure and increasing lipid levels. Kidney Int. 2012;82(9):990–9.
159. Deighan CJ, et al. Patients with nephrotic-range proteinuria have apolipoprotein C and E deficient VLDL1. Kidney Int. 2000;58(3):1238–46.
160. Furukawa S, et al. Catabolic defect of triglyceride is associated with abnormal very-low-density lipoprotein in experimental nephrosis. Metabolism. 1990;39(1):101–7.
161. Han S, et al. Hepatic fatty acid and cholesterol metabolism in nephrotic syndrome. Am J Transl Res. 2013;5(2):246–53.
162. Vaziri ND, et al. Up-regulation of hepatic Acyl CoA: diacylglycerol acyltransferase-1 (DGAT-1) expression in nephrotic syndrome. Kidney Int. 2004;66(1):262–7.
163. Zhou Y, et al. Expression profiling of hepatic genes associated with lipid metabolism in nephrotic rats. Am J Physiol Renal Physiol. 2008;295(3):F662–71.
164. Clement LC, et al. Circulating angiopoietin-like 4 links proteinuria with hypertriglyceridemia in nephrotic syndrome. Nat Med. 2014;20(1):37–46.
165. Clement LC, et al. The proteinuria-hypertriglyceridemia connection as a basis for novel therapeutics for nephrotic syndrome. Transl Res. 2015;165(4):499–504.
166. Clement LC, et al. Podocyte-secreted angiopoietin-like-4 mediates proteinuria in glucocorticoid-sensitive nephrotic syndrome. Nat Med. 2011;17(1):117–22.
167. Herman-Edelstein M, et al. Altered renal lipid metabolism and renal lipid accumulation in human diabetic nephropathy. J Lipid Res. 2014;55(3):561–72.
168. Vaziri ND, Moradi H. Dual role of circulating angiopoietin-like 4 (ANGPTL4) in promoting hypertriglyceridemia and lowering proteinuria in nephrotic syndrome. Am J Kidney Dis. 2014;64(4):495–8.
169. Jin K, Norris K, Vaziri ND. Dysregulation of hepatic fatty acid metabolism in chronic kidney disease. Nephrol Dial Transplant. 2013;28(2):313–20.
170. Kim HJ, et al. Renal mass reduction results in accumulation of lipids and dysregulation of lipid regulatory proteins in the remnant kidney. Am J Physiol Renal Physiol. 2009;296(6):F1297–306.

13 Drugs for Treatment of Dyslipidemia Available in the USA

Elani Streja and Dan A. Streja

Clinical Guidelines for Management of Dyslipidemia

Management of dyslipidemia has been the core of pharmacological intervention for cardiovascular (CV) prevention for over 30 years [1]. In spite of this, it has remained an area of continuous controversy. In the past 5 years, 11 guidelines for management of hyperlipidemia were published in the English language. All included recommendations, as summarized in Table 13.1, were applicable to dyslipidemia in non-dialysis-dependent chronic kidney disease (NDD-CKD). However, treatment of dyslipidemia after renal replacement therapy has not been included in these guidelines because of failure of clinical trials to show benefit.

Although evidence from clinical studies was similarly available to all guideline-writing committees, there are major differences in recommendation approaches resulting in major differences in guidelines, which have not yet been reconciled. Guidelines can be classified into three types according to their specificity for chronic kidney disease (CKD) patients: guidelines specific for CKD patients, guidelines who identify CKD as a high-risk group, and guidelines for whom CKD patients are no different from the rest of the population they are addressing.

Specific CKD Guidelines

Kidney Disease: Improving Global Outcomes (*KDIGO*), an international foundation, recommends a "fire and forget" approach [2]. The authors consider patients with CKD over age 50 to be at high risk of developing CV disease (CVD) and therefore recommend statin with or without ezetimibe treatment, irrespective of baseline serum cholesterol. They advise that baseline cholesterol should be determined only to rule out low-density lipoprotein cholesterol (LDLc) higher than 190 mg/dL, which is considered indicative of a familial hyperlipidemia. No follow-up determination of lipid levels is necessary in the majority of the patients, and no target for lipoprotein goal was established. There is no upper age treatment limit recommended. In addition, in patients of age below 50, treatment is recommended if the patient has diabetes and atherosclerotic CVD (ASCVD) or if a 10-year global risk is in excess of 10%. There is no

E. Streja (✉)
Division of Nephrology and Hypertension, University of California Irvine School of Medicine, Orange, CA, USA

Tibor Rubin Veterans Affairs Medical Center, Long Beach, CA, USA
e-mail: estreja@uci.edu

D. A. Streja
Department of Medicine, David Geffen School of Medicine at UCLA, VA Greater Los Angeles Health Care System, Los Angeles, CA, USA

C. M. Rhee et al. (eds.), *Endocrine Disorders in Kidney Disease*,
https://doi.org/10.1007/978-3-319-97765-2_13

Table 13.1 Differences between guidelines in recommendations for management of dyslipidemia

Guidelines	ACC/ AHA-2013	VA-DOD	KDIGO	KDOQI	ADA-2016	AACE	C-CHANGE	NICE	JAS	NLA	ACC/ AHA-2016
Specificity	General population	General population	CKD	CKD	Diabetes	Diabetes	General population	General population	General population	General population	General population
Global risk evaluation	Calculator or ASCVD	Calculator or ASCVD	No	No	No	ASCVD or risk factors	No	No	NIPPON-DATA80	ASCVD or risk factors	Calculator or ASCVD or high risk
Global risk threshold	7.50%	12%	10%	Stage of CKD	LDLc >100 is a "risk factor"	No	No	No	2% 10-year CAD-Death	No	7.50%
Goal	No	No	No	No	No	For LDLc, ApoB and particle number	LDLc<70 or nonHDLc <100 or ApoB <80	No	LDLc<100 or nonHDLc <130	LDLc<70 or nonHDLc <100 or ApoB <80	LDLc<70 or nonHDLc <100
Statin dose	High dose for ASCVD or diabetes	Moderate dose initially	Moderate dose only	High dose for ACS or stage 3a CKD	High dose preferred	No	Over 50% LDLc decrease	Over 40% nonHDLc decrease	No	No	High dose for ASCVD or high risk
Non-statin drugs	No	No	Ezetimibe only	Ezetimibe only	No	Yes	Yes	No	Yes	Yes	Yes

Abbreviations: *AACE* American Association of Clinical Endocrinologists, *ACC/AHA* American College of Cardiology/American Heart Association, *ACS* acute coronary syndrome, *ADA* American Diabetes Association, *ApoB* apolipoprotein B, *ASCVD* atherosclerotic cardiovascular disease, *CAD* coronary artery disease, *CKD* chronic kidney disease, *JAS* Japanese Atherosclerosis Society, *KDIGO* Kidney Disease: Improving Global Outcomes, *KDOQI* Kidney Disease Outcomes Quality Initiative, *LDLc* low-density lipoprotein cholesterol, *NICE* National Clinical Guideline Centre of the United Kingdom, *NLA* National Lipid Association, *nonHDLc* non-highdensity lipoprotein cholesterol, and *VA-DOD* Veteran Administration-Department of Defense specification for differences in the ethnicity of the patient. Irrespective of estimated glomerular filtration rate (eGFR) and comorbidity, the guidelines advise the patient should be treated with a moderate-dose statin.

Conversely, a group of authors representing the US National Kidney Foundation and its Kidney Disease Outcomes Quality Initiative *(KDOQI)* has published a few revisions of the KDIGO guidelines [3], observing that (1) for achieving benefit from statins, LDLc lowering must exceed 30%; (2) that in patients younger than age 40, global risk is difficult to evaluate so individualization should be implemented; and (3) that patients could be treated with high-dose statins if the eGFR is higher than 45 mL/min/1.73m^2 or if the risk of ASCVD is very high.

Guidelines Specifying that Patients with CKD Are at High Risk of ASCVD Outcomes

The National Clinical Guideline Centre of the United Kingdom (*NICE*) [4] recommends treatment of all patients with CKD, irrespective of age, with atorvastatin 20 mg/day. This is similar to their treatment recommendation for general population patients who have a 10% or greater 10-year risk of developing CVD. They also state that plant stanols and sterols, fibrates, niacin, bile acid-binding resins, and omega-3 fatty acids are specifically not to be recommended for CKD patients. Additionally, in CKD patients, the dose of statins should be increased, if the goal of at least 40% decrease in non-high-density lipoprotein cholesterol (nonHDLc) is not achieved. In patients with stage 4 CKD, the guidelines recommend consultation with a kidney specialist to discuss prescribing a higher-dose statin.

The Canadian CV Society (*CCS*) [5] recommends specific goals to be achieved in terms of levels of LDLc (<70 mg/dL), nonHDLc (<100 mg/dL), or apolipoprotein B (ApoB) <80 mg/dL in patients at high risk. The guidelines state that patients with CKD are at increased risk of ASCVD, if they have eGFR<45 mL/min/1.73m^2 or albumin/creatinine ratio (ACR) of >30 mg/mmol.

The European Atherosclerosis Society and European Society of Cardiology (*EAS/ESC*) [6] consider patients with moderate to severe CKD (eGFR <60 mL/min/1.73 m^2) to be at high risk of ASCVD. Consequently they recommend a treatment target for LDLc <70 mg/dL or a ≥50% reduction from baseline LDLc. This would imply use of a high-dose statin or addition of a non-statin drug to a moderate-dose statin in all patients. These guidelines accept targeting to goals other than LDLc. They also recommend use of statins eliminated mostly by hepatic route such as atorvastatin, fluvastatin, and pitavastatin.

The Japanese Atherosclerosis Society *(JAS)* guidelines [7] are distinctly characterized by its targeting of triglycerides and high-density lipoprotein cholesterol (HDLc) for cardiovascular prevention. They advise that statin use in elderly patients is to be individualized. However, in these guidelines, drugs other than statins are recommended in order to target all components of dyslipidemia. The goals in term of LDLc and nonHDLc are <100 mg/dL and <130 mg/dL, respectively, which makes these guidelines less aggressive.

For the National Lipid Association (*NLA*) [8], similar goals are expressed in terms of LDLc and nonHDLc. LDL particle number could be determined, but no goal is recommended. For these recommendations, CKD is considered high risk only if eGFR is <45 mL/min/1.73 m^2.

In July 2016, the ACC published new guidelines in which CKD was added to conditions conferring a high risk of cardiovascular events and recommended aggressive cholesterol-lowering therapy in all patients [9].

Guidelines for Which Patients with CKD Are No Different from the General Population

The 2013 American College of Cardiology and American Heart Association (*ACC/AHA*) guidelines [10] have been the subject of wide controversy, with respect to treatment of dyslipidemia in CKD patients. They emphatically state that low eGFR and increased albumin excretion rate have not been proven to contribute to evaluation of CV risk. Consequently, the risk of patients with CKD is therefore evaluated according to the same risk calculator as the general population. The calculator takes into consideration age, smoking status, presence of hypertension and its control, diabetes, ethnicity, total cholesterol, and HDLc. In patients with documented ASCVD and diabetes, who represent the majority of patients with CKD, the guidelines recommend the use of high-dose statins. In the rest of the patients, moderate-dose statins are recommended if the global 10-year risk exceeds 7.5%. No drug other than statins is recommended, and no goal is recommended for treatment. In patients over the age of 75 or under 40, they suggest treatment should be individualized.

In 2015 the Veteran Affairs and the Department of Defense (*VA-DOD*) [11] published their own guidelines, which are characterized by their emphasis on safety. They are similar with the ACC/AHA guidelines, but they recommend initiation of statins with moderate dose in all patients, and the threshold for initiation is a 10-year global risk of 12%.

In 2015 the American Diabetes Association (*ADA*) [12] adopted most of the ACC/AHA guidelines for patients with diabetes. In these guidelines, since the recommendations pertain to patients with diabetes, all diabetic CKD patients are to be treated with high-dose statins. Patients under age 40 are to be treated if ASCVD or risk factors are present, but there is no specification for upper limit of age.

The American Association of Clinical Endocrinologists (*AACE*) [13], as opposed to the ADA, maintained its prior to 2013 guidelines for patients with diabetes. In patients with diabetes and either ASCVD or one or more risk factors, which includes most patients with CKD, statins should be initiated. They also advise that lipid-lowering drugs, not limited to statins, should be added to obtain an LDLc <70 mg/dL, nonHDLc <100 mg/dL, ApoB <80 mg/dL, or LDL particle number <1000 mmol/L.

In summary the details of the approaches and consequently the recommendations are so different that no harmonization is possible without additional evidence. In spite of the differences between the guidelines, an analysis of the decisions for treatment with statins showed acceptable concordance [14]. From a practical point of view, the main remaining questions are:

1. Are high-dose statins safe in all stages of CKD?
2. Which NDD-CKD patients should be treated with high-dose statins?
3. Should there be a goal for atherogenic particles?
4. Should other drugs than statins be added to achieve the goal?

Statin Use in Non-Dialysis-Dependent CKD Patients

In 2009, Nakamura et al. conducted a post hoc analysis of patients included in the Management of Elevated Cholesterol in the Primary Prevention Group of Adult Japanese (MEGA) study and evaluated the effect of pravastatin (10–20 mg) vs. placebo in 1471 treated and 1507 placebo-treated controls with moderate kidney disease (eGFR 30 – <60 mL/min/1.73m^2), mild to moderate hypercholesterolemia, and no past history of ischemic heart disease and/or stroke. Results of the post hoc analysis showed that over 5 years of follow-up, the pravastatin patients had reduced coronary heart disease by 48% and stroke by 73% and had a 51% lower risk of all-cause mortality.

In 2010 Ridker et al. conducted a post hoc analysis of the Justification for the Use of Statins in Primary Prevention: An Intervention Trial Evaluating Rosuvastatin (JUPITER) trial, which included patients with a low-density lipoprotein cholesterol (LDLc) >130 mg/dL and high-sensitivity C-reactive protein (hsCRP) ≥2 mg/L. They compared 1638 patients treated with 20 mg with rosuvastatin and 1629 patients treated with placebo (both groups with 30 – <60 mL/min/1.73m^2) and found statin-treated patients had a 45% risk reduction in myocardial infarction, stroke, hospital stay for unstable angina, arterial revascularization, or confirmed CV death and a 43% lower risk of all-cause mortality.

Conversely, in a number of post hoc analysis studies evaluating the effect of statin on CV outcomes and all-cause mortality in NDD-CKD patients, although associations trended toward lower risk, no significant effect of statins on preventing all-cause mortality was observed. These studies include post hoc analyses of pravastatin (PREVEND-IT [15], ALLHAT [16], PPP-WOSCOPS, CARE, LIPID [17]), atorvastatin (CARDS [18], ALLIANCE [19]), and fluvastatin (LIPS) [20]. However, in the post hoc analysis of the Air Force/Texas Coronary Atherosclerosis Prevention (AFCAP) study, which compared the effect of 20 mg lovastatin vs. placebo on clinical outcomes in analyses of 304 men with eGFR<60 mL/min/1.73m^2 at baseline, statin therapy significantly reduced fatal and nonfatal CV events [RR 0.40, 95%CI 0.18–0.91] in unadjusted models.

To date, two large meta-analyses have pooled the results of these as well as other studies to investigate the benefits of statin therapy in CKD patients. Palmer et al. [21] as part of the Cochrane collaboration reviewed over 50 studies in over 45,000 CKD patients and found that statin therapy, compared with placebo, reduced the risk of major CV events by 18%, risk of all-cause mortality by 21%, risk of CV mortality by 23%, and risk of myocardial infarction by 45%. However, there was only a nonsignificant reduction of stroke risk in statin-treated CKD patients. Their meta-analyses included pooled results of the largest statin clinical trial to date in CKD patients, namely, the Study of Heart and Renal Protection (SHARP). Although results in their meta-analyses examined effects of statin therapy by specific outcome, their report did not examine potential effect modification by staging of CKD.

In 2013, Hou et al. [22] also conducted a meta-analysis including 31 trials and over 40,000 CKD patients examining the effects of statin therapy in CKD patients and similarly found that treatment with statin therapy in these patients reduced major CV events by 23%, including a 22% reduction in coronary events and a 9% reduction in CV or all-cause death but also found no significant effect on stroke outcomes. Moreover, they found that each mmol/L reduction of LDLc lowering with a statin could yield an 18% reduction in CV events in CKD patients, which is similar and consistent with results observed in the general population of non-CKD patients. However, the most notable finding of this meta-analysis concluded that the effects of statin therapy in CKD patients differed by staging of the disease, where statins are most effective in earlier stages of NDD-CKD. For stage 3 CKD (which also included two small studies of stage 2 CKD patients), CV outcomes were reduced by 31% in the statin treated vs. placebo group, while stage 4 CKD patients showed a 22% reduction in composite CV risk. Analyses in the stage 5 CKD patients (mostly on-dialysis subgroup) showed only an 8% risk reduction.

Most studies included in Palmer's and Hou's meta-analyses included post hoc analyses of larger clinical trials, where each study included only less than 1000 NDD-CKD patients. To date, the SHARP is the largest trial to evaluate the effect of statin therapy (simvastatin plus ezetimibe) vs. placebo on clinical outcomes in patients with CKD. SHARP randomized 9270 patients with CKD (3023 dialysis-dependent and 6247 NDD-CKD) with no known history of myocardial infarction or coronary revascularization. Patients were assigned to simvastatin 20 mg plus ezetimibe 10 mg daily or matching placebo. After 4.9 years, there was a significant 17% reduction in major atherosclerotic events, 25% reduction in non-hemorrhagic stroke, and 21% reduction in arterial revascularization procedure. The trial also evaluated effect according to CKD stage estimated by the Modification of Diet in Renal Disease (MDRD) equation for glomerular filtration rate. In their subgroup analyses, a linear trend according to CKD stage appeared to be present, where the effects of statin treatment appeared to be more potent in earlier stages of NDD-CKD. Patients with stage 4 CKD had a 22% reduction of the primary endpoint, while the decrease in risk for stage 5 CKD was not significant, but the number of patients in which these data were obtained was very small. Moreover, no significant heterogeneity of effect (p = 0.73) was observed across CKD stages. Similarly, no heterogeneity of effect was observed in comparison of results for patients on dialysis vs. not on dialysis. However, due to the insignificant findings in the dialysis population, clinicians believe these study results show that statins are ineffective in dialysis-dependent patients.

Statin Use in Dialysis Patients

The all-cause mortality rate in US dialysis patients is 230 deaths per 1000 patient-years [23]. Cardiac disease is the major cause of death in dialysis patients and accounts for 43% of all-cause mortality. Sixty two percent of cardiac deaths (or 27% of all deaths) are attributable to arrhythmic mechanisms. The estimated rate of sudden cardiac death in US dialysis patients is 7% per year. Among patients initiating dialysis, the main cardiac abnormality is left ventricular hypertrophy [24, 25]. This is associated with other vascular abnormalities, including arterial stiffening and prominent generalized and aortocoronary calcification. Myocardial infarction is in part attributed to reperfusion injury [26]. Plaques are more likely to be fibrotic and calcified and less likely to have a "vulnerable" lipid core. Serum cholesterol is reported to be paradoxically associated with improved survival. In this context the plaque stabilizing effect of statins is expected to be less efficient in dialysis patients [27].

The Stegmayr et al. [28] study included 97 hemodialysis and 13 peritoneal dialysis patients, randomized to atorvastatin 10 mg/day or placebo for a mean of 31 months. Although atorvastatin reduced LDLc by 35%, it was not beneficial regarding CV endpoints or survival.

During the same year, a larger trial was published: the Deutsche Diabetes Dialyse Studie (4D study) [29]. It enrolled 1255 subjects with type 2 diabetes mellitus, receiving maintenance hemodialysis, randomly assigned to receive 20 mg of atorvastatin per day or matching placebo. During a median follow-up period of 4 years, 469 patients reached the primary endpoint (composite of death from cardiac causes, nonfatal myocardial infarction, and stroke), of which 226 were assigned to atorvastatin and 243 to placebo (RR 0.92, 95% CI 0.77–1.10). Atorvastatin significantly reduced the rate of all cardiac events combined (RR 0.82, 95% CI 0.68–0.99) but also significantly increased the risk of fatal stroke (RR 2.03, 95%CI 1.05–3.93). There was no benefit in terms of all-cause mortality. Atorvastatin significantly reduced the rates of adverse outcomes in the highest quartile of LDLc (>145 mg/dL) with a 31% reduction in the primary endpoint, 42% reduction in cardiac death, 52% reduction in sudden death, 38% reduction in nonfatal myocardial infarction, 32% reduction in cardiac events combined, and 28% reduction in all-cause mortality [30]. There was no treatment effect on CV events if the LDLc was <145 mg/dL.

The Study to Evaluate the Use of Rosuvastatin in Subjects on Regular Hemodialysis: An Assessment of Survival and CV Events (AURORA) was designed to investigate the effects of rosuvastatin 20 mg/day vs. placebo therapy in patients undergoing regular hemodialysis treatment [31]. The combined primary endpoint was death from CV causes, nonfatal MI, or nonfatal stroke. During a median follow-up period of 3.8 years, 396 patients in the rosuvastatin group and 408 patients in the placebo group reached the primary endpoint (HR 0.96, 95%CI 0.84–1.11) Rosuvastatin had no effect on the individual components of the primary endpoint and no significant effect on all-cause mortality. Lipoproteins were not independent predictors of mortality in these patients [32].

The SHARP trial included 3023 dialysis patients randomized to simvastatin 20 mg/day + ezetimibe 10 mg/day [33]. As opposed to the success of the intervention in NDD-CKD patients, there was no significant reduction in ASCVD events or mortality in this predefined subgroup (HR 0.90, 95%CI 0.75–1.08).

In summary, intervention with statins with or without ezetimibe appears to be ineffective in hemodialysis patients with the exception of patients with very high LDLc levels who presumably are more likely to experience an ASCVD associated with a plaque rupture.

Peritoneal Dialysis

Compared to hemodialysis patients, peritoneal dialysis patients have higher levels of ApoB-containing lipoproteins across their entire spectrum [34]. Although a small subgroup (<500) of peritoneal dialysis patients was evaluated in the SHARP trial showing nonsignificant results [33], to date no study has specifically addressed CV event reduction with statins in patients with peritoneal dialysis. A retrospective study using USRDS data and propensity score methodology analyzed the outcomes in 1053 patients receiving peritoneal dialysis [35]. Use of lipid-modifying medications was associated with decreased all-cause (HR 0.74, 95%CI 0.56–0.98) and CV (HR 0.67, 95%CI 0.47–0.95) mortality. In subgroup analyses, use of lipid-modifying medications was associated with significantly decreased all-cause and CV mortality in the subgroups with cholesterol levels of 226–275 mg/dL and all-cause mortality in the subgroup with cholesterol >275 mg/dL. Use of lipid-modifying medications also was associated with significantly decreased CV mortality (by 36%) in patients with diabetes and decreased all-cause (by 35%) and CV mortality (by 45%) in those with Charlson Comorbidity Index score higher than two. In another study analyzing 1024 Korean peritoneal dialysis patients, after propensity score matching, the use of statins was associated with improved survival (HR 0.55, 95%CI 0.38–0.79) [36]. In view of the differences in lipid profile between hemodialysis and peritoneal dialysis, a large clinical trial addressing statin intervention in peritoneal dialysis should be undertaken.

Statin Use in Renal Transplant Patients

Renal transplant recipients have also markedly shortened life expectancy [24]. Premature CVD is the leading cause of death in patients with a functioning renal graft. Many transplant recipients have preexisting CVD at the time of transplantation, and immunosuppressive therapy may accelerate the progression of vascular pathology.

Statin intervention for prevention of CV events was tested only in one trial. The Assessment of Lescol in Renal Transplantation (ALERT) trial [37] was a multicenter, randomized, double-blind, placebo-controlled trial in 2102 renal transplant recipients with total cholesterol 4.0–9.0 mmol/L (150–350 mg/dL). Patients were randomly assigned to fluvastatin 80 mg/day ($n = 1050$) or placebo ($n = 1052$) and followed up for a mean of 5.1 years. The primary endpoint was the occurrence of a major adverse cardiac event, defined as cardiac death, nonfatal myocardial infarction, or coronary revascularization. Secondary endpoints were individual cardiac events, combined cardiac death or nonfatal myocardial infarction, cerebrovascular events, non-CV death, all-cause mortality, and graft loss or doubling of serum creatinine. Analysis was by intention to treat. Fluvastatin lowered LDLc by 32%. Risk reduction with fluvastatin for the primary endpoint was not significant (RR 0.83, 95%CI 0.64–1.06). There were, however, fewer cardiac deaths or nonfatal myocardial infarction events (70 vs. 104, RR 0.65, 95%CI 0.48–0.88) in the fluvastatin group than in the placebo group. Coronary intervention procedures and other secondary endpoints did not differ significantly between groups. The authors performed multiple analyses for the endpoint of cardiac deaths or nonfatal myocardial infarction. Fluvastatin use was associated with reduction of risk in many subgroups with no heterogeneity. Statistical significance was achieved in patients who were younger, nondiabetic, nonsmokers, and without preexisting CVD. Multiple sclerosis was diagnosed in 32% of the patients enrolled in this study. CVD risk was 74% higher in patients with metabolic syndrome ($p = 0.012$), and the benefit of statin treatment in reducing CVD risk appeared to be attributable exclusively to those with metabolic syndrome.

The data were also analyzed according to the time after transplant or the time after renal replacement therapy (dialysis followed by transplant) [38]. The frequency of cardiac death and nonfatal myocardial infarction was 3.2%, 5.1%, 9.6%, and 8.2% with fluvastatin treatment as compared to 6%, 10.4%, 13.4%, and 9.6% with placebo when therapy was initiated at 0–2, 2–4, 4–6, and >6 years after the last transplant, respectively. The risk reduction for patients initiating therapy with fluvastatin at years 0–2 (compared with >6 years) following transplantation was 59% (RR 0.41, 95%CI 0.18–0.92). This is also reflected in total time on renal replacement therapy: in patients in the first quartile (<47 months), fluvastatin use was associated with a risk reduction of 64%, compared with 19% for patients in the fourth quartile (>120 months). These data were interpreted to support the early introduction of statins following renal transplantation.

An extension study offered open-label fluvastatin for two additional years to all patients. Patients randomized to fluvastatin had a 29% reduction in cardiac death or definite nonfatal myocardial infarction (HR 0.71, 95%CI 0.55–0.93) [39].

In summary, the ALERT study, in spite of the negative primary outcome, appears to support statin use in renal transplant patients.

Statins and Progression of CKD

The effect of statins on the rate of decrease of eGFR with time has been investigated in most randomized clinical trials of statin therapy in the hope that significant beneficial effects will be reported. An early meta-analysis [40] showed statin-treated patients compared with controls had a slower rate of decline in glomerular filtration rate. This effect appeared to be significant independent of study quality, percentage change in cholesterol, and cause of renal disease. However, statin effects on improvement in glomerular filtration rate were more likely observed in studies with longer follow-up. There was also a tendency for a favorable effect of statin treatment on protein excretion; however, the results were statistically heterogeneous between studies. Further meta-analyses confirmed these findings [41–43], and the impression was reinforced by the belief that decrease in albumin excretion rate is usually associated with decrease of the rate of progression of CKD [44].

Since the SHARP study was the only trial of cholesterol lowering to specifically address benefit in CKD patients, it had a strong influence on the beliefs of clinicians on the effect of statins on eGFR change [45]. In this study, there was no effect of simvastatin and ezetimibe on progression of CKD. However, after the publication of these study data, three meta-analyses and systematic reviews published contradictory results. One study showed that statins moderately decreased the rate of reduction of eGFR and slowed the progression of proteinuria [46]. Another study concluded that the effect of statins on the progression of CKD is uncertain [21]. The most recent systematic review reported a small but statistically significant decrease in the rate of eGFR decline in statin-treated patients. In a subgroup analysis, those who received high-intensity statins had a significant difference in eGFR decrease with a mean of 3.35 (95%CI 0.91–5.79) mL/min/1.73 m^2 compared to control [47]. There was no significant change in eGFR with moderate- and low-intensity statin therapy. Additionally, compared with the control group, the statin group did not have a significant difference in reduction of proteinuria.

Some studies have reported differences in statin effect on renal function irrespective of LDLc lowering. One study reported that pravastatin was more effective than atorvastatin, rosuvastatin, and pitavastatin in preserving renal function in patients with type 2 diabetes [48]. Another study reported that pitavastatin is more effective than pravastatin for the reduction of albuminuria in type 2 diabetic patients with early stages of diabetic nephropathy [49]. In a large trial, in patients with diabetic nephropathy, despite high-dose rosuvastatin (40 mg/day) lowering plasma lipid concentrations to a greater extent than did high-dose atorvastatin (80 mg/day), atorvastatin had more renoprotective effects for the patients studied [50].

Studies addressing specific subgroups of CKD patients have also published positive results of statin benefit on renal function, but publication bias is possible. In patients with diabetic nephropathy, rosuvastatin 10 mg/day significantly reduced albumin excretion rate and cystatin C levels [51]. This is in keeping with the results of CARDS, which showed benefit in reduction of progression of CKD from atorvastatin limited to patients with type 2 diabetes with proteinuria [18]. In a post hoc analysis of SPARCL, in patients with diabetes mellitus, with and without CKD, atorvastatin treatment prevented eGFR decline in patients with stroke [52]. In another study, pravastatin reduced total kidney volume, left ventricular mass index, and microalbuminuria in pediatric autosomal dominant polycystic kidney disease [53]. Fluvastatin was shown to decrease proteinuria in patients with immunoglobulin A nephropathy [54]. In HIV-infected subjects on antiretroviral therapy, rosuvastatin was shown to preserve renal function and lower cystatin C [55].

In summary, the effects of statins on progression of CKD and on albumin excretion rate are variable and likely not to be clinically significant. Additional data are necessary to select populations for which clinical benefit of a certain statin in a certain dose will be confirmed to extend to renoprotection.

Statin Therapy and Adverse Outcomes/Safety in CKD

The safety of statins has been a subject of debate from the appearance of this class of therapeutic agents. Early assessment of the reports of adverse events has resulted in an opinion that statin therapy should be used with caution in CKD patients. This opinion was based mostly on the theoretical consideration that metabolite accumulation and uremia-related muscle injury could increase the risk of myopathy [56]. To date, there is no epidemiological confirmation of this opinion or that statin-treated patients across any CKD stage including dialysis had a higher risk of adverse events [22]. Moreover in studies using high-dose atorvastatin [57] or high-dose rosuvastatin [58] in NDD-CKD patients, the risk of adverse events was no higher than in patients with normal renal function.

More recently a large number of studies have addressed the association between statin therapy and incident diabetes as well as acute kidney injury (AKI).

Statins and Incident Diabetes

In 2001, Freeman et al. reported a 30% reduction of incident diabetes in pravastatin-treated patients [59]. Subsequently, randomized clinical trials focused on this possible outcome. The hypothesis was reversed after Ridker et al. reported that rosuvastatin-treated patients had a 28% increase in incident diabetes [60]. A large amount of research has been published on this subject and was summarized in a few meta-analyses [61–65], showing that there is a significant increase in risk of incident diabetes in statin-treated patients. The magnitude of risk is different from one study to another depending on the definition of diabetes and the percent of each statin included in the analysis [61–65]. The size of the effect reported could be magnified by bias, attributable to differences in survival between statin- and placebo-treated patients in randomized trials [66].

There are differences in risk between statins with rosuvastatin, atorvastatin, and simvastatin studies showing statistically significant increases in incident diabetes, while in published pravastatin, fluvastatin, and pitavastatin studies, statistical significance is not achieved for this outcome [65, 67]. Some authors have concluded that the effect is limited to "powerful statins" [68]. In addition, randomized trials of high-dose vs. moderate-dose statins indicate a higher risk of diabetes incidence for high-dose statins [63, 64].

The risk of statin-induced diabetes increases with age [69] and is higher in women [60]. There is also a possibility that the risk is increased by prolonged exposure to statin therapy [69]. The risk of statin-induced incident diabetes is likely to be confined in patients with prediabetes [70] or patients who gain weight during the exposure to statin [71]. The definition of "patients at risk" seems to be best defined by triglyceride level [59] or liver fat content [72], but not by the number of components of the metabolic syndrome [73].

All authors reporting on this outcome conclude, however, that the benefits of statins outweigh the risk conferred by incident diabetes. In long-term studies, attempts have been made to quantify this risk-benefit ratio [74]. Of course the ratio depended on the risk of incident diabetes in the individual patients and the absolute risk reduction induced by statins. In patients without high liver fat content, the effect of statin therapy was more favorable in patients with high coronary calcium [72].

The mechanism of action by which statins increase the risk of incident diabetes is not clear. Most authors have implicated an induced decrease in beta cell function associated with inhibition of beta cell glucose transporters, delayed ATP production, pro-inflammatory and oxidative intracellular effects of plasma-derived cholesterol, inhibition of calcium channel-dependent insulin secretion and beta cell apoptosis [75], statin-induced decrease in circulating adiponectin and coenzyme Q10 [76], and suppressed insulin secretion stimulated by muscarinic M3 or GPR40 receptor agonists [77]. One study attributed the differences between statins in incident diabetes induction to differences in insulin sensitivity [78].

The effect of statins on glycemic control in patients with preexistent type 2 diabetes is minimal and likely not clinically significant [79].

There is no study to date that has focused directly on the incidence of diabetes in statin-treated patients with NDD-CKD. It is known, however, that diabetes worsens the prognosis of these patients [80]. Until further evidence is available, one should recommend statin therapy in these patients because of high risk of CV events and good evidence of statin benefit. Conversely, in dialysis patients, initiation of statin therapy cannot be recommended in absence of clear cardioprotective benefit.

Statins and Acute Kidney Injury

There is controversy concerning the association of statin therapy with AKI. Some studies showed an increase in AKI in statin-treated patients, others showed no effect, and others showed a beneficial effect in prevention of AKI. Special attention was given to attempts to prevent contrast-induced AKI with statin therapy.

Increased risk of AKI in statin-treated patients usually occurs in the context of induced rhabdomyolysis [81]. In addition, tubular proteinuria can be seen with all statins [82]. An increased AKI incidence was reported for high-dose statins [83]. The authors reported a 54% increase risk of AKI in the first 6 months after initiation of high-dose statins. In another study [84], in non-CKD patients, current users of high-potency statins were 34% more likely to be hospitalized with AKI within 120 days after starting treatment. However, this effect was not statistically significant in CKD patients.

No change in risk of AKI was reported by meta-analyses of large long-term clinical trials including patients with and without coronary artery disease, with and without diabetes, and some with stage 3 CKD [85]. The same negative results were reported by analyses of statin trials after acute coronary syndromes [86] or in studies including patients undergoing vascular and endovascular surgery [87].

Decrease in risk of AKI in statin-treated patients was reported by one analysis to be present in observational studies but not in randomized clinical trials [88]. A recent large meta-analysis showed an 11% decrease in the incidence of postoperative renal dysfunction after cardiac surgery in preoperative statin-treated patients [89]. AKI was reduced by 13%, and there was a 24% reduction in the postoperative need for renal replacement therapy. A Cochrane review published almost simultaneously concluded that an analysis of currently available data did not suggest that preoperative statin use is associated with decreased incidence of AKI in adults undergoing coronary bypass [90].

The benefit of statin therapy for prevention of contrast-induced AKI has been confirmed by multiple authors. The mechanism of this protective effect seems to be related to statin reduction of contrast media-induced activation of caspase-3, c-Jun N-terminale kinase (JNK), and p53, through preventing induction of renal cell apoptosis, as well as restoration of the survival signals mediated by Akt and extracellular-signal-regulated kinase (ERK) pathways [91]. The extent and limitations of the clinical benefit have been also characterized. Statins are effective in preventing contrast-induced AKI in patients with diabetes [91, 92]. Their effectiveness is independent of the age of the patients [93, 94], of the level of hydration, and of the use of N-acetylcysteine [93, 95]. They are effective in preventing AKI if the contrast agent is administered in moderate volume, but not in high volume [96]. The effectiveness seems to be independent of the osmolality of the contrast media [93].

Statins decrease the risk of contrast agent-induced AKI when the procedure is performed in the setting of an acute coronary syndrome [97], and the benefit is higher in patients with elevated C-reactive protein (CRP) [94, 98]. High-dose but not moderate-dose statins are effective in preventing this outcome [99, 100]. Atorvastatin and rosuvastatin are equally effective [101].

The protective effect is present in patients with CKD [91, 92, 101, 102], with the caveat being that most studies have included predominantly or exclusively CKD stage 3 patients. The benefit might be attenuated when CKD patients are compared with non-CKD patients [95] and is absent in patients with CKD undergoing elective angiography [100].

In summary high-dose statins have a definite protective effect in CKD patients with and without diabetes receiving contrast agents and may protect against AKI in CKD patients undergoing cardiac or vascular surgery. The overall safety of high-dose statins in CKD patients needs to be addressed in future studies.

Fibrates in Patients with CKD

Fibrates have been used in clinical practice to decrease triglycerides and increase HDLc, although increases in HDLc are small. Two fibrates are available on the US market, gemfibrozil and fenofibrate. They have both been tested in clinical trials for reduction of CV events.

The Helsinki Heart Study (HHS) [103] enrolled 4081 middle-aged men with nonHDLc >200 mg/dL to receive gemfibrozil 600 mg twice a day or placebo for 5 years. Treatment resulted in a 34% reduction in fatal and nonfatal myocardial infarction. The Veterans Affairs High-Density Lipoprotein Cholesterol Intervention Trial (VA-HIT) [104] enrolled 2531 men with coronary heart disease, an HDLc level of 40 mg per deciliter or less, and an LDLc level of 140 mg per deciliter (3.6 mmol per liter) or less. The primary study outcome was nonfatal myocardial infarction or death from coronary causes. After 5.1 years, there was a 22% reduction in the primary endpoint and a 31% reduction in adjudicated stroke [104, 105]. The success of these clinical trials was not translated in clinical practice because of the emphasis of clinical guidelines on LDLc reduction, particularly with statin therapy. Concurrent use of gemfibrozil and statins resulted in marked increases in the risk of rhabdomyolysis [106].

Fenofibrate was introduced on the US market in order to be used with statins. In pharmacokinetic studies, fenofibrate was tested against each statin, and its presence resulted in no changes in statin kinetic parameters [107–109]. It is used in a once-a-day dosage (120–200 mg/day depending on brand name, in patients with normal renal function). Large randomized clinical trials enrolling patients with diabetes have reported the effect on CV endpoints by fenofibrate. In the Diabetes Atherosclerosis Intervention Study (DAIS) trial [110], 418 patients were randomized between placebo and fenofibrate monotherapy. The fenofibrate group showed a significantly smaller increase in percentage diameter stenosis than the placebo group and a significantly smaller decrease in minimum lumen diameter. In the much larger Fenofibrate Intervention and Event Lowering in Diabetes (FIELD) trial [111], 9795 patients were also randomized between fenofibrate monotherapy and placebo. Fenofibrate did not reduce the primary endpoint (coronary heart disease death or nonfatal myocardial infarction) but significantly reduced nonfatal myocardial infarction by 24%, total CVD events by 11%, and coronary revascularizations by 21%. The authors also stated that the higher rate of off-protocol initiation of statin therapy in patients allocated to placebo might have masked a moderately larger treatment benefit.

A meta-analysis addressed data concerning patients with CKD enrolled in VA-HIT and FIELD [112]. In 918 patients enrolled, the intervention with a fibrate significantly decreased total CV events by 30% and CV death by 40%. However, there was no reduction in all-cause mortality and stroke.

The Action to Control CV Risk in Diabetes (ACCORD) study [113] enrolled 5518 patients with type 2 diabetes who were being treated with open-label simvastatin to receive either masked fenofibrate or placebo. There were no differences in the first occurrence of nonfatal MI, nonfatal stroke, or death from CV causes or any prespecified secondary clinical endpoint. To date there is no evidence that fenofibrate adds CV benefit to patients treated with a moderate-dose statin. Only 141 patients in this trial had an eGFR<50 mL/min/1.73 m^2.

Fenofibrate, but not gemfibrozil, has a reversible negative effect on eGFR [114], and this has caused safety concerns [115]. The effect is present shortly after the initiation of treatment [116]. Guidelines recommend decrease in the dose of fenofibrate in CKD patients, [117] usually to one third of the dose used in patients with normal renal function.

As opposed to the short-term demonstrable effect on eGFR, fenofibrate has shown a renoprotective effect in long-term clinical trials. In the DAIS trial [110], the treated arm had a lower likelihood of developing an increased albumin excretion rate [116]. In the much larger FIELD trial [111], fenofibrate reduced the albumin excretion rate and significantly reduced eGFR decline over 5 years, despite initially and reversibly increasing plasma creatinine [118]. In the ACCORD trial [113], the authors reported a reduction of increased albumin excretion rate and a reduction of GFR decline in patients who did not have a marked initial increase in creatinine [119]. The initial rise in creatinine was confirmed to be reversible upon completion of the drug therapy intervention [120].

In summary, additional studies are necessary to document the long-term risks and benefits of fenofibrate added to statin therapy in CKD patients.

Niacin in Patients with CKD

Niacin is the oldest drug available for treatment of dyslipidemia [121]. In pharmacological doses, niacin's effects on lipids and lipoproteins are fairly well known [122], and its relative safety in patients with CKD has been documented [123]. The drug is used in clinical practice predominantly to increase HDLc and reduce triglyceride concentration. Niacin used in combination with other lipid-lowering drugs has consistently resulted in reversal of atherosclerosis expressed as carotid intima thickness and coronary stenosis [124–127]. Two meta-analyses reported that niacin significantly reduced major coronary events, stroke, CV events, and any of the composite endpoints of any CVD [128, 129].

The results of two recent studies, Atherothrombosis Intervention in Metabolic Syndrome With Low HDL/High Triglycerides and Impact on Global Health Outcomes (AIM-HIGH) [130] and Treatment of HDL to Reduce the Incidence of Vascular Events (HPS-THRIVE) [131] have casted doubt on the safety and the efficacy of niacin for reducing CVD events in high-risk patients. The AIM-HIGH study enrolled 3414 patients with coronary artery disease, low HDLc (men below 40 mg/dL and women below 50 mg/dL), and high triglycerides (over 150 mg/dL) with LDLc lowered to 40–80 mg/dL with simvastatin and ezetimibe. There was no incremental clinical benefit from the addition of niacin to statin therapy during a 36-month follow-up period, despite significant improvements in HDLc and triglyceride levels. A subgroup analysis from the AIM-HIGH trial showed a significant decrease in primary events in 439 patients with triglycerides ≥200 mg/dL and HDLc ≤32 mg/dL [132] suggesting that in order to demonstrate benefit from niacin in a trial, the threshold for enrollment should be higher for triglycerides and lower for HDLc. Another subgroup analysis addressed the outcomes in patients with stage 3 CKD enrolled in this study [133]. The authors concluded that the intervention improved triglyceride and HDLc concentrations but did not improve CV outcomes or kidney function and was associated with higher all-cause mortality.

HPS-THRIVE used niacin/laropiprant vs. placebo in statin-treated patients with ASCVD who were recruited without regard for their lipid levels and failed to show incremental benefit with treatment [131]. This study included patients with mean normal HDLc (44 mg/dL) and triglyceride levels (126 mg/dL) but whose LDLc were controlled with simvastatin. In the past or now, these patients with such a lipid profile would not have been treated with niacin.

The hope that further clinical trials will show benefit for niacin in CKD patients was not abandoned [134, 135]. Niacin has properties that could be beneficial in CKD patients, mostly through its effect on HDL function and concentration. HDL in patients with CKD is not only reduced but also dysfunctional, mostly through reduced antioxidant capacity [136]. Dysfunctional HDL predicts a poor outcome in end-stage renal disease (ESRD) [137]. Niacin significantly decreases the release of myeloperoxidase by leukocytes and prevents HDL from becoming dysfunctional [138]. Consequently niacin has demonstrated an anti-inflammatory potential by decreasing fibrinogen [139, 140], CRP [141, 142], and soluble CD40 ligand (sCD40L) [143] and improved endothelial function in patients with coronary artery disease who had low HDLc [144].

Another property of niacin, which has been well documented, is its effect on serum phosphorous. Niacin decreased serum phosphorous in patients without CKD [145–147], stage 3 CKD [147, 148], and ESRD [149–152]. This property might add benefit in CKD patients.

The effect of niacin on renal function and albumin excretion rate has been studied in experimental kidney disease. Cho et al. [153, 154] reported that niacin-treated partially nephrectomized rats had marked reduction of 24-h protein excretion and rate of GFR decline.

In summary, large clinical trials of niacin should be undertaken to explore the potential benefit of niacin in CKD patients.

Bile Acid-Binding Resins in CKD

Bile acid-binding resins are used as adjuvants to statins to increase cholesterol lowering. They can be used also in statin-intolerant patients. The mechanism of action is an interruption of enterohepatic circulation of bile salts [155]. This interruption is referred by the authors as "medical" as opposed to "surgical interruption" which is the result of partial ileal bypass [156]. This interruption results in a reduction as well as qualitative changes in the bile acid pool [157], resulting in a decrease in the activation of farnesoid X receptor (FXR) receptors with widespread metabolic consequences. The metabolic effect of this intervention is a decrease in total cholesterol and LDLc associated with an increase in triglycerides as well as an improvement in glycemic control in patients with type 2 diabetes [158].

Cholestyramine, colestipol, and colesevelam are the only drugs classified as bile acid-binding resins in the USA. Colesevelam is less effective in maximum dose but better tolerated and associated with less drug interaction [159].

Interruption of enterohepatic circulation of bile acids has been tested in randomized clinical trials with clinical endpoints in hypercholesterolemic patients. The Lipid Research Clinics Coronary Primary Prevention Trial (LRC-CPPT) enrolled 3806 men free of coronary artery disease with an LDLc >175 mg/dL [1]. Patients were randomized between cholestyramine with an intended dose of 24 g/day and placebo. After 7.1 years there was a significant 19% reduction in the incidence of non-fatal myocardial infarction or coronary death. The Program On the Surgical Control of the Hyperlipidemias (POSCH) [160] study was designed to test whether cholesterol lowering induced by partial ileal bypass would decrease the incidence of fatal and nonfatal coronary events. The study enrolled 838 men and women, myocardial infarction survivors with an LDLc >140 mg/dL. After 9.7 years there was a highly significant 35% reduction in nonfatal myocardial infarction and coronary death and a 62% reduction in coronary artery bypass graft. At 18-year follow-up, there was a significant difference in overall survival reported as an average survival advantage of 2.7 years [161]. These studies, however, excluded patients with CKD at enrollment.

Sevelamer used as a phosphate binder was shown to act as a bile acid binder in patients with CKD [162]. Shortly after that, colestimide [163] and colestilan [164], bile acid-binding resins used in Japan, with a chemical structure similar to sevelamer, were shown to be useful as phosphate binders in ESRD patients. This expanded the knowledge of use of bile acid sequestrants in CKD. Colestilan was shown to be equivalent to sevelamer in phosphate-binding and LDLc-lowering efficacy [165] and non-inferior to simvastatin in LDLc lowering [166].

Sevelamer therapy has been tested for clinical and surrogate CV endpoints, mostly on the assumption that it will be superior to calcium-based phosphate binders. A meta-analysis of 11 randomized trials (4622 patients) showed that patients assigned to noncalcium-based phosphate binders (sevelamer or lanthanum) had a 22% reduction in all-cause mortality compared with those assigned to calcium-based phosphate binders [167]. Another meta-analysis reported a beneficial effect of sevelamer on multiple all-cause hospitalizations and hospital days [168]. A cross-sectional study reported an association between sevelamer treatment and a lower carotid intima-media thickness suggesting an impact on atherosclerosis progression [169]. A meta-analysis of studies comparing the effects of sevelamer- and calcium-based phosphate binders on coronary artery and aortic calcification in dialysis patients showed significant benefit favoring sevelamer. The fact that this benefit might be associated with the lipid-lowering effect of sevelamer is supported by data reporting that the effect is absent if the control group is treated with atorvastatin [170]. However, these data should not be extrapolated to mean clinical benefit in dialysis patients, in view of the clinical trials showing lack of benefit of lipid lowering in dialysis patients. In addition, the results of studies of sevelamer on arterial stiffness are conflicting [171, 172].

In summary, the CV benefit of bile acid-binding resins including sevelamer has not been adequately tested in CKD patients.

Ezetimibe in CKD

Ezetimibe has been adequately tested in CKD in the SHARP trial [33] and is recommended by some but not all of the guidelines. The argument is rooted in the belief of need for a target LDLc in cholesterol-lowering intervention or lack thereof. Ezetimibe is used in addition to statin therapy in order to achieve lower LDLc. Addition of ezetimibe to simvastatin in high-risk patients has resulted in a small but statistically significant benefit [173]. The arguments in favor of a target are multiple. The association of cholesterol and of cholesterol lowering with CV events is continuous, and lower levels could provide better outcomes. The POSCH study has demonstrated that it produces benefit irrespective of the method used for cholesterol lowering [160]. Consequently, if dissatisfied with the results of LDLc lowering, a clinician should increase the intensity of the therapy. In addition, in studies of regression of atherosclerosis using statins for LDLc lowering, a threshold LDLc (~75 mg/dL) should be exceeded in order to achieve regression [174, 175]. Finally, recent studies using proprotein convertase subtilisin/kexin 9 (PCSK9) inhibitors have shown benefit from LDLc lowering at levels considered unachievable until now [176, 177] and might have a strong impact on the future guidelines.

PCSK9 Inhibitors in CKD

PCSK9 inhibitors have not been tested in patients with CKD. In proteinuric patients, PCSK9 is elevated, which might contribute to the hypercholesterolemia present in these patients [178, 179]. The levels drop after renal replacement therapy [180] and are below the level of general population in dialysis patients [181]. View of the controversies concerning the safety and efficacy of statins in CKD results of clinical trials are awaited. In 2017 the data of the FOURIER study showed that lowering the cholesterol to an average of 30 mg/dL using evolocumab in addition to standard lipid-lowering therapy reduced the primary endpoint (CV death, myocardial infarction, stroke, hospitalization for unstable angina, or coronary revascularization) by 15% and the secondary endpoint (CV death, myocardial infarction, or stroke) [182] by 20%. The study included CKD patients with eGFR >20 mL/min/1.73m^2; however, to date subgroup analysis for these patients has not yet been presented.

N-3 Fatty Acids in CKD

The biological activity of N-3 fatty acids depends on two products: eicosapentaenoic acid (EPA) and docosahexaenoic acid (DHA). There are two prescription strength preparations on the US market: Lovaza[R] containing 375 mg DHA and 465 mg EPA and Vascepa[R], containing 1 g purified EPA per capsule. Omega-3 fatty acids decrease triglyceride concentrations by reducing VLDL production. Vascepa decreases LDLc, while Lovaza increases it [183].

Clinical trials of N-3 fatty acids for CV endpoints have yielded mixed results. For EPA + DHA preparations, low-dose monotherapy improved survival in patients with previous myocardial infarction [184, 185]. A significant reduction in mortality in heart failure patients was also documented in a study [186]. Studies of this preparation as an add-on to statin therapy, however, were negative [187–189]. For purified EPA, a successful trial as add-on to statin therapy was undertaken in Japan. The investigators of the Japan EPA Lipid Intervention Study (JELIS) randomized 18,645 patients with or without preexisting coronary artery disease and a serum cholesterol higher than 250 mg/dL to statin + a preparation containing 1800 mg EPA or statin + placebo [190]. After 4.6 years, there was a significant reduction in the risk of major coronary events and nonfatal coronary events, each of 19%, a 28% decrease in the risk of unstable angina, and a 20% reduction in stroke [191, 192].

There is a high level of interest in the research of N-3 fatty acids in CKD and particularly in ESRD. Hemodialysis patients have markedly lower levels of plasma EPA and DHA when compared with NDD-CKD patients [193]. In hemodialysis, DHA is an independent predictor of all-cause mortality [194] and of sudden cardiac death [195]. A small trial randomized 206 hemodialysis patients between low-dose N-3 fatty acids and placebo [196]. A significant reduction was seen in the number of myocardial infarctions (4 vs. 13; $P = 0.036$). The Fish Oil Inhibition of Stenosis in Hemodialysis Grafts (FISH) study enrolled 201 patients for 12 months. In the fish oil group, there were half as many thrombosis and fewer corrective interventions, and 57% improved CV event-free survival [197].

N-3 fatty acids were reported to decrease albumin excretion rate in patients already treated with renin-angiotensin system blockers who have IgA nephropathy [198]. A subsequent meta-analysis confirmed this effect but could not confirm that this effect leads to preservation of renal function [199].

The cardioprotective and renoprotective effect as well as the effect on graft patency of omega-3 fatty acid supplementation in CKD patients are not yet clarified and require additional larger studies.

Probucol in CKD

Probucol was withdrawn from the US market in the 1990s after a clinical trial showed no efficacy of improvement in femoral atherosclerosis [200]. It acts as an antioxidant and moderately lowers LDLc. It may improve reverse cholesterol transport, in spite of decreasing HDLc levels. It is used in Japan where it has been shown to cause marked regression of cutaneous and tendon xanthomata [201]. The drug has been tested in small clinical endpoint trials. In the Probucol Angioplasty Restenosis Trial (PART), therapy was a negative predictor of repeat revascularization ($p = 0.034$) [202]. In the Fukuoka Atherosclerosis Trial (FAST), probucol decreased significantly the rate of intima-media thickness increase and significantly reduced CV events (2.4% vs. 13.6%; $p = 0.0136$) [203, 204].

In CKD, probucol has been successfully tested, also in small studies, as a renoprotective agent: in diabetic nephropathy [205, 206], IgA nephropathy [207], and contrast-induced AKI [208, 209]. This drug has, however, a long way before returning to the US market.

Conclusion

Although there are different guidelines and recommendations for use of statin therapy in CKD patients, clinical trial evidence to date demonstrates that statins are effective in reducing CV outcome risk in patients with NDD-CKD. So far, cholesterol-lowering trials do not show support of a statin benefit in dialysis-treated patients, but the current guidelines suggest continuing statin therapy in patients who were already on a statin prior to transition to dialysis. Statins have also been shown to be safe across all stages of CKD and independent of statin dose. However, this conclusion is based on a limited amount of data and more studies are needed to fully address these concerns. Nonetheless, the clinical benefit of statin therapy outweighs the risk of adverse events, including incident development of diabetes and AKI. There have been a number of drugs that have shown additional benefit when added to a statin for achieving CV risk reduction; however, more studies are needed to evaluate the effectiveness of these drugs across stages of CKD and in dialysis patients.

References

1. LRC-CPPT. The lipid research clinics coronary primary prevention trial results. I. Reduction in incidence of coronary heart disease. JAMA. 1984;251:351–64.
2. Tonelli M, Wanner C, Kidney Disease: Improving Global Outcomes Lipid Guideline Development Work Group, M. Lipid management in chronic kidney disease: synopsis of the kidney disease: improving global outcomes 2013 clinical practice guideline. Ann Intern Med. 2014;160:182.
3. Sarnak MJ, Bloom R, Muntner P, Rahman M, Saland JM, Wilson PW, Fried L. KDOQI US commentary on the 2013 KDIGO clinical practice guideline for lipid management in CKD. Am J Kidney Dis. 2015;65:354–66.
4. NICE 2014. Cardiovascular risk assessment and the modification of blood lipids for the primary and secondary prevention of cardiovascular disease. http://www.nice.org.uk/guidance/CG181.
5. Anderson TJ, Gregoire J, Hegele RA, Couture P, Mancini GB, Mcpherson R, Francis GA, Poirier P, Lau DC, Grover S, Genest J, Carpentier AC, Dufour R, Gupta M, Ward R, Leiter LA, Lonn E, Ng DS, Pearson GJ, Yates GM, Stone JA, Ur E. 2012 update of the Canadian Cardiovascular Society guidelines for the diagnosis and treatment of dyslipidemia for the prevention of cardiovascular disease in the adult. Can J Cardiol. 2013;29:151–67.
6. European Association for Cardiovascular, P., Rehabilitation, Reiner Z, Catapano AL, De Backer G, Graham I, Taskinen MR, Wiklund O, Agewall S, Alegria E, Chapman MJ, Durrington P, Erdine S, Halcox J, Hobbs R, Kjekshus J, Filardi PP, Riccardi G, Storey RF, Wood D, Guidelines, E. S. C. C. F. P. & Committees. ESC/EAS Guidelines for the management of dyslipidaemias: the Task Force for the management of dyslipidaemias of the European Society of Cardiology (ESC) and the European Atherosclerosis Society (EAS). Eur Heart J. 2011;32:1769–818.
7. Teramoto T, Sasaki J, Ishibashi S, Birou S, Daida H, Dohi S, Egusa G, Hiro T, Hirobe K, Iida M, Kihara S, Kinoshita M, Maruyama C, Ohta T, Okamura T, Yamashita S, Yokode M, Yokote K, Japan Atherosclerosis, S. Executive summary of the Japan Atherosclerosis Society (JAS) guidelines for the diagnosis and prevention of atherosclerotic cardiovascular diseases in Japan –2012 version. J Atheroscler Thromb. 2013;20:517–23.
8. Jacobson TA, Ito MK, Maki KC, Orringer CE, Bays HE, Jones PH, Mckenney JM, Grundy SM, Gill EA, Wild RA, Wilson DP, Brown WV. National Lipid Association recommendations for patient-centered management of dyslipidemia: part 1 - executive summary. J Clin Lipidol. 2014;8:473–88.
9. Writing C, Lloyd-Jones DM, Morris PB, Ballantyne CM, Birtcher KK, Daly DD, Depalma SM, Minissian MB, Orringer CE, Smith SC. 2016 ACC expert consensus decision pathway on the role of non-statin therapies for LDL-Cholesterol lowering in the management of atherosclerotic cardiovascular disease risk: a report of the American College of Cardiology Task Force on Clinical Expert Consensus Documents. J Am Coll Cardiol. 2016;68:92–125.
10. Stone, N. J., Robinson, J., Lichtenstein, A. H., Merz, C. N., Blum, C. B., Eckel, R. H., Goldberg, A. C., Gordon, D., Levy, D., Lloyd-Jones, D. M., Mcbride, P., Schwartz, J. S., Shero, S. T., Smith, S. C., Watson, K. & Wilson, P. W. 2013. 2013 ACC/AHA Guideline on the Treatment of Blood Cholesterol to Reduce Atherosclerotic Cardiovascular Risk in Adults:. Circulation, 129, S1-72.
11. Downs JR, O'malley PG. Management of dyslipidemia for cardiovascular disease risk reduction: synopsis of the 2014 U.S. Department of Veterans Affairs and U.S. Department of Defense Clinical Practice Guideline. Ann Intern Med. 2015;163:291.
12. ADA 2015. Standards of medical care in diabetes--2015: summary of revisions. Diabetes Care. 38(Suppl):S4.
13. Handelsman Y, Bloomgarden ZT, Grunberger G, Umpierrez G, Zimmerman RS, Bailey TS, Blonde L, Bray GA, Cohen AJ, Dagogo-Jack S, Davidson JA, Einhorn D, Ganda OP, Garber AJ, Garvey WT, Henry RR, Hirsch IB, Horton ES, Hurley DL, Jellinger PS, Jovanovic L, Lebovitz HE, Leroith D, Levy P, Mcgill JB, Mechanick JI, Mestman JH, Moghissi ES, Orzeck EA, Pessah-Pollack R, Rosenblit PD, Vinik AI, Wyne K, Zangeneh F. American association of clinical endocrinologists and american college of endocrinology - clinical practice guidelines for developing a diabetes mellitus comprehensive care plan - 2015. Endocr Pract. 2015;21:1–87.
14. Colantonio LD, Baber U, Banach M, Tanner RM, Warnock DG, Gutierrez OM, Safford MM, Wanner C, Howard G, Muntner P. Contrasting cholesterol

management guidelines for adults with CKD. J Am Soc Nephrol. 2015;26:1173–80.
15. Atthobari J, Brantsma AH, Gansevoort RT, Visser ST, Asselbergs FW, Van Gilst WH, De Jong PE, De Jong-Van Den Berg LT. The effect of statins on urinary albumin excretion and glomerular filtration rate: results from both a randomized clinical trial and an observational cohort study. Nephrol Dial Transplant. 2006;21:3106–14.
16. Rahman M, Yang W, Akkina S, Alper A, Anderson AH, Appel LJ, He J, Raj DS, Schelling J, Strauss L, Teal V, Rader DJ, For the, C. S. I. Relation of serum lipids and lipoproteins with progression of CKD: the CRIC Study. Clin J Am Soc Nephrol. 2014;9:1190.
17. Tonelli M, Isles C, Craven T, Tonkin A, Pfeffer MA, Shepherd J, Sacks FM, Furberg C, Cobbe SM, Simes J, West M, Packard C, Curhan GC. Effect of pravastatin on rate of kidney function loss in people with or at risk for coronary disease. Circulation. 2005;112:171–8.
18. Colhoun HM, Betteridge DJ, Durrington PN, Hitman GA, Neil HA, Livingstone SJ, Charlton-Menys V, Demicco DA, Fuller JH, Investigators, C. Effects of atorvastatin on kidney outcomes and cardiovascular disease in patients with diabetes: an analysis from the Collaborative Atorvastatin Diabetes Study (CARDS). Am J Kidney Dis. 2009;54:810–9.
19. Koren MJ, Hunninghake DB. Clinical outcomes in managed-care patients with coronary heart disease treated aggressively in lipid-lowering disease management clinics: the alliance study. J Am Coll Cardiol. 2004;44:1772–9.
20. Lemos PA, Serruys PW, De Feyter P, Mercado NF, Goedhart D, Saia F, Arampatzis CA, Soares PR, Ciccone M, Arquati M, Cortellaro M, Rutsch W, Legrand V. Long-term fluvastatin reduces the hazardous effect of renal impairment on four-year atherosclerotic outcomes (a LIPS substudy). Am J Cardiol. 2005;95:445–51.
21. Palmer SC, Navaneethan SD, Craig JC, Johnson DW, Perkovic V, Hegbrant J, Strippoli GF. HMG CoA reductase inhibitors (statins) for people with chronic kidney disease not requiring dialysis. Cochrane Database Syst Rev. 2014;5:CD007784.
22. Hou W, Lv J, Perkovic V, Yang L, Zhao N, Jardine MJ, Cass A, Zhang H, Wang H. Effect of statin therapy on cardiovascular and renal outcomes in patients with chronic kidney disease: a systematic review and meta-analysis. Eur Heart J. 2013;34:1807–17.
23. Herzog CA. Sudden cardiac death and acute myocardial infarction in dialysis patients: perspectives of a cardiologist. Semin Nephrol. 2005;25:363–6.
24. Baigent C, Burbury K, Wheeler D. Premature cardiovascular disease in chronic renal failure. Lancet. 2000;356:147–52.
25. Sarnak MJ. Cardiovascular complications in chronic kidney disease. Am J Kidney Dis. 2003;41:11–7.
26. Sniderman AD, Solhpour A, Alam A, Williams K, Sloand JA. Cardiovascular death in dialysis patients: lessons we can learn from AURORA. Clin J Am Soc Nephrol. 2010;5:335–40.
27. Palmer SC, Navaneethan SD, Craig JC, Johnson DW, Perkovic V, Nigwekar SU, Hegbrant J, Strippoli GF. HMG CoA reductase inhibitors (statins) for dialysis patients. Cochrane Database Syst Rev. 2013;9:CD004289.
28. Stegmayr BG, Brannstrom M, Bucht S, Crougneau V, Dimeny E, Ekspong A, Eriksson M, Granroth B, Grontoft KC, Hadimeri H, Holmberg B, Ingman B, Isaksson B, Johansson G, Lindberger K, Lundberg L, Mikaelsson L, Olausson E, Persson B, Stenlund H, Wikdahl AM, NEDIAT Study, G. Low-dose atorvastatin in severe chronic kidney disease patients: a randomized, controlled endpoint study. Scand J Urol Nephrol. 2005;39:489–97.
29. Wanner C, Krane V, Marz W, Olschewski M, Mann JF, Ruf G, Ritz E. Atorvastatin in patients with type 2 diabetes mellitus undergoing hemodialysis. N Engl J Med. 2005;353:238–48.
30. Marz W, Genser B, Drechsler C, Krane V, Grammer TB, Ritz E, Stojakovic T, Scharnagl H, Winkler K, Holme I, Holdaas H, Wanner C, German D, Dialysis Study, I. Atorvastatin and low-density lipoprotein cholesterol in type 2 diabetes mellitus patients on hemodialysis. Clin J Am Soc Nephrol. 2011;6:1316–25.
31. Fellstrom BC, Jardine AG, Schmieder RE, Holdaas H, Bannister K, Beutler J, Chae DW, Chevaile A, Cobbe SM, Gronhagen-Riska C, de Lima JJ, Lins R, Mayer G, Mcmahon AW, Parving HH, Remuzzi G, Samuelsson O, Sonkodi S, Sci D, Suleymanlar G, Tsakiris D, Tesar V, Todorov V, Wiecek A, Wuthrich RP, Gottlow M, Johnsson E, Zannad F. Rosuvastatin and cardiovascular events in patients undergoing hemodialysis. N Engl J Med. 2009;360:1395–407.
32. Holme I, Fellstrom BC, Jardin AG, Schmieder RE, Zannad F, Holdaas H. Prognostic model for total mortality in patients with haemodialysis from the Assessments of Survival and Cardiovascular Events (AURORA) study. J Intern Med. 2012;271:463–71.
33. Baigent C, Landray MJ, Reith C, Emberson J, Wheeler DC, Tomson C, Wanner C, Krane V, Cass A, Craig J, Neal B, Jiang L, Hooi LS, Levin A, Agodoa L, Gaziano M, Kasiske B, Walker R, Massy ZA, Feldt-Rasmussen B, Krairittichai U, Ophascharoensuk V, Fellstrom B, Holdaas H, Tesar V, Wiecek A, Grobbee D, de Zeeuw D, Gronhagen-Riska C, Dasgupta T, Lewis D, Herrington W, Mafham M, Majoni W, Wallendszus K, Grimm R, Pedersen T, Tobert J, Armitage J, Baxter A, Bray C, Chen Y, Chen Z, Hill M, Knott C, Parish S, Simpson D, Sleight P, Young A, Collins R, Investigators S. The effects of lowering LDL cholesterol with simvastatin plus ezetimibe in patients with chronic kidney disease (Study of Heart and Renal Protection): a randomised placebo-controlled trial. Lancet. 2011;377:2181–92.

34. Attman PO, Samuelsson O, Johansson AC, Moberly JB, Alaupovic P. Dialysis modalities and dyslipidemia. Kidney Int Suppl. 2003;(84):S110–2.
35. Goldfarb-Rumyantzev AS, Habib AN, Baird BC, Barenbaum LL, Cheung AK. The association of lipid-modifying medications with mortality in patients on long-term peritoneal dialysis. Am J Kidney Dis. 2007;50:791–802.
36. Lee JE, Oh KH, Choi KH, Kim SB, Kim YS, Do JY, Kim YL, Kim DJ. Statin therapy is associated with improved survival in incident peritoneal dialysis patients: propensity-matched comparison. Nephrol Dial Transplant. 2011a;26:4090–4.
37. Holdaas H, Fellstrom B, Jardine AG, Holme I, Nyberg G, Fauchald P, Gronhagen-Riska C, Madsen S, Neumayer HH, Cole E, Maes B, Ambuhl P, Olsson AG, Hartmann A, Solbu DO, Pedersen TR. Effect of fluvastatin on cardiac outcomes in renal transplant recipients: a multicentre, randomised, placebo-controlled trial. Lancet. 2003;361:2024–31.
38. Holdaas H, Fellstrom B, Jardine AG, Nyberg G, Gronhagen-Riska C, Madsen S, Neumayer HH, Cole E, Maes B, Ambuhl P, Logan JO, Staffler B, Gimpelewicz C, Group, A. S. Beneficial effect of early initiation of lipid-lowering therapy following renal transplantation. Nephrol Dial Transplant. 2005;20:974–80.
39. Holdaas H, Fellstrom B, Cole E, Nyberg G, Olsson AG, Pedersen TR, Madsen S, Gronhagen-Riska C, Neumayer HH, Maes B, Ambuhl P, Hartmann A, Staffler B, Jardine AG. Long-term cardiac outcomes in renal transplant recipients receiving fluvastatin: the ALERT extension study. Am J Transplant. 2005;5:2929–36.
40. Fried LF, Orchard TJ, Kasiske BL. Effect of lipid reduction on the progression of renal disease: a meta-analysis. Kidney Int. 2001;59:260–9.
41. Douglas K, O'malley PG, Jackson JL. Meta-analysis: the effect of statins on albuminuria. Ann Intern Med. 2006;145:117–24.
42. Sandhu S, Wiebe N, Fried LF, Tonelli M. Statins for improving renal outcomes: a meta-analysis. J Am Soc Nephrol. 2006;17:2006–16.
43. Strippoli GF, Navaneethan SD, Johnson DW, Perkovic V, Pellegrini F, Nicolucci A, Craig JC. Effects of statins in patients with chronic kidney disease: meta-analysis and meta-regression of randomised controlled trials. BMJ. 2008;336:645–51.
44. Heerspink HJ, Kropelin TF, Hoekman J, de Zeeuw D, Reducing Albuminuria As Surrogate Endpoint, C. Drug-induced reduction in albuminuria is associated with subsequent renoprotection: a meta-analysis. J Am Soc Nephrol. 2015;26:2055–64.
45. Haynes R, Lewis D, Emberson J, Reith C, Agodoa L, Cass A, Craig JC, De Zeeuw D, Feldt-Rasmussen B, Fellstrom B, Levin A, Wheeler DC, Walker R, Herrington WG, Baigent C, Landray MJ, Group, S. C. & Group, S. C. Effects of lowering LDL cholesterol on progression of kidney disease. J Am Soc Nephrol. 2014;25:1825–33.
46. Geng Q, Ren J, Song J, Li S, Chen H. Meta-analysis of the effect of statins on renal function. Am J Cardiol. 2014;114:562–70.
47. Sanguankeo A, Upala S, Cheungpasitporn W, Ungprasert P, Knight EL. Effects of statins on renal outcome in chronic kidney disease patients: a systematic review and meta-analysis. PLoS One. 2015;10:e0132970.
48. Hanai K, Babazono T, Takemura S, Toyonaga A, Yoshida N, Uchigata Y. Comparative effects of statins on the kidney function in patients with type 2 diabetes. J Atheroscler Thromb. 2015;22:618–27.
49. Kimura S, Inoguchi T, Yokomizo H, Maeda Y, Sonoda N, Takayanagi R. Randomized comparison of pitavastatin and pravastatin treatment on the reduction of urinary albumin in patients with type 2 diabetic nephropathy. Diabetes Obes Metab. 2012;14:666–9.
50. DE Zeeuw D, Anzalone DA, Cain VA, Cressman MD, Heerspink HJ, Molitoris BA, Monyak JT, Parving HH, Remuzzi G, Sowers JR, Vidt DG. Renal effects of atorvastatin and rosuvastatin in patients with diabetes who have progressive renal disease (PLANET I): a randomised clinical trial. Lancet Diabetes Endocrinol. 2015;3:181–90.
51. Abe M, Maruyama N, Okada K, Matsumoto S, Matsumoto K, Soma M. Effects of lipid-lowering therapy with rosuvastatin on kidney function and oxidative stress in patients with diabetic nephropathy. J Atheroscler Thromb. 2011;18:1018–28.
52. Amarenco, P., Callahan, A., Campese, V. M., Goldstein, L. B., Hennerici, M. G., Messig, M., Sillesen, H., Welch, K. M., Wilson, D. J. & Zivin, J. A. 2014. Effect of high-dose atorvastatin on renal function in subjects with stroke or transient ischemic attack in the SPARCL trial. Stroke, 45, 2974-2982.
53. Cadnapaphornchai MA, George DM, Mcfann K, Wang W, Gitomer B, Strain JD, Schrier RW. Effect of pravastatin on total kidney volume, left ventricular mass index, and microalbuminuria in pediatric autosomal dominant polycystic kidney disease. Clin J Am Soc Nephrol. 2014;9:889–96.
54. Buemi M, Allegra A, Corica F, Aloisi C, Giacobbe M, Pettinato G, Corsonello A, Senatore M, Frisina N. Effect of fluvastatin on proteinuria in patients with immunoglobulin A nephropathy. Clin Pharmacol Ther. 2000;67:427–31.
55. Longenecker CT, Hileman CO, Funderburg NT, Mccomsey GA. Rosuvastatin preserves renal function and lowers cystatin C in HIV-infected subjects on antiretroviral therapy: the SATURN-HIV trial. Clin Infect Dis. 2014;59:1148–56.
56. Wanner C. HMG-CoA reductase inhibitor treatment in renal insufficiency. Nephrol Dial Transplant. 1996;11:1951–2.
57. Shepherd J, Kastelein JJ, Bittner V, Deedwania P, Breazna A, Dobson S, Wilson DJ, Zuckerman A, Wenger NK. Intensive lipid lowering with atorvastatin in patients with coronary heart disease

and chronic kidney disease: the TNT (Treating to New Targets) study. J Am Coll Cardiol. 2008;51:1448–54.
58. Ridker PM, Macfadyen J, Cressman M, Glynn RJ. Efficacy of rosuvastatin among men and women with moderate chronic kidney disease and elevated high-sensitivity C-reactive protein. *J Am Coll Cardiol*. 2010;55:1266–73.
59. Freeman DJ, Norrie J, Sattar N, Neely RD, Cobbe SM, Ford I, Isles C, Lorimer AR, Macfarlane PW, Mckillop JH, Packard CJ, Shepherd J, Gaw A. Pravastatin and the development of diabetes mellitus: evidence for a protective treatment effect in the West of Scotland Coronary Prevention Study. Circulation. 2001;103:357–62.
60. Ridker PM, Pradhan A, Macfadyen JG, Libby P, Glynn RJ. Cardiovascular benefits and diabetes risks of statin therapy in primary prevention: an analysis from the JUPITER trial. Lancet. 2012;380:565–71.
61. Rajpathak SN, Kumbhani DJ, Crandall J, Barzilai N, Alderman M, Ridker PM. Statin therapy and risk of developing type 2 diabetes: a meta-analysis. Diabetes Care. 2009;32:1924–9.
62. Mills EJ, Wu P, Chong G, Ghement I, Singh S, Akl EA, Eyawo O, Guyatt G, Berwanger O, Briel M. Efficacy and safety of statin treatment for cardiovascular disease: a network meta-analysis of 170,255 patients from 76 randomized trials. QJM. 2011;104:109–24.
63. Preiss D, Seshasai SR, Welsh P, Murphy SA, Ho JE, Waters DD, Demicco DA, Barter P, Cannon CP, Sabatine MS, Braunwald E, Kastelein JJ, De Lemos JA, Blazing MA, Pedersen TR, Tikkanen MJ, Sattar N, Ray KK. Risk of incident diabetes with intensive-dose compared with moderate-dose statin therapy: a meta-analysis. JAMA. 2011;305:2556–64.
64. Navarese EP, Buffon A, Andreotti F, Kozinski M, Welton N, Fabiszak T, Caputo S, Grzesk G, Kubica A, Swiatkiewicz I, Sukiennik A, Kelm M, de Servi S, Kubica J. Meta-analysis of impact of different types and doses of statins on new-onset diabetes mellitus. Am J Cardiol. 2013;111:1123–30.
65. Sattar N, Preiss D, Murray HM, Welsh P, Buckley BM, de Craen AJ, Seshasai SR, Mcmurray JJ, Freeman DJ, Jukema JW, Macfarlane PW, Packard CJ, Stott DJ, Westendorp RG, Shepherd J, Davis BR, Pressel SL, Marchioli R, Marfisi RM, Maggioni AP, Tavazzi L, Tognoni G, Kjekshus J, Pedersen TR, Cook TJ, Gotto AM, Clearfield MB, Downs JR, Nakamura H, Ohashi Y, Mizuno K, Ray KK, Ford I. Statins and risk of incident diabetes: a collaborative meta-analysis of randomised statin trials. Lancet. 2010;375:735–42.
66. Blackburn DF, Chow JY, Smith AD. Statin use and incident diabetes explained by bias rather than biology. Can J Cardiol. 2015;31:966–9.
67. Vallejo-Vaz AJ, Kondapally Seshasai SR, Kurogi K, Michishita I, Nozue T, Sugiyama S, Tsimikas S, Yoshida H, Ray KK. Effect of pitavastatin on glucose, HbA1c and incident diabetes: a meta-analysis of randomized controlled clinical trials in individuals without diabetes. Atherosclerosis. 2015;241:409–18.
68. Steen DL, Bhatt DL. Statin potency associated with incident diabetes in a real-world evaluation. Evid Based Med. 2014;19:68.
69. Zaharan NL, Williams D, Bennett K. Statins and risk of treated incident diabetes in a primary care population. Br J Clin Pharmacol. 2013;75:1118–24.
70. Kohli P, Waters DD, Nemr R, Arsenault BJ, Messig M, Demicco DA, Laskey R, Kastelein JJ. Risk of new-onset diabetes and cardiovascular risk reduction from high-dose statin therapy in pre-diabetics and non-pre-diabetics: an analysis from TNT and IDEAL. J Am Coll Cardiol. 2015;65:402–4.
71. Ong KL, Waters DD, Messig M, Demicco DA, Rye KA, Barter PJ. Effect of change in body weight on incident diabetes mellitus in patients with stable coronary artery disease treated with atorvastatin (from the treating to new targets study). Am J Cardiol. 2014;113:1593–8.
72. Shah RV, Allison MA, Lima JA, Bluemke DA, Abbasi SA, Ouyang P, Jerosch-Herold M, Ding J, Budoff MJ, Murthy VL. Liver fat, statin use, and incident diabetes: the multi-ethnic study of Atherosclerosis. *Atherosclerosis*. 2015;242:211–7.
73. van de Woestijne AP, van der Graaf Y, Westerink J, Nathoe HM, Visseren FL. Effect of statin therapy on incident type 2 diabetes mellitus in patients with clinically manifest vascular disease. Am J Cardiol. 2015;115:441–6.
74. Wang KL, Liu CJ, Chao TF, Huang CM, Wu CH, Chen SJ, Chen TJ, Lin SJ, Chiang CE. Statins, risk of diabetes, and implications on outcomes in the general population. J Am Coll Cardiol. 2012;60:1231–8.
75. Jahangir E, Fazio S, Sampson UK. Incident diabetes and statins: the blemish of an undisputed heavy weight champion? Br J Clin Pharmacol. 2013;75:955–8.
76. Chan DC, Pang J, Watts GF. Pathogenesis and management of the diabetogenic effect of statins: a role for adiponectin and coenzyme Q10? Curr Atheroscler Rep. 2015;17:472.
77. Yaluri N, Modi S, Lopez Rodriguez M, Stancakova A, Kuusisto J, Kokkola T, Laakso M. Simvastatin impairs insulin secretion by multiple mechanisms in MIN6 Cells. PLoS One. 2015;10:e0142902.
78. Baker WL, Talati R, White CM, Coleman CI. Differing effect of statins on insulin sensitivity in non-diabetics: a systematic review and meta-analysis. Diabetes Res Clin Pract. 2010;87:98–107.
79. Erqou S, Lee CC, Adler AI. Statins and glycaemic control in individuals with diabetes: a systematic review and meta-analysis. Diabetologia. 2014;57:2444–52.
80. Foley RN, Murray AM, Li S, Herzog CA, Mcbean AM, Eggers PW, Collins AJ. Chronic kidney disease and the risk for cardiovascular disease, renal replacement, and death in the United States Medicare population, 1998 to 1999. J Am Soc Nephrol. 2005;16:489–95.

81. Antons KA, Williams CD, Baker SK, Phillips PS. Clinical perspectives of statin-induced rhabdomyolysis. Am J Med. 2006;119:400–9.
82. Kiortsis DN, Filippatos TD, Mikhailidis DP, Elisaf MS, Liberopoulos EN. Statin-associated adverse effects beyond muscle and liver toxicity. Atherosclerosis. 2007;195:7–16.
83. Corrao G, Soranna D, Casula M, Merlino L, Porcellini MG, Catapano AL. High-potency statins increase the risk of acute kidney injury: evidence from a large population-based study. Atherosclerosis. 2014;234:224–9.
84. Dormuth CR, Hemmelgarn BR, Paterson JM, James MT, Teare GF, Raymond CB, Lafrance JP, Levy A, Garg AX, Ernst P, Canadian Network for Observational Drug Effect, S. Use of high potency statins and rates of admission for acute kidney injury: multicenter, retrospective observational analysis of administrative databases. BMJ. 2013;346:f880.
85. Bangalore S, Fayyad R, Hovingh GK, Laskey R, Vogt L, Demicco DA, Waters DD, Treating To New Targets Steering, C. & investigators. Statin and the risk of renal-related serious adverse events: Analysis from the IDEAL, TNT, CARDS, ASPEN, SPARCL, and other placebo-controlled trials. Am J Cardiol. 2014;113:2018–20.
86. Sarma A, Cannon CP, de Lemos J, Rouleau JL, Lewis EF, Guo J, Mega JL, Sabatine MS, O'donoghue ML. The incidence of kidney injury for patients treated with a high-potency versus moderate-potency statin regimen after an acute coronary syndrome. J Am Heart Assoc. 2014;3:e000784.
87. Antoniou GA, Hajibandeh S, Hajibandeh S, Vallabhaneni SR, Brennan JA, Torella F. Meta-analysis of the effects of statins on perioperative outcomes in vascular and endovascular surgery. J Vasc Surg. 2015;61:519–532 e1.
88. Pan SY, Wu VC, Huang TM, Chou HC, Ko WJ, Wu KD, Lee C, C. & GROUP, N. Effect of preoperative statin therapy on postoperative acute kidney injury in patients undergoing major surgery: systemic review and meta-analysis. Nephrology (Carlton). 2014;19:750–63.
89. Wang L, Peng P, Zhang O, Xu X, Yang S, Zhao Y, Zhou Y. High-dose statin pretreatment decreases periprocedural myocardial infarction and cardiovascular events in patients undergoing elective percutaneous coronary intervention: a meta-analysis of twenty-four randomized controlled trials. PLoS One. 2014;9:e113352.
90. Lewicki M, Ng I, Schneider AG. HMG CoA reductase inhibitors (statins) for preventing acute kidney injury after surgical procedures requiring cardiac bypass. Cochrane Database Syst Rev. 2015;3:CD010480.
91. Quintavalle C, Fiore D, de Micco F, Visconti G, Focaccio A, Golia B, Ricciardelli B, Donnarumma E, Bianco A, Zabatta MA, Troncone G, Colombo A, Briguori C, Condorelli G. Impact of a high loading dose of atorvastatin on contrast-induced acute kidney injury. Circulation. 2012;126:3008–16.
92. Han Y, Zhu G, Han L, Hou F, Huang W, Liu H, Gan J, Jiang T, Li X, Wang W, Ding S, Jia S, Shen W, Wang D, Sun L, Qiu J, Wang X, Li Y, Deng J, Li J, Xu K, Xu B, Mehran R, Huo Y. Short-term rosuvastatin therapy for prevention of contrast-induced acute kidney injury in patients with diabetes and chronic kidney disease. J Am Coll Cardiol. 2014;63:62–70.
93. Lee JM, Park J, Jeon KH, Jung JH, Lee SE, Han JK, Kim HL, Yang HM, Park KW, Kang HJ, Koo BK, Jo SH, Kim HS. Efficacy of short-term high-dose statin pretreatment in prevention of contrast-induced acute kidney injury: updated study-level meta-analysis of 13 randomized controlled trials. PLoS One. 2014;9:e111397.
94. Tropeano F, Leoncini M, Toso A, Maioli M, Dabizzi L, Biagini D, Villani S, Bellandi F. Impact of Rosuvastatin in contrast-induced acute kidney injury in the elderly: Post Hoc analysis of the PRATO-ACS trial. J Cardiovasc Pharmacol Ther. 2015;21:159.
95. Giacoppo D, Capodanno D, Capranzano P, Aruta P, Tamburino C. Meta-analysis of randomized controlled trials of preprocedural statin administration for reducing contrast-induced acute kidney injury in patients undergoing coronary catheterization. Am J Cardiol. 2014;114:541–8.
96. Zhang J, Li Y, Tao GZ, Chen YD, Hu TH, Cao XB, Jing QM, Wang XZ, Ma YY, Wang G, Liu HW, Wang B, Xu K, Li J, Deng J, Han YL. Short-term rosuvastatin treatment for the prevention of contrast-induced acute kidney injury in patients receiving moderate or high volumes of contrast media: a sub-analysis of the TRACK-D study. Chin Med J. 2015;128:784–9.
97. Li W, Fu X, Wang Y, Li X, Yang Z, Wang X, Geng W, Gu X, Hao G, Jiang Y, Fan W, Wu W, Li S. Beneficial effects of high-dose atorvastatin pretreatment on renal function in patients with acute ST-segment elevation myocardial infarction undergoing emergency percutaneous coronary intervention. Cardiology. 2012;122:195–202.
98. Toso A, Leoncini M, Maioli M, Tropeano F, Di Vincenzo E, Villani S, Bellandi F. Relationship between inflammation and benefits of early high-dose rosuvastatin on contrast-induced nephropathy in patients with acute coronary syndrome: the pathophysiological link in the PRATO-ACS study (Protective effect of Rosuvastatin and antiplatelet therapy on contrast-induced nephropathy and myocardial damage in patients with acute coronary Syndrome undergoing coronary intervention). JACC Cardiovasc Interv. 2014;7:1421–9.
99. Peruzzi M, de Luca L, Thomsen HS, Romagnoli E, D'ascenzo F, Mancone M, Sardella G, Lucisano L, Abbate A, Frati G, Biondi-Zoccai G. A network meta-analysis on randomized trials focusing on the preventive effect of statins on contrast-induced nephropathy. Biomed Res Int. 2014;2014:213239.

100. Ukaigwe A, Karmacharya P, Mahmood M, Pathak R, Aryal MR, Jalota L, Donato AA. Meta-analysis on efficacy of statins for prevention of contrast-induced acute kidney injury in patients undergoing coronary angiography. Am J Cardiol. 2014;114:1295–302.
101. Liu YH, Liu Y, Duan CY, Tan N, Chen JY, Zhou YL, Li LW, He PC. Statins for the prevention of contrast-induced nephropathy after coronary angiography/percutaneous interventions: a meta-analysis of randomized controlled trials. J Cardiovasc Pharmacol Ther. 2015;20:181–92.
102. Qiao B, Deng J, Li Y, Wang X, Han Y. Rosuvastatin attenuated contrast-induced nephropathy in diabetes patients with renal dysfunction. Int J Clin Exp Med. 2015;8:2342–9.
103. Frick MH, Elo O, Haapa K, Heinonen OP, Heinsalmi P, Helo P, Huttunen JK, Kaitaniemi P, Koskinen P, Manninen V, et al. Helsinki heart study: primary-prevention trial with gemfibrozil in middle-aged men with dyslipidemia. Safety of treatment, changes in risk factors, and incidence of coronary heart disease. N Engl J Med. 1987;317:1237–45.
104. Rubins HB, Robins SJ, Collins D, Fye CL, Anderson JW, Elam MB, Faas FH, Linares E, Schaefer EJ, Schectman G, Wilt TJ, Wittes J. Gemfibrozil for the secondary prevention of coronary heart disease in men with low levels of high-density lipoprotein cholesterol. Veterans Affairs High-Density Lipoprotein Cholesterol Intervention Trial Study Group. N Engl J Med. 1999;341:410–8.
105. Bloomfield Rubins H, Davenport J, Babikian V, Brass LM, Collins D, Wexler L, Wagner S, Papademetriou V, Rutan G, Robins SJ, Group, V.-H. S. Reduction in stroke with gemfibrozil in men with coronary heart disease and low HDL cholesterol: The Veterans Affairs HDL Intervention Trial (VA-HIT). Circulation. 2001;103:2828–33.
106. Pierce LR, Wysowski DK, Gross TP. Myopathy and rhabdomyolysis associated with lovastatin-gemfibrozil combination therapy. JAMA. 1990;264:71–5.
107. Pan WJ, Gustavson LE, Achari R, Rieser MJ, Ye X, Gutterman C, Wallin BA. Lack of a clinically significant pharmacokinetic interaction between fenofibrate and pravastatin in healthy volunteers. J Clin Pharmacol. 2000;40:316–23.
108. Bergman AJ, Murphy G, Burke J, Zhao JJ, Valesky R, Liu L, Lasseter KC, He W, Prueksaritanont T, Qiu Y, Hartford A, Vega JM, Paolini JF. Simvastatin does not have a clinically significant pharmacokinetic interaction with fenofibrate in humans. J Clin Pharmacol. 2004;44:1054–62.
109. Whitfield LR, Porcari AR, Alvey C, Abel R, Bullen W, Hartman D. Effect of gemfibrozil and fenofibrate on the pharmacokinetics of atorvastatin. J Clin Pharmacol. 2011;51:378–88.
110. DAIS. Effect of fenofibrate on progression of coronary-artery disease in type 2 diabetes: the Diabetes Atherosclerosis Intervention Study, a randomised study. Lancet. 2001;357:905–10.
111. Keech A, Simes RJ, Barter P, Best J, Scott R, Taskinen MR, Forder P, Pillai A, Davis T, Glasziou P, Drury P, Kesaniemi YA, Sullivan D, Hunt D, Colman P, D'emden M, Whiting M, Ehnholm C, Laakso M. Effects of long-term fenofibrate therapy on cardiovascular events in 9795 people with type 2 diabetes mellitus (the FIELD study): randomised controlled trial. Lancet. 2005;366:1849–61.
112. Jun M, Zhu B, Tonelli M, Jardine MJ, Patel A, Neal B, Liyanage T, Keech A, Cass A, Perkovic V. Effects of fibrates in kidney disease: a systematic review and meta-analysis. J Am Coll Cardiol. 2012;60:2061–71.
113. Group, A. S, Ginsberg HN, Elam MB, Lovato LC, Crouse JR, Leiter LA, Linz P, Friedewald WT, Buse JB, Gerstein HC, Probstfield J, Grimm RH, Ismail-Beigi F, Bigger JT, Goff DC, Cushman WC, Simons-Morton DG, Byington RP. Effects of combination lipid therapy in type 2 diabetes mellitus. N Engl J Med. 2010;362:1563–74.
114. Broeders N, Knoop C, Antoine M, Tielemans C, Abramowicz D. Fibrate-induced increase in blood urea and creatinine: is gemfibrozil the only innocuous agent? Nephrol Dial Transplant. 2000;15:1993–9.
115. Nissen SE, Nicholls SJ, Wolski K, Howey DC, Mcerlean E, Wang MD, Gomez EV, Russo JM. Effects of a potent and selective PPAR-alpha agonist in patients with atherogenic dyslipidemia or hypercholesterolemia: two randomized controlled trials. JAMA. 2007;297:1362–73.
116. Ansquer JC, Foucher C, Rattier S, Taskinen MR, Steiner G. Fenofibrate reduces progression to microalbuminuria over 3 years in a placebo-controlled study in type 2 diabetes: results from the Diabetes Atherosclerosis Intervention Study (DAIS). Am J Kidney Dis. 2005;45:485–93.
117. Mcpherson R, Frohlich J, Fodor G, Genest J, Canadian Cardiovascular, S. Canadian Cardiovascular Society position statement--recommendations for the diagnosis and treatment of dyslipidemia and prevention of cardiovascular disease. Can J Cardiol. 2006;22:913–27.
118. Davis TM, Ting R, Best JD, Donoghoe MW, Drury PL, Sullivan DR, Jenkins AJ, O'connell RL, Whiting MJ, Glasziou PP, Simes RJ, Kesaniemi YA, Gebski VJ, Scott RS, Keech AC, Fenofibrate I, Event Lowering in Diabetes Study, I. Effects of fenofibrate on renal function in patients with type 2 diabetes mellitus: the Fenofibrate Intervention and Event Lowering in Diabetes (FIELD) Study. Diabetologia. 2011;54:280–90.
119. Mychaleckyj JC, Craven T, Nayak U, Buse J, Crouse JR, Elam M, Kirchner K, Lorber D, Marcovina S, Sivitz W, Sperl-Hillen J, Bonds DE, Ginsberg HN. Reversibility of fenofibrate therapy-induced renal function impairment in ACCORD type 2 diabetic participants. Diabetes Care. 2012;35:1008–14.
120. Bonds DE, Craven TE, Buse J, Crouse JR, Cuddihy R, Elam M, Ginsberg HN, Kirchner K, Marcovina S, Mychaleckyj JC, O'connor PJ, Sperl-Hillen

JA. Fenofibrate-associated changes in renal function and relationship to clinical outcomes among individuals with type 2 diabetes. Diabetologia. 2012;55:1641–50.
121. Altschul RA, Hoffer A, Stephen JD. Influence of nicotinic acid on serum cholesterol in man. Arch Biochem. 1955;54:558.
122. Kamanna VS, Ganji SH, Kashyap ML. Recent advances in niacin and lipid metabolism. Curr Opin Lipidol. 2013;24:239–45.
123. Reiche I, Westphal S, Martens-Lobenhoffer J, Troger U, Luley C, Bode-Boger SM. Pharmacokinetics and dose recommendations of Niaspan(R) in chronic kidney disease and dialysis patients. Nephrol Dial Transplant. 2011;26:276–82.
124. Blankenhorn DH, Nessim SA, Johnson RL, Sanmarco ME, Azen SP, Cashin-Hemphill L. Beneficial effects of combined colestipol-niacin therapy on coronary atherosclerosis and coronary venous bypass grafts. JAMA. 1987;257:3233–40.
125. Thoenes M, Oguchi A, Nagamia S, Vaccari CS, Hammoud R, Umpierrez GE, Khan BV. The effects of extended-release niacin on carotid intimal media thickness, endothelial function and inflammatory markers in patients with the metabolic syndrome. Int J Clin Pract. 2007;61:1942–8.
126. Taylor AJ, Lee HJ, Sullenberger LE. The effect of 24 months of combination statin and extended-release niacin on carotid intima-media thickness: ARBITER 3. Curr Med Res Opin. 2006;22:2243–50.
127. Taylor AJ, Villines TC, Stanek EJ, Devine PJ, Griffen L, Miller M, Weissman NJ, Turco M. Extended-release niacin or ezetimibe and carotid intima-media thickness. N Engl J Med. 2009;361:2113–22.
128. Bruckert E, Labreuche J, Amarenco P. Meta-analysis of the effect of nicotinic acid alone or in combination on cardiovascular events and atherosclerosis. Atherosclerosis. 2010;210:353–61.
129. Lavigne PM, Karas RH. The current state of niacin in cardiovascular disease prevention: a systematic review and meta-regression. J Am Coll Cardiol. 2013;61:440–6.
130. Investigators A-H, Boden WE, Probstfield JL, Anderson T, Chaitman BR, Desvignes-Nickens P, Koprowicz K, Mcbride R, Teo K, Weintraub W. Niacin in patients with low HDL cholesterol levels receiving intensive statin therapy. N Engl J Med. 2011;365:2255–67.
131. Group, H. T. C, Landray MJ, Haynes R, Hopewell JC, Parish S, Aung T, Tomson J, Wallendszus K, Craig M, Jiang L, Collins R, Armitage J. Effects of extended-release niacin with laropiprant in high-risk patients. N Engl J Med. 2014;371:203–12.
132. Guyton JR, Slee AE, Anderson T, Fleg JL, Goldberg RB, Kashyap ML, Marcovina SM, Nash SD, O'brien KD, Weintraub WS, Xu P, Zhao XQ, Boden WE. Relationship of lipoproteins to cardiovascular events: the AIM-HIGH Trial. J Am Coll Cardiol. 2013;62:1580–4.
133. Kalil RS, Wang JH, de Boer IH, Mathew RO, Ix JH, Asif A, Shi X, Boden WE. Effect of extended-release niacin on cardiovascular events and kidney function in chronic kidney disease: a post hoc analysis of the AIM-HIGH trial. Kidney Int. 2015;87:1250.
134. Streja E, Kovesdy CS, Streja DA, Moradi H, Kalantar-Zadeh K, Kashyap ML. Niacin and the progression of chronic kidney disease. Am J Kidney Dis. 2015;65 (in print)
135. Taketani Y, Masuda M, Yamanaka-Okumura H, Tatsumi S, Segawa H, Miyamoto K, Takeda E, Yamamoto H. Niacin and Chronic Kidney Disease. J Nutr Sci Vitaminol (Tokyo). 2015;61(Suppl):S173–5.
136. Moradi H, Pahl MV, Elahimehr R, Vaziri ND. Impaired antioxidant activity of high-density lipoprotein in chronic kidney disease. Transl Res. 2009;153:77–85.
137. Kalantar-Zadeh K, Kopple JD, Kamranpour N, Fogelman AM, Navab M. HDL-inflammatory index correlates with poor outcome in hemodialysis patients. Kidney Int. 2007;72:1149–56.
138. Ganji SH, Kamanna VS, Kashyap ML. Niacin decreases leukocyte myeloperoxidase: mechanistic role of redox agents and Src/p38MAP kinase. Atherosclerosis. 2014;235:554–61.
139. Chesney CM, Elam MB, Herd JA, Davis KB, Garg R, Hunninghake D, Kennedy JW, Applegate WB. Effect of niacin, warfarin, and antioxidant therapy on coagulation parameters in patients with peripheral arterial disease in the Arterial Disease Multiple Intervention Trial (ADMIT). Am Heart J. 2000;140:631–6.
140. Lin TH, Voon WC, Yen HW, Huang CH, Su HM, Lai WT, Sheu SH. Randomized comparative study of the effects of treatment with once-daily, niacin extended-release/lovastatin and with simvastatin on lipid profile and fibrinolytic parameters in Taiwan. Kaohsiung J Med Sci. 2006;22:257–65.
141. Ferguson JF, Patel PN, Shah RY, Mulvey CK, Gadi R, Nijjar PS, Usman HM, Mehta NN, Shah R, Master SR, Propert KJ, Reilly MP. Race and gender variation in response to evoked inflammation. J Transl Med. 2013;11:63.
142. Wi J, Kim JY, Park S, Kang SM, Jang Y, Chung N, Shim WH, Cho SY, Lee SH. Optimal pharmacologic approach to patients with hypertriglyceridemia and low high-density lipoprotein-cholesterol: randomized comparison of fenofibrate 160 mg and niacin 1500 mg. Atherosclerosis. 2010;213:235–40.
143. Lee K, Ahn TH, Kang WC, Han SH, Choi IS, Shin EK. The effects of statin and niacin on plaque stability, plaque regression, inflammation and oxidative stress in patients with mild to moderate coronary artery stenosis. Korean Circ J. 2011b;41:641–8.
144. Warnholtz A, Wild P, Ostad MA, Elsner V, Stieber F, Schinzel R, Walter U, Peetz D, Lackner K, Blankenberg S, Munzel T. Effects of oral niacin on endothelial dysfunction in patients with coronary artery disease: results of the randomized, double-blind, placebo-controlled INEF study. Atherosclerosis. 2009;204:216–21.
145. Maccubbin D, Tipping D, Kuznetsova O, Hanlon WA, Bostom AG. Hypophosphatemic effect of nia-

cin in patients without renal failure: a randomized trial. Clin J Am Soc Nephrol. 2010;5:582–9.
146. Hu S, Shearer GC, Steffes MW, Harris WS, Bostom AG. Once-daily extended-release niacin lowers serum phosphorus concentrations in patients with metabolic syndrome dyslipidemia. Am J Kidney Dis. 2011;57:181.
147. Bostom AG, Maclean AA, Maccubbin D, Tipping D, Giezek H, Hanlon WA. Extended-release niacin/laropiprant lowers serum phosphorus concentrations in patients with type 2 diabetes. J Clin Lipidol. 2011;5:281–7.
148. Ix, J. H., Ganjoo, P., Tipping, D., Tershakovec, A. M. & Bostom, A. G. 2011. Sustained hypophosphatemic effect of once-daily niacin/laropiprant in dyslipidemic CKD stage 3 patients. Am J Kidney Dis57963
149. Sampathkumar K, Selvam M, Sooraj YS, Gowthaman S, Ajeshkumar RN. Extended release nicotinic acid - a novel oral agent for phosphate control. Int Urol Nephrol. 2006;38:171–4.
150. Muller D, Mehling H, Otto B, Bergmann-Lips R, Luft F, Jordan J, Kettritz R. Niacin lowers serum phosphate and increases HDL cholesterol in dialysis patients. Clin J Am Soc Nephrol. 2007;2:1249–54.
151. Restrepo Valencia CA, Cruz J. Safety and effectiveness of nicotinic acid in the management of patients with chronic renal disease and hyperlipidemia associated to hyperphosphatemia. Nefrologia. 2008;28:61–6.
152. Ahmadi F, Shamekhi F, Lessan-Pezeshki M, Khatami MR. Comparison of efficacy of the phosphate binders nicotinic acid and sevelamer hydrochloride in hemodialysis patients. Saudi J Kidney Dis Transpl. 2012;23:934–8.
153. Cho KH, Kim HJ, Kamanna VS, Vaziri ND. Niacin improves renal lipid metabolism and slows progression in chronic kidney disease. Biochim Biophys Acta. 2010;1800:6–15.
154. Cho KH, Kim HJ, Rodriguez-Iturbe B, Vaziri ND. Niacin ameliorates oxidative stress, inflammation, proteinuria, and hypertension in rats with chronic renal failure. Am J Physiol Renal Physiol. 2009;297:F106–13.
155. Packard CJ, Shepherd J. The hepatobiliary axis and lipoprotein metabolism: effects of bile acid sequestrants and ileal bypass surgery. J Lipid Res. 1982;23:1081–98.
156. Moore RB, Buchwald H, Varco RL. The effect of partial ileal bypass on plasma lipoproteins. Circulation. 1980;62:469–76.
157. Out C, Groen AK, Brufau G. Bile acid sequestrants: more than simple resins. Curr Opin Lipidol. 2012;23:43–55.
158. Bays HE. Colesevelam hydrochloride added to background metformin therapy in patients with type 2 diabetes mellitus: a pooled analysis from 3 clinical studies. Endocr Pract. 2011;17:933–8.
159. Bays H, Dujovne C. Colesevelam HCl: a non-systemic lipid-altering drug. Expert Opin Pharmacother. 2003;4:779–90.
160. Buchwald H, Varco RL, Matts JP, Long JM, Fitch LL, Campbell GS, Pearce MB, Yellin AE, Edmiston WA, Smink RD, et al. Effect of partial ileal bypass surgery on mortality and morbidity from coronary heart disease in patients with hypercholesterolemia. Report of the Program on the Surgical Control of the Hyperlipidemias (POSCH). N Engl J Med. 1990;323:946–55.
161. Buchwald H, Williams SE, Matts JP, Nguyen PA, Boen JR. Overall mortality in the program on the surgical control of the hyperlipidemias. J Am Coll Surg. 2002;195:327–31.
162. Chertow GM, Burke SK, Dillon MA, Slatopolsky E. Long-term effects of sevelamer hydrochloride on the calcium x phosphate product and lipid profile of haemodialysis patients. Nephrol Dial Transplant. 1999;14:2907–14.
163. Date T, Shigematsu T, Kawashita Y, Satake N, Morita K. Colestimide can be used as a phosphate binder to treat uraemia in end-stage renal disease patients. Nephrol Dial Transplant. 2003;18(Suppl 3):iii90–3.
164. Kurihara S, Tsuruta Y, Akizawa T. Effect of MCI-196 (colestilan) as a phosphate binder on hyperphosphataemia in aemodialysis patients: a double-blind, placebo-controlled, short-term trial. Nephrol Dial Transplant. 2005;20:424–30.
165. Locatelli F, Spasovski G, Dimkovic N, Wanner C, Dellanna F, Pontoriero G. The effects of colestilan versus placebo and sevelamer in patients with CKD 5D and hyperphosphataemia: a 1-year prospective randomized study. Nephrol Dial Transplant. 2014;29:1061–73.
166. Wanner C, Marz W, Varushchanka A, Apanasovich N, Dosta N, Yakubtsevich R, Locatelli F. Dyslipidemia in chronic kidney disease: randomized controlled trial of colestilan versus simvastatin in dialysis patients. Clin Nephrol. 2014;82:163–72.
167. Jamal SA, Vandermeer B, Raggi P, Mendelssohn DC, Chatterley T, Dorgan M, Lok CE, Fitchett D, Tsuyuki RT. Effect of calcium-based versus non-calcium-based phosphate binders on mortality in patients with chronic kidney disease: an updated systematic review and meta-analysis. Lancet. 2013;382:1268–77.
168. St Peter WL, Liu J, Weinhandl E, Fan Q. A comparison of sevelamer and calcium-based phosphate binders on mortality, hospitalization, and morbidity in hemodialysis: a secondary analysis of the Dialysis Clinical Outcomes Revisited (DCOR) randomized trial using claims data. Am J Kidney Dis. 2008;51:445–54.
169. Boaz M, Katzir Z, Schwartz D, Gafter U, Biro A, Shtendik L, Kon V, Chernin G, Weinstein T. Effect of sevelamer hydrochloride exposure on carotid intima media thickness in hemodialysis patients. Nephron Clin Pract. 2011;117:c83–8.
170. Qunibi W, Moustafa M, Muenz LR, He DY, Kessler PD, Diaz-Buxo JA, Budoff M, Investigators, C. A 1-year randomized trial of calcium acetate versus sevelamer on progression of coronary artery cal-

cification in hemodialysis patients with comparable lipid control: the Calcium Acetate Renagel Evaluation-2 (CARE-2) study. Am J Kidney Dis. 2008;51:952–65.
171. Iimori S, Mori Y, Akita W, Takada S, Kuyama T, Ohnishi T, Shikuma S, Ishigami J, Tajima M, Asai T, Okado T, Kuwahara M, Sasaki S, Tsukamoto Y. Effects of sevelamer hydrochloride on mortality, lipid abnormality and arterial stiffness in hemodialyzed patients: a p ropensity-matched observational study. Clin Exp Nephrol. 2012;16:930–7.
172. Chue CD, Townend JN, Moody WE, Zehnder D, Wall NA, Harper L, Edwards NC, Steeds RP, Ferro CJ. Cardiovascular effects of sevelamer in stage 3 CKD. J Am Soc Nephrol. 2013;24:842–52.
173. Cannon CP, Blazing MA, Giugliano RP, Mccagg A, White JA, Theroux P, Darius H, Lewis BS, Ophuis TO, Jukema JW, De Ferrari GM, Ruzyllo W, De Lucca P, Im K, Bohula EA, Reist C, Wiviott SD, Tershakovec AM, Musliner TA, Braunwald E, Califf RM, Investigators, I.-I. Ezetimibe Added to Statin Therapy after Acute Coronary Syndromes. N Engl J Med. 2015;372:2387–97.
174. Von Birgelen C, Hartmann M, Mintz GS, Baumgart D, Schmermund A, Erbel R. Relation between progression and regression of atherosclerotic left main coronary artery disease and serum cholesterol levels as assessed with serial long-term (> or =12 months) follow-up intravascular ultrasound. Circulation. 2003;108:2757–62.
175. Puri R, Nissen SE, Shao M, Kataoka Y, Uno K, Kapadia SR, Tuzcu EM, Nicholls SJ. The beneficial effects of raising high-density lipoprotein cholesterol depends upon achieved levels of low-density lipoprotein cholesterol during statin therapy: Implications for coronary atheroma progression and cardiovascular events. Eur J Prev Cardiol. 2015;23:474.
176. Robinson JG, Farnier M, Krempf M, Bergeron J, Luc G, Averna M, Stroes ES, Langslet G, Raal FJ, El Shahawy M, Koren MJ, Lepor NE, Lorenzato C, Pordy R, Chaudhari U, Kastelein JJ, Investigators, O. L. T. Efficacy and safety of alirocumab in reducing lipids and cardiovascular events. N Engl J Med. 2015;372:1489–99.
177. Sabatine MS, Giugliano RP, Wiviott SD, Raal FJ, Blom DJ, Robinson J, Ballantyne CM, Somaratne R, Legg J, Wasserman SM, Scott R, Koren MJ, Stein EA, Open-Label Study of Long-Term Evaluation Against, L. D. L. C. I. Efficacy and safety of evolocumab in reducing lipids and cardiovascular events. N Engl J Med. 2015;372:1500–9.
178. Kwakernaak AJ, Lambert G, Slagman MC, Waanders F, Laverman GD, Petrides F, Dikkeschei BD, Navis G, Dullaart RP. Proprotein convertase subtilisin-kexin type 9 is elevated in proteinuric subjects: relationship with lipoprotein response to antiproteinuric treatment. Atherosclerosis. 2013;226:459–65.
179. Jin K, Park BS, Kim YW, Vaziri ND. Plasma PCSK9 in nephrotic syndrome and in peritoneal dialysis: a cross-sectional study. Am J Kidney Dis. 2014;63:584–9.
180. Konarzewski M, Szolkiewicz M, Sucajtys-Szulc E, Blaszak J, Lizakowski S, Swierczynski J, Rutkowski B. Elevated circulating PCSK-9 concentration in renal failure patients is corrected by renal replacement therapy. Am J Nephrol. 2014;40:157–63.
181. Abujrad H, Mayne J, Ruzicka M, Cousins M, Raymond A, Cheesman J, Taljaard M, Sorisky A, Burns K, Ooi TC. Chronic kidney disease on hemodialysis is associated with decreased serum PCSK9 levels. Atherosclerosis. 2014;233:123–9.
182. Sabatine MS, Giugliano RP, Keech AC, Honarpour N, Wiviott SD, Murphy SA, Kuder JF, Wang H, Liu T, Wasserman SM, Sever PS, Pedersen TR, Committee, F. S. & Investigators. Evolocumab and clinical outcomes in patients with cardiovascular disease. N Engl J Med. 2017;376:1713.
183. Ito MK. A comparative overview of prescription omega-3 fatty acid products. P T. 2015;40:826–57.
184. GISSI-PREVENZIONE. Dietary supplementation with n-3 polyunsaturated fatty acids and vitamin E after myocardial infarction: results of the GISSI-Prevenzione trial. Gruppo Italiano per lo Studio della Sopravvivenza nell'Infarto miocardico. Lancet. 1999;354:447–55.
185. Marchioli R, Barzi F, Bomba E, Chieffo C, DI Gregorio D, Di Mascio R, Franzosi MG, Geraci E, Levantesi G, Maggioni AP, Mantini L, Marfisi RM, Mastrogiuseppe G, Mininni N, Nicolosi GL, Santini M, Schweiger C, Tavazzi L, Tognoni G, Tucci C, Valagussa F. Early protection against sudden death by n-3 polyunsaturated fatty acids after myocardial infarction: time-course analysis of the results of the Gruppo Italiano per lo Studio della Sopravvivenza nell'Infarto Miocardico (GISSI)-Prevenzione. Circulation. 2002;105:1897–903.
186. Tavazzi L, Maggioni AP, Marchioli R, Barlera S, Franzosi MG, Latini R, Lucci D, Nicolosi GL, Porcu M, Tognoni G. Effect of n-3 polyunsaturated fatty acids in patients with chronic heart failure (the GISSI-HF trial): a randomised, double-blind, placebo-controlled trial. Lancet. 2008;372:1223–30.
187. Rauch B, Schiele R, Schneider S, Diller F, Victor N, Gohlke H, Gottwik M, Steinbeck G, del Castillo U, Sack R, Worth H, Katus H, Spitzer W, Sabin G, Senges J. OMEGA, a randomized, placebo-controlled trial to test the effect of highly purified omega-3 fatty acids on top of modern guideline-adjusted therapy after myocardial infarction. Circulation. 2010;122:2152–9.
188. Kromhout D, Giltay EJ, Geleijnse JM. n-3 fatty acids and cardiovascular events after myocardial infarction. N Engl J Med. 2010;363:2015–26.
189. Galan P, Kesse-Guyot E, Czernichow S, Briancon S, Blacher J, Hercberg S. Effects of B vitamins and omega 3 fatty acids on cardiovascular diseases: a randomised placebo controlled trial. BMJ. 341:c6273.
190. Yokoyama M, Origasa H, Matsuzaki M, Matsuzawa Y, Saito Y, Ishikawa Y, Oikawa S, Sasaki J, Hishida H, Itakura H, Kita T, Kitabatake A, Nakaya N, Sakata T, Shimada K, Shirato K. Effects of eicosapentaenoic acid on major coronary events in hyper-

cholesterolaemic patients (JELIS): a randomised open-label, blinded endpoint analysis. Lancet. 2007;369:1090–8.
191. Tanaka K, Ishikawa Y, Yokoyama M, Origasa H, Matsuzaki M, Saito Y, Matsuzawa Y, Sasaki J, Oikawa S, Hishida H, Itakura H, Kita T, Kitabatake A, Nakaya N, Sakata T, Shimada K, Shirato K. Reduction in the recurrence of stroke by eicosapentaenoic acid for hypercholesterolemic patients: subanalysis of the JELIS trial. Stroke. 2008;39:2052–8.
192. Oikawa S, Yokoyama M, Origasa H, Matsuzaki M, Matsuzawa Y, Saito Y, Ishikawa Y, Sasaki J, Hishida H, Itakura H, Kita T, Kitabatake A, Nakaya N, Sakata T, Shimada K, Shirato K. Suppressive effect of EPA on the incidence of coronary events in hypercholesterolemia with impaired glucose metabolism: Sub-analysis of the Japan EPA Lipid Intervention Study (JELIS). Atherosclerosis. 2009;206:535–9.
193. Nakamura N, Fujita T, Kumasaka R, Murakami R, Shimada M, Shimaya Y, Osawa H, Yamabe H, Okumura K. Serum lipid profile and plasma fatty acid composition in hemodialysis patients--comparison with chronic kidney disease patients. In Vivo. 2008;22:609–11.
194. Hamazaki K, Terashima Y, Itomura M, Sawazaki S, Inagaki H, Kuroda M, Tomita S, Hirata H, Inadera H, Hamazaki T. Docosahexaenoic acid is an independent predictor of all-cause mortality in hemodialysis patients. Am J Nephrol. 2011;33:105–10.
195. Friedman AN, Yu Z, Denski C, Tamez H, Wenger J, Thadhani R, Li Y, Watkins B. Fatty acids and other risk factors for sudden cardiac death in patients starting hemodialysis. Am J Nephrol. 2013;38:12–8.
196. Svensson M, Schmidt EB, Jorgensen KA, Christensen JH, Group, O. S. N-3 fatty acids as secondary prevention against cardiovascular events in patients who undergo chronic hemodialysis: a randomized, placebo-controlled intervention trial. Clin J Am Soc Nephrol. 2006;1:780–6.
197. Lok CE, Moist L, Hemmelgarn BR, Tonelli M, Vazquez MA, Dorval M, Oliver M, Donnelly S, Allon M, Stanley K, Fish oil Inhibition of Stenosis in Hemodialysis Grafts Study, G. Effect of fish oil supplementation on graft patency and cardiovascular events among patients with new synthetic arteriovenous hemodialysis grafts: a randomized controlled trial. JAMA. 2012;307:1809–16.
198. Ferraro PM, Ferraccioli GF, Gambaro G, Fulignati P, Costanzi S. Combined treatment with renin-angiotensin system blockers and polyunsaturated fatty acids in proteinuric IgA nephropathy: a randomized controlled trial. Nephrol Dial Transplant. 2009;24:156–60.
199. Chou HH, Chiou YY, Hung PH, Chiang PC, Wang ST. Omega-3 fatty acids ameliorate proteinuria but not renal function in IgA nephropathy: a meta-analysis of randomized controlled trials. Nephron Clin Pract. 2012;121:c30–5.
200. Walldius G, Erikson U, Olsson AG, Bergstrand L, Hadell K, Johansson J, Kaijser L, Lassvik C, Molgaard J, Nilsson S, et al. The effect of probucol on femoral atherosclerosis: the Probucol Quantitative Regression Swedish Trial (PQRST). Am J Cardiol. 1994;74:875–83.
201. Miyagawa F, Fukumoto T, Kobayashi N, Asada H. Successful treatment of diffuse normolipemic plane xanthoma with probucol. Case Rep Dermatol. 2013;5:148–51.
202. Daida H, Kuwabara Y, Yokoi H, Nishikawa H, Takatsu F, Nakata Y, Kutsumi Y, Oshima S, Nishiyama S, Ishiwata S, Kato K, Nishimura S, Miyauchi K, Kanoh T, Yamaguchi H. Effect of probucol on repeat revascularization rate after percutaneous transluminal coronary angioplasty (from the Probucol Angioplasty Restenosis Trial [PART]). Am J Cardiol. 2000;86:550 2, A9.
203. Sawayama Y, Shimizu C, Maeda N, Tatsukawa M, Kinukawa N, Koyanagi S, Kashiwagi S, Hayashi J. Effects of probucol and pravastatin on common carotid atherosclerosis in patients with asymptomatic hypercholesterolemia. Fukuoka Atherosclerosis Trial (FAST). J Am Coll Cardiol. 2002;39:610–6.
204. Sawayama Y, Maeda S, Ohnishi H, Okada K, Hayashi J. Effect of probucol on elderly hypercholesterolemic patients in the FAST study. Fukuoka Igaku Zasshi. 2006;97:15–24.
205. Endo K, Miyashita Y, Sasaki H, Ohira M, Saiki A, Koide N, Otsuka M, Oyama T, Takeyoshi M, Ito Y, Shirai K. Probucol delays progression of diabetic nephropathy. Diabetes Res Clin Pract. 2006;71:156–63.
206. Endo K, Saiki A, Yamaguchi T, Sakuma K, Sasaki H, Ban N, Kawana H, Nagayama D, Nagumo A, Ohira M, Oyama T, Murano T, Miyashita Y, Yamamura S, Suzuki Y, Shirai K, Tatsuno I. Probucol suppresses initiation of chronic hemodialysis therapy and renal dysfunction-related death in diabetic nephropathy patients: Sakura study. J Atheroscler Thromb. 2013;20:494–502.
207. Ye Z, Zhang L, Xu L, Shi W, Hu H, Shi X, Zhong W, Hou S, Yan H, Zhang B, Xia Y, Wang W, Feng Z, Wang L, Liang Y. Probucol combined with valsartan in immunoglobulin A nephropathy: a multicentre, open labelled, randomized controlled study. Nephrology (Carlton). 2014;19:40–6.
208. Li G, Yin L, Liu T, Zheng X, Xu G, Xu Y, Yuan R, Che J, Liu H, Zhou L, Chen X, He M, Li Y, Wu L, Liu E. Role of probucol in preventing contrast-induced acute kidney injury after coronary interventional procedure. Am J Cardiol. 2009;103:512–4.
209. Yin L, Li G, Liu T, Yuan R, Zheng X, Xu G, Xu Y, Che J, Liu X, Ma X, Li F, Liu E, Chen X, Wu L, Fan Z, Ruan Y, He M, Li Y. Probucol for the prevention of cystatin C-based contrast-induced acute kidney injury following primary or urgent angioplasty: a randomized, controlled trial. Int J Cardiol. 2013;167:426–9.

Part V

Mineral Bone Disorders

14 Calcium Homeostasis in Kidney Disease

Michel Chonchol and Jessica Kendrick

Calcium Homeostasis in Kidney Disease

Calcium ion homeostasis is an important factor as calcium is essential to many vital physiologic functions including neuromuscular activity, preservation of the integrity of cellular membranes, blood coagulation, hormone secretion, and bone metabolism. Approximately 99% of body calcium resides in bone. The other 1% is present in the extracellular and intracellular spaces either in diffusible nonionized form (10%) or in ionized form (45%) [1]. Free ionized calcium (Ca^{2+}) is the biologically active component, and the nonionized form is called complexed calcium. The total amount of calcium in the human body ranges from 1000 to 1200 g. The serum calcium concentration is held in a very narrow range in both the intracellular and extracellular spaces [1]. Calcium homeostasis is dependent on three components: (1) the kidney, intestine, and bone (re)absorbing or storing calcium; (2) hormones that regulate the transport of calcium; and (3) the calcium-sensing receptor that controls the transport of calcium in the tissues.

Intestinal Absorption of Calcium

Dietary calcium intake varies widely. Generally, in a well-balanced diet, approximately 800–1000 mg of calcium is ingested daily. Gastrointestinal absorption of calcium is a highly selective process. Only 20–25% of total dietary calcium is absorbed. Calcium is absorbed along the small intestine by two transport processes: transcellular (i.e., through the cell) and paracellular (i.e., between the cells) [2–4]. Transcellular absorption is an active process, is saturable, and is physiologically regulated. This process involves three steps: (1) transport of calcium from the lumen into the cell through apical calcium channels, (2) movement of calcium within the cell, and (3) movement of calcium from the cell into the interstitial fluid by a Ca^{2+}-ATPase. Paracellular absorption is passive and is nonsaturable. It is determined by concentration gradients between the luminal and serosal spaces. Hence, it is the predominant route of absorption when the luminal concentration of calcium is high. Many factors regulate intestinal calcium absorption including (a) age, (b) calcium and vitamin D intake, and (c) circulating levels of calcitriol and parathyroid hormone (PTH) [3, 6]. Calcitriol is the most important hormonal regulatory factor

M. Chonchol (✉)
Division of Renal Diseases and Hypertension, University of Colorado Hospital, Department of Medicine, Aurora, CO, USA
e-mail: Michel.Chonchol@ucdenver.edu

J. Kendrick
Division of Renal Diseases and Hypertension, Department of Medicine, Denver Health Medical Center and University of Colorado, Denver, CO, USA

C. M. Rhee et al. (eds.), *Endocrine Disorders in Kidney Disease*,
https://doi.org/10.1007/978-3-319-97765-2_14

and primarily controls the active absorption of calcium. Calcitriol induces the expression of calcium channels, calbindin (which binds calcium and removes calcium from the microvilli region), and increases the Ca^{2+}-ATPase [6].

Increased calcium absorption occurs with low calcium intake to ensure that adequate amounts of calcium are delivered to the body. Calcium absorption also increases in direct proportion to the requirements; for example, calcium absorption increases during puberty, pregnancy, and lactation. It is important to note that many substances (e.g., oxalate, citrate) may interfere with calcium absorption in the gastrointestinal tract by chelating, precipitating, or forming complexes with oral calcium. Certain medications such as glucocorticoids and colchicine also interfere with calcium absorption.

Renal Regulation of Calcium

The kidneys play a critical role in the regulation of serum calcium. In humans who have a glomerular filtration rate of 170 liters per 24 h, roughly 10 g of calcium is filtered per day. The amount of calcium excreted in the urine varies considerably in normal subjects, but the upper normal range of calcium excretion per day is <300 mg for men and <250 mg for women. Ninety-eight percent to 99% of the filtered load of calcium is reabsorbed by the renal tubules [6]. The kidney reabsorbs ionized calcium more easily than complexed calcium. The complexed calcium is bound to molecules such as phosphate, citrate, and sulfate. Approximately 60% to 70% of the filtered calcium is reabsorbed in the proximal convoluted tubule, 20% in the loop of Henle, 10% by the distal convoluted tubule, and 5% by the collecting system. The terminal nephron, although responsible for the reabsorption of only 5–10% of the filtered calcium load, is the major site for regulation of calcium excretion [1].

In the proximal tubule, 80% of calcium is reabsorbed passively by diffusion paralleling that of sodium and water. The remaining 10–15% of proximal tubule calcium reabsorption is through an active two-step transport mechanism. Calcium enters from the tubular fluid across the apical membrane and exits through the basolateral membrane. This active reabsorption is regulated by PTH and calcitonin [5]. There is no reabsorption of calcium in the thin segment of the loop of Henle. In the thick ascending limb of the loop of Henle (TAL), 20% of the filtered calcium is reabsorbed. The majority of calcium reabsorption is through the paracellular pathway and is proportional to the transtubular electrochemical driving force. Apical Na^+-K^+-$2Cl^-$ cotransporter and the renal outer medullary potassium (ROMK) channel generate a lumen-positive transepithelial voltage, which drives calcium reabsorption. Calcium transport in the TAL is influenced by PTH and the calcium-sensing receptor (CaSR). PTH increases paracellular permeability resulting in increased calcium reabsorption. Stimulation of the CaSR by increased serum calcium levels results in decreased calcium reabsorption by decreasing the paracellular permeability to calcium [6].

The distal tubule reabsorbs 5–10% of the filtered calcium exclusively via the transcellular route. The distal tubule is the major site of calcium reabsorption. Calcium is transported across the apical membrane toward the basolateral membrane where calcium is reabsorbed via a sodium-calcium exchanger and a Ca^{2+}-ATPase. Both PTH and calcitriol regulate calcium reabsorption in the distal tubule.

Factors that Regulate the Absorption of Calcium

There are numerous factors that control the absorption of calcium. The most important regulator of serum calcium is PTH, which stimulates calcium absorption. PTH is a polypeptide secreted from the parathyroid gland in response to a decrease in the plasma concentration of ionized calcium. The key physiological role of the parathyroid gland is to regulate calcium homeostasis. PTH increases serum calcium levels by (1) stimulating bone resorption, (2) promoting the formation of calcitriol in the kidney to enhance intestinal calcium absorption, and (3) increasing active renal calcium absorption. These effects are reversed by small changes in the serum calcium concentration which lower PTH secretion.

Calcitriol is another key factor controlling calcium absorption. Calcitriol (1,25-dihydroxyvitamin D_3) is made in the kidney, enters the circulation, and is transported to the small intestine where it enhances intestinal calcium absorption. Calcitriol also increases calcium absorption in the distal tubule. Metabolic acidosis is associated with a decrease in calcium absorption and an increase in calcium excretion, independent of changes in PTH. Expansion of the extracellular fluid is associated with increased calcium excretion, whereas decreased excretion is seen with volume contraction. Diuretics also influence calcium absorption. Loop diuretics decrease absorption by inhibiting transport in the TAL. Thiazide diuretics result in decreased calcium excretion presumably through increasing proximal sodium and water reabsorption and increasing distal calcium reabsorption in the distal tubule.

Consequences of Changes in Calcium Balance

Hypercalcemia

Hypercalcemia is a common disorder that presents a challenge to clinicians. The normal range of calcium is between 8.5–10.5 mg/dL and 2.12–2.62 mmol/L. Hypercalcemia occurs when the serum level of ionized calcium increases. The two most common causes of hypercalcemia are malignancy and primary hyperparathyroidism, accounting for almost 90% of cases [7, 8]. The diagnostic approach to new cases of hypercalcemia is focused on distinguishing between these two common causes. A careful history and physical examination should be performed to identify the etiology. Malignancy often results in more severe hypercalcemia requiring hospitalization, whereas primary hyperparathyroidism usually results in asymptomatic hypercalcemia. Primary hyperparathyroidism is more common in women, and the incidence increases after menopause [9]. Hypercalcemia is less common in children than adults but is more likely to be clinically significant in children. Idiopathic infantile hypercalcemia is a disorder characterized by transiently high serum calcium levels in infancy. It is usually a benign disorder, but there is a severe form associated with somatic deformations called Williams syndrome which is characterized by mental deficiency, "elfin face," epicanthal folds, renal disease, heart defects, and bladder diverticuli. Seventeen percent of patients with sarcoidosis develop hypercalcemia, and it is more common in males [10]. Patients with a family history of hypercalcemia are more likely to have primary hyperparathyroidism or familial hypocalciuric hypercalcemia (FHH). FHH is an autosomal dominant disorder in which patients have hypocalciuria and hypercalcemia. The hypercalcemia is mild and usually does not require treatment. Patients may also have a family history or personal history of multiple endocrine neoplasia type 1 (MEN 1) or type 2A (MEN 2A). A family history of recurrent kidney stones is also suggestive of a familial cause of hypercalcemia. Many medications may result in hypercalcemia so a careful medication history must be obtained. There are other endocrine disorders that can be associated with hypercalcemia including hyperthyroidism, acromegaly, and pheochromocytoma. Hypercalcemia develops in 10–22% of patients with hyperthyroidism, but the hypercalcemia is usually mild and reverses with antithyroid therapy [11]. Rarely, hypercalcemia results in patients with pheochromocytomas either from the pheochromocytoma itself or in combination with hyperparathyroidism (i.e., MEN 2A) [12]. Immobilization may also result in hypercalcemia primarily in states of rapid bone turnover (e.g., normal children and adolescents and bone abnormalities such as Paget's). The most common causes of hypercalcemia are listed in Fig. 14.1.

There are three basic pathophysiologic mechanisms contributing to hypercalcemia: increased intestinal calcium absorption, increased bone resorption, and decreased urinary calcium excretion. Increased bone resorption by neoplastic processes is the predominant cause in most cases of hypercalcemia. The tumors cause bone resorption either directly by invasion of the bone or by producing factors that stimulate osteoclastic activity, e.g., parathyroid hormone-related protein [13].

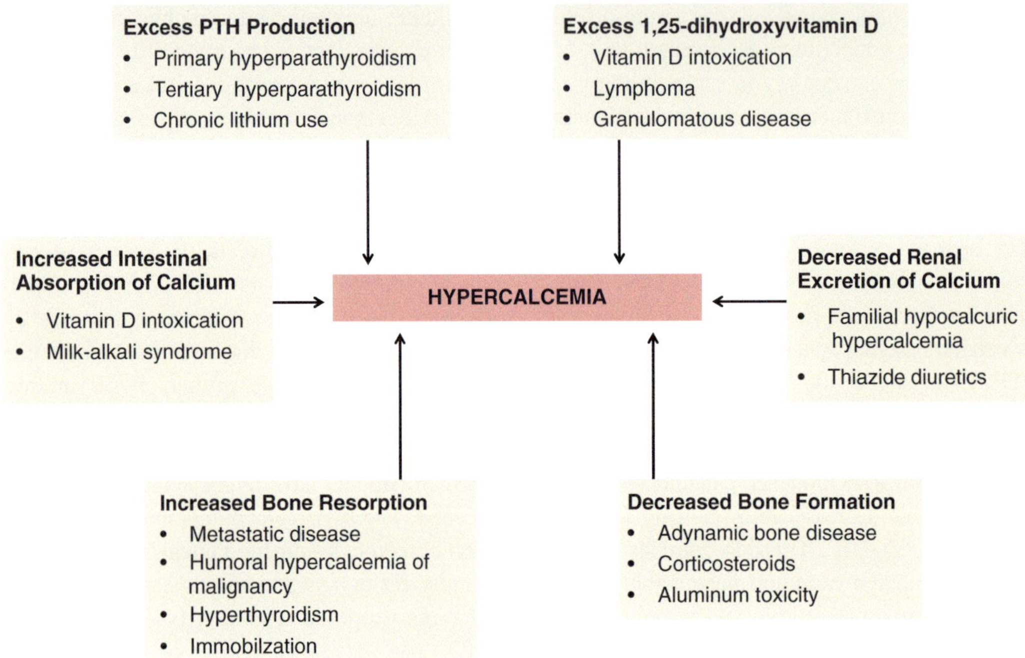

Fig. 14.1 Causes of hypercalcemia

Excess calcitriol (e.g., sarcoidosis, vitamin D intoxication) results in hypercalcemia by increasing intestinal absorption of calcium and increasing calcium release from the bone. Many medications can result in hypercalcemia by either increasing intestinal absorption of calcium (e.g., vitamin D, milk-alkali syndrome) or by decreasing renal excretion of calcium (e.g., thiazide diuretics).

Clinical Manifestations of Hypercalcemia

The severity of clinical symptoms depends on the level and rate of rise of serum calcium. Patients with serum calcium levels <12 mg/dL are often asymptomatic and do not require emergent treatment. Severe hypercalcemia may have few clinical manifestations if it developed slowly, whereas much less severe hypercalcemia can lead to significant symptoms. Levels >14 mg/dL are not well tolerated and may result in severe symptoms including coma. The first symptoms that occur are usually general and nonspecific and include fatigue, muscle weakness, nervousness, difficulty concentrating, and depression. As hypercalcemia persists, other symptoms begin to manifest. Gastrointestinal symptoms include nausea, vomiting, and constipation. Renal-related symptoms include polyuria, kidney stones, and acute and chronic kidney failure. Neuropsychiatric manifestations include headache, mild cognitive dysfunction, lethargy, and rarely stupor and coma. Cardiac arrhythmias have been reported in patients with severe hypercalcemia (levels >14 mg/dL) but are rare.

Diagnosis

The approach to hypercalcemia involves a careful history and clinical examination and additional laboratory testing. As discussed earlier, oftentimes, the diagnosis can be ascertained based on the history and clinical examination. However, when a diagnosis cannot be made by history and physical, additional laboratory testing is warranted. Hypercalcemia should be confirmed by repeat testing if there is only one elevated serum calcium level. Additionally, serum calcium should always be corrected for albumin, and a direct measurement of ionized calcium should be performed if it is available. Once hypercalcemia is confirmed, the next step is to measure the serum intact parathyroid hormone level (iPTH). Measurement of the iPTH is critical to differentiate PTH-mediated from non-PTH-mediated causes of hypercalcemia. Even though primary hyperparathyroidism is only the second most common cause of hypercalcemia, its laboratory diagnosis is easier to make than hypercalcemia from malignancy. If the serum iPTH is high, this is indicative of primary hyperparathyroidism. If iPTH is low-normal or low in the setting of hypercalcemia, other causes should be considered, and the patient should undergo measurement of PTH-related peptide (PTHrP) and vitamin D metabolites. If PTHrP is negative and vitamin D metabolite levels (25-hydroxyvitamin D [25(OH) D] and 1,25-dihydroxyvitamin D [1,25$(OH)_2$D]) are normal, other non-PTH-related causes of hypercalcemia should be considered. Given the large number of diseases associated with hypercalcemia, one should use patient factors and symptoms to guide further testing. All patients with hypercalcemia should have a creatinine checked to evaluate for acute or chronic kidney dysfunction.

Treatment

The main goal of treatment is to treat the underlying disorder. Whether the patient requires immediate treatment of hypercalcemia depends on symptoms and the level of serum calcium. Patients that are asymptomatic with calcium levels <14 mg/dL do not usually require immediate treatment. Patients with severe (defined as >14 mg/dL) and/or symptomatic hypercalcemia require rapid correction. Initially, the patient must be treated with isotonic saline as they are often markedly volume depleted due to urinary losses of sodium and water. Isotonic saline results in increased urinary calcium excretion and decreased proximal tubule calcium reabsorption. Since large volumes of isotonic saline are often required, there is a risk of volume overload so patients must be monitored closely. Contraindications to the use of large amounts of volume resuscitation include severe cardiac failure and advanced chronic kidney disease. Loop diuretics can be used as an adjunct therapy to facilitate urinary excretion of calcium once euvolemia is established [13, 14].

If hypercalcemia persists despite volume resuscitation or if patients have contraindications to saline therapy, then pharmacologic therapies should be used. Bisphosphonates are often first choice, especially in hypercalcemia associated with cancer. Bisphosphonates inhibit calcitriol synthesis and bone resorption. In severe disease, these drugs should be given intravenously. Pamidronate (60–90 mg IV over 4 h) and zoledronate (4 mg over 15 min) are frequently used agents. Zoledronate is more potent than pamidronate at reversing hypercalcemia. These medications should be used with caution in patients with significant renal impairment, and the dose should be reduced. A single dose of these medications usually corrects hypercalcemia within 2–4 days. These drugs are well tolerated, and very rare side effects of these medications are osteonecrosis of the jaw and acute renal failure. Calcitonin can also be used for hypercalcemia as it increases urinary calcium excretion and decreases bone resorption. The recommended dose is 4 international units/kg of salmon calcitonin given subcutaneously or intramuscularly every 12 h. It works within 4–6 h, but its use is limited by its short duration of action and the rapid development of tachyphylaxis [13, 14].

Glucocorticoids are effective for hypercalcemia resulting from malignancy, vitamin D intoxication, and sarcoidosis. The dose is usually around 0.5–1 mg/kg daily, and the decrease in serum calcium usually occurs 1–2 days after starting therapy.

Mithramycin is a cytostatic drug that lowers serum calcium level by inhibiting bone resorption. Administration of a single dose of 25 μg/kg intravenously effectively lowers serum calcium within a few hours, and the effect lasts several days. Serious side effects including bone marrow suppression and liver and renal toxicity occur and have limited its use in clinical practice. Patients with refractory severe hypercalcemia should be considered for dialysis [13, 14].

Hypocalcemia

Hypocalcemia can either be false hypocalcemia (due to reduced serum albumin level) or true hypocalcemia (decrease in ionized calcium). False hypocalcemia can be excluded by correcting the calcium for the albumin or by directly measuring the ionized calcium level. False hypocalcemia should be considered in patients with chronic illness, malnutrition, cirrhosis, and/or nephrotic syndrome as these disorders result in hypoalbuminemia.

There are numerous causes of hypocalcemia [15]. Hypocalcemia spans all ages, and the incidence is equal in males and females. The differential diagnosis will vary depending on the patient's age and other comorbidities. Hypocalcemia can be divided into that associated with high and that associated with low/normal PTH levels (Fig. 14.2). Hypocalcemia associated with low PTH is usually due to decreased/inadequate PTH secretion (hypoparathyroidism). Hypoparathyroidism may be acquired (e.g., after surgery or radiation, secondary to autoimmune damage or amyloidosis, etc.), hereditary (autosomal dominant hypocalcemia and familial isolated hypoparathyroidism), or idiopathic. Hypomagnesemia results in decreased serum ionized calcium levels by inducing PTH resistance and decreasing PTH secretion.

Hypocalcemia associated with high PTH results from many different causes but primarily results from vitamin D-deficient states (Fig. 14.2). Most cases of 25(OH)D deficiency do not result in hypocalcemia unless the deficiency is severe. Vitamin D deficiency can occur from decreased intake, decreased absorption (e.g., from gastrointestinal surgery, intestinal malabsorption, or hepatobiliary disease), or decreased formation (e.g., liver disease). Decreased $1{,}25(OH)_2D$ formation or resistance to $1{,}25(OH)_2D$ also results in low calcium levels (e.g., vitamin D-dependent rickets). Pseudohypoparathyroidism (parathyroid hormone resistance) is a familial disease that causes hypocalcemia as well as short stature, hypothyroidism, hypogonadism, and developmental delay. Chronic kidney disease is also a common cause of hypocalcemia due to secondary hyperparathyroidism. Acute pancreatitis is a frequent cause of hypocalcemia due to precipitation of calcium in the retroperitoneum. Osteoblastic metastases can also result in hypocalcemia. Occasionally, hypocalcemia occurs acutely as a result of either extravascular calcium deposition or intravascular binding.

Clinical Manifestations of Hypocalcemia

Similar to hypercalcemia, the symptoms of hypocalcemia depend on how quickly it develops and how severe it is. The hallmark of acute hypocalcemia is neuromuscular irritability including perioral numbness, carpopedal spasms of the hands and feet, tetany, altered mental status, and seizures. Tetany usually only occurs when the total serum calcium level falls below 7.0 mg/dL. Chvostek's sign (tapping on the facial nerve near the temporal mandibular joint leads to twitching of facial muscle) and Trousseau's sign (carpal spasm in response to inflation of a blood pressure cuff in the forearm) are signs of neuromuscular irritability [15]. Grand mal, petit mal, and focal seizures all can occur as a result of hypocalcemia. Patients who develop seizures usually also have tetany, but seizures can occur

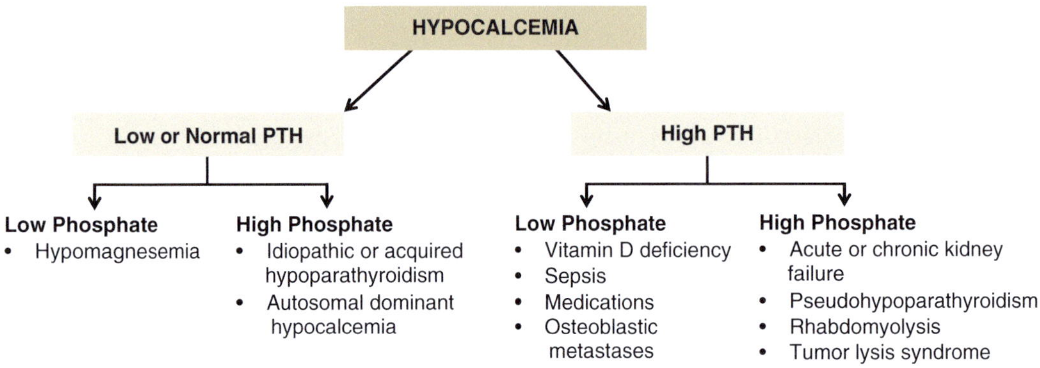

Fig. 14.2 Causes of hypocalcemia

without tetany. Cardiovascular manifestations (prolongation of the QT interval, arrhythmias) may be present as a sign or symptom of hypocalcemia. Patients with chronic hypocalcemia are often asymptomatic. However, chronic hypocalcemia is associated with brittle nails, dry skin, coarse hair, cataracts, skeletal abnormalities, and basal ganglia calcifications.

Diagnosis

Hypocalcemia should be confirmed if there is only one low serum calcium value and the value needs to be corrected for the albumin level. The laboratory evaluation of hypocalcemia should be guided by the history and clinical examination. If the cause of the hypocalcemia is not obvious from the patient's history, the first step in the evaluation is to measure PTH. A low PTH is essentially diagnostic of hypoparathyroidism (hereditary or acquired), but autosomal dominant hypocalcemia (activating mutation of the calcium-sensing receptor) must be ruled out. Chronic hypomagnesemia also results in low or normal PTH. A high PTH level is the normal response to hypocalcemia. Hence, an elevated PTH level is seen in patients with hypocalcemia from chronic kidney disease, pseudohypoparathyroidism, vitamin D deficiency, osteoblastic metastases, sepsis, etc. Most of these causes are obvious from the patient's history and physical examination. In addition to PTH, other important measurements include serum creatinine, phosphate, magnesium, 25(OH)D, $1,25(OH)_2D$, and alkaline phosphatase. Imaging studies should be ordered based on the history and physical examination. For example, plain films are useful for identifying osteoblastic metastases.

Treatment

Treatment is aimed at the underlying cause. Urgent management of hypocalcemia depends on the severity and rapidity with which the hypocalcemia develops. Patients with acute hypocalcemia may have severe symptoms (tetany, seizures, QT prolongation), which require aggressive treatment with intravenous calcium [15, 16]. An intravenous bolus of 1–2 g (93–186 mg elemental calcium) of calcium gluconate diluted in 50–100 mL of 5% dextrose should be infused over 10–20 min. If hypocalcemia persists, a slow calcium infusion should be started at 0.5–1.5 mg/kg/hour. Calcium gluconate is preferred over calcium chloride as calcium chloride can lead to skin necrosis if accidentally extravasated. Serum magnesium must also be repleted if low.

Patients with chronic hypocalcemia are often asymptomatic and should be treated with oral calcium and vitamin D supplementation. One to three grams of elemental calcium should be given in two to three divided doses daily. There are numerous preparations of oral calcium available. Calcium carbonate is the most common formulation used, and it contains 40% elemental calcium. Vitamin D may need to be added if the oral calcium administration does not correct the hypocalcemia. Vitamin D supplementation ($1,25(OH)_2D$) is needed for the treatment of hypoparathyroidism. Concurrent magnesium deficiency should be treated with oral magnesium oxide or by magnesium infusion. The goal of therapy in chronic hypocalcemia is to restore and maintain the serum calcium level in the low-normal range. Higher targets increase the risk of hypercalciuria, which can lead to nephrolithiasis and/or nephrocalcinosis. Calcium levels need to be monitored to avoid hypercalcemia.

References

1. Kumar R. Calcium metabolism. In: Jacobson HR, Striker GE, Klahr S, editors. The principles and practice of nephrology. 2nd ed. St. Louis: Mosby-Year Book; 1995. p. 964–71.
2. Borke JL, Caride A, Verma AK, Penniston JT, Kumar R. Cellular and segmental distribution of Ca++ pump epitopes in rat intestine. Pflugers Arch. 1990;417:120–2.
3. Kumar R. Calcium transport in epithelial cells of the intestine and kidney. J Cell Biochem. 1995;57:392–8.
4. Johnson JA, Kumar R. Renal and intestinal calcium transport: roles of vitamin D and vitamin D-dependent calcium binding proteins. Semin Nephrol. 1994;14:119–28.
5. Felsenfeld A, Rodriguez M, Levine B. New insights in regulation of calcium homeostasis. Curr Opin Nephrol Hypertens. 2013;22:371–6.
6. Blaine J, Chonchol M, Levi M. Renal control of calcium, phosphate and magnesium homeostasis. Clin J Am Soc Neprhol. 2015;10:1257–72.

7. Lafferty FW. Differential diagnosis of hypercalcemia. J Bone Miner Res. 1991;6(Suppl 2):S51–9. discussion S61
8. Burtis WJ, Wu TL, Insogna KL, Stewart AF. Humoral hypercalcemia of malignancy. Ann Intern Med. 1988;108:454–7.
9. Minisola S, Pepe J, Piemonte S, Cipriani C. The diagnosis and management of hypercalcemia. BMJ. 2015;350:h2723.
10. Renier M, Sjurdsson G, Nunziata V, Malik MA, Pople GW, Joplin GF. Abnormal calcium metabolism in normocalcemic sarcoidosis. Br Med J. 1976;2:1473–6.
11. Calcium metabolism and bone in hyperthyroidism. Lancet. 1970;2:1300–2.
12. Garbini A, Mainardi M, Grimi M, Repaci G, Nanni G, Bragherio G. Pheochromocytoma and hypercalcemia due to ectopic production of parathyroid hormone. N Y State J Med. 1986;86:25–7.
13. Mirrakhimov AE. Hypercalcemia of malignancy: an update on pathogenesis and management. N Am J Med Sci. 2015;7:483–93.
14. Bilezikian JP. Management of acute hypercalcemia. N Engl J Med. 1992;326:1196–203.
15. Cooper MS. Diagnosis and management of hypocalcemia. BMJ. 2008;336:1298–302.
16. Tohme JF, Bilezikian JP. Hypocalcemic emergencies. Endocrinol Metab Clin N Am. 1993;22:363–75.

15 Phosphorus Retention and Elevated FGF-23 in Chronic Kidney Disease

Yoshitsugu Obi and Connie M. Rhee

Background

Cardiovascular disease is a major cause of morbidity and mortality in patients with chronic kidney disease (CKD), especially in those with end-stage renal disease (ESRD) [1], and the risk of cardiovascular mortality is 10–20-fold higher among hemodialysis patients. However, some of the traditional risk factors of cardiovascular disease such as African-American race, hypertension, hypercholesterolemia, and obesity are paradoxically associated with better outcomes in CKD and ESRD patients [2–7], and these observations point to the presence of novel cardiovascular risk factors in CKD. In addition to the fact that decreased kidney function itself is a strong and independent predictor of cardiovascular events, CKD is characterized by a complex metabolic milieu that consists of multiple biochemical and hormonal abnormalities. Those abnormalities in mineral and bone metabolism have also been associated with worse cardiovascular outcomes and mortality independent of traditional risk factors [8–14]. These findings have led to the emergence of a framework termed CKD-related mineral and bone disorders (CKD-MBD) [15].

Congestive heart failure is the leading cardiovascular condition among patients with CKD, and the terminal events in congestive heart failure are pump failure and sudden arrhythmic death [16]. Indeed, unlike the general population, in whom ischemic heart disease is the primary cause of cardiovascular mortality, many patients with advanced CKD expire from chronic heart failure and sudden cardiac death [17–19]. This is consistent with the fact that left ventricular hypertrophy (LVH) and vascular calcification are the most apparent cardiovascular abnormalities in patients with CKD [20]. In particular, hyperphosphatemia and elevated fibroblast growth factor (FGF)-23 are common and have been strongly and consistently linked to those abnormalities among patients with CKD. Excesses in phosphorus and FGF23 are potential therapeutic targets in CKD, and a better understanding of the physiological and pathologic processes may help develop therapeutic strategies and guide patient care for the treatment of CKD-mineral and bone disorders (MBDs).

Y. Obi
Division of Nephrology and Hypertension, Department of Medicine, University of California Irvine School of Medicine, Orange, CA, USA

C. M. Rhee (✉)
Division of Nephrology and Hypertension, Departments of Medicine and Public Health, University of California Irvine School of Medicine, Orange, CA, USA
e-mail: crhee1@uci.edu

C. M. Rhee et al. (eds.), *Endocrine Disorders in Kidney Disease*,
https://doi.org/10.1007/978-3-319-97765-2_15

Physiology

Phosphorus is an essential macronutrient for the survival of living organisms and play major roles on the maintenance of its biological functions. It constitutes hydroxyapatite in skeleton, phospholipids in cell membrane, adenosine triphosphate (ATP) as a major source of cellular energy, and nuclear acids (i.e., DNA and RNA). Furthermore, posttranslational modifications through phosphorylation and dephosphorization regulate a wide variety of enzymes and proteins in pathways of intracellular signal transduction. Serum phosphate levels are maintained by delicate multi-organ cross talks among the kidney, parathyroid, bone, and intestine through several hormones such as 1α,25-dihydroxyvitamin D [1α,25$(OH)_2$D], parathyroid hormone (PTH), and FGF23 (Fig. 15.1), and their concentrations are regulated by a negative feedback loop among each of them [21–34].

Secreted FGF23 is a 32 kDa hormone derived from the bone (i.e., osteocytes and osteoblasts) and regulates phosphorus and vitamin D homeostasis [35, 36]. It belongs to the FGF family; thus far a total of 22 FGFs with diverse biological activities have been identified in humans and grouped into seven subfamilies according to their mechanisms of action [37]. Among them, the FGF19 subfamily (i.e., FGF19, FGF21, and FGF23) has hormone-like characteristics due to the reduced affinity to heparin sulfate which enable them to avoid being captured in the extracellular matrices [38, 39]. They have also low binding ability to heparin resulting in diminished affinity to FGF receptors (FGFR), and hence, require the coexistence of a co-receptor Klotho to activate FGFR [37, 40]. Specifically, FGF23 interacts with α-Klotho via its C-terminus, and the physiologic actions of FGF23 are predominantly exerted through the FGFR-α-Klotho complex [41–43]. The tissue-specificity of FGF23 actions is explained by the limited distribution of the full-length transmembrane α-Klotho molecule to certain tissues with its expression highest in the renal distal tubule followed by the brain and the pituitary gland and to a lower extent in placenta, skeletal muscle, urinary bladder, aorta, pancreas, testis, ovary, colon, and the thyroid gland [44].

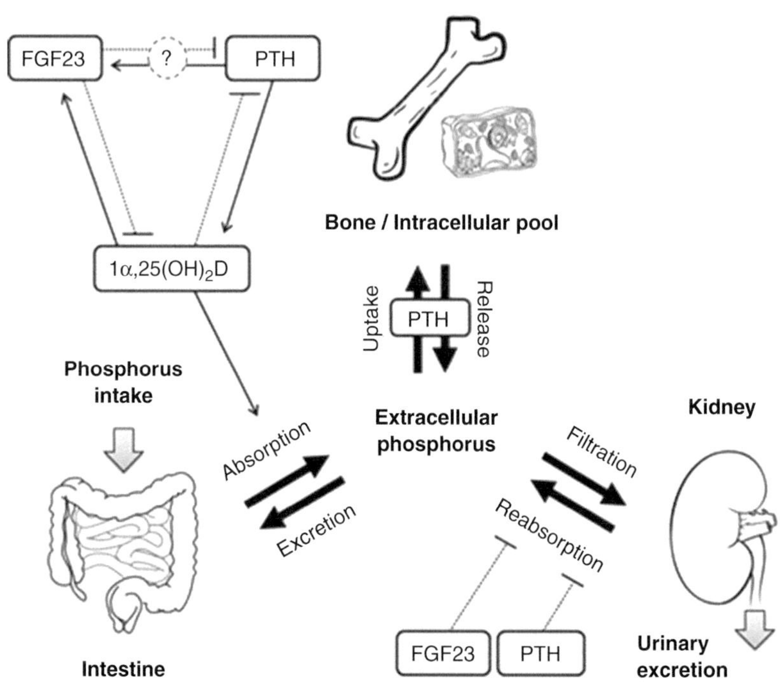

Fig. 15.1 Phosphorus homeostasis. (Modified from reference [34]). Extracellular phosphate levels are maintained by intestinal phosphate absorption, renal phosphate handling, and equilibrium of phosphate between extracellular fluid and phosphate in the bone or the intracellular pool. PTH, 1α,25$(OH)_2$D, and FGF23 regulate serum phosphate by modulating intestinal phosphate absorption, renal phosphate reabsorption, and/or bone metabolism

The primary physiologic actions of FGF23 are (1) suppression of the type II sodium- phosphate (NaPi) cotransporters and (2) inhibition of Cyp27b1 (1α-hydroxylase) in renal proximal tubular cells, leading to decreased reabsorption of phosphate and reduced activation of vitamin D in the kidney, respectively [21–25, 45, 46]. Nevertheless, it remains largely unknown how FGF23 interacts with the renal proximal tubule because α-Klotho is mainly expressed in the distal tubules. The proximal tubules express α-Klotho at low level [47], but a mouse model with the proximal tubule-specific α-Klotho deletion resulted in at most mild hyperphosphatemia [48], while another mouse model with partial deletion of Klotho in distal tubular segments exhibited apparent hyperphosphatemia [49]. Other actions of FGF23 include enhancement of the vitamin D degradation via stimulation of Cyp24A1 (24-hydroxylase) [21], stimulation of distal tubular sodium and calcium reabsorption [50, 51], and suppression of α-klotho and angiotensin-converting enzyme (ACE)-2 transcription in the kidney [52, 53]. FGF23 also interacts with PTH through negative feedback loops involving 1α,25$(OH)_2$D as described above, but in a direct manner, FGF23 decreases the synthesis and secretion of PTH and increases calcium-sensing receptor (CaSR) and vitamin D receptor (VDR) expression in normal parathyroid glands [24, 29, 30].

The regulatory mechanism of FGF23 is complex and not yet fully understood. PTH and 1α,25$(OH)_2$D appear to be important stimulators for FGF23 secretion and synthesis by osteocytes and osteoblasts [25–27, 54], but there are several studies demonstrating conflicting results regarding PTH [55–57]. Direct regulation of FGF23 production by extracellular phosphate levels has been difficult to demonstrate because several hormones regulate extracellular phosphate levels [58, 59], but high phosphate alone does not appear to directly affect FGF23 levels [49, 60, 61]. The activation of the renin-angiotensin-aldosterone system (RAAS), which is known to induce proteinuria through hemodynamic factors [62], appears to induce phosphate retention and FGF23 elevation in part via downregulation of renal Klotho expression [63–65]. Other regulatory factors include calcium [22, 66], metabolic acidosis [67], leptin/sympathetic nervous system [68, 69], bone mineralization-related proteins (i.e., PHEX and DMP1) [70–73], and importantly, factors affecting iron metabolism such as iron deficiency, inflammation, and intravenous iron administration [74–78].

The biological activity of FGF23 is also regulated by its intracellular posttranslational processing. The secretion of FGF23 requires O-glycosylation by polypeptide N-acetylgalactosaminyltransferase 3 (GALNT3) [79]. Additionally, the O-glycosylation also plays a pivotal role in the proteolytic inactivation of FGF23 [79, 80]. Intact FGF23 is cleaved into inactive fragments between 179Arg and 180Ser by a family of calcium-dependent cleavage enzymes (i.e., subtilisin-like protein convertases including furin and PC5/6) that recognize the RXXR motif at the boundary between the core homology region and the carboxy (C)-terminal region (Fig. 15.2) [81, 82]. The resultant C-terminal fragments may also inhibit the effective binding of intact FGF23 to FGFRs as an antagonist [83]. This cleavage is prevented by the GALNT3-mediated O-glycosylation in the RXXR motif [84, 85], and O-glycosylation of FGF23 is inhibited by the ubiquitous Golgi secretory kinase FAM20c that directs phosphorylation of FGF23 on three serines within the C-terminal fragment [86, 87]. Therefore, unglycosylated, phosphorylated FGF23 is the substrate of cleavage enzymes. Intact FGF23 may also be degraded by the kidney because the proportion of circulating c-terminal versus intact FGF23 decreases as CKD progresses [88–90]. Furthermore, iron deficiency and inflammation do not only increase FGF23 expression in the bone but also enhance FGF23 degradation through upregulating hypoxia-inducible factor (HIF) 1α [78, 91]. However, it is yet to be clarified the mechanisms by which these conditions alter the activity of the cleavage enzymes.

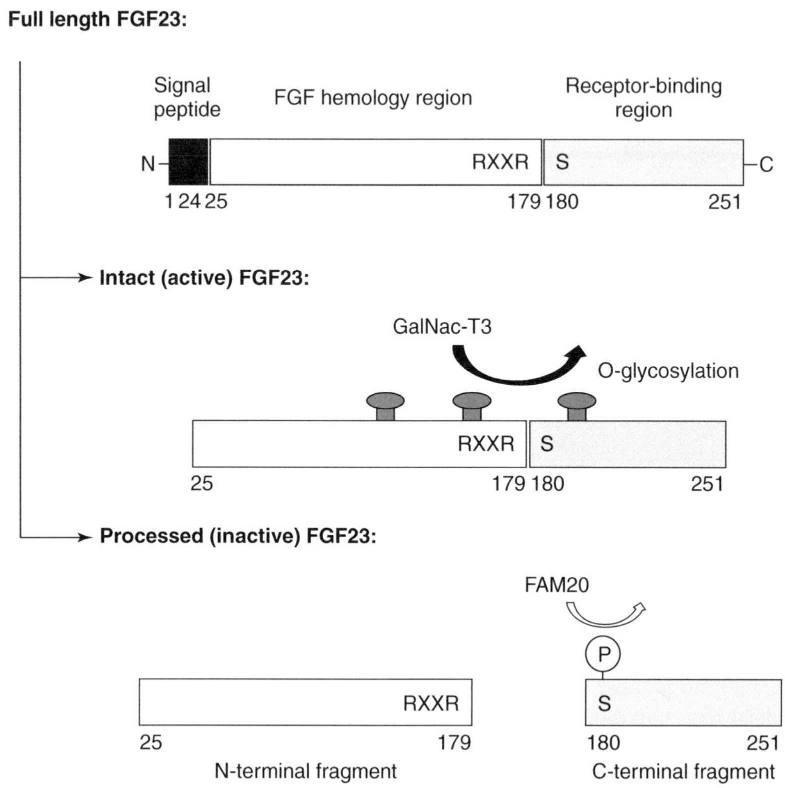

Fig. 15.2 Schematic diagram showing the structure of the FGF23 protein with 251 amino acids. The FGF protein has a signal peptide with 24 amino acids (aa 1–24), and the secreted FGF23 protein consists of the remaining 227 amino acids, which can be cleaved into the amino (N)-terminal region (aa 25–179; 18 kDa) homologous to other known FGFs and the carboxyl (C)-terminal receptor-binding region (aa 180–251; 14 kDa) that might have possible klotho-interacting site. O-glycosylation of Thr^{178} by polypeptide N-acetylgalactosaminyltransferase 3 (GalNac-T3) inhibits this cleavage, while phosphorylation of Ser^{180} inhibits O-glycosylation by GalNac-T3 and enhances the processing of FGF23 protein

Longitudinal Change in the Course of Chronic Kidney Disease

Taken together, trajectories of mineral and bone disorders in the course of CKD (Fig. 15.3) [92] can be explained as follows. At the early stage of CKD, as the expression of α-Klotho decreases in the damaged kidney [93–95], FGF23 levels start to rise earlier than other parameters such as calcium, phosphorus, and PTH [92, 96, 97]. Elevated FGF23 inhibits its renal 1α-hydroxylase expression, leading to concomitant decrease in $1\alpha,25(OH)_2D$ levels. Suboptimal VDR activation in the parathyroid glands leads to higher expression and release of PTH as CKD progresses, and decreased renal PTH clearance also results in accumulation of PTH [98]. Increases in PTH maintain serum calcium levels within the physiological range through bone resorption. Despite the decreased functioning nephron, elevation in serum phosphate levels is not observed in moderate CKD owing to high levels of two phosphaturic hormones (i.e., FGF23 and PTH) and low $1\alpha,25(OH)_2D$. In the late stages of CKD, however, serum phosphorus starts to increase when FGF23 and PTH fail to compensate for decreased urinary phosphorus excretion, and hyperphosphatemia then exacerbates hyperparathyroidism [99–101]. Renal tubular damage and elevated FGF23 blunt the response of renal 1α-hydroxylase against PTH

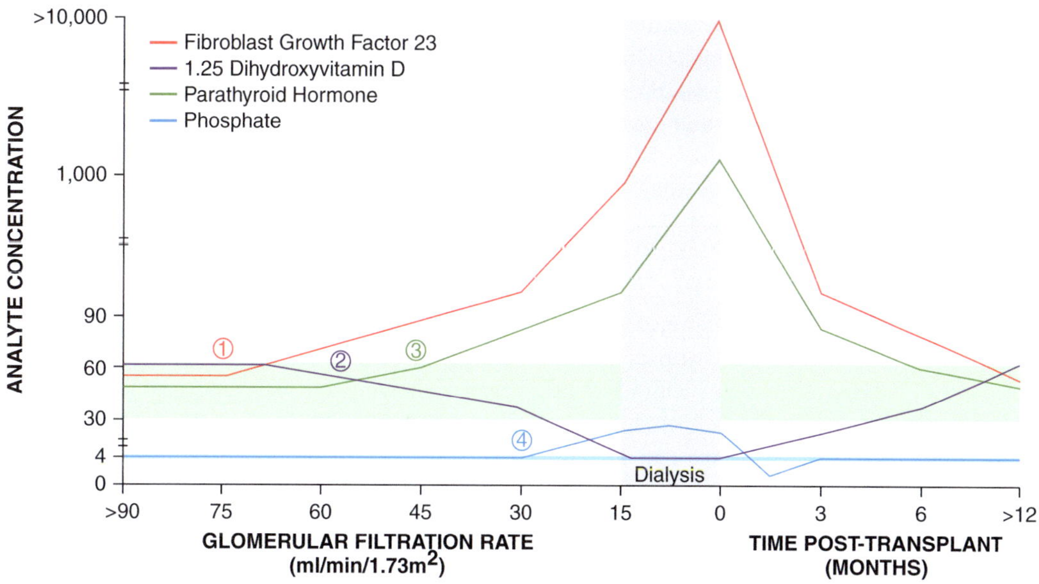

Fig. 15.3 Temporal aspects of disordered phosphorus metabolism in progressive CKD and after kidney transplantation. (Adopted from reference [92])

and further decrease 1α,25(OH)$_2$D. Resultant inclination towards hypocalcemia additively stimulates the parathyroid gland, accelerating the development of secondary hyperparathyroidism. Hyperplastic parathyroid glands have low expressions of CaSR, VDR, FGFR1, and α-klotho and, hence, show resistance against FGF23 and VDR activators [30, 102–105]. Aggravated secondary hyperparathyroidism then enhances the expression of FGF23 in osteocytes and osteoblasts. Thus, both diminished renal clearance and increased bone expression contribute to exponential elevation in FGF23 among patients with advanced CKD.

It still remains unclear why FGF23 rises when serum levels of calcium and phosphorus are unchanged and when 1α,25(OH)$_2$D is even declining. Recent cumulative data, however, suggest a key role of the kidney on FGF23 homeostasis by clearing FGF23 from blood [89, 98, 106]. Several studies also demonstrated FGF23 production in diseased kidneys [107, 108], but further studies are necessary to reveal the whole mechanisms of early FGF23 elevation in the course of CKD.

Epidemiology and Potential Pathophysiology

Phosphate and Cardiovascular Toxicity

Hyperphosphatemia is a well-known risk factor of cardiovascular events and mortality among patients with a wide range of CKD, and it should be noted that higher serum phosphorus levels are incrementally associated with greater mortality risk even within its normal range [109]. With respect to underlying pathways, research by Giachelli et al. has shown that elevated extracellular phosphorous directly stimulates vascular smooth muscle cells to undergo phenotypic changes leading to vascular calcification vis-à-vis increasing osteogenic gene expression, decreasing smooth muscle specific gene expression, and stimulating secretion of potential mineral nucleating molecules (e.g., alkaline phosphatase) [110]. It has also been suggested that phosphate disorders may lead to vascular calcification through the regulation of bone matrix proteins such as osteopontin, and work by Chen et al. has shown that phosphorus induces expression of the bone matrix osteopontin and calcification of vascular smooth muscle cells [111]. In in vivo models, phosphorus loading has been shown to inhibit endothelium-dependent vasodilation, and in humans, high dietary phosphorus loads have been shown to increase serum phosphorus and decrease flow-mediated vasodilation [112].

Adverse Effects of FGF23

FGF23 levels are exponentially elevated as kidney function declines and associated with worse renal outcomes in pre-dialysis patients with CKD [97, 113–117]. Elevated FGF23 levels are also associated with cardiovascular events and mortality across CKD stages and even in community-based populations with mostly normal kidney function, independent of potential risk factors including serum phosphorus [116–123]. While the elevation in FGF23 is an adaptive response in the course of CKD, there is still controversy regarding whether high FGF23 also has maladaptive pathologic effects in advanced CKD (Fig. 15.4).

Interestingly, in a US-based national cohort of pre-dialysis patients with CKD, the risk associated with high FGF23 levels appeared stronger and more robust for heart failure than atherosclerotic events such as myocardial infarction and ischemic stroke [118]. Similar findings were observed in other cohorts of elderly community-dwelling adults and in patients with coronary artery disease [119, 120]. These results indicate that there may be a certain phenotype of cardiovascular disease where FGF23 plays a key pathogenic role on its development and progression. Indeed, there are cumulative evidence showing the link between high FGF23 and LVH [125–128], an established risk factor for heart failure. Although the heart expresses little or no α-Klotho protein, the causal relationship of FGF23 on LVH is supported by in vitro studies demonstrating FGF23-induced hypertrophy of cardiomyocytes and also by in vivo studies showing the development of concentric LVH by both intravenous and intramyocardial FGF23 infusion [128, 129]. This noncanonical, klotho-independent effect of high FGF23 on cardiac hypertrophy is shown to be mediated through FGFR4 in the heart [128, 129].

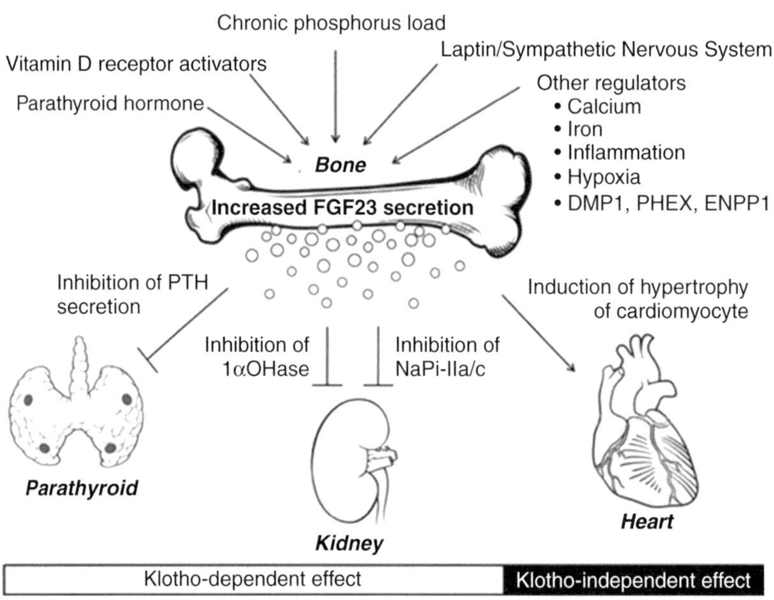

Fig. 15.4 Klotho-dependent and Klotho-independent effects of FGF23 in ESRD. Circulating FGF23 levels are markedly elevated among patients with ESRD due to multiple factors including response to chronic phosphate load, active vitamin D therapy, and PTH hypersecretion. In this setting, Klotho-dependent effects of FGF23 are largely attenuated by the loss of kidney function and the downregulation of αKlotho in the parathyroid gland, but FGF23 potentially exerts a hypertrophic effect on cardiomyocytes in a Klotho-independent manner. (Modified from reference [124])

Indeed, the activation of FGFR4/calcineurin/NFAT signaling induced cardiac hypertrophy, which was inhibited by a FGFR4-specific inhibitor or a calcineurin inhibitor [128, 129]. A retrospective, case-control study of myocardial autopsy also confirmed a strong association of LVH with enhanced expression levels of FGF23, FGFR4 and calcineurin, activation of NFAT, and reduced levels of soluble Klotho in the myocardium in patients with CKD [130]. However, super-physiological levels of FGF23 may be necessary to exert its hypertrophic action given the low affinity of FGF23 to FGFRs [40–42], and indeed Klotho knockout mice also have extremely high FGF23 levels and exhibit cardiac hypertrophy [44], a consistent observation in advanced CKD. Nevertheless, the associations of FGF23 with LVH and adverse outcomes have been reported even in populations where FGF23 levels were not very high [119, 120, 125], and no clear difference in phenotypes between Klotho and FGF23 knockout mice has been reported so far [43]. Furthermore, anti-FGF23 antibody treatment did not decrease the increased gene expression of the heart hypertrophy markers in 5/6-nephrectomized mice although it certainly improved hyperparathyroidism [131].

FGF23 may also exert a direct stimulatory effect on the renin-angiotensin system (RAS) through suppression of angiotensin-converting enzyme (ACE)-2 [53], a homologue of the ACE enzyme which cleaves angiotensin II to generate angiotensin 1–7 [132]. ACE2 and angiotensin 1–7 counteract the unfavorable effects of angiotensin (i.e., vasoconstriction, sodium retention, fibrosis, oxidative stress, and inflammation) [133–135] and participate in maintaining the normal functions of heart and endothelium [136, 137]. ACE2 insufficiency has been linked to the development and progression of atherosclerosis, heart failure, LVH, and kidney disease [138–143]. FGF23 also indirectly stimulates the RAS by decreasing $1,25(OH)_2D$ levels which suppresses the renin activity [144]. These data suggest an alternative mechanism, whereby FGF23 could exert negative effects on various adverse clinical outcomes including not only heart failure [118–120] but also atherosclerotic events [117–119] and the progression of CKD [113–115].

Analytical Considerations of Measurement

Phosphorus is routinely measured in clinical laboratories by colorimetric methods with automated machines, and the results are generally precise and reproducible. Its serum concentrations are maintained approximately between 2.5 and 4.5 mg/dL, with a small variation in the reference range depending on the laboratory. A majority of phosphorus in the body is stored in the bone and intracellular pool, and factors such as acid-base balance disorders and glucose/insulin can induce transcellular shifts of phosphate, changing serum concentrations despite the same total body phosphorus content. Hemolysis during sample collection results in falsely increased phosphorus levels. There is a diurnal and postprandial variation in serum phosphorus levels among individuals without CKD [145, 146]. No such diurnal variation was observed among hemodialysis patients on non-dialysis days [147], but phosphate levels are higher after a longer period of dialysis. In an international cohort study of hemodialysis patients, samples collected before Monday or Tuesday sessions vs a Wednesday or Thursday sessions were higher only by 0.08 mg/dL [148]. However, another study showed that when compared within individuals, serum phosphorus levels were 1.3 mg/dL higher after 3-day vs. 2-day intervals between hemodialysis sessions [149]. Therefore, trends of progressive increases or decreases, rather than individual values or their small variations, may be preferable for clinical decision-making [150].

Several FGF23 assays are currently available but limited to research purposes. The intact assays use monoclonal antibodies directed to the N- and C-terminal portions and thus detect only the intact molecule, while the C-terminal assay uses two polyclonal antibodies directed exclusively to the C-terminal portion and detects both the intact molecule and the cleaved C-terminal fragments [151–153]. Although different FGF23 assays yield highly correlated results, their absolute values cannot be directly compared even among intact assays because of differences in the calibration [154, 155]. As with serum phosphorus levels, diurnal variation is observed in intact FGF23 levels among healthy subjects; intact

FGF23 peaks in the early morning and reaches its nadir in the evening with a mean decrease of 30% [90]. Meanwhile, C-terminal FGF23 does not show such diurnal variation in both healthy subjects and pre-dialysis CKD patients [90, 156], suggesting that FGF23 actions are mainly regulated by degradation rather than the production of FGF23 at least in the short term.

The values of FGF23 are also variably affected by ex vivo proteolytic degradation of intact hormone after blood draw, depending on several factors such as the assay, sample type (plasma vs. serum), time to measurement, and temperature. Plasma samples show decreasing intact FGF23 levels and increasing C-terminal FGF23 levels after blood draw when kept at room temperature [91, 92]. Unfortunately, so far there have been no clear reasons why C-terminal FGF23 levels increase over time. These changes can be prevented by adding broad-spectrum protease inhibitor cocktail but not by a furin inhibitor, suggesting that proteases other than furin are involved in FGF23 degradation [157, 158]. When samples were stored at 4 or 22 °C, FGF23 levels, whichever intact or C-terminal, are stable in both serum and plasma samples up to 48 h with the caveat that serum samples stored at 22 °C show increased C-terminal FGF23 levels after 24 h [158]. Both plasma and serum FGF23 levels are stable against freezing and thawing up to 5 cycles, but long-term storage at −80 °C for 40 months induces some variability.

Treatment

In the management of hyperphosphatemia, the mainstays of treatment include dietary phosphorus restriction, phosphate-binding drugs, and other medications that modulate the CKD-MBD axis, as well as adjustment of the dialysis prescription [159].

Dietary Phosphorus Restriction

Among non-dialysis-dependent CKD and ESRD patients receiving dialysis, the National Kidney Foundation Kidney Disease Outcomes Quality Initiative, European Best Practice Guidelines, and International Society of Renal Nutrition and Metabolism guidelines recommend daily phosphorus intake of 800–1000 mg per day [160–162]. The net absorption of phosphorus in the gastrointestinal tract is approximately 40–80% per day, depending on an individual's diet and modulation of intestinal absorption by hormones (e.g., calcitriol) [159].

Sources of dietary phosphorus largely exist in two forms, namely, (1) organic phosphorus present in animal (e.g., casein) or plant (e.g., phytate) protein sources and (2) inorganic phosphate (e.g., phosphorus additives in processed foods) [159]. While animal protein sources of phosphorus have a bioavailability of 40–60%, the bioavailability of plant sources is lower (20–40%) given that humans lack the degrading enzyme phytase. In contrast, the bioavailability of inorganic phosphorus is as high as 100%.

There is a strong positive relationship between dietary protein and phosphorus intake [163]. Among 73 Israeli CKD patients who underwent food frequency questionnaire, the following regression equation was developed to characterize the relationship between dietary protein and phosphorus intake in this population: Dietary P (mg) = 128 mg P + (dietary protein in g) × 14 mg P/g protein [164]. Similarly, among 107 US maintenance hemodialysis patients who underwent 3-day diet diaries, the following formula was derived to characterize the association between dietary protein and phosphorus intake in this group: Dietary Phosphorus (P) (mg) = 78 mg P + (dietary protein) × 11.8 mg P/g protein [165]. While dietary protein restriction is typically advised among pre-dialysis CKD patients (0.6–0.8 g/kg/day), it should be cautioned that the risk of restricting phosphorus intake by protein restriction may outweigh the benefit among dialysis patients in whom higher dietary protein is recommended giving their underlying hypercatabolic states (>1.2 g/kg/day) [162]. While there are a number of benefits with respect to food additives (i.e., extension of shelf life, improvement in color and flavor, retaining moisture), restriction of processed food sources that have little to no protein may be preferable [159].

Phosphate Binders and Calcimimetics

Phosphate binders are a mainstay in the management of hyperphosphatemia, particularly among dialysis patients with higher dietary protein targets. However randomized controlled trials comparing specific or combined classes of phosphate binders upon hard outcomes in pre-dialysis CKD and ESRD patients receiving dialysis have shown mixed findings [166]. Among three meta-analyses, sevelamer vs. calcium-containing phosphate binders were shown to demonstrate significantly lower death rates in pre-dialysis CKD and ESRD patients [167–169]. While these comparative effectiveness studies suggest lower mortality risk with sevelamer, there is lack of data showing that any phosphate binder reduces the risk for mortality compared to placebo [166]. Hence, rigorous trials are needed to determine whether sevelamer or any other phosphate binder is superior to placebo or another class of binders in improving hard outcomes.

Dialysis

The amount of phosphate removed during conventional thrice-weekly in-center hemodialysis with 4 h sessions ranges from 600 to 1200 mg per treatment session (i.e., 1800–3600 mg per week) [170]. In contrast, nocturnal hemodialysis may remove approximately 600 to 1200 mg per session (i.e., 3000 to 8400 mg per week). As a continuous modality, it is estimated that peritoneal dialysis removal is 300 to 360 mg per day (i.e., 2100–2520 mg per week). Given that ESRD patients are advised to consume 800 to 1000 mg of phosphate per day (i.e., 5600–7000 mg) and likely ingest higher amounts (i.e., 1500 mg per day or 10,500 mg per week), the limited amount of phosphorus removal by dialysis alone is unlikely to achieve target phosphorus levels.

References

1. Foley RN, Murray AM, Li S, et al. Chronic kidney disease and the risk for cardiovascular disease, renal replacement, and death in the United States Medicare population, 1998 to 1999. J Am Soc Nephrol. 2005;16:489–95.
2. Kalantar-Zadeh K, Block G, Humphreys MH, et al. Reverse epidemiology of cardiovascular risk factors in maintenance dialysis patients. Kidney Int. 2003;63:793–808.
3. Kalantar-Zadeh K, Abbott KC, Salahudeen AK, et al. Survival advantages of obesity in dialysis patients. Am J Clin Nutr. 2005;81:543–54.
4. Kovesdy CP, Trivedi BK, Kalantar-Zadeh K, et al. Association of low blood pressure with increased mortality in patients with moderate to severe chronic kidney disease. Nephrol Dial Transplant. 2006;21:1257–62.
5. Kovesdy CP, Anderson JE, Kalantar-Zadeh K. Paradoxical association between body mass index and mortality in men with CKD not yet on dialysis. Am J Kidney Dis. 2007;49:581 91.
6. Kovesdy CP, Anderson JE, Kalantar-Zadeh K. Inverse association between lipid levels and mortality in men with chronic kidney disease who are not yet on dialysis: effects of case mix and the malnutrition-inflammation-cachexia syndrome. J Am Soc Nephrol. 2007;18:304–11.
7. Kovesdy CP, Quarles LD, Lott EH, et al. Survival advantage in black versus white men with CKD: effect of estimated GFR and case mix. Am J Kidney Dis. 2013;62:228–35.
8. Kalantar-Zadeh K, Kuwae N, Regidor DL, et al. Survival predictability of time-varying indicators of bone disease in maintenance hemodialysis patients. Kidney Int. 2006;70:771–80.
9. Regidor DL, Kovesdy CP, Mehrotra R, et al. Serum alkaline phosphatase predicts mortality among maintenance hemodialysis patients. J Am Soc Nephrol. 2008;19:2193–203.
10. Kovesdy CP, Kuchmak O, Lu JL, et al. Outcomes associated with serum calcium level in men with non-dialysis-dependent chronic kidney disease. Clin J Am Soc Nephrol. 2010;5:468–76.
11. Kovesdy CP, Anderson JE, Kalantar-Zadeh K. Outcomes associated with serum phosphorus level in males with non-dialysis dependent chronic kidney disease. Clin Nephrol. 2010;73:268–75.
12. Kalantar-Zadeh K, Shah A, Duong U, et al. Kidney bone disease and mortality in CKD: revisiting the role of vitamin D, calcimimetics, alkaline phosphatase, and minerals. Kidney Int Suppl. 2010;78:S10–21.
13. Streja E, Wang HY, Lau WL, et al. Mortality of combined serum phosphorus and parathyroid hormone concentrations and their changes over time in hemodialysis patients. Bone. 2014;61:201–7.
14. Rivara MB, Ravel V, Kalantar-Zadeh K, et al. Uncorrected and albumin-corrected calcium, phosphorus, and mortality in patients undergoing maintenance dialysis. J Am Soc Nephrol. 2015;26:1671.
15. Moe S, Drueke T, Cunningham J, et al. Definition, evaluation, and classification of renal osteodystrophy: a position statement from kidney disease:

improving global outcomes (KDIGO). Kidney Int. 2006;69:1945–53.
16. Herzog CA, Asinger RW, Berger AK, et al. Cardiovascular disease in chronic kidney disease. A clinical update from kidney disease: improving global outcomes (KDIGO). Kidney Int. 2011;80:572–86.
17. Wanner C, Krane V, Marz W, et al. Atorvastatin in patients with type 2 diabetes mellitus undergoing hemodialysis. N Engl J Med. 2005;353:238–48.
18. Drechsler C, Kalim S, Wenger JB, et al. Protein carbamylation is associated with heart failure and mortality in diabetic patients with end-stage renal disease. Kidney Int. 2015;87:1201–8.
19. Quarles LD. Reducing cardiovascular mortality in chronic kidney disease: something borrowed, something new. J Clin Invest. 2013;123:542–3.
20. Foley RN, Parfrey PS, Harnett JD, et al. The prognostic importance of left ventricular geometry in uremic cardiomyopathy. J Am Soc Nephrol. 1995;5:2024–31.
21. Shimada T, Hasegawa H, Yamazaki Y, et al. FGF-23 is a potent regulator of vitamin D metabolism and phosphate homeostasis. J Bone Miner Res. 2004;19:429–35.
22. Shimada T, Yamazaki Y, Takahashi M, et al. Vitamin D receptor-independent FGF23 actions in regulating phosphate and vitamin D metabolism. Am J Physiol Renal Physiol. 2005;289:F1088–95.
23. Perwad F, Zhang MY, Tenenhouse HS, et al. Fibroblast growth factor 23 impairs phosphorus and vitamin D metabolism in vivo and suppresses 25-hydroxyvitamin D-1alpha-hydroxylase expression in vitro. Am J Physiol Renal Physiol. 2007;293:F1577–83.
24. Krajisnik T, Bjorklund P, Marsell R, et al. Fibroblast growth factor-23 regulates parathyroid hormone and 1alpha-hydroxylase expression in cultured bovine parathyroid cells. J Endocrinol. 2007;195:125–31.
25. Liu S, Tang W, Zhou J, et al. Fibroblast growth factor 23 is a counter-regulatory phosphaturic hormone for vitamin D. J Am Soc Nephrol. 2006;17:1305–15.
26. Lavi-Moshayoff V, Wasserman G, Meir T, et al. PTH increases FGF23 gene expression and mediates the high-FGF23 levels of experimental kidney failure: a bone parathyroid feedback loop. Am J Physiol Renal Physiol. 2010;299:F882–9.
27. Lopez I, Rodriguez-Ortiz ME, Almaden Y, et al. Direct and indirect effects of parathyroid hormone on circulating levels of fibroblast growth factor 23 in vivo. Kidney Int. 2011;80:475.
28. Kolek OI, Hines ER, Jones MD, et al. 1alpha,25-Dihydroxyvitamin D3 upregulates FGF23 gene expression in bone: the final link in a renal-gastrointestinal-skeletal axis that controls phosphate transport. Am J Physiol Gastrointest Liver Physiol. 2005;289:G1036–42.
29. Ben-Dov IZ, Galitzer H, Lavi-Moshayoff V, et al. The parathyroid is a target organ for FGF23 in rats. J Clin Invest. 2007;117:4003–8.
30. Canalejo R, Canalejo A, Martinez-Moreno JM, et al. FGF23 fails to inhibit uremic parathyroid glands. J Am Soc Nephrol. 2010;21:1125–35.
31. Brenza HL, DeLuca HF. Regulation of 25-hydroxyvitamin D3 1alpha-hydroxylase gene expression by parathyroid hormone and 1,25-dihydroxyvitamin D3. Arch Biochem Biophys. 2000;381:143–52.
32. Murayama A, Takeyama K, Kitanaka S, et al. Positive and negative regulations of the renal 25-hydroxyvitamin D3 1alpha-hydroxylase gene by parathyroid hormone, calcitonin, and 1alpha,25(OH)2D3 in intact animals. Endocrinology. 1999;140:2224–31.
33. Kong XF, Zhu XH, Pei YL, et al. Molecular cloning, characterization, and promoter analysis of the human 25-hydroxyvitamin D3-1alpha-hydroxylase gene. Proc Natl Acad Sci U S A. 1999;96:6988–93.
34. Fukumoto S. Phosphate metabolism and vitamin D. BoneKEy Rep. 2014;3:497.
35. Kovesdy CP, Quarles LD. FGF23 from Bench to Bedside. Am J Physiol Renal Physiol. 2016.; ajprenal 00606 02015.
36. Kovesdy CP, Quarles LD. Fibroblast growth factor-23: what we know, what we don't know, and what we need to know. Nephrol Dial Transplant. 2013;28:2228–36.
37. Itoh N. Hormone-like (endocrine) Fgfs: their evolutionary history and roles in development, metabolism, and disease. Cell Tissue Res. 2010;342:1–11.
38. Harmer NJ, Pellegrini L, Chirgadze D, et al. The crystal structure of fibroblast growth factor (FGF) 19 reveals novel features of the FGF family and offers a structural basis for its unusual receptor affinity. Biochemistry (Mosc). 2004;43:629–40.
39. Goetz R, Ohnishi M, Kir S, et al. Conversion of a paracrine fibroblast growth factor into an endocrine fibroblast growth factor. J Biol Chem. 2012;287:29134–46.
40. Zhang X, Ibrahimi OA, Olsen SK, et al. Receptor specificity of the fibroblast growth factor family. The complete mammalian FGF family. J Biol Chem. 2006;281:15694–700.
41. Urakawa I, Yamazaki Y, Shimada T, et al. Klotho converts canonical FGF receptor into a specific receptor for FGF23. Nature. 2006;444:770–4.
42. Kurosu H, Ogawa Y, Miyoshi M, et al. Regulation of fibroblast growth factor-23 signaling by klotho. J Biol Chem. 2006;281:6120–3.
43. Nakatani T, Sarraj B, Ohnishi M, et al. In vivo genetic evidence for klotho-dependent, fibroblast growth factor 23 (Fgf23) -mediated regulation of systemic phosphate homeostasis. FASEB J. 2009;23:433–41.
44. Kuro-o M, Matsumura Y, Aizawa H, et al. Mutation of the mouse klotho gene leads to a syndrome resembling ageing. Nature. 1997;390:45–51.
45. Quarles LD. Role of FGF23 in vitamin D and phosphate metabolism: implications in chronic kidney disease. Exp Cell Res. 2012;318:1040–8.
46. Gattineni J, Bates C, Twombley K, et al. FGF23 decreases renal NaPi-2a and NaPi-2c expression and induces hypophosphatemia in vivo predominantly via FGF receptor 1. Am J Physiol Renal Physiol. 2009;297:F282–91.

47. Andrukhova O, Zeitz U, Goetz R, et al. FGF23 acts directly on renal proximal tubules to induce phosphaturia through activation of the ERK1/2-SGK1 signaling pathway. Bone. 2012;51:621–8.
48. Ide N, Olauson H, Sato T, et al. In vivo evidence for a limited role of proximal tubular Klotho in renal phosphate handling. Kidney Int. 2016;90:348.
49. Olauson H, Lindberg K, Amin R, et al. Targeted deletion of klotho in kidney distal tubule disrupts mineral metabolism. J Am Soc Nephrol. 2012;23:1641.
50. Andrukhova O, Smorodchenko A, Egerbacher M, et al. FGF23 promotes renal calcium reabsorption through the TRPV5 channel. EMBO J. 2014;33:229–46.
51. Andrukhova O, Slavic S, Smorodchenko A, et al. FGF23 regulates renal sodium handling and blood pressure. EMBO Mol Med. 2014;6:744.
52. Krajisnik T, Olauson H, Mirza MA, et al. Parathyroid klotho and FGF-receptor 1 expression decline with renal function in hyperparathyroid patients with chronic kidney disease and kidney transplant recipients. Kidney Int. 2010;78:1024–32.
53. Dai B, David V, Martin A, et al. A comparative transcriptome analysis identifying FGF23 regulated genes in the kidney of a mouse CKD model. PLoS One. 2012;7:e44161.
54. Ohnishi M, Nakatani T, Lanske B, et al. Reversal of mineral ion homeostasis and soft-tissue calcification of klotho knockout mice by deletion of vitamin D 1alpha-hydroxylase. Kidney Int. 2009;75:1166–72.
55. Samadfam R, Richard C, Nguyen-Yamamoto L, et al. Bone formation regulates circulating concentrations of fibroblast growth factor 23. Endocrinology. 2009;150:4835–45.
56. Gutierrez OM, Smith KT, Barchi-Chung A, et al. (1-34) parathyroid hormone infusion acutely lowers fibroblast growth factor 23 concentrations in adult volunteers. Clin J Am Soc Nephrol. 2012;7:139–45.
57. Saji F, Shigematsu T, Sakaguchi T, et al. Fibroblast growth factor 23 production in bone is directly regulated by 1{alpha},25-dihydroxyvitamin D, but not PTH. Am J Physiol Renal Physiol. 2010;299:F1212–7.
58. Mirams M, Robinson BG, Mason RS, et al. Bone as a source of FGF23: regulation by phosphate? Bone. 2004;35:1192–9.
59. Saito H, Maeda A, Ohtomo S, et al. Circulating FGF-23 is regulated by 1alpha,25-dihydroxyvitamin D3 and phosphorus in vivo. J Biol Chem. 2005;280:2543–9.
60. Ito M, Sakai Y, Furumoto M, et al. Vitamin D and phosphate regulate fibroblast growth factor-23 in K-562 cells. Am J Physiol Endocrinol Metab. 2005;288:E1101–9.
61. Ito N, Fukumoto S, Takeuchi Y, et al. Effect of acute changes of serum phosphate on fibroblast growth factor (FGF)23 levels in humans. J Bone Miner Metab. 2007;25:419–22.
62. Bohrer MP, Deen WM, Robertson CR, et al. Mechanism of angiotensin II-induced proteinuria in the rat. Am J Phys. 1977;233:F13–21.
63. Mitani H, Ishizaka N, Aizawa T, et al. In vivo klotho gene transfer ameliorates angiotensin II-induced renal damage. Hypertension. 2002;39:838–43.
64. Tang R, Zhou QL, Ao X, et al. Fosinopril and losartan regulate klotho gene and nicotinamide adenine dinucleotide phosphate oxidase expression in kidneys of spontaneously hypertensive rats. Kidney Blood Press Res. 2011;34:350–7.
65. Yoon HE, Ghee JY, Piao S, et al. Angiotensin II blockade upregulates the expression of klotho, the anti-ageing gene, in an experimental model of chronic cyclosporine nephropathy. Nephrol Dial Transplant. 2011;26:800–13.
66. Rodriguez-Ortiz ME, Lopez I, Munoz-Castaneda JR, et al. Calcium deficiency reduces circulating levels of FGF23. J Am Soc Nephrol. 2012;23:1190–7.
67. Krieger NS, Culbertson CD, Kyker-Snowman K, et al. Metabolic acidosis increases fibroblast growth factor 23 in neonatal mouse bone. Am J Physiol Renal Physiol. 2012;303:F431–6.
68. Fajol A, Chen H, Umbach AT, et al. Enhanced FGF23 production in mice expressing PI3K-insensitive GSK3 is normalized by beta-blocker treatment. FASEB J. 2016;30:994–1001.
69. Tsuji K, Maeda T, Kawane T, et al. Leptin stimulates fibroblast growth factor 23 expression in bone and suppresses renal 1alpha,25-dihydroxyvitamin D3 synthesis in leptin-deficient mice. J Bone Miner Res. 2010;25:1711–23.
70. Bowe AE, Finnegan R, Jan de Beur SM, et al. FGF-23 inhibits renal tubular phosphate transport and is a PHEX substrate. Biochem Biophys Res Commun. 2001;284:977–81.
71. Martin A, Liu S, David V, et al. Bone proteins PHEX and DMP1 regulate fibroblastic growth factor Fgf23 expression in osteocytes through a common pathway involving FGF receptor (FGFR) signaling. FASEB J. 2011;25:2551–62.
72. Shimada T, Mizutani S, Muto T, et al. Cloning and characterization of FGF23 as a causative factor of tumor-induced osteomalacia. Proc Natl Acad Sci U S A. 2001;98:6500–5.
73. Pereira RC, Juppner H, Azucena-Serrano CE, et al. Patterns of FGF-23, DMP1, and MEPE expression in patients with chronic kidney disease. Bone. 2009;45:1161–8.
74. Shimizu Y, Tada Y, Yamauchi M, et al. Hypophosphatemia induced by intravenous administration of saccharated ferric oxide: another form of FGF23-related hypophosphatemia. Bone. 2009;45:814–6.
75. Schouten BJ, Hunt PJ, Livesey JH, et al. FGF23 elevation and hypophosphatemia after intravenous iron polymaltose: a prospective study. J Clin Endocrinol Metab. 2009;94:2332–7.
76. Takeda Y, Komaba H, Goto S, et al. Effect of intravenous saccharated ferric oxide on serum FGF23 and mineral metabolism in hemodialysis patients. Am J Nephrol. 2011;33:421–6.

77. Wolf M, Koch TA, Bregman DB. Effects of iron deficiency anemia and its treatment on fibroblast growth factor 23 and phosphate homeostasis in women. J Bone Miner Res. 2013;28:1793–803.
78. David V, Martin A, Isakova T, et al. Inflammation and functional iron deficiency regulate fibroblast growth factor 23 production. Kidney Int. 2016;89:135–46.
79. Kato K, Jeanneau C, Tarp MA, et al. Polypeptide GalNAc-transferase T3 and familial tumoral calcinosis. Secretion of fibroblast growth factor 23 requires O-glycosylation. J Biol Chem. 2006;281:18370–7.
80. Bhattacharyya N, Wiench M, Dumitrescu C, et al. Mechanism of FGF23 processing in fibrous dysplasia. J Bone Miner Res. 2012;27:1132–41.
81. Benet-Pages A, Lorenz-Depiereux B, Zischka H, et al. FGF23 is processed by proprotein convertases but not by PHEX. Bone. 2004;35:455–62.
82. Yamamoto H, Ramos-Molina B, Lick AN, et al. Posttranslational processing of FGF23 in osteocytes during the osteoblast to osteocyte transition. Bone. 2016;84:120–30.
83. Goetz R, Nakada Y, Hu MC, et al. Isolated C-terminal tail of FGF23 alleviates hypophosphatemia by inhibiting FGF23-FGFR-klotho complex formation. Proc Natl Acad Sci U S A. 2010;107:407–12.
84. Bergwitz C, Banerjee S, Abu-Zahra H, et al. Defective O-glycosylation due to a novel homozygous S129P mutation is associated with lack of fibroblast growth factor 23 secretion and tumoral calcinosis. J Clin Endocrinol Metab. 2009;94:4267–74.
85. Schjoldager KT, Vester-Christensen MB, Goth CK, et al. A systematic study of site-specific GalNAc-type O-glycosylation modulating proprotein convertase processing. J Biol Chem. 2011;286:40122–32.
86. Tagliabracci VS, Engel JL, Wiley SE, et al. Dynamic regulation of FGF23 by Fam20C phosphorylation, GalNAc-T3 glycosylation, and furin proteolysis. Proc Natl Acad Sci U S A. 2014;111:5520–5.
87. Lindberg I, Pang HW, Stains JP, et al. FGF23 is endogenously phosphorylated in bone cells. J Bone Miner Res. 2015;30:449–54.
88. Shimada T, Urakawa I, Isakova T, et al. Circulating fibroblast growth factor 23 in patients with end-stage renal disease treated by peritoneal dialysis is intact and biologically active. J Clin Endocrinol Metab. 2010;95:578–85.
89. Stubbs JR, He N, Idiculla A, et al. Longitudinal evaluation of FGF23 changes and mineral metabolism abnormalities in a mouse model of chronic kidney disease. J Bone Miner Res. 2012;27:38–46.
90. Smith ER, Cai MM, McMahon LP, et al. Biological variability of plasma intact and C-terminal FGF23 measurements. J Clin Endocrinol Metab. 2012;97:3357.
91. Farrow EG, Yu X, Summers LJ, et al. Iron deficiency drives an autosomal dominant hypophosphatemic rickets (ADHR) phenotype in fibroblast growth factor-23 (Fgf23) knock-in mice. Proc Natl Acad Sci U S A. 2011;108:E1146–55.
92. Wolf M. Forging forward with 10 burning questions on FGF23 in kidney disease. J Am Soc Nephrol. 2010;21:1427–35.
93. Hu MC, Shi M, Zhang J, et al. Klotho deficiency causes vascular calcification in chronic kidney disease. J Am Soc Nephrol. 2011;22:124–36.
94. Asai O, Nakatani K, Tanaka T, et al. Decreased renal alpha-klotho expression in early diabetic nephropathy in humans and mice and its possible role in urinary calcium excretion. Kidney Int. 2012;81:539–47.
95. Sakan H, Nakatani K, Asai O, et al. Reduced renal alpha-klotho expression in CKD patients and its effect on renal phosphate handling and vitamin D metabolism. PLoS One. 2014;9:e86301.
96. Isakova T, Wahl P, Vargas GS, et al. Fibroblast growth factor 23 is elevated before parathyroid hormone and phosphate in chronic kidney disease. Kidney Int. 2011;79:1370–8.
97. Nakano C, Hamano T, Fujii N, et al. Combined use of vitamin D status and FGF23 for risk stratification of renal outcome. Clin J Am Soc Nephrol. 2012;7:810–9.
98. van Ballegooijen AJ, Rhee EP, Elmariah S, et al. Renal clearance of mineral metabolism biomarkers. J Am Soc Nephrol. 2016;27:392–7.
99. Slatopolsky E, Finch J, Denda M, et al. Phosphorus restriction prevents parathyroid gland growth. High phosphorus directly stimulates PTH secretion in vitro. J Clin Invest. 1996;97:2534–40.
100. Almaden Y, Canalejo A, Hernandez A, et al. Direct effect of phosphorus on PTH secretion from whole rat parathyroid glands in vitro. J Bone Miner Res. 1996;11:970–6.
101. Almaden Y, Hernandez A, Torregrosa V, et al. High phosphate level directly stimulates parathyroid hormone secretion and synthesis by human parathyroid tissue in vitro. J Am Soc Nephrol. 1998;9:1845–52.
102. Fukuda N, Tanaka H, Tominaga Y, et al. Decreased 1,25-dihydroxyvitamin D3 receptor density is associated with a more severe form of parathyroid hyperplasia in chronic uremic patients. J Clin Invest. 1993;92:1436–43.
103. Kifor O, Moore FD Jr, Wang P, et al. Reduced immunostaining for the extracellular Ca2+−sensing receptor in primary and uremic secondary hyperparathyroidism. J Clin Endocrinol Metab. 1996;81:1598–606.
104. Brown AJ, Ritter CS, Finch JL, et al. Decreased calcium-sensing receptor expression in hyperplastic parathyroid glands of uremic rats: role of dietary phosphate. Kidney Int. 1999;55:1284–92.
105. Komaba H, Goto S, Fujii H, et al. Depressed expression of klotho and FGF receptor 1 in hyperplastic parathyroid glands from uremic patients. Kidney Int. 2010;77:232–8.
106. Mace ML, Gravesen E, Hofman-Bang J, et al. Key role of the kidney in the regulation of fibroblast growth factor 23. Kidney Int. 2015;88:1304–13.
107. Zanchi C, Locatelli M, Benigni A, et al. Renal expression of FGF23 in progressive renal disease of

diabetes and the effect of ACE inhibitor. PLoS One. 2013;8:e70775.
108. Spichtig D, Zhang H, Mohebbi N, et al. Renal expression of FGF23 and peripheral resistance to elevated FGF23 in rodent models of polycystic kidney disease. Kidney Int. 2014;85:1340–50.
109. Palmer SC, Hayen A, Macaskill P, et al. Serum levels of phosphorus, parathyroid hormone, and calcium and risks of death and cardiovascular disease in individuals with chronic kidney disease. a systematic review and meta-analysis. JAMA. 2011;305:1119–27.
110. Giachelli CM, Jono S, Shioi A, Nishizawa Y, Mori K, Morii H. Vascular calcification and inorganic phosphate. Am J Kidney Dis. 2001;38(4 Suppl 1):S34–7.
111. Chen NX, O'Neill KD, Duan D, Moe SM. Phosphorus and uremic serum up-regulate osteopontin expression in vascular smooth muscle cells. Kidney Int. 2002;62:1724–31.
112. Shuto E, Taketani Y, Tanaka R, et al. Dietary phosphorus acutely impairs endothelial function. J Am Soc Nephrol. 2009;20:1504–12.
113. Fliser D, Kollerits B, Neyer U, et al. Fibroblast growth factor 23 (FGF23) predicts progression of chronic kidney disease: the mild to moderate kidney disease (MMKD) study. J Am Soc Nephrol. 2007;18:2600–8.
114. Titan SM, Zatz R, Graciolli FG, et al. FGF-23 as a predictor of renal outcome in diabetic nephropathy. Clin J Am Soc Nephrol. 2011;6:241–7.
115. Hamano T, Nakano C, Obi Y, et al. Fibroblast growth factor 23 and 25-hydroxyvitamin D levels are associated with estimated glomerular filtration rate decline. Kidney Int Suppl. 2013;3:469–75.
116. Isakova T, Xie H, Yang W, et al. Fibroblast growth factor 23 and risks of mortality and end-stage renal disease in patients with chronic kidney disease. JAMA. 2011;305:2432–9.
117. Kendrick J, Cheung AK, Kaufman JS, et al. FGF-23 associates with death, cardiovascular events, and initiation of chronic dialysis. J Am Soc Nephrol. 2011;22:1913–22.
118. Scialla JJ, Xie H, Rahman M, et al. Fibroblast growth Factor-23 and cardiovascular events in CKD. J Am Soc Nephrol. 2014;25:349–60.
119. Parker BD, Schurgers LJ, Brandenburg VM, et al. The associations of fibroblast growth factor 23 and uncarboxylated matrix Gla protein with mortality in coronary artery disease: the heart and soul study. Ann Intern Med. 2010;152:640–8.
120. Ix JH, Katz R, Kestenbaum BR, et al. Fibroblast growth factor-23 and death, heart failure, and cardiovascular events in community-living individuals: CHS (cardiovascular health study). J Am Coll Cardiol. 2012;60:200–7.
121. Jean G, Terrat JC, Vanel T, et al. High levels of serum fibroblast growth factor (FGF)-23 are associated with increased mortality in long haemodialysis patients. Nephrol Dial Transplant. 2009;24:2792–6.
122. Nakano C, Hamano T, Fujii N, et al. Intact fibroblast growth factor 23 levels predict incident cardiovascular event before but not after the start of dialysis. Bone. 2012;50:1266–74.
123. Gutierrez OM, Mannstadt M, Isakova T, et al. Fibroblast growth factor 23 and mortality among patients undergoing hemodialysis. N Engl J Med. 2008;359:584–92.
124. Komaba H, Fukagawa M. The role of FGF23 in CKD--with or without klotho. Nat Rev Nephrol. 2012;8:484 90.
125. Mirza MA, Larsson A, Melhus H, et al. Serum intact FGF23 associate with left ventricular mass, hypertrophy and geometry in an elderly population. Atherosclerosis. 2009;207:546–51.
126. Gutierrez OM, Januzzi JL, Isakova T, et al. Fibroblast growth factor 23 and left ventricular hypertrophy in chronic kidney disease. Circulation. 2009;119:2545–52.
127. Kirkpantur A, Balci M, Gurbuz OA, et al. Serum fibroblast growth factor-23 (FGF-23) levels are independently associated with left ventricular mass and myocardial performance index in maintenance haemodialysis patients. Nephrol Dial Transplant. 2011;26:1346–54.
128. Faul C, Amaral AP, Oskouei B, et al. FGF23 induces left ventricular hypertrophy. J Clin Invest. 2011;121:4393–408.
129. Grabner A, Amaral AP, Schramm K, et al. Activation of cardiac fibroblast growth factor receptor 4 causes left ventricular hypertrophy. Cell Metab. 2015;22:1020–32.
130. Leifheit-Nestler M, Große Siemer R, Flasbart K, Richter B, Kirchhoff F, Ziegler WH, Klintschar M, Becker JU, Erbersdobler A, Aufricht C, Seeman T, Fischer DC, Faul C, Haffner D. Induction of cardiac FGF23/FGFR4 expression is associated with left ventricular hypertrophy in patients with chronic kidney disease. Nephrology Dialysis Transplantation. 2016;31(7):1088–99.
131. Shalhoub V, Shatzen EM, Ward SC, et al. FGF23 neutralization improves chronic kidney disease-associated hyperparathyroidism yet increases mortality. J Clin Invest. 2012;122:2543–53.
132. Donoghue M, Hsieh F, Baronas E, et al. A novel angiotensin-converting enzyme-related carboxypeptidase (ACE2) converts angiotensin I to angiotensin 1-9. Circ Res. 2000;87:E1–9.
133. Wysocki J, Ye M, Rodriguez E, et al. Targeting the degradation of angiotensin II with recombinant angiotensin-converting enzyme 2: prevention of angiotensin II-dependent hypertension. Hypertension. 2010;55:90–8.
134. Gurley SB, Allred A, Le TH, et al. Altered blood pressure responses and normal cardiac phenotype in ACE2-null mice. J Clin Invest. 2006;116:2218–25.
135. Zhong J, Guo D, Chen CB, et al. Prevention of angiotensin II-mediated renal oxidative stress, inflammation, and fibrosis by angiotensin-converting enzyme 2. Hypertension. 2011;57:314–22.

136. Crackower MA, Sarao R, Oudit GY, et al. Angiotensin-converting enzyme 2 is an essential regulator of heart function. Nature. 2002;417:822–8.
137. Rentzsch B, Todiras M, Iliescu R, et al. Transgenic angiotensin-converting enzyme 2 overexpression in vessels of SHRSP rats reduces blood pressure and improves endothelial function. Hypertension. 2008;52:967–73.
138. Lovren F, Pan Y, Quan A, et al. Angiotensin converting enzyme-2 confers endothelial protection and attenuates atherosclerosis. Am J Physiol Heart Circ Physiol. 2008;295:H1377–84.
139. Lieb W, Graf J, Gotz A, et al. Association of angiotensin-converting enzyme 2 (ACE2) gene polymorphisms with parameters of left ventricular hypertrophy in men. Results of the MONICA Augsburg echocardiographic substudy. J Mol Med (Berl). 2006;84:88–96.
140. Zhong J, Basu R, Guo D, et al. Angiotensin-converting enzyme 2 suppresses pathological hypertrophy, myocardial fibrosis, and cardiac dysfunction. Circulation. 2010;122:717–28. 718 p following 728.
141. Wong DW, Oudit GY, Reich H, et al. Loss of angiotensin-converting enzyme-2 (Ace2) accelerates diabetic kidney injury. Am J Pathol. 2007;171: 438–51.
142. Oudit GY, Herzenberg AM, Kassiri Z, et al. Loss of angiotensin-converting enzyme-2 leads to the late development of angiotensin II-dependent glomerulosclerosis. Am J Pathol. 2006;168:1808–20.
143. Oudit GY, Liu GC, Zhong J, et al. Human recombinant ACE2 reduces the progression of diabetic nephropathy. Diabetes. 2010;59:529–38.
144. Zhou C, Lu F, Cao K, et al. Calcium-independent and 1,25(OH)2D3-dependent regulation of the renin-angiotensin system in 1alpha-hydroxylase knockout mice. Kidney Int. 2008;74:170–9.
145. Portale AA, Halloran BP, Morris RC. Dietary-intake of phosphorus modulates the circadian-rhythm in serum concentration of phosphorus - implications for the renal production of 1,25-Dihydroxyvitamin-D. J Clin Invest. 1987;80:1147–54.
146. de Boer IH, Rue TC, Kestenbaum B. Serum phosphorus concentrations in the third National Health and nutrition examination survey (NHANES III). Am J Kidney Dis. 2009;53:399–407.
147. Trivedi H, Moore H, Atalla J. Lack of significant circadian and post-prandial variation in phosphate levels in subjects receiving chronic hemodialysis therapy. J Nephrol. 2005;18:417–22.
148. Tentori F, Blayney MJ, Albert JM, et al. Mortality risk for dialysis patients with different levels of serum calcium, phosphorus, and PTH: the Dialysis outcomes and practice patterns study (DOPPS). Am J Kidney Dis. 2008;52:519–30.
149. Yokoyama K, Katoh N, Kubo H, et al. Clinical significance of the K/DOQI bone guidelines in Japan. Am J Kidney Dis. 2004;44:383–4. author reply 384
150. Kidney Disease: Improving Global Outcomes (KDIGO) CKD-MBD Work Group. KDIGO clinical practice guideline for the diagnosis, evaluation, prevention, and treatment of Chronic Kidney Disease-Mineral and Bone Disorder (CKD-MBD). Kidney Int Suppl. 2009;113:S1–130.
151. Yamazaki Y, Okazaki R, Shibata M, et al. Increased circulatory level of biologically active full-length FGF-23 in patients with hypophosphatemic rickets/osteomalacia. J Clin Endocrinol Metab. 2002;87:4957–60.
152. Jonsson KB, Zahradnik R, Larsson T, et al. Fibroblast growth factor 23 in oncogenic osteomalacia and X-linked hypophosphatemia. N Engl J Med. 2003;348:1656–63.
153. Fukumoto S, Martin TJ. Bone as an endocrine organ. Trends Endocrinol Metab. 2009;20:230–6.
154. Smith ER, McMahon LP, Holt SG. Method-specific differences in plasma fibroblast growth factor 23 measurement using four commercial ELISAs. Clin Chem Lab Med. 2013;51:1971–81.
155. Sinha MD, Turner C, Goldsmith DJ. FGF23 concentrations measured using "intact" assays similar but not interchangeable. Int Urol Nephrol. 2013;45:1821–3.
156. Isakova T, Xie H, Barchi-Chung A, et al. Daily variability in mineral metabolites in CKD and effects of dietary calcium and calcitriol. Clin J Am Soc Nephrol. 2012;7:820–8.
157. Smith ER, Ford ML, Tomlinson LA, et al. Instability of fibroblast growth factor-23 (FGF-23): implications for clinical studies. Clin Chim Acta. 2011; 412:1008–11.
158. El-Maouche D, Dumitrescu CE, Andreopoulou P, et al. Stability and degradation of fibroblast growth factor 23 (FGF23): the effect of time and temperature and assay type. Osteoporos Int. 2016;27:2345–53.
159. Kalantar-Zadeh K, Gutekunst L, Mehrotra R, et al. Understanding sources of dietary phosphorus in the treatment of patients with chronic kidney disease. Clin J Am Soc Nephrol. 2010;5:519–30.
160. National Kidney Foundation. K/DOQI clinical practice guidelines for bone metablism and disease on chronic kidney disease. Am J Kidney Dis. 2003;42:S1–S201.
161. Fouque D, Vennegoor M, ter Wee P, et al. EBPG guideline on nutrition. Nephrol Dial Transplant. 2007;22:ii45–87.
162. Ikizler TA, Cano NJ, Franch H, et al. International Society of Renal Nutrition and Metabolism. Prevention and treatment of protein energy wasting in chronic kidney disease patients: a consensus statement by the International Society of Renal Nutrition and Metabolism. Kidney Int. 2013;6:1096–107.
163. Shinaberger CS, Greenland S, Kopple JD, et al. Ratio of paricalcitol dosage to serum parathyroid hormone level and survival in maintenance hemodialysis patients. Clin J Am Soc Nephrol. 2008;6:1769–76.
164. Boaz M, Smetana S. Regression equation predicts dietary phosphorus intake from estimate of dietary protein intake. J Am Diet Assoc. 1996;96:1268–70.

165. Rambod M, Kovesdy CP, Bross R, et al. Association of serum prealbumin and its changes over time with clinical outcomes and survival in patients receiving hemodialysis. Am J Clin Nutr. 2008;88:1485–94.
166. St Peter WL, Wazny LD, Weinhandl ED. Phosphate-binder use in US Dialysis patients: prevalence, costs, evidence, and policies. Am J Kidney Dis. 2018;71:246–53.
167. Palmer SC, Gardner S, Tonelli M, et al. Phosphate-binding agents in adults with CKD: a network meta-analysis of randomized trials. Am J Kidney Dis. 2016;68:691–702.
168. Sekercioglu N, Thabane L, Diaz Martinez JP, et al. Comparative effectiveness of phosphate binders in patients with chronic kidney disease: a systematic review and network meta-analysis. PLoS One. 2016;11:e0156891.
169. Patel L, Bernard LM, Elder GJ. Sevelamer versus calcium based binders for treatment of hyperphosphatemia in CKD: a meta-analysis of randomized controlled trials. Clin J Am Soc Nephrol. 2016;11:232–44.
170. Waheed AA, Pedraza F, Lenz O, et al. Phosphate control in end-stage renal disease: barriers and opportunities. Nephrol Dial Transplant. 2013;28:2961–8.

Vitamin D and Parathyroid Hormone in Kidney Disease

16

Sagar U. Nigwekar

Introduction

Chronic kidney disease (CKD) is a modern-day global epidemic [1]. CKD affects over 20 million adults in the United States. CKD is associated with significant morbidity and mortality, and unfortunately the outcomes for patients with CKD and particularly for those with end-stage renal disease (ESRD) remain poor. Mineral and bone metabolism disarray, referred to as chronic kidney disease-mineral bone disease (CKD-MBD), is common in CKD and is focused around the important roles of vitamin D and parathyroid hormone (PTH) [2, 3]. One of the great debates has centered around whether correcting the abnormalities in vitamin D and PTH in CKD will improve outcomes in these patients. To understand this debate, it is important to review the epidemiology and pathophysiology of CKD-MBD along with relevant clinical and research aspects of the diagnosis and treatment. In this chapter, we specifically focus on vitamin D and PTH as they relate to CKD.

S. U. Nigwekar
Department of Medicine, Division of Nephrology, Massachusetts General Hospital, Boston, MA, USA
e-mail: snigwekar@mgh.harvard.edu

Pathophysiology

Serum calcium and phosphorous are mainly regulated by vitamin D and PTH. Relatively recently, another hormone fibroblast growth factor 23 (FGF-23) has also been discovered to play a critical role in phosphorous regulation [4]. Altered mineral bone metabolism in CKD is collectively known as CKD-MBD, and it encompasses (1) biochemical abnormalities in calcium, phosphorous, PTH, vitamin D, and FGF-23, (2) alterations in bone morphological features (bone volume, turnover, and mineralization), and (3) soft tissue and vascular calcification (Fig. 16.1) [2, 5].

In healthy individuals, ultraviolet rays convert 7-dehydrocholesterol to cholecalciferol in the

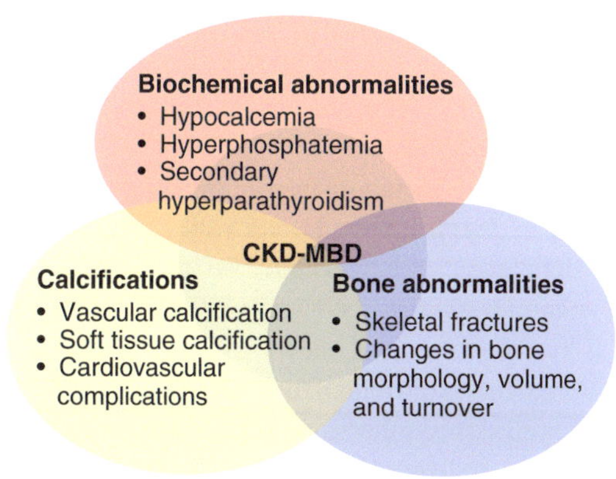

Fig. 16.1 Biochemical and clinical components of chronic kidney disease-mineral bone disease (CKD-MBD)

C. M. Rhee et al. (eds.), *Endocrine Disorders in Kidney Disease*,
https://doi.org/10.1007/978-3-319-97765-2_16

skin tissue [6–8]. The dietary forms of vitamin D are incorporated into chylomicrons and are transported into the venous circulation via the lymphatic system. In the liver, vitamin D undergoes hydroxylation to become 25-hydroxyvitamin D. 25-Hydroxyvitamin D is a major circulating form of vitamin D, and almost all of it is in the bound form (bound to vitamin D-binding protein [DBP] and albumin). This complex dissociates in the kidney tissue where 25-hydroxyvitamin D is converted to 1,25-dihyroxyvitamin D by the 1α-hydroxylase enzyme. The 1α-hydroxylase enzyme is present in multiple extrarenal sites including the pancreas, brain, lymph nodes, heart, gastrointestinal tract, adrenal glands, and prostate gland.

The actions of 1, 25-dihyroxyvitamin D are mediated by binding to the intracellular vitamin D receptor. The main actions of active vitamin D include increasing enteric calcium and phosphorous absorption, stimulating bone osteoclast activity, and stimulating calcium reabsorption in the kidneys [8]. Renal 1α-hydroxylase is tightly regulated by PTH, serum concentrations of calcium and phosphorous, and FGF-23. Hypocalcemia, hypophosphatemia, and hyperparathyroidism stimulate renal 1α-hydroxylase to increase the synthesis of active vitamin D that in turn suppresses PTH production. FGF-23 inhibits the expression of renal 1α-hydroxylase and blocks the production of active vitamin D.

CKD is characterized by abnormalities in vitamin D metabolism, hypocalcemia, hyperphosphatemia, secondary hyperparathyroidism, and elevations in FGF-23 [6]. The abnormalities in vitamin D metabolism encompass deficiency of 25-hydroxyvitamin D, 1,25-dihyroxyvitamin D deficiency, and resistance to the actions of vitamin D. As early as in stage 2 CKD, the serum 25-hydroxyvitamin D levels begin to decline. This decline is attributed to reduced sun exposure, impaired skin synthesis of endogenous vitamin D partly due to hyperpigmentation and partly due to uremia, reduced intake of vitamin D rich foods, and impaired gastrointestinal absorption of vitamin D. Proteinuric kidney diseases may lead to renal loss of vitamin D-binding protein, and in peritoneal dialysis patients, there may be a loss of vitamin D-binding protein in the peritoneal fluid. In addition to the deficiency of 25-hydroxyvitamin D, CKD is also characterized by reduced renal and extrarenal 1-α hydroxylase activity. In addition to the deficiencies of 25-hydroxyvitamin D and 1,25-dihyroxyvitamin D, advancing CKD leads to a progressive loss of vitamin D receptor on the parathyroid gland inducing resistance to the actions of vitamin D. Alterations explained above in vitamin D metabolism accompanied by hyperphosphatemia and hypocalcemia lead to increased synthesis and increased secretion of PTH leading to secondary hyperparathyroidism. Osteocyte secretion of FGF-23 is increased in early stages of CKD and that reduces PTH expression.

Considering the high prevalence of cardiovascular disease in patients with CKD and presence of CKD-MBD abnormalities, attention needs to be paid to the possible underlying pathophysiology between CKD-MBD and cardiovascular disease [9]. Animals with vitamin D deficiency develop hypertension and cardiomegaly [10]. Vitamin D receptor deficient mice demonstrate increases in renin and angiotensin [11]. In animal models, vitamin D treatment attenuates cardiac hypertrophy, reduces end-diastolic pressures, attenuates inflammation, and improves cardiac contractility [12]. However, the concern for vascular calcification is relevant to CKD and ESRD [13, 14]. In that regard, it is important to consider the dose–response relationship and differential effects of active vitamin D compounds on the biology of vascular calcification independent of increases in serum calcium and phosphorous. It is notable that a recent small study reported that the risk of calciphylaxis, a severe vascular calcification disorder, is increased in patients treated with calcitriol but not in patients treated with selective vitamin D analogues such as paricalcitol or doxercalciferol [15].

Epidemiological Data

The epidemiological data regarding vitamin D and clinical outcomes suffer from the conundrum regarding definition of vitamin D deficiency.

Table 16.1 Definition of vitamin D status

Category	Serum 25-hydroxyvitamin D level
Normal	30–80 ng/mL
Insufficient	20–30 ng/mL
Deficient	<20 ng/mL
Toxic	>80 ng/mL

The most recognized definitions of vitamin D status are tabulated in Table 16.1. The prevalence of vitamin D deficiency ranges between 20% and 40% in the general population [16].

The history of medical application of vitamin D dates back to the industrial revolution in Europe. As the work patterns evolved from being predominantly outdoors to indoors and the cities filled with smog, the sun exposure of populations was reduced. Many children and young adults began to develop skeletal deformities characteristic of rickets such as bowed legs and pigeon chest. These patients also demonstrated high mortality. In the 1900s, two important observations opened the doors for vitamin D investigation. One was an epidemiological observation that rickets was predominantly seen in persons from cities and not from rural areas suggesting that exposure to sun played an important role in its development. The second one was that cod liver oil supplementation cured abnormalities of rickets in some patients suggesting that a micronutrient/vitamin that is present in diet was responsible for the resolution of skeletal abnormalities. These observations were subsequently followed by derivation of structure and molecular functions of vitamin D and its receptor. Later on it was realized that it is the interplay between PTH and vitamin D that was necessary for maintaining adequate body and circulating calcium levels. Recent attention has focused on bioavailable 25-hydroxyvitamin D (comprised of the free fraction plus albumin-bound vitamin D) as bioavailable 25-hydroxyvitamin D has been shown to be more strongly associated with serum calcium and parathyroid hormone levels than total 25-hydroxyvitamin D [17, 18]. Racial differences in genetic polymorphisms likely explain the differences in 25-hydroxyvitamin D levels between white and black patients [19].

Multiple observational studies have reported an inverse association between 25-hydroxyvitamin D and clinical outcomes in populations without CKD [20–22]. When compared to vitamin D sufficient patients, patients with vitamin D deficiency are reported to carry a two to three times increased risk of cardiovascular outcomes. However, these strong epidemiological observations have not translated to better outcomes in patients. Despite significant association between vitamin D deficiency and risk of hypertension, supplementation with vitamin D did not reduce blood pressure, and despite significant association between vitamin D deficiency and risk of diabetes mellitus, supplementation with vitamin D did not reduce the risk and/or complications of diabetes mellitus [3, 6, 9, 23, 24].

In the ESRD population, vitamin D deficiency is present in 70–80% of patients [6]. Vitamin D deficiency is reported to have even higher prevalence in the CKD population with estimates as high as 70–80% in some studies. Over 75% of incident dialysis patients have deficiency of vitamin D, and over 20% of these patients have 25-hydroxyvitamin D levels below 10 ng/mL [25]. Vitamin D deficiency begins in earlier stages of CKD even before other abnormalities such as hyperparathyroidism become detectable [26].

Observational studies have reported an association between vitamin D deficiency and poor clinical outcomes in patients with CKD and ESRD. Each 10 ng/ml reduction in serum 25-hydroxyvitamin D level is associated with a 10–20% increase in mortality with most deaths attributed to cardiovascular disease [6, 27]. Among the dialysis patients, combination of low 25-hydroxyvitamin D and elevated PTH was associated with even higher mortality compared to low 25-hydroxyvitamin D alone demonstrating the influence of reduced conversion to 1,25-hydroxyvitamin D in the presence of elevated PTH in this population [28]. Although 1,25-hydroxyvitamin D levels were not reported in this study, the association with cardiovascular mortality was most prominent in patients with high parathyroid hormone levels suggesting that low conversion from

25-hydroxyvitamin D to 1,25-hydroxyvitamin D may predispose patients to the highest risks from adverse consequences of 25-hydroxyvitamin D deficiency.

In observational studies, elevated serum levels of phosphorus, calcium, parathyroid hormone, and fibroblast growth factor 23 (FGF23) have also been associated with increased risk of cardiovascular events and increased mortality in dialysis patients. In addition to the cardiovascular complications, CKD-MBD is also associated with a number of non-cardiovascular complications. Dialysis patients have a greater than twofold increased risk of skeletal fractures compared to general population, and this higher fracture rate is attributed to abnormalities in bone morphology due to vitamin D deficiency and secondary hyperparathyroidism. It is interesting to note that despite these observational data with clinical outcomes, studies examining associations between 25-hydrxyvitamin D levels and abnormalities in calcium, phosphorous, and PTH have not shown consistent associations [29]. One possible explanation for this discrepancy is based on the fact that 25-hydroxyvitamin D is a highly protein bound hormone with <1% in free form and the majority bound to DBP and a smaller fraction bound to albumin. Serum bioavailable 25-hydroxyvitamin D (albumin-bound and free fraction combined) levels have been shown to have a better association with serum calcium and PTH than total 25-hydroxyvitamin D in dialysis patients.

Randomized Controlled Trials

Considering the associations observed between CKD-MBD and poor outcomes, a natural question is whether correcting these CKD-MBD biochemical abnormalities will provide clinical benefits. The potential limitations of observational studies can be best addressed by randomized controlled trials. In fact, the CKD and ESRD populations, with higher rates of cardiovascular events and skeletal complications, represent an optimal clinical setting to test the efficacy of interventions.

Nutritional Vitamin D

Nutritional vitamin D includes the fungal-derived ergocalciferol and the animal-based cholecalciferol. In a meta-analysis of five randomized controlled trials, nutritional vitamin D treatment was associated with a significant increase in serum 25-hydroxyvitamin D levels and an associated decline in PTH levels [30]. However, none of the studies reported outcomes related to cardiovascular events, bone disease, or survival. In a recent randomized controlled trial of incident dialysis patients, nutritional vitamin D supplementation was associated with a nonsignificant reduction in all-cause mortality. In proteinuric CKD patients, nutritional vitamin D treatment led to a significant reduction in proteinuria, an indirect measure of cardiovascular and endothelial health [31]. Thus, recent data indicate possible benefit on endothelial dysfunction and albuminuria and argue for the need for larger studies.

Active Vitamin D

In the setting of diabetic nephropathy, paricalcitol administration has been shown to reduce albuminuria and systolic blood pressure compared with placebo [32]. Whether the improvements in proteinuria seen with active vitamin D correspond with improved clinical outcomes needs further investigation [33].

Important insights into the actions of active vitamin D on cardiac function and structure are available from the Paricalcitol Capsule Benefits in Renal Failure–Induced Cardiac Morbidity (PRIMO) trial [34]. This study aimed to examine the effects of paricalcitol on left ventricular mass index in patients with moderate CKD who had left ventricular hypertrophy. Active vitamin D treatment in the PRIMO trial did not alter left ventricular mass index. Interestingly, paricalcitol treatment was associated with fewer cardiovascular-related hospitalizations and attenuated the increase in brain natriuretic peptide levels.

The effects of active vitamin D treatment on clinically relevant skeletal outcomes such as falls and fractures are also limited, and studies suffer from the limitation of small sample size. In a meta-analysis, rates of fractures, bone pain, and surgical parathyroidectomy were not altered by active vitamin D treatment.

Cinacalcet

Cinacalcet, a calcimimetic agent, reduces PTH levels by binding to the calcium-sensing receptor on the parathyroid gland and simulating a hypercalcemic state in the setting of normal serum calcium levels. Cinacalcet offers the potential to control PTH without the risk of hypercalcemia or hyperphosphatemia. In the EVOLVE trial, maintenance hemodialysis patients with moderate-to-severe secondary hyperparathyroidism were randomized to cinacalcet or placebo [35]. This trial found that PTH levels were more suppressed in the calcimimetic arm; however, no differences were noted for mortality and other cardiovascular events (except calciphylaxis). A high rate of treatment crosses over limits conclusions, but overall the promise was not fulfilled.

Surgical Parathyroidectomy

There are no data from randomized controlled trials regarding parathyroidectomy vs. cinacalcet in ESRD patients. The observational data regarding parathyroidectomy and outcomes in the ESRD patients are exciting and warrant further investigation. In a Japanese study, >30% reduction in 1-year mortality was noted following parathyroidectomy [36].

Practical Considerations for Treatment

The target values for serum calcium, phosphorous, and PTH for CKD and ESRD patients are summarized in Table 16.2. In the absence of consistent evidence for treatments to control PTH and vitamin D, the medical community has relied on guidelines and expert opinions to manage patients with and at risk for CKD-MBD [37]. It is worth noting that the guidelines are constantly evolving in this area and emphasize the uncertainty that clinicians face as they treat patients [38].

Table 16.2 Target values for chronic kidney disease-mineral bone disease (CKD-MBD) parameters per Kidney Disease: Improving Global Outcomes (KDIGO) guidelines

Category	Target for CKD patients	Target for ESRD patients
Serum calcium	Normal range	Normal range
Serum phosphorous	Normal range	Normal range
Serum PTH	No target but begin therapy when progressive rise in PTH	2–9 times the upper limit of normal

Abbreviations: *CKD* chronic kidney disease, *ESRD* end-stage renal disease, *PTH* parathyroid hormone

Nutritional Vitamin D

Guidelines and expert opinion suggest treatment with nutritional vitamin D for stage 3 and 4 CKD patients with secondary hyperparathyroidism if 25-hydroxyvitamin D levels are <30 ng/mL.

- Measure serum 25-hydroxyvitamin D levels annually.
- Dose – Ergocalciferol 50,000 units of once a week for 4 weeks followed by the same dose once a month for 4 months if 25-hydroxyvitamin D levels are below 15 ng/mL; 50,000 units once a month for 6 months if levels are 20–30 ng/mL. Patients with levels ≥30 ng/ml should be continued on a maintenance dose of oral ergocalciferol at 50,000 IU once per month. Oral cholecalciferol at 1000–2000 IU daily can be used as an alternative maintenance dose.
- Monitoring – Serum calcium and phosphorus should be monitored every 3 months. The need for continuing therapy with ergocalciferol is to be reevaluated annually.
- Nutritional vitamin D supplements should be held if the serum 25(OH) vitamin D level is >100 ng/mL or serum calcium level >10.5 mg/dl.

Active Vitamin D

Expert recommendations and guidelines suggest adding active vitamin D analogues in the management of CKD-MBD in ESRD patients if PTH elevation persists despite dietary phosphate restriction, phosphate binders, and nutritional vitamin D treatment. A recent Kidney Disease: Improving Global Outcomes (KDIGO) controversies conference suggests treatment with active vitamin D in patients with CKD stages 3–5 not on dialysis when there is progressive rise in serum PTH.

Cinacalcet and Surgical Parathyroidectomy

Cinacalcet is typically administered in patients with ESRD with persistent hyperparathyroidism despite active vitamin D treatment or when hyperphosphatemia and/or hypercalcemia limit application of vitamin D treatment. Surgical parathyroidectomy is reserved for hyperparathyroidism that is refractory to medical therapies in ESRD patients. However, the threshold PTH for surgery is not clearly established, and patients who undergo parathyroidectomy in this setting typically have PTH elevations exceeding 1000 pg/mL. The European Renal Best Practice group recommends against the routine use of cinacalcet in the ESRD patients noting the risks do not justify benefits.

Conclusion

A cascade of alterations in calcium, phosphorous, FGF-23, PTH, and vitamin D lead to a disordered state of mineral metabolism in CKD. Despite the exciting experimental and observational data, randomized controlled trials have not convinced the community regarding the efficacy of currently available treatments. However, considering the risk of metabolic bone disease and cardiovascular complications associated with CKD-MBD, attempts to regulate the biochemical abnormalities remain central to the management of CKD.

References

1. Nwankwo E, Bello AK, El Nahas AM. Chronic kidney disease: stemming the global tide. Am J Kidney Dis. 2005;45(1):201–8.
2. Moe SM, Radcliffe JS, White KE, et al. The pathophysiology of early-stage chronic kidney disease-mineral bone disorder (CKD-MBD) and response to phosphate binders in the rat. J Bone Miner Res. 2011;26(11):2672–81.
3. Nigwekar SU, Tamez H, Thadhani RI. Vitamin D and chronic kidney disease-mineral bone disease (CKD-MBD). Bonekey Rep. 2014;3:498.
4. Larsson TE. The role of FGF-23 in CKD-MBD and cardiovascular disease: friend or foe? Nephrol Dial Transplant. 2010;25(5):1376–81.
5. Hruska KA, Choi ET, Memon I, Davis TK, Mathew S. Cardiovascular risk in chronic kidney disease (CKD): the CKD-mineral bone disorder (CKD-MBD). Pediatr Nephrol. 2010;25(4):769–78.
6. Nigwekar SU, Bhan I, Thadhani R. Ergocalciferol and cholecalciferol in CKD. Am J Kidney Dis. 2012;60(1):139–56.
7. Slatopolsky E, Hruska K, Rutherford WE. Current concepts of parathyroid hormone and vitamin D metabolism: perturbations in chronic renal disease. Kidney Int Suppl. 1975;(2):90–6.
8. Holick MF, DeLuca HF. Vitamin D metabolism. Annu Rev Med. 1974;25:349–67.
9. Nigwekar SU, Thadhani R. Vitamin D receptor activation: cardiovascular and renal implications. Kidney Int Suppl (2011). 2013;3(5):427–30.
10. Weishaar RE, Simpson RU. Vitamin D3 and cardiovascular function in rats. J Clin Invest. 1987;79(6):1706–12.
11. Li YC, Kong J, Wei M, Chen ZF, Liu SQ, Cao LP. 1,25-Dihydroxyvitamin D(3) is a negative endocrine regulator of the renin-angiotensin system. J Clin Invest. 2002;110(2):229–38.
12. Bodyak N, Ayus JC, Achinger S, et al. Activated vitamin D attenuates left ventricular abnormalities induced by dietary sodium in Dahl salt-sensitive animals. Proc Natl Acad Sci U S A. 2007;104(43):16810–5.
13. Floege J, Ketteler M. Vascular calcification in patients with end-stage renal disease. Nephrol Dial Transplant. 2004;19(Suppl 5):V59–66.
14. Moe SM. Vascular calcification: Hardening of the evidence. Kidney Int. 2006;70(9):1535–7.
15. Nigwekar SU, Bhan I, Turchin A, et al. Statin use and calcific uremic arteriolopathy: a matched case-control study. Am J Nephrol. 2013;37(4):325–32.
16. Holick MF. Vitamin D deficiency. N Engl J Med. 2007;357(3):266–81.
17. Bhan I, Powe CE, Berg AH, et al. Bioavailable vitamin D is more tightly linked to mineral metabolism than total vitamin D in incident hemodialysis patients. Kidney Int. 2012;82(1):84–9.
18. Powe CE, Evans MK, Wenger J, et al. Vitamin D-binding protein and vitamin D status of black

Americans and white Americans. N Engl J Med. 2013;369(21):1991–2000.
19. Holick MF. Bioavailability of vitamin D and its metabolites in black and white adults. N Engl J Med. 2013;369(21):2047–8.
20. Ford ES, Ajani UA, McGuire LC, Liu S. Concentrations of serum vitamin D and the metabolic syndrome among U.S. adults. Diabetes Care. 2005;28(5):1228–30.
21. Liu S, Song Y, Ford ES, Manson JE, Buring JE, Ridker PM. Dietary calcium, vitamin D, and the prevalence of metabolic syndrome in middle-aged and older U.S. women. Diabetes Care. 2005;28(12):2926–32.
22. Pittas AG, Lau J, Hu FB, Dawson-Hughes B. The role of vitamin D and calcium in type 2 diabetes. A systematic review and meta-analysis. J Clin Endocrinol Metab. 2007;92(6):2017–29.
23. Wolf M, Thadhani R. Vitamin D in patients with renal failure: a summary of observational mortality studies and steps moving forward. J Steroid Biochem Mol Biol. 2007;103(3–5):487–90.
24. Tamez H, Kalim S, Thadhani RI. Does vitamin D modulate blood pressure? Curr Opin Nephrol Hypertens. 2013;22(2):204–9.
25. Wolf M, Shah A, Gutierrez O, et al. Vitamin D levels and early mortality among incident hemodialysis patients. Kidney Int. 2007;72(8):1004–13.
26. Wolf M, Thadhani R. Beyond minerals and parathyroid hormone: role of active vitamin D in end-stage renal disease. Semin Dial. 2005;18(4):302–6.
27. Bhan I, Thadhani R. Vitamin D therapy for chronic kidney disease. Semin Nephrol. 2009;29(1):85–93.
28. Drechsler C, Verduijn M, Pilz S, et al. Vitamin D status and clinical outcomes in incident dialysis patients: results from the NECOSAD study. Nephrol Dial Transplant. 2011;26(3):1024–32.
29. Thadhani RI, Manson JE. Vitamin D: too soon to turn out the lights? Arterioscler Thromb Vasc Biol. 2013;33(11):2467–9.
30. Kandula P, Dobre M, Schold JD, Schreiber MJ, Mehrotra R, Navaneethan SD. Vitamin D supplementation in chronic kidney disease: a systematic review and meta-analysis of observational studies and randomized controlled trials. Clin J Am Soc Nephrol 2011;6(1):50–62.
31. Zhao J, Dong J, Wang H, Shang H, Zhang D, Liao L. Efficacy and safety of vitamin D3 in patients with diabetic nephropathy: a meta-analysis of randomized controlled trials. Chin Med J. 2014;127(15):2837–43.
32. de Zeeuw D, Agarwal R, Amdahl M, et al. Selective vitamin D receptor activation with paricalcitol for reduction of albuminuria in patients with type 2 diabetes (VITAL study): a randomised controlled trial. Lancet. 2010;376(9752):1543–51.
33. de Borst MH, Hajhosseiny R, Tamez H, Wenger J, Thadhani R, Goldsmith DJ. Active vitamin D treatment for reduction of residual proteinuria: a systematic review. J Am Soc Nephrol. 2013;24(11):1863 71.
34. Thadhani R, Appelbaum E, Pritchett Y, et al. Vitamin D therapy and cardiac structure and function in patients with chronic kidney disease: the PRIMO randomized controlled trial. JAMA. 2012;307(7):674–84.
35. Investigators ET, Chertow GM, Block GA, et al. Effect of cinacalcet on cardiovascular disease in patients undergoing dialysis. N Engl J Med. 2012;367(26):2482–94.
36. Lundquist AL, Nigwekar SU. Optimal management of bone mineral disorders in chronic kidney disease and end stage renal disease. Curr Opin Nephrol Hypertens. 2016;25(2):120–6.
37. Moe S, Drueke T, Cunningham J, et al. Definition, evaluation, and classification of renal osteodystrophy: a position statement from Kidney Disease: Improving Global Outcomes (KDIGO). Kidney Int. 2006;69(11):1945–53.
38. Ketteler M, Elder GJ, Evenepoel P, et al. Revisiting KDIGO clinical practice guideline on chronic kidney disease-mineral and bone disorder: a commentary from a Kidney Disease: Improving Global Outcomes controversies conference. Kidney Int. 2015;87(3):502–28.

Management of Bone Disorders in Kidney Disease

17

Stuart M. Sprague

Introduction

In healthy individuals, normal serum concentrations of phosphorus and calcium are maintained through the interaction of three hormones: parathyroid hormone (PTH), calcitriol ($1,25(OH)_2D_3$), and fibroblast growth factor 23 (FGF-23). These hormones act on four primary target organs: bone, kidney, intestine, and parathyroid glands. The kidneys play a critical role in the regulation of serum calcium and phosphorus concentrations as well as these three hormones. In patients with chronic kidney disease (CKD), increased PTH concentrations are generally the first clinically measured abnormality observed in patients with evolving CKD; however, FGF-23 increases prior to PTH [1, 2]. Shortly following the increases in FGF-23 and PTH, calcitriol concentrations will fall [1]. Changes in these hormones in the early stages of the CKD are an adaptive mechanism to help maintain the serum phosphorus and calcium concentrations in the normal range. It is not until the development of CKD stages 4–5 (glomerular filtration rate less than 30 mL/min/1.73m^2) that measurable abnormalities of calcium and phosphorus become apparent [1].

With progression of CKD, these compensatory responses become unable to maintain normal mineral homeostasis, resulting in [1] altered concentrations of calcium, phosphorus, PTH, calcitriol, and FGF-23, [2] disturbances in bone remodeling and mineralization (renal osteodystrophy) and/or impaired linear growth in children, and [3] extra-skeletal calcification in soft tissues and arteries. In 2006, the term chronic kidney disease-mineral and bone disorder (CKD-MBD) was developed by the Kidney Disease Improving Global Outcomes (KDIGO) work group to describe this triad of abnormalities in biochemical measures, skeletal abnormalities, and extra-skeletal calcification [3]. Of note, osteoporosis was not defined as an independent skeletal disorder and should not be treated without considering the other metabolic disorders associated with CKD-MBD [3, 4]. The updated 2017 guidelines do recommend obtaining bone mineral densitometry in patients with CKD stages 3–5 if they have other risk factors for osteoporotic fractures; however, the results do not predict the specific bone lesion but may be useful for deciding to proceed with a bone biopsy [5]. The abnormalities that constitute CKD-MBD are interrelated in both the pathophysiology of the disease and the response to treatment. All three components of CKD-MBD are associated with increased risk of fractures, cardiovascular disease, and mortality in

S. M. Sprague (✉)
Division of Nephrology and Hypertension, NorthShore University HealthSystem, Evanston, IL, USA

University of Chicago Pritzker School of Medicine, Chicago, IL, USA
e-mail: ssprague@northshore.org

C. M. Rhee et al. (eds.), *Endocrine Disorders in Kidney Disease*,
https://doi.org/10.1007/978-3-319-97765-2_17

patients with advanced CKD. Treatment of CKD-MBD focuses on the prevention and correction of these hormonal abnormalities.

Pathophysiology of Chronic Kidney Disease-Mineral Bone Disorder

Parathyroid hormone, calcitriol, and FGF-23 work together to maintain normal phosphate and calcium homeostasis to achieve appropriate balance in the blood and urine so as to avoid extra-skeletal calcification and ensure adequate availability of these ions for bone remodeling. This response is a very complex system of multiple integrated feedback loops and is easier to understand if broken into loops that regulate phosphate, calcium, and calcitriol. Both PTH and FGF-23 have similar effects in stimulating renal phosphate excretion [6]. However, these hormones differ in their effects on vitamin D metabolism. Parathyroid hormone stimulates CYP27B1 activity, thus increasing the production of calcitriol, which in turn negatively feeds back on the parathyroid gland to decrease PTH secretion. In contrast, FGF-23 inhibits CYP27B1 and stimulates CYP24, thereby decreasing the production and increasing the deactivation of calcitriol and which results in limiting further secretion of FGF-23, as calcitriol normally stimulates FGF-23 production [7].

As CKD progresses, there is decreased renal phosphate excretion resulting in an increased phosphate load causing increases in both PTH and FGF-23 [1, 2]. Both the elevated PTH and FGF-23 increase urinary phosphate excretion through downregulation of the sodium-phosphate (NaPi) transporters [6]. Parathyroid hormone also increases renal calcium reabsorption preventing the worsening of hypocalcemia as well as minimizing the possibility of high urinary calcium and phosphate concentrations. Parathyroid hormone also stimulates the secretion of FGF-23 from osteocytes, and the increased FGF-23 inhibits PTH gene expression and secretion [7–9].

Hypocalcemia is a potent stimulator of PTH and blunts FGF-23 release [10]. Thus, the decrease in FGF-23 release would result in less FGF-23 inhibition of both PTH and calcitriol synthesis thus offsetting the development of hypocalcemia. This process would maximize both the PTH effects to increase renal calcium reabsorption, increase bone resorption, and enhance calcitriol stimulation of intestinal calcium absorption with the goal of normalizing serum calcium concentrations. Hypercalcemia would stimulate FGF-23 (which reduces PTH and calcitriol synthesis) as well as directly inhibit calcitriol synthesis and PTH secretion [7]. The result is decreased intestinal calcium absorption, renal calcium reabsorption, and bone resorption.

Diagnosis of Chronic Kidney Disease-Mineral Bone Disorder

Parathyroid Hormone

Parathyroid hormone concentration in plasma or serum serves not only as an indicator of abnormal mineral metabolism in CKD-MBD but also as a noninvasive biochemical sign for the initial diagnosis of renal osteodystrophy, the bone component of CKD-MBD. Parathyroid hormone measurements also can be a useful index for monitoring the evolution of renal osteodystrophy and can serve as a surrogate measure of bone turnover in patients with CKD. Although the sensitivity and specificity of PTH as a marker of bone remodeling are not ideal, it appears to be the best biomarker currently available [11]. Unfortunately, it is not clear what the optimal PTH concentration should be at each stage of CKD. Thus, guidelines recommend using the same PTH assay for all measurements and evaluating trends rather than targeting precise levels [4, 5].

Vitamin D

Calcidiol concentrations are generally measured by immunoassays, although the gold standard for calcidiol measurement is high-performance liquid chromatography (HPLC), which is not widely available clinically. Similar to PTH, the optimal concentration of calcidiol in CKD-MBD is not well defined. Vitamin D deficiency is associated with hyperparathyroidism in patients with normal kidney function and plays a role in CKD. Higher concentrations of calcidiol are required to maximally inhibit PTH with worsening CKD [12]. Calcitriol concentrations are universally low [1] and are generally not measured, except in the setting of hypercalcemia.

FGF-23

FGF-23 is currently measured primarily with two different assays: one which measures the intact hormone as well as C-terminal fragments and a second assay that detects the intact hormone. Although these two assays appear comparable in the association with clinical events at this time, they have poor agreement because of differences in FGF-23 fragment detection, antibody specificity, and calibration. From a clinical perspective, more data are required prior to the use of FGF-23 measurements for routine clinical management.

Bone-Specific Alkaline Phosphatase

Bone-specific alkaline phosphatase (BALP) is not renally cleared. BALP concentrations have relatively good correlation with bone formation in CKD and may be additive to the interpretation of parathyroid hormone measurements [4]. However, its concentration has limited ability as an independent measurement [11].

Bone Biopsy Assessment in Chronic Kidney Disease-Mineral Bone Disorder

The definitive method for establishing the specific type of renal osteodystrophy in individual patients requires bone biopsy [3–5, 11], an invasive diagnostic procedure, and access to specialized laboratory personnel and equipment capable of providing assessments of bone histology. Abnormalities of bone quality and quantity are common in CKD-MBD, leading to fractures and impaired growth in children. Clinically, bone biopsies are most useful for differentiating bone turnover as well as bone volume and mineralization. KDIGO recommends that the definition of renal osteodystrophy be limited to describing the alterations of bone morphology in patients with CKD and is one measure of the skeletal component of the systemic disorder of CKD-MBD that can be quantifiable by histomorphometry [3–5]. Three key histologic descriptors—bone turnover, mineralization, and volume (TMV system)—with any combination of each of the descriptors possible in a given specimen were developed to classify bone biopsies and help guide therapy [3].

Turnover reflects the rate of skeletal remodeling, which is normally the coupled process of bone resorption and bone formation. Bone turnover is affected mainly by hormones, cytokines, mechanical stimuli, and growth factors that influence the recruitment, differentiation, and activity of osteoclasts and osteoblasts. Mineralization reflects how well bone collagen becomes calcified during the formation phase of skeletal remodeling. Causes of impaired mineralization include inadequate vitamin D, mineral (calcium or phosphate) deficiency, acidosis, and bone aluminum toxicity. Volume indicates the amount of bone per unit volume of tissue, and an imbalance in bone resorption and formation can affect bone volume. For example, if resorption exceeds formation, negative bone balance and decreased bone volume result. Determinants of bone volume include age, sex, race, genetic factors, nutrition, endocrine disorders, mechanical stimuli, toxicities, neurologic function, vascular supply, growth factors, and cytokines. Osteoporosis would indicate low bone volume and could be diagnosed via a biopsy. Two large-scale analyses utilizing the TMV system revealed that this classification system provides clinically relevant information [11, 13].

Dual-Energy X-Ray Absorptiometry

Dual-energy X-ray absorptiometry (DXA) measures areal bone mineral density (aBMD) in g/cm^2 using minimal radiation and rapid scan times. Bone mineral density assessment by DXA has good reproducibility (<1–2% coefficient variation) and reliable reference ranges for age, sex, and race. In the general population, aBMD measured by DXA can be used clinically to define osteoporosis and is an accepted surrogate end point after prospective studies demonstrated an age-dependent predictive value of DXA for fractures [14]. However, DXA has not been found to be as sensitive and specific to assess fracture risk across the spectrum of CKD, in part as it cannot assess bone quality [15, 16]. The KDIGO guidelines recommend DXA to assess fracture risk in patients with CKD stage 1 through stage 3a, as long as biochemical testing does not suggest CKD-MBD [3, 5]. However, for patients with CKD stages 3b through 5, the current guidelines recommend DXA testing to assess fracture risk if results will impact treatment decisions [5]. Although previous studies and a meta-analysis demonstrated that DXA testing may have been lower in patients with CKD and a history of fracture, there is considerable overlap in aBMD results such that aBMD provides poor fracture discrimination in individuals [17]. Subsequent studies have demonstrated that aBMD was able to predict fractures in patients with CKD G3 to G5 [18, 19]. However, DXA cannot make a specific diagnosis as to why there is low bone density. Unlike patients with normal kidney function and a low DXA being classified as having osteoporosis, patients with CKD and low bone density should not be routinely treated with anti-osteoporosis therapies [3–5, 15].

Management of Chronic Kidney Disease-Mineral Bone Disorder

The primary objective of therapy is to correct the underlying pathophysiologic disturbances in mineral metabolism with the goal to prevent the development of severe hyperparathyroidism, fractures, and extra-skeletal mineralization. The KDIGO working group has published guidelines for managing CKD-MBD [4, 5].

Hyperparathyroidism

Most recently the KDIGO guidelines recommend measuring the serum calcium, phosphorus, alkaline phosphatase, and PTH at least once in persons with a glomerular filtration rate (GFR) <45 ml/min/1.73m^2. In people with GFR <45 ml/min/1.73 m^2 (GFR categories 3B–5/5D), the optimal PTH level is not known. In non-dialysis-dependent patients, it is suggested that levels of intact PTH above the upper normal limit of the assay are first evaluated for hyperphosphatemia, hypocalcemia, and vitamin D deficiency. If any of these metabolic disorders are present, then initial therapy would be directed at correcting them [5]. In patients with CKD stage 5 undergoing dialysis, it is suggested to maintain PTH concentrations in the range of approximately two to nine times the upper normal limit for the specific assay. If there are marked changes in PTH levels in either direction within this range, therapy should either be initiated or altered to prevent progression to levels outside of this range [5]. An important element of the recent KDIGO guidelines is the recommendation to make clinical decisions on managing the PTH level on the change in PTH "trend over time" rather than a single measurement. This suggestion is in part due to the variability in PTH levels from day to day or from time of day and in part due to the variability among laboratories in the PTH immunoassay [20]. Thus, the clinical decisions in the management of a chronic disease such as secondary hyperparathyroidism should be made over time as well. Options for the treatment of hyperparathyroidism in CKD include controlling the serum phosphorus and/or serum calcium concentration, pharmacological use of agents that reduce PTH secretion by altering the calcium-sensing receptor which includes specific active vitamin D analogs or the calcimimetics, or surgical parathyroidectomy. Thus, the updated clinical guidelines recommend that PTH-lowering therapy should include the use of calcimimetics, calcitriol, or other active vitamin D analogs or a combination of calcimimetics with calcitriol or active vitamin D analogs, without prioritizing therapy other than parathyroidectomy being considered when medical therapy fails [5].

Phosphate Management

Practice guidelines suggest maintaining serum calcium and phosphorous with the normal range via dietary restriction and/or administration of phosphate binders [4, 5]. The use of vegetarian products as well as protein restriction is commonly suggested to limit phosphate intake [4]. However, diet is often insufficient to reach a desirable control of serum phosphate levels, and a wide range of phosphate binders are now available (Table 17.1). Aluminum-based binders are very effective; however, due to their potential toxicity, they have been replaced by other mineral-based and polymer-based phosphate

Table 17.1 Phosphate binders

Phosphate binder	Clinical considerations	Relative phosphate binding[a] (per gram binder)
Aluminum hydroxide	Very effective Well tolerated Liquid Low cost Risk of aluminum intoxication	1.9
Calcium carbonate	Effective High pill burden Risk of hypercalcemia Not recommended for patients with low PTH or vascular calcifications	1.0
Calcium acetate	Similar to calcium carbonate Slightly lower calcium load than calcium carbonate	1.0
Magnesium carbonate	Effective Anti-constipating Diarrhea Hypermagnesemia	1.7
Sevelamer hydrochloride	Effective Calcium-free resin High pill burden Lipid and uric acid lowering May bind bile acids and fat-soluble substances May worsen metabolic acidosis	0.75
Sevelamer carbonate	Effective Calcium-free resin High pill burden Lipid and uric acid lowering May bind bile acids and fat-soluble substances	0.75
Lanthanum carbonate	Effective Low pill burden Must be chewed GI side effects	2.0
Sucroferric oxyhydroxide	Effective Low pill burden Must be chewed Diarrhea	3.0
Ferric citrate	Effective High pill burden Iron absorption, may require less IV iron Diarrhea	0.9

[a]Relative phosphate binding capacity relative to calcium carbonate

binders [21]. Thus, guidelines suggest limiting the use of aluminum-based phosphate binders for cases of severe hyperphosphatemia and for a short period of time [4]. When compared to placebo, all available phosphate binders have been shown to lower serum phosphate to a similar extent [22–26]. However, differences among the drugs exist, which includes changes in serum calcium, effect on PTH control, and pill burden [22, 24–26]. Preliminary data also suggest that phosphate restriction and calcium-free phosphate binders may reduce FGF-23 [21, 27]. Although the clinical relevance of different biochemical profiles still needs to be elucidated, some lines of evidence suggest that calcium-based phosphate binders may accelerate vascular calcification deposition and progression when compared to calcium-free phosphate binders [28]. There is some evidence that calcium-free phosphate binders are associated with better survival when compared to calcium-based phosphate binders [29], and current guidelines advise restricting the use of calcium-containing binders [5].

Vitamin D

Nutritional vitamin D, calcifediol, calcitriol, and other vitamin D analogs are used in patients with CKD to prevent and treat secondary hyperparathyroidism (Table 17.2). Despite theoretical benefits of raising 25-hydroxyvitamin D levels with nutritional vitamin D (e.g., ergocalciferol and cholecalciferol) in CKD stage 3–4 patients, there has been limited effectiveness in correcting hyperparathyroidism [30, 31]. However extended release calcifediol has been shown to effectively increase vitamin D levels and correct hyperparathyroidism in these pre-dialysis patients [32]. Unfortunately, there are no trials in dialysis patients nor large long-term randomized controlled trials in patients with earlier stages of CKD supporting an improvement in PTH [33, 34]. Calcitriol and other active analogs, alphacalcidol, doxercalciferol, and paricalcitol, have all been demonstrated to effectively treat hyperparathyroidism in CKD stages 3–4 [35–38]. It was claimed that these analogs provided effective control of PTH without causing hypercalcemia or hyperphosphatemia compared to calcitriol [35, 36]. However, in the only prospective study comparing one of these analogs (paricalcitol) with calcitriol, there was equivalent control of PTH with no difference in the development of hypercalcemia or hyperphosphatemia [39]. Thus, guidelines do not differentiate the use of any of these compounds in CKD stages 3–4 [5].

In patients undergoing chronic dialysis, calcitriol and the other active analogs, alphacalcidol, doxercalciferol, and paricalcitol, have all been shown to lower PTH concentrations. Among patients undergoing chronic hemodialysis, the use of intravenous doses given thrice weekly during each dialysis session became a common practice, especially in the United States. This practice was supported by a meta-analysis which found that the parenteral forms of active vitamin D analogs were superior to the oral form in reducing PTH

Table 17.2 Comparison of vitamin D therapies

Class	Sterol	Comment	Effect on blood levels		
			25-D	Ca/Phos	PTH
Nutritional vitamin D	Cholecalciferol	D_3 animal source	Mild Inc	None	Mild Dec
	Ergocalciferol	D_2 plant source	Mild Inc	None	Mild Dec
Vitamin D	Calcifediol $25(OH)D_3$	D_3 prohormone	Mod Inc	None	Mod Dec
Vitamin D receptor agonists (VDRA)	Calcitriol $1,25(OH)_2D_3$	D_3 natural analog	Mild Dec	Mod Inc	Marked Dec
	Alphacalcidol $1(OH)D_3$	D_3 synthetic prohormone	Mild Dec	Mod Inc	Marked Dec
	Doxercalciferol $1(OH)D_2$	D_2 synthetic prohormone	Mild Dec	Mod Inc	Marked Dec
	Paricalcitol $19nor,1,25(OH)_2D_2$	D_2 synthetic analog	Mild Dec	Mod Inc	Marked Dec

concentrations [40]. However, when one study that used very high doses of intravenous analogs was removed from the meta-analysis, there were no differences in the PTH concentrations. Thus, the evidence supporting the use of large intermittent intravenous doses of vitamin D analogs is limited. Thus, the recent therapeutic trend is to use oral forms of calcitriol and its analogs. As previously discussed, KDIGO guidelines recommend maintaining PTH concentrations between two and nine times the upper limit of normal in dialysis patients [4, 5]. Both the oral and intravenous formulations of the active vitamin D analogs increase the risk of hypercalcemia, especially as the PTH decreases and the updated guidelines recommend decreasing or stopping analogs as the calcium increases [5].

Calcimimetics

Calcimimetics are agents for the treatment of hyperparathyroidism that bind to and activate the calcium-sensing receptor (CaSR) resulting in a decrease in PTH production and release [41–44]. Currently available calcimimetics include cinacalcet hydrochloride which is a small organic molecule that is orally administered with a relatively short half-life [41, 42, 45], whereas etelcalcetide is a parenterally administered synthetic peptide with a longer half-life which can be administered thrice weekly at the end of hemodialysis [43, 44]. As opposed to the active vitamin D analogs, these agents are effective in lowering PTH concentrations while also decreasing serum and phosphate concentrations. In the pivotal phase 3 study, treatment of uncontrolled secondary hyperparathyroidism with cinacalcet or placebo for 26 weeks resulted in a greater proportion of patients in the cinacalcet arm achieving PTH concentrations ≤250 pg/mL with better control of serum calcium and phosphorous [41]. Subsequent studies further demonstrated efficacy of cinacalcet as monotherapy to suppress PTH when compared with active vitamin D analogs [46]. Furthermore, cinacalcet therapy was associated with a decrease in FGF-23 as opposed to an increase seen in those treated with the active vitamin D analogs [47]. Clinical studies with etelcalcetide demonstrated similar results as those with cinacalcet when compared to placebo [44] and were non-inferior to cinacalcet [43]. Notably, in all these studies, mild-to-moderate hypocalcemia, nausea, and vomiting were common, albeit easily managed, side effects. Unfortunately, the EVOLVE study, which was the largest placebo-controlled, double-blind clinical trial with cinacalcet conducted in dialysis patients with secondary hyperparathyroidism designed to evaluate hard outcomes, was not able to meet the primary endpoint (i.e., time until death, myocardial infarction, hospitalization for unstable angina, heart failure, or peripheral vascular event) [48]. However, serum concentrations of PTH, calcium, phosphate, and FGF-23 were better controlled among patients allocated to cinacalcet [48]. Current recommendations are that calcimimetics should only be used in dialysis patients as when administered to pre-dialysis CKD patients they will increase serum phosphorus and decrease serum calcium [5, 49, 50].

Parathyroidectomy

In both CKD and dialysis patients with severe hyperparathyroidism who fail to respond to medical therapy, parathyroidectomy is recommended [5]. Successful parathyroidectomy can yield a dramatic reduction in PTH concentrations and clinical symptoms. Furthermore, some investigators have reported that parathyroidectomy may be more cost-effective than calcimimetics in treating patients with uncontrolled hyperparathyroidism [51]. However, an analysis of 4435 hemodialysis patients undergoing parathyroidectomy demonstrated a 2% perioperative mortality rate and a 39% increase in overall hospitalizations in the subsequent year [52]. Another retrospective review of dialysis patients with severe and unresponsive hyperparathyroidism indicated that parathyroidectomy did not improve cardiovascular outcomes compared with standard medical treatment [53]. Furthermore, in some instances hyperparathyroidism may persist after parathyroidectomy because of incomplete resection or because of ongoing PTH secretion from autotransplanted parathyroid tissue. Thus, recommendations are that parathyroidectomy be reserved to when medical therapy fails [5].

Treatment of Osteoporosis in CKD

Clinical studies evaluating all the approved pharmacologic therapies for osteoporosis included subjects with CKD stages 1–3a (GFR >45 ml/min/1.73m^2). Thus, osteoporosis management should not differ in CKD stages 1–3a as it is in persons without CKD, as long as there are no biochemical markers suggestive of the presence of CKD-MBD [3, 5, 54]. There is a lack of data demonstrating fracture risk reduction in patients with CKD stages 3b–5, with the exception of a few post hoc analyses in a small number of patients from the registered cohorts for postmenopausal osteoporosis. Approved anti-osteoporosis agents include calcitonin, estrogens, selective estrogen receptor modulators, bisphosphonates, teriparatide, abaloparatide, and denosumab (Table 17.3).

Table 17.3 Use of osteoporosis therapeutic agents in chronic kidney disease-mineral bone disorder

Estrogen
Potential use in hypogonadism
Safety data lacking
Increased drug half-life
Increases BMD, no fracture data
Selective estrogen receptor modulators (SERMs)
Safety data lacking
Efficacy unknown
Post hoc analysis appears to be similar vertebral fracture protection in CKD 3
Calcitonin
Efficacy unknown
Probably safe
Bisphosphonates
Post hoc analysis efficacious for stabilizing/increasing BMD in CKD 3–4
Effect on fracture rate in advanced CKD subset is unknown
May be useful in treating calciphylaxis
Theoretically dangerous in low-turnover bone disease
Safety data not available
Prolonged T1/2
Removed by dialysis
Consider bone biopsy prior to use to further evaluate CKD-MBD
Teriparatide (1–34 parathyroid hormone analog)
Limited data
Improved BMD in patients with low bone turnover
Abaloparatide (1–34 parathyroid hormone-related protein analog)
No data in CKD
Likely the same as teriparatide
Denosumab (monoclonal antibody to RANK-L)
Women with CKD 3 had similar vertebral fracture reduction as normal
May have exaggerated increase in PTH
Safety data are not available
Romosozumab (monoclonal antibody to sclerostin)
No published data in CKD

Anti-resorptive Agents

Anti-resorptive agents have a common pathway resulting in the inhibition of bone resorption. Available anti-resorptive agents include calcitonin, estrogens, selective estrogen receptor modulators, bisphosphonates, and denosumab. Each anti-resorptive agent has its own unique mechanism of action. Since bisphosphonates and denosumab are the most widely used anti-resorptive agents for osteoporosis, these agents will be further discussed. Bisphosphonates are biological analogs of naturally occurring pyrophosphates (P-O-P), degradation products of adenosine triphosphate (ATP) metabolism. Pyrophosphates are rapidly metabolized by the ubiquitous presence of pyrophosphatases, while bisphosphonates (P-C-P) are not metabolized [55]. Bisphosphonates are rapidly taken up by the bone and inhibit bone resorption by two mechanisms: a physiochemical one by stabilizing the calcium-phosphorus surface and a cellular one by inhibiting osteoclast activity. Bisphosphonates are cleared by the kidney by both glomerular filtration and active proximal tubular secretion. Bisphosphonates are retained in the bone in the remodeling resorption cavity, and the amount of bisphosphonate retained is probably a function of the rate of bone turnover and the GFR. While oral bisphosphonates are poorly (<1%) absorbed, approximately 50% is renally excreted. Intravenous bisphosphonates have a

100% bioavailability, also with 50% being renally excreted [55, 56]. Thus, in patients with CKD stage 3 who have a low bone mineral density and/or fragility fractures, bisphosphonate therapy should be considered after addressing the biochemical abnormalities associated with CKD-MBD [5]. Whereas in patients with CKD stages 4–5, limited data suggests that bisphosphonates have no effect on bone density [57], however, there are no clinical studies in which CKD-MBD abnormalities are addressed; thus, a bone biopsy should be considered prior to initiating bisphosphonate therapy [4, 5].

Denosumab is a fully humanized monoclonal antibody that binds to an osteoblast (and osteocyte)-derived glycoprotein and receptor activator of nuclear factor kappa-B ligand (RANK-L), inhibiting RANK-L from binding to an osteoclast membrane receptor, RANK, and, thereby, inhibiting osteoclastogenesis [58]. In clinical studies, similar fracture reduction was noted in patients with CKD stages 3–4 as to those with normal kidney function; however, in order to be included in the studies, all subjects had normal PTH concentrations [59]. There was also the observation that in patients with advanced CKD, denosumab may produce marked increases in PTH as well as profound hypocalcemia [60, 61]. This hypocalcemic and hyperparathyroid effect may be mitigated by ensuring adequate vitamin D and calcium intake [60]. Furthermore, since denosumab decreases bone turnover, until further data are available, it should be avoided in subjects with advanced kidney disease who are at risk for low bone turnover.

Anabolic Agents

Currently available anabolic agents include teriparatide which is a recombinant human 1–34 PTH analog [62] and abaloparatide which is 1–34 analog of human parathyroid hormone-related protein (PTHrP) [63]. Abaloparatide effectively improves bone density and decreases fractures in postmenopausal women. However, it has not been studied in men or analyzed in patients with decreasing GFR [64, 65]. In both women and men with osteoporosis, treatment with teriparatide compared with placebo increased bone mineral density as well as decreased the risk of vertebral and nonvertebral fractures [62, 66, 67]. Furthermore, teriparatide has also been shown to be effective in steroid-induced osteoporosis [68, 69]. The teriparatide trials did not randomize subjects with known CKD stages 4–5. However, during subsequent analysis, it was noted that these studies had subsets of patients with eGFR down to 30 ml/min [70, 71]. In these subsets, there were similar increases in bone mineral density across tertiles of eGFR. Fracture numbers were too small to have power for statistical analysis across these three tertiles. There were no changes in renal function as assessed by changes in serum creatinine or serum calcium concentrations as a function of eGFR. There are no studies on the effect of teriparatide or patients with advanced CKD stages 4–5 or in subjects with bone biopsy-proven low-turnover bone disease, other than a few case reports which demonstrate a positive effect on both bone mineral density and fractures [57, 72, 73]. Thus, it is possible, though unproven, that teriparatide may have a beneficial role in patients with advanced CKD and low-turnover bone disease.

Summary

The management of patients with fragility fractures across the spectrum of CKD should not differ between persons without reductions in GFR or persons with CKD stages 1–3, at least as it pertains to patients with age-related reductions in GFR with normal mineral metabolism [5]. This suggestion is predicated on the absence of information that could suggest the presence of CKD-MBD. In patients with CKD stages 4–5 and who have fragility fractures, the first management step is making the correct diagnosis. Diagnosis of osteoporosis in CKD stages 4–5 is an exclusionary one. Exclusion is best made by bone biopsy, a clinical service that is not widely available. Biochemical markers of bone turnover, in particular serum PTH and bone-specific alkaline phosphatase, may help provide differentiation between biopsy-proven low-turnover and high-turnover disease; however, as previously discussed, these measurements do not have high specificity [11]. The exclusion, in particular, of low-turnover bone disease is especially important as the use of anti-resorptive agents may not be beneficial and in fact could worsen the low bone turnover state. There is a great need to gain knowledge and evidence for the appropriate use of traditional anti-osteoporosis treatments in patients with CKD stages 4–5 who have low bone density or have sustained a low-trauma fracture.

References

1. Levin A, Bakris GL, Molitch M, Smulders M, Tian J, Williams LA, et al. Prevalence of abnormal serum vitamin D, PTH, calcium, and phosphorus in patients with chronic kidney disease: results of the study to evaluate early kidney disease. Kidney Int. 2007;71(1):31–8.
2. Isakova T, Wahl P, Vargas GS, Gutiérrez OM, Scialla J, Xie H, et al. Fibroblast growth factor 23 is elevated before parathyroid hormone and phosphate in chronic kidney disease. Kidney Int. 2011;79(12):1370–8.
3. Moe S, Drüeke T, Cunningham J, Goodman W, Martin K, Olgaard K, et al. Definition, evaluation, and classification of renal osteodystrophy: a position statement from Kidney Disease: Improving Global Outcomes (KDIGO). Kidney Int. 2006;69(11):1945–53.
4. Group KDIGOKC-MW. KDIGO clinical practice guideline for the diagnosis, evaluation, prevention, and treatment of Chronic Kidney Disease-Mineral and Bone Disorder (CKD-MBD). Kidney Int Suppl. 2009;113:S1–130.
5. Ketteler M, Block GA, Evenepoel P, Fukagawa M, Herzog CA, McCann L, et al. Executive summary of the 2017 KDIGO Chronic Kidney Disease-Mineral and Bone Disorder (CKD-MBD) guideline update: what's changed and why it matters. Kidney Int. 2017;92(1):26–36.
6. Bergwitz C, Jüppner H. Regulation of phosphate homeostasis by PTH, vitamin D, and FGF23. Annu Rev Med. 2010;61:91–104.
7. Blau JE, Collins MT. The PTH-vitamin D-FGF23 axis. Rev Endocr Metab Disord. 2015;16(2):165–74.
8. Ben-Dov IZ, Galitzer H, Lavi-Moshayoff V, Goetz R, Kuro-o M, Mohammadi M, et al. The parathyroid is a target organ for FGF23 in rats. J Clin Invest. 2007;117(12):4003–8.
9. Lavi-Moshayoff V, Wasserman G, Meir T, Silver J, Naveh-Many T. PTH increases FGF23 gene expression and mediates the high-FGF23 levels of experimental kidney failure: a bone parathyroid feedback loop. Am J Physiol Renal Physiol. 2010;299(4):F882–9.
10. Rodriguez-Ortiz ME, Lopez I, Muñoz-Castañeda JR, Martinez-Moreno JM, Ramírez AP, Pineda C, et al. Calcium deficiency reduces circulating levels of FGF23. J Am Soc Nephrol. 2012;23(7):1190–7.
11. Sprague SM, Bellorin-Font E, Jorgetti V, Carvalho AB, Malluche HH, Ferreira A, et al. Diagnostic accuracy of bone turnover markers and bone histology in patients with CKD treated by Dialysis. Am J Kidney Dis. 2016;67(4):559–66.
12. Ennis JL, Worcester EM, Coe FL, Sprague SM. Current recommended 25-hydroxyvitamin D targets for chronic kidney disease management may be too low. J Nephrol. 2016;29(1):63–70.
13. Malluche HH, Mawad HW, Monier-Faugere MC. Renal osteodystrophy in the first decade of the new millennium: analysis of 630 bone biopsies in black and white patients. J Bone Miner Res. 2011;26(6):1368–76.
14. Hui SL, Slemenda CW, Johnston CC. Age and bone mass as predictors of fracture in a prospective study. J Clin Invest. 1988;81(6):1804–9.
15. Sprague SM. Is bone mineral density measurement of any value in a dialysis patient? Semin Dial. 2011;24(4):433–4.
16. Alexander AJ, Jahangir D, Lazarus M, Sprague SM. Imaging in chronic kidney disease-metabolic bone disease. Semin Dial. 2017;30(4):361–8.
17. Jamal SA, Hayden JA, Beyene J. Low bone mineral density and fractures in long-term hemodialysis patients: a meta-analysis. Am J Kidney Dis. 2007;49(5):674–81.
18. Iimori S, Mori Y, Akita W, Kuyama T, Takada S, Asai T, et al. Diagnostic usefulness of bone mineral density and biochemical markers of bone turnover in predicting fracture in CKD stage 5D patients – a single-center cohort study. Nephrol Dial Transplant. 2012;27(1):345–51.
19. West SL, Lok CE, Langsetmo L, Cheung AM, Szabo E, Pearce D, et al. Bone mineral density predicts fractures in chronic kidney disease. J Bone Miner Res. 2015;30(5):913–9.
20. Sturgeon CM, Sprague SM, Metcalfe W. Variation in parathyroid hormone immunoassay results – a critical governance issue in the management of chronic kidney disease. Nephrol Dial Transplant. 2011;26(11):3440–5.
21. Cozzolino M, Tomlinson J, Walsh L, Bellasi A. Emerging drugs for secondary hyperparathyroidism. Expert Opin Emerg Drugs. 2015;20(2):197–208.
22. Sekercioglu N, Angeliki Veroniki A, Thabane L, Busse JW, Akhtar-Danesh N, Iorio A, et al. Effects of different phosphate lowering strategies in patients with CKD on laboratory outcomes: a systematic review and NMA. PLoS One. 2017;12(3):e0171028.
23. Sekercioglu N, Thabane L, Diaz Martinez JP, Nesrallah G, Longo CJ, Busse JW, et al. Comparative effectiveness of phosphate binders in patients with chronic kidney disease: a systematic review and network meta-analysis. PLoS One. 2016;11(6):e0156891.

24. Daugirdas JT, Finn WF, Emmett M, Chertow GM. Frequent hemodialysis network trial G. The phosphate binder equivalent dose. Semin Dial. 2011;24(1):41–9.
25. Floege J, Covic AC, Ketteler M, Rastogi A, Chong EM, Gaillard S, et al. A phase III study of the efficacy and safety of a novel iron-based phosphate binder in dialysis patients. Kidney Int. 2014;86(3):638–47.
26. Van Buren PN, Lewis JB, Dwyer JP, Greene T, Middleton J, Sika M, et al. The phosphate binder ferric citrate and mineral metabolism and inflammatory markers in maintenance dialysis patients: results from prespecified analyses of a randomized clinical trial. Am J Kidney Dis. 2015;66(3):479–88.
27. Yilmaz MI, Sonmez A, Saglam M, Yaman H, Kilic S, Eyileten T, et al. Comparison of calcium acetate and sevelamer on vascular function and fibroblast growth factor 23 in CKD patients: a randomized clinical trial. Am J Kidney Dis. 2012;59(2):177–85.
28. Cozzolino M, Mazzaferro S, Brandenburg V. The treatment of hyperphosphataemia in CKD: calcium-based or calcium-free phosphate binders? Nephrol Dial Transplant. 2011;26(2):402–7.
29. Palmer SC, Gardner S, Tonelli M, Mavridis D, Johnson DW, Craig JC, et al. Phosphate-binding agents in adults with CKD: a network meta-analysis of randomized trials. Am J Kidney Dis. 2016;68(5):691–702.
30. Zisman AL, Hristova M, Ho LT, Sprague SM. Impact of ergocalciferol treatment of vitamin D deficiency on serum parathyroid hormone concentrations in chronic kidney disease. Am J Nephrol. 2007;27(1):36–43.
31. Chandra P, Binongo JN, Ziegler TR, Schlanger LE, Wang W, Someren JT, et al. Cholecalciferol (vitamin D3) therapy and vitamin D insufficiency in patients with chronic kidney disease: a randomized controlled pilot study. Endocr Pract. 2008;14(1):10–7.
32. Sprague SM, Crawford PW, Melnick JZ, Strugnell SA, Ali S, Mangoo-Karim R, et al. Use of extended-release calcifediol to treat secondary hyperparathyroidism in stages 3 and 4 chronic kidney disease. Am J Nephrol. 2016;44(4):316–25.
33. Bhan I, Dobens D, Tamez H, Deferio JJ, Li YC, Warren HS, et al. Nutritional vitamin D supplementation in dialysis: a randomized trial. Clin J Am Soc Nephrol. 2015;10(4):611–9.
34. Massart A, Debelle FD, Racape J, Gervy C, Husson C, Dhaene M, et al. Biochemical parameters after cholecalciferol repletion in hemodialysis: results from the VitaDial randomized trial. Am J Kidney Dis. 2014;64(5):696–705.
35. Coburn JW, Maung HM, Elangovan L, Germain MJ, Lindberg JS, Sprague SM, et al. Doxercalciferol safely suppresses PTH levels in patients with secondary hyperparathyroidism associated with chronic kidney disease stages 3 and 4. Am J Kidney Dis. 2004;43(5):877–90.
36. Coyne D, Acharya M, Qiu P, Abboud H, Batlle D, Rosansky S, et al. Paricalcitol capsule for the treatment of secondary hyperparathyroidism in stages 3 and 4 CKD. Am J Kidney Dis. 2006;47(2):263–76.
37. Nordal KP, Dahl E. Low dose calcitriol versus placebo in patients with predialysis chronic renal failure. J Clin Endocrinol Metab. 1988;67(5):929–36.
38. Rix M, Eskildsen P, Olgaard K. Effect of 18 months of treatment with alfacalcidol on bone in patients with mild to moderate chronic renal failure. Nephrol Dial Transplant. 2004;19(4):870–6.
39. Coyne DW, Goldberg S, Faber M, Ghossein C, Sprague SM. A randomized multicenter trial of paricalcitol versus calcitriol for secondary hyperparathyroidism in stages 3-4 CKD. Clin J Am Soc Nephrol. 2014;9(9):1620–6.
40. Palmer SC, McGregor DO, Macaskill P, Craig JC, Elder GJ, Strippoli GF. Meta-analysis: vitamin D compounds in chronic kidney disease. Ann Intern Med. 2007;147(12):840–53.
41. Block GA, Martin KJ, de Francisco AL, Turner SA, Avram MM, Suranyi MG, et al. Cinacalcet for secondary hyperparathyroidism in patients receiving hemodialysis. N Engl J Med. 2004;350(15):1516–25.
42. Goodman WG, Hladik GA, Turner SA, Blaisdell PW, Goodkin DA, Liu W, et al. The calcimimetic agent AMG 073 lowers plasma parathyroid hormone levels in hemodialysis patients with secondary hyperparathyroidism. J Am Soc Nephrol. 2002;13(4):1017–24.
43. Block GA, Bushinsky DA, Cheng S, Cunningham J, Dehmel B, Drueke TB, et al. Effect of etelcalcetide vs cinacalcet on serum parathyroid hormone in patients receiving hemodialysis with secondary hyperparathyroidism: a randomized clinical trial. JAMA. 2017;317(2):156–64.
44. Block GA, Bushinsky DA, Cunningham J, Drueke TB, Ketteler M, Kewalramani R, et al. Effect of etelcalcetide vs placebo on serum parathyroid hormone in patients receiving hemodialysis with secondary hyperparathyroidism: two randomized clinical trials. JAMA. 2017;317(2):146–55.
45. Lindberg JS, Moe SM, Goodman WG, Coburn JW, Sprague SM, Liu W, et al. The calcimimetic AMG 073 reduces parathyroid hormone and calcium x phosphorus in secondary hyperparathyroidism. Kidney Int. 2003;63(1):248–54.
46. Wetmore JB, Gurevich K, Sprague S, Da Roza G, Buerkert J, Reiner M, et al. A randomized trial of cinacalcet versus vitamin D analogs as monotherapy in secondary hyperparathyroidism (PARADIGM). Clin J Am Soc Nephrol. 2015;10(6):1031–40.
47. Sprague SM, Wetmore JB, Gurevich K, Da Roza G, Buerkert J, Reiner M, et al. Effect of cinacalcet and vitamin D analogs on fibroblast growth factor-23 during the treatment of secondary hyperparathyroidism. Clin J Am Soc Nephrol. 2015;10(6):1021–30.
48. Investigators ET, Chertow GM, Block GA, Correa-Rotter R, Drueke TB, Floege J, et al. Effect of cinacalcet on cardiovascular disease in patients undergoing dialysis. N Engl J Med. 2012;367(26):2482–94.
49. Chonchol M, Locatelli F, Abboud HE, Charytan C, de Francisco AL, Jolly S, et al. A randomized, double-blind, placebo-controlled study to assess the efficacy and safety of cinacalcet HCl in participants

with CKD not receiving dialysis. Am J Kidney Dis. 2009;53(2):197–207.
50. Charytan C, Coburn JW, Chonchol M, Herman J, Lien YH, Liu W, et al. Cinacalcet hydrochloride is an effective treatment for secondary hyperparathyroidism in patients with CKD not receiving dialysis. Am J Kidney Dis. 2005;46(1):58–67.
51. Narayan R, Perkins RM, Berbano EP, Yuan CM, Neff RT, Sawyers ES, et al. Parathyroidectomy versus cinacalcet hydrochloride-based medical therapy in the management of hyperparathyroidism in ESRD: a cost utility analysis. Am J Kidney Dis. 2007;49(6):801–13.
52. Ishani A, Liu J, Wetmore JB, Lowe KA, Do T, Bradbury BD, et al. Clinical outcomes after parathyroidectomy in a nationwide cohort of patients on hemodialysis. Clin J Am Soc Nephrol. 2015;10(1):90–7.
53. Conzo G, Perna AF, Savica V, Palazzo A, Della Pietra C, Ingrosso D, et al. Impact of parathyroidectomy on cardiovascular outcomes and survival in chronic hemodialysis patients with secondary hyperparathyroidism. A retrospective study of 50 cases prior to the calcimimetics era. BMC Surg. 2013;13(Suppl 2):S4.
54. Zangeneh F, Clarke BL, Hurley DL, Watts NB, Miller PD. Chronic Kidney Disease-Mineral and Bone Disorders (CKD-MBDs): what the endocrinologist needs to know. Endocr Pract. 2014;20(5):500–16.
55. Russell RG, Watts NB, Ebetino FH, Rogers MJ. Mechanisms of action of bisphosphonates: similarities and differences and their potential influence on clinical efficacy. Osteoporos Int. 2008;19(6):733–59.
56. Rogers MJ, Crockett JC, Coxon FP, Monkkonen J. Biochemical and molecular mechanisms of action of bisphosphonates. Bone. 2011;49(1):34–41.
57. Mitsopoulos E, Ginikopoulou E, Economidou D, Zanos S, Pateinakis P, Minasidis E, et al. Impact of long-term cinacalcet, ibandronate or teriparatide therapy on bone mineral density of hemodialysis patients: a pilot study. Am J Nephrol. 2012;36(3):238–44.
58. Miller PD. Denosumab: anti-RANKL antibody. Curr Osteoporos Rep. 2009;7(1):18–22.
59. Jamal SA, Ljunggren O, Stehman-Breen C, Cummings SR, McClung MR, Goemaere S, et al. Effects of denosumab on fracture and bone mineral density by level of kidney function. J Bone Miner Res. 2011;26(8):1829–35.
60. Block GA, Bone HG, Fang L, Lee E, Padhi D. A single-dose study of denosumab in patients with various degrees of renal impairment. J Bone Miner Res. 2012;27(7):1471–9.
61. Ivanov P, Khedr M. Prolonged hypocalcaemia following a single dose of 60 mg denosumab in two patients with CKD 4/5 on cinacalcet treatment for tertiary hyperparathyroidism. Clin Kidney J. 2013;6(2):245.
62. Miller PD, Bilezikian JP, Deal C, Harris ST, Ci RP. Clinical use of teriparatide in the real world: initial insights. Endocr Pract. 2004;10(2):139–48.
63. Leder BZ, O'Dea LS, Zanchetta JR, Kumar P, Banks K, McKay K, et al. Effects of abaloparatide, a human parathyroid hormone-related peptide analog, on bone mineral density in postmenopausal women with osteoporosis. J Clin Endocrinol Metab. 2015;100(2):697–706.
64. Miller PD, Hattersley G, Riis BJ, Williams GC, Lau E, Russo LA, et al. Effect of abaloparatide vs placebo on new vertebral fractures in postmenopausal women with osteoporosis: a randomized clinical trial. JAMA. 2016;316(7):722–33.
65. Cosman F, Hattersley G, Hu MY, Williams GC, Fitzpatrick LA, Black DM. Effects of abaloparatide-SC on fractures and bone mineral density in subgroups of postmenopausal women with osteoporosis and varying baseline risk factors. J Bone Miner Res. 2017;32(1):17–23.
66. Neer RM, Arnaud CD, Zanchetta JR, Prince R, Gaich GA, Reginster JY, et al. Effect of parathyroid hormone (1-34) on fractures and bone mineral density in postmenopausal women with osteoporosis. N Engl J Med. 2001;344(19):1434–41.
67. Kaufman JM, Orwoll E, Goemaere S, San Martin J, Hossain A, Dalsky GP, et al. Teriparatide effects on vertebral fractures and bone mineral density in men with osteoporosis: treatment and discontinuation of therapy. Osteoporos Int. 2005;16(5):510–6.
68. Saag KG, Shane E, Boonen S, Marin F, Donley DW, Taylor KA, et al. Teriparatide or alendronate in glucocorticoid-induced osteoporosis. N Engl J Med. 2007; 357(20):2028–39.
69. Gluer CC, Marin F, Ringe JD, Hawkins F, Moricke R, Papaioannu N, et al. Comparative effects of teriparatide and risedronate in glucocorticoid-induced osteoporosis in men: 18-month results of the EuroGIOPs trial. J Bone Miner Res. 2013;28(6):1355–68.
70. Nishikawa A, Yoshiki F, Taketsuna M, Kajimoto K, Enomoto H. Safety and effectiveness of daily teriparatide for osteoporosis in patients with severe stages of chronic kidney disease: post hoc analysis of a post-marketing observational study. Clin Interv Aging. 2016;11:1653–9.
71. Miller PD, Schwartz EN, Chen P, Misurski DA, Krege JH. Teriparatide in postmenopausal women with osteoporosis and mild or moderate renal impairment. Osteoporos Int. 2007;18(1):59–68.
72. Cejka D, Kodras K, Bader T, Haas M. Treatment of hemodialysis-associated adynamic bone disease with Teriparatide (PTH1-34): a pilot study. Kidney Blood Press Res. 2010;33(3):221–6.
73. Palcu P, Dion N, Ste-Marie LG, Goltzman D, Radziunas I, Miller PD, et al. Teriparatide and bone turnover and formation in a hemodialysis patient with low-turnover bone disease: a case report. Am J Kidney Dis. 2015;65(6):933–6.

Mineral and Bone Disorders Following Renal Transplantation

18

Hatem Amer and Rajiv Kumar

Introduction

Bone disease and abnormalities in calcium and phosphorus metabolism frequently occur in patients who have received a renal allograft [1]. Changes seen in transplant recipients reflect, in part, antecedent renal osteodystrophy that develops on account of chronic renal failure and end-stage renal disease (ESRD) [2–5]. Many transplant recipients with ESRD will have been maintained on dialysis for varying periods of time prior to receiving a transplant and will have alterations in bone mineral metabolism that are influenced by the amount of time that they have been on dialysis and therapy that they have received while on hemodialysis or peritoneal dialysis. Additionally, changes in bone mineral metabolism develop as a result of therapy required to prevent organ rejection. Antirejection therapy with various drugs, especially glucocorticoids [6–16], but also other antirejection agents such as calcineurin inhibitors (cyclosporine or tacrolimus) [17–19], influences bone and mineral metabolism, and phenotypic abnormalities seen in patients at any given time reflect many of the variables mentioned above. It should be remembered that antirejection therapy is rapidly evolving with the use of biologic agents such thymoglobulin [20], anti-CD3 antibodies [21, 22], and anti-CD52 antibody (*alemtuzumab*) [23–27] and the amount of corticosteroids used for antirejection therapy have been decreasing. Finally, many transplant programs proactively treat bone disease with defined treatment protocols thereby influencing outcomes. Hence, one can anticipate that the changes seen in bone and mineral metabolism in the future may be different than those seen in the past.

Changes in bone and mineral metabolism also occur in subjects who have donated a kidney. Each year approximately 30,000 people worldwide become living kidney donors [28–30]. In the USA in 2016, about 30% of all transplants performed were from living donors [28]. Living kidney donation is not without health risks to the donor. Although it is appreciated that the risk of ESRD is increased following kidney donation [31–33], it is less well appreciated that there are abnormalities in bone and mineral metabolism seen within six months of kidney donation

H. Amer (✉)
Division of Nephrology and Hypertension, Department of Internal Medicine, Mayo Clinic, Rochester, MN, USA
e-mail: amer.hatem@mayo.edu

R. Kumar (✉)
Division of Nephrology and Hypertension, Departments of Internal Medicine, Biochemistry, and Molecular Biology, Mayo Clinic, Rochester, MN, USA
e-mail: rkumar@mayo.edu

C. M. Rhee et al. (eds.), *Endocrine Disorders in Kidney Disease*,
https://doi.org/10.1007/978-3-319-97765-2_18

[34, 35]. The changes are sustained for at least three years and perhaps longer. Hence, healthy volunteers who have donated a kidney are at risk for bone disease as they age. The study of this population of patients will yield new information regarding the effects of reductions in glomerular filtration rate (GFR) in the absence of disease on bone turnover.

Bone Disease and Mineral Abnormalities in Renal Transplant Recipients

Prior to transplantation, well-defined skeletal abnormalities and extra-osseous mineral changes (chronic kidney disease-mineral bone disorder, CKD-MBD) are present in patients with CKD and ESRD [36–39]. These skeletal abnormalities may be ameliorated following transplantation. They do, however, persist for several months following transplantation. The bone is, however, altered as a result of the administration of anti-rejection drugs, predominantly glucocorticoids, which have unique effects on the bone and that are responsible for the altered bone architecture that is observed at later times following transplantation.

Renal osteodystrophy in CKD and ESRD patients prior to transplantation comprises several groups including secondary hyperparathyroidism of varying severity, mixed uremic osteodystrophy, osteomalacia, and adynamic bone disease, which are best assessed by quantitative bone histomorphometry and the analysis of bone turnover following the administration of tetracycline to label bone [40–46]. Hyperparathyroidism, the most frequent type of renal osteodystrophy in CKD and ESRD prior to transplantation [41, 47–52], is generally detectable by the time GFR reaches 40–50 mL/minute/1.73m^2 [42, 45, 53–56]. Phosphate retention [19, 42, 57–63], a decline in concentrations of 1α,25 dihydroxyvitamin D_3 (1α,25$(OH)_2$D) [38, 39, 64–71] with an attendant decrease in intestinal calcium absorption and hypocalcemia [72–75], increased concentrations of parathyroid hormone (PTH), increased fibroblast growth factor 23 (FGF-23) concentrations [76–81], and diminished acid excretion by the kidney [82–84] occur when the GFR has decreased to 30–50 mL/min/1.73m^2 and contribute to the pathogenesis of CKD-MBD. An analysis of bone histomorphometry of 630 patients with renal osteodystrophy and CKD/ESRD showed racial differences in the type of osteodystrophy observed [52]. Malluche et al. reported that 62% of whites had low bone turnover, whereas 68% of blacks had high turnover. A mineralization defect was observed in only 3% of patients. Cancellous bone volume was low, normal, or high in approximately the same number of white patients, whereas in blacks, cancellous bone volume was high in two-thirds. Low cancellous bone volume and thin trabeculae occurred in blacks and whites with low bone formation. Seventy-five percent of blacks had normal cortical thickness compared to 50% of whites. Cortical porosity was high in 50% of whites and 75% of blacks. Despite these findings, bone mineral density assessed by dual-energy X-ray absorptiometry has been quite variable [85–90]. The incidence of hip and vertebral fractures is increased in patients with CKD/ESRD and is reduced in these patients following parathyroidectomy [91–100].

Characteristics and Pathophysiology of Bone Prior to and Following Renal Transplantation

Many of the pathophysiological abnormalities driving the occurrence of renal osteodystrophy disappear or are diminished following kidney transplantation. Phosphate retention disappears as GFR is restored, 1α,25$(OH)_2$D concentrations normalize, and PTH and FGF-23 concentrations decrease [101–103]. These changes have dramatic effects on bone remodeling in the immediate transplant period. Rojas et al. examined early alterations in osteoblast number and surfaces, 22–160 days following renal transplantation [2]. A decrease in osteoid and osteoblast surfaces, adjusted bone formation rate, and prolonged mineralization lag time were observed.

Peritrabecular fibrosis markedly decreased. Posttransplant osteoblast surface correlated positively with PTH levels and negatively with glucocorticoid cumulative dose. Lehmann et al. performed bone biopsies in 57 patients an average of 53.5 months following transplantation. Of note, these biopsies were not samples obtained in random patients, but were performed for specific clinical indications such as hypercalcemia and persistent elevations of PTH. Patients had been on hemodialysis for a mean of 43 months prior to transplant. The cumulative dose of glucocorticoid received in these individuals was approximately 5.5 grams. Mild osteitis fibrosa and more marked osteitis fibrosa were the most frequent forms of renal osteodystrophy and were observed in 13 (22.8%) and 14 patients (24.6%), respectively. Mixed uremic osteodystrophy was found in seven patients (12.3%), and adynamic renal bone disease was observed in three patients (5.3%). Osteomalacia was noted in two patients (3.5%). In 13 patients (22.8%), reduced bone mass and structural damage without typical signs of renal osteodystrophy, such as endosteal fibrosis or osteoclasia, were detected, and 5 patients (8.7%) showed normal histomorphometric parameters. Carlini et al. examined bone biopsies by bone histomorphometry in 25 asymptomatic men with normal renal function approximately 7.5 years following renal transplantation [104]. Serum intact parathyroid hormone (PTH) levels were elevated in about half of the subjects. Mean BMD at the lumbar spine and femoral neck was low in the entire group. Bone histomorphometric analysis showed higher than normal bone resorption, osteoid volume, and osteoid surfaces in the majority of patients. However, bone formation rate and mineralization surface were low, and mineralization time was delayed in most patients. These lesions were more severe in patients after 3–4 years of transplantation but improved with time and approached normal values after a period of 10 years. Borchhardt et al. examined bone biopsy specimens in 17 patients with hypercalcemic hyperparathyroidism in the posttransplant state [105]. High-turnover renal osteodystrophy (ROD) was present in nine and low-turnover ROD in eight patients. The bone formation rate was significantly associated with bone alkaline phosphatase, c-telopeptide, and osteocalcin. Interestingly, lumbosacral and femoral neck T-scores did not differ significantly between the patients with low- or high-turnover disease. Monier-Faugere et al. examined bone biopsies in 57 adult posttransplant (32 men and 25 women) who had received a kidney transplant 5.6 +/− 0.8 years before biopsy [106]. Bone pain, fractures, and avascular necrosis were present in 38.5, 21.0, and 12% of patients. 21% of patients were hypercalcemic, 63.2% had elevated PTH (>65 pg/ml), and 91.2% had normal calcitriol levels. Cancellous bone volume/tissue volume, bone turnover, and bone formation rate were reduced in about half of all patients. Mineralization was prolonged in 87.5% of patients, including nine patients with osteomalacia and 12 patients with focal osteomalacia. The dose of prednisone and time elapsed since transplantation correlated negatively with bone volume and bone turnover, whereas cumulative doses of cyclosporine or azathioprine, age, gender, or serum PTH levels did not. In summary, bone biopsy findings are dependent upon whether the patients have symptomatic bone disease or changes in serum calcium and PTH and are dependent upon the time since transplantation. Most patients have bone disease that is characterized by low bone turnover and low bone volume.

The changes in bone histomorphometry are associated with reductions in bone mineral density [9, 13, 19, 104, 107–126]. The change in bone mineral density occurs relatively rapidly following renal transplantation [127] (Fig. 18.1). The decrease is associated with an increase in the fracture rate as well as the rate of aseptic necrosis of the hip [94, 108, 109, 114, 116, 128–137].

Factors associated with changes in bone histology, bone density, and fracture rate include the duration of dialysis prior to transplantation, elevated PTH concentrations, elevated FGF-23, the duration and dose of corticosteroid therapy, the administration of calcineurin inhibitors, vitamin D receptor polymorphisms, and the presence of diabetes [110, 111, 138–149].

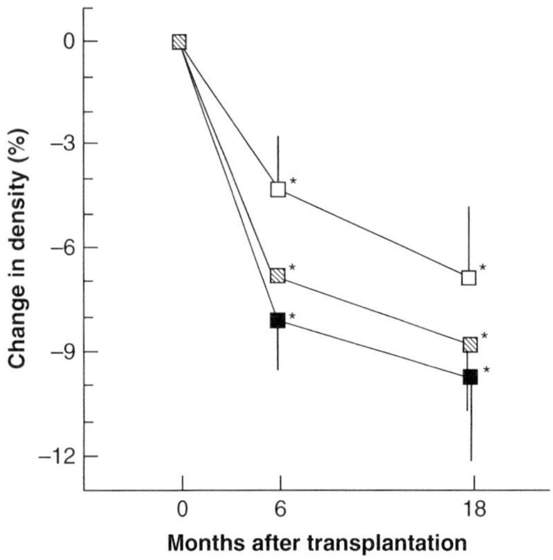

Fig. 18.1 Mean (±SE) percent changes in bone mineral density of the second, third, and fourth lumbar vertebrae after transplantation in all patients (hatched squares), male patients (solid squares), and female patients (open squares). (Julian et al. [127])

Role of Immunosuppressive Agents in Posttransplant Bone Disease

Immunosuppressive agents are needed for the life of renal allografts [150]. In addition to the side effects of generalized immunosuppression, many of these agents have an impact on bone mineral metabolism and bone health.

Corticosteroids

Of the current immunosuppressive agents, corticosteroids have been used the longest being the backbone of immunosuppressive regimens from the earliest times of allotransplantation [150]. The dose used and duration of varying regimens of corticosteroids have varied over the years [151–154]. Even in corticosteroid avoidance regimens, corticosteroids are frequently used in high doses early on as part of the immunosuppressive induction regimen.

Several studies have confirmed that glucocorticoids increase the incidence of posttransplant bone loss, reduce the quality of trabecular bone, and correlate with an increased risk of bone fractures. A significant part of the negative impact of glucocorticoids on the bone occurs in the first few months posttransplant and are likely related to the higher doses used in the early posttransplant period [155–159]. Immunosuppressive regimens that avoid the use of glucocorticoids have been associated with improved bone density and reduced fractures post-kidney transplantation, albeit with a higher incidence of rejection and subclinical inflammation [151, 160–165].

The effects of glucocorticoids on bone metabolism are varied. They exert effects on the various cells involved in bone integrity (osteoblasts, osteoclasts, and osteocytes) resulting in uncoupling of bone resorption and formation with a decrease in overall bone density and decreased quality of trabecular bone (Fig. 18.2) [166].

Improved bone density and decreased fracture risk have been the most compelling findings favoring glucocorticoid avoidance regimens in transplant populations [103, 152, 154, 165]. Identifying patients who would benefit from these regimens and not be at a clinically significant risk of rejection is the challenge. In our kidney/pancreas transplant program, we utilize a corticosteroid-free regimen in patients of low immunologic risk and couple this with a surveillance biopsy program to identify grafts with subclinical inflammation, thus hoping to reap the benefit of corticosteroid avoidance and mitigate the risk of their absence.

Calcineurin Inhibitors

The introduction of cyclosporine in the 1980s revolutionized solid organ transplantation [150]. It increased the one-year survival of kidney allografts to greater than 80% and allowed the adoption of liver and heart transplantation as plausible treatment modalities for end-stage liver and heart failure, respectively. Patients treated with cyclosporine have an increased fracture risk [113, 114, 167]. This increased risk has been attributed to increased bone turnover, with bone loss increasing over bone formation due to uncoupling of the normal bone turnover. Several molecular mechanisms have been implicated in this [149, 168]. Some studies have found that if cyclosporine is used without glucocorticoids, there is either no change in bone density or there is in fact an increase in bone density [169]. The newer and more commonly used calcineurin inhibitor, tacrolimus, has

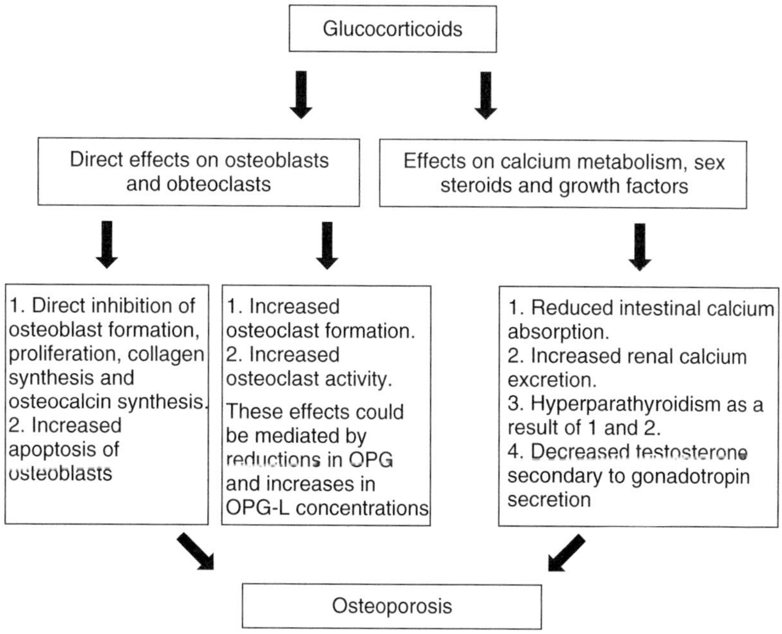

Fig. 18.2 Direct and indirect effects of glucocorticoids on the bone. (Adapted from Kumar [166])

been found to have similar effects to cyclosporine. Animal models have shown a less deleterious effect of tacrolimus over cyclosporine, a finding that may be substantiated in human liver transplant recipients [170]. How much of the favorable findings in humans are due to a difference in pharmacodynamics of the drugs vs. the reduced exposure to corticosteroids given the higher immunosuppressive potency of tacrolimus is not known.

A rare but serious complication of calcineurin inhibitors is the calcineurin inhibitor pain syndrome (CIPS). This is believed to be due to intraosseous hypertension and/or ischemia brought about by the vasoconstrictive effects of calcineurin inhibitors that can be reversed with calcium channel blockers [171–173].

mTOR Inhibitors (Mammalian Target of Rapamycin)

These agents were introduced in the 1990s with the hope that their antiproliferative, anti-fibrotic properties coupled with their immunosuppressive effects will provide the same benefit of calcineurin inhibitors but avoid the calcineurin inhibitor nephrotoxic effects. Both available agents, sirolimus and everolimus, have been found to exert effects on bone remodeling [174]. One study showed a possible beneficial effect in human renal transplant recipients with reduced markers of osteoclast activity [175]. Several animal studies have provided some evidence that these agents may be protective to bones but can have a negative impact on growth plates [19, 176].

The Antimetabolites

Both azathioprine and mycophenolate have not been shown to have any effects on bone metabolism and are believed to be neutral in that regard. We should note, however, that with the introduction of mycophenolate, first as the mofetil form and then the enteric-coated sodium salt, the reduced risk of rejection has encouraged the wider use of corticosteroid avoidance regimens and reduced the incidence of acute cellular rejections and, as such, may have contributed indirectly to better bone health of the transplant populations.

Co-stimulatory Blockade

The first of this new class of agents, belatacept, was approved in 2011. The effects on bone remodeling are yet unknown but are thought to be neutral [177–183].

Therapy of Posttransplant Hyperparathyroidism

Hyperparathyroidism persists for many months after transplantation and contributes to significant derangements in bone mineral metabolism [101, 184–187]. During the pre-transplant period with decreased renal function, phosphate retention, and vitamin D deficiency, the parathyroid glands undergo hypertrophy and hyperplasia. There is an obligate basal rate of release of parathyroid hormone from each parathyroid gland cell. Following restoration of renal function with transplantation, these hypertrophied glands result in a protracted period of excess parathyroid hormone. The prevalence of persistent hyperparathyroidism, defined as an intact PTH level > or = 2.5 times the upper normal limit or the need for parathyroidectomy following transplantation, was 17% up to four years after transplantation [101].

Treating this posttransplant hyperparathyroidism is a major target of interventional therapies to minimize the posttransplant bone morbidity.

Parathyroidectomy

Surgical excision of a substantial portion of parathyroid glandular tissue will result in abrupt decrease in PTH production and correction of posttransplant secondary hyperparathyroidism. This approach has been associated with an increased risk of allograft loss though this has been questioned [188–199]. Pre-transplant parathyroidectomy in patients with markedly elevated PTH levels may be an underutilized intervention at this time [200–202].

Vitamin D and Vitamin D Receptor Analogs

Similar to their use in hyperparathyroidism of chronic renal disease, these have been used in the therapy of posttransplant hyperparathyroidism as vitamin D deficiency persists following transplantation [203]. We noted previous studies showing the improved survival of dialysis patients treated with paricalcitol as compared to calcitriol [204]. We hypothesized that paricalcitol, a synthetic vitamin D receptor analog, would be effective in lowering posttransplant hyperparathyroidism and would be well-tolerated with a lower incidence of hypercalcemia. To examine this, we conducted the first trial of paricalcitol in renal transplant recipients [103]. This trial enrolled de novo renal transplant recipients and randomized patients 1:1 to standard Mayo Clinic posttransplant care vs. Mayo Clinic posttransplant care plus 2 micrograms of paricalcitol orally daily for the first year posttransplant. Fifty one patients were randomized to the paricalcitol arm and 49 to the control arm. Paricalcitol was well-tolerated. Calcium supplementation was discontinued due to hypercalcemia in two control subjects and in 15 treated patients. The dose of paricalcitol was reduced in two patients due to hypercalcemia/hypercalciuria, and in four, it was discontinued. One year from transplant, hyperparathyroidism (primary end point) was present in 63% of controls and in only 29% of treated patients (p = 0.005). Figure 18.3 shows the trends in PTH over the study period. Bone density improved similarly in both groups. Of note, patients in this trial were maintained on corticosteroid-free immunosuppressive regimen. These findings were confirmed in another trial [205].

An additional interesting finding in our trial was the salutary effect of paricalcitol on renal histology examined by surveillance biopsies. We observed a statistically significant difference in moderate to severe fibrosis at one-year posttransplant favoring therapy—4 (10.5%) vs. 0 (0%) had ci score ≥ 2 $p = 0.04$. There was also numerically fewer allografts exhibiting any inflammation at one year in the paricalcitol-treated patients: four (10.5%) vs. nine (23.7%) $p = 0.22$.

Calcimimetics

Sensipar® (cinacalcet) activates the calcium-sensing receptor on the parathyroid cells, simulating hypercalcemia and decreasing PTH secretion [206–215]. Calcimimetics have been used predominantly in situations where there is hypercalcemic hyperparathyroidism posttransplant

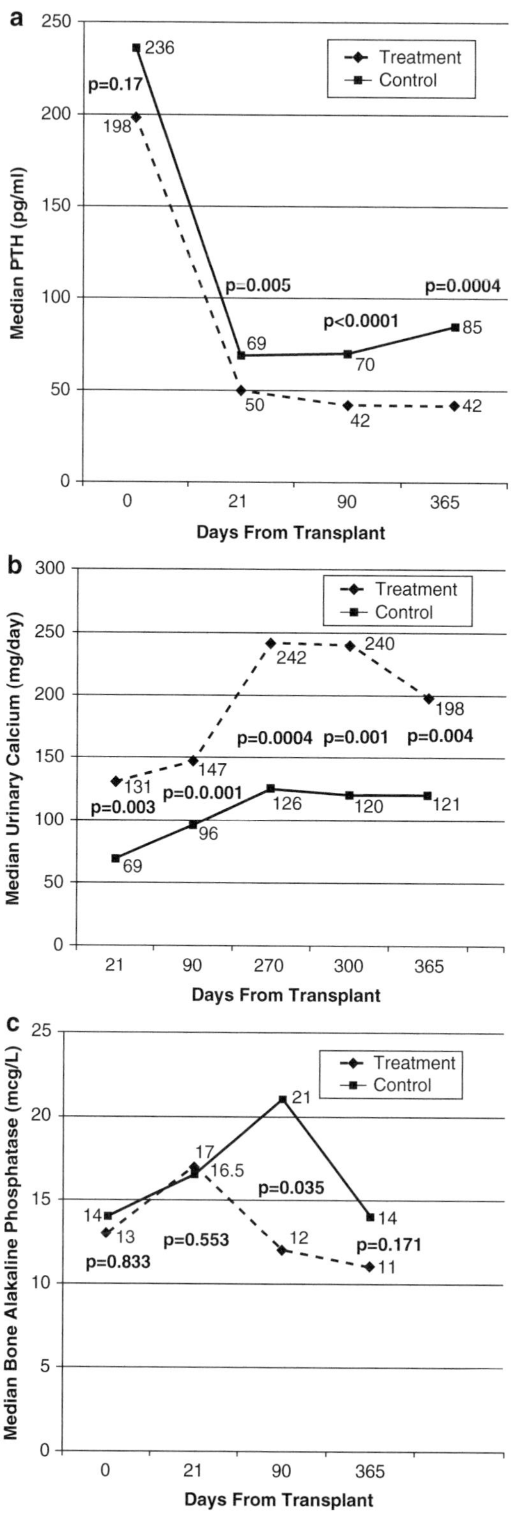

Fig. 18.3 The change in (**a**) median parathyroid levels, (**b**) 24-h urine calcium levels, (**c**) bone alkaline phosphatase at various time points during the study. P values are between groups (treatment vs. control) [103]

[216–223]. Uniformly they decrease PTH and serum calcium levels. The effects of cinacalcet on bone mineral density after transplantation have been varied. There is also a concern regarding the associated hypercalciuria that accompanies therapy. As with other agents, careful monitoring of serum and urine calcium and phosphorus is warranted in our opinion [195, 224–244].

Bisphosphonates in Renal Transplant Recipients

There have been several trials of bisphosphonates in renal transplant recipients (Table 18.1) [1]. These have shown a beneficial effect on bone density, but as of yet, have not shown a decrease in bone fracture rates [124, 126, 245–251]. There is also a concern that excessive use may result in development of, or worsening of, adynamic bone disease [1].

In our kidney/pancreas program, we have a structured and protocol-driven approach to posttransplant bone disease. This involved the minimization of corticosteroids in selected individuals; surveillance of bone mineral density on an annual or semiannual basis depending on therapy undertaken; supplementation with vitamin D analogs; encouraging adequate dietary calcium intake and physical exercise, with judicious, time-limited use of bisphosphonates with monitoring of bone turnover; and in selected individuals measurement of anabolic hormones.

Bone Disease in Living Kidney Donors

Each year approximately 30,000 people worldwide become living kidney donors [28–30]. In the USA in 2016, 5631 living donor transplants were performed from a total of 19,062 kidney transplants [28]. Living kidney donation is not without health risks to the donor. For example, the 15-year observed risk of ESRD in kidney donors is 3.5 to 5.3 times higher than the projected risk in the absence of donation [31–33]. In a definitive prospective study, we measured markers of mineral and bone metabolism in

Table 18.1 Studies reporting the effects of bisphosphonate or vitamin D analog use in prevention and treatment of posttransplantation osteopenia/osteoporosis

Study/reference	Therapy	Outcome
Grotz et al. [245]	Ibandronate	Less bone loss, spinal deformation in ibandronate
Fan et al. [124]	Pamidronate	Preserved lumbar and femoral neck BMD in pamidronate treated group
Haas et al. [246]	Zoledronic acid	Improved LS BMD, stable femoral neck BMD
Coco et al. [247]	Pamidronate + vitamin D/Ca or vitamin D/Ca alone	Preserved spine BMD with increased risk of adynamic bone disease with pamidronate
Jeffery et al. [126]	Alendronate and Ca versus calcitriol and Ca	Improved LS and femoral neck BMD in both groups; alendronate preserved BMD better than calcitriol and Ca
El-Agroudy et al. [248]	Alendronate or alphacalcidol or calcitonin vs. control	Improved LS and femoral neck BMD with treatment
Nowacka-Cieciura et al. [249]	Alendronate or risedronate or no drug	Improved BMD in femoral neck in bisphosphonate-treated group
Torregrosa et al. [250]	Residronate + daily vitamin D/Ca or vitamin D/Ca alone	Increased LS BMD in risedronate-treated group
Abediazar et al. [251]	Alendronate plus daily vitamin D or of daily vitamin D alone	Increased distal radius and LS BMD in alendronate-treated group

Modified from Alshayeb et al. [1]
Abbreviations: *BMD* bone mineral density, *LS* lumbar spine, *Ca* calcium

182 kidney donors and 173 paired normal controls after kidney donation [35]. Donors had significantly higher serum intact PTH and FGF-23 concentrations and significantly lower serum $1,25(OH)_2D$ and inorganic phosphate (Pi) concentrations and measured GFR and reduced tubular reabsorption of phosphate, six and 36 months after donation compared to healthy controls. Higher concentrations of bone resorption markers, carboxyterminal cross-linking telopeptide of collagen (CTX) and aminoterminal cross-linking telopeptide of collagen (NTX), and the bone formation markers, osteocalcin (OC) and procollagen type I N-terminal propeptide (P1NP), were observed in donors compared to healthy controls (Table 18.2). Small retrospective/prospective studies have shown similar findings [140, 252–256]. Note that bone formation was increased due to the well-recognized "coupling" of bone formation to bone resorption [257]; however, in adults, increased bone turnover is uniformly associated with an increase in bone resorption relative to formation, bone microarchitectural deterioration, and bone loss [258]. Figure 18.4 summarizes the mechanism by which we believe changes in bone quality may occur. The studies suggest that bone quality might be impaired in kidney donors, predisposing them to fractures. Further studies in this regard will be important in establishing the risk of bone disease in living kidney donors.

Summary and Conclusions

Bone disease in the context of renal transplantation is a significant clinical problem that can be ameliorated by several approaches including limitation of steroid usage and the judicious use of vitamin D analogs, calcium supplements, and anti-resorptive agents such as calcitonin and bisphosphonates. One should also be aware of the fact that mineral metabolism is altered in kidney donors and might be a harbinger of increased bone loss especially as subjects age.

Table 18.2 The effect of kidney donation on mineral and bone disorder biomarkers

		Visits			*P* values donors versus controls		
Test	Group	Baseline before	6 months after	36 months after	Baseline	6 months	36 months
Serum calcium (mg/dl)	Controls	9.14 (9.08–9.19) [169]	9.19 (9.13–9.25) [165]	9.21 (9.15–9.27) [170]	0.02	0.24	0.26
	Donors	9.24 (9.19–9.30) [164]	9.24 (9.18–9.30) [174]	9.26 (9.20–9.32) [179]			
Tubular resorption of calcium %	Controls	99.3 (99.2–99.4) [166]	99.3 (99.2–99.4) [162]	99.2 (99.2–99.3) [165]	0.16	0.19	0.36
	Donors	99.2 (99.1–99.3) [158]	99.2 (99.1–99.3) [172]	99.2 (99.1–99.3) [176]			
Serum phosphate (mg/dl)	Controls	3.48 (3.40–3.56) [167]	3.51 (3.43–3.58) [165]	3.51 (3.44–3.57) [169]	0.66	<0.001	0.12
	Donors	3.51 (3.43–3.58) [164]	3.28 (3.21–3.35) [174]	3.42 (3.35–3.50) [175]			
Tubular resorption of phosphate %	Controls	90.3 (89.6–91.0) [164]	90.3 (89.6–91.0) [162]	90.1 (89.4–90.8) [164]	0.54	<0.001	<0.001
	Donors	89.9 (891–90.7) [164]	84.0 (83.1–85.0) [172]	85.6 (84.7–86.5) [172]			
Serum parathyroid hormone (pg/ml)	Controls	32.9 (30.9–34.9) [169]	32.7 (30.9–34.6) [165]	32.9 (30.7–35.2) [170]	0.44	<0.001	<0.001
	Donors	31.9 (29.8–34.0) [164]	40.7 (38.3–43.1) [174]	39.3 (36.7–42.0) [179]			
Serum FGF-23 (pg/ml)	Controls	49.7 (40.9–59.5) [169]	50.3 (40.6–60.2) [165]	53.2 (42.6–61.5) [170]	0.04[b]	0.02[b]	0.02[b]
	Donors	45.1 (38.7–55.4) [164]	55.1 (43.9–66.2) [174]	54.9 (42.6–61.5) [179]			
Serum aminoterminal cross-linking telopeptide of bone type I collagen (ng/ml)	Controls	12.6 (9.9–16.0) [169]	13.4 (10.4–16.4) [165]	13.5 (10.9–17.8) [170]	0.69[b]	<0.001[b]	0.001[b]
	Donors	12.8 (10.2–16.0) [164]	15.3 (11.6–19.7) [174]	15.3 (11.7–20.1 [179]			
Serum carboxyterminal cross-linking telopeptide of bone type I collagen (ng/ml)	Controls	0.33 (0.27–0.49) [169]	0.36 (0.28–0.48) [165]	0.37 (0.28–0.48) [170]	0.47[b]	<0.001[b]	0.002[b]
	Donors	0.36 [0.27–0.52] [164]	0.46 [0.32–0.58] [173]	0.42 [0.31–0.63] [179]			
Serum tartrate-resistant acid phosphatase 5b (U/l)	Controls	2.40 (2.31–2.49) [169]	2.36 (2.27–2.44) [165]	2.46 (2.37–2.56) [170]	0.10	0.03	0.21
	Donors	2.53 (2.42–2.64) [164]	2.49 (2.39–2.59) [174]	2.55 (2.45–2.66) [179]			
Serum osteocalcin (ng/ml)	Controls	19.1 [15.4–24.2] [169]	19.2 [15.6–23.7] [165]	20.3 [15.8–24.6] [170]	0.36[b]	<0.001[b]	<0.001[b]
	Donors	19.8 [16.0–25.0] [164]	23.8 [18.7–31.1] [174]	22.1 [17.2–29.6] [179]			
Serum alkaline phosphatase (U/l)	Controls	68.7 (65.2–72.1) [164]	66.4 (63.2–69.7) [161]	65.3 (62.5–68.0) [169]	0.45	0.03	0.13
	Donors	71.2 (67.9–74.5) [159]	71.7 (68.4–75.1) [173]	68.2 (65.3–71.0) [177]			
Serum bone alkaline phosphatase (U/l)	Controls	21.2 [17.3–25.3] [169]	21.1 [18.0–26.3] [165]	21.4 [17.4–25.7] [170]	0.012[b]	0.002[b]	0.011[b]
	Donors	23.4 [19.1–28.3] [164]	24.8 [19.4–29.5] [174]	23.7 [19.1–28.4] [179]			
Serum procollagen type I (μg/l)	Controls	47.2 [35.7–57.1] [166]	43.6 [36.8–60.2] [161]	46.5 [35.2–62.4] [165]	0.38[b]	0.001[b]	0.11[b]
	Donors	49.5 [36.5–63.4] [159]	55.0 [39.7–70.3] [166]	47.7 [36.0–69.0] [172]			
Serum 1,25(OH)$_2$D$_3$ (pg/ml)	Controls	51.1 (49.1–53.1) [163]	53.0 (50.6–55.3) [164]	50.7 (48.4–52.9) [161]	0.75	<0.001	<0.001
	Donors	51.7 (49.2–54.2) [164]	43.9 (41.8–46.0) [170]	44.3 (42.2–46.3) [173]			
Serum 25(OH)D$_3$ (ng/ml)	Controls	26.4 (24.9–27.9) [169]	27.5 (26.1–28.9) [165]	28.8 (27.0–30.6) [170]	0.71	<0.001	<0.001
	Donors	27.1 (25.5–28.6) [164]	33.3 (31.4–35.1) [174]	34.4 (32.7–36.2) [179]			
Serum 25(OH)D total (ng/ml)	Controls	27.1 (25.5–28.6) [168]	28.0 (26.7–29.4) [165]	29.4 (27.7–31.1) [170]	0.55	<0.001	<0.001
	Donors	28.0 (26.4–29.6) [164]	34.0 (32.2–35.9) [174]	35.1 (33.3–36.9) [179]			

Kasiske et al. [35]

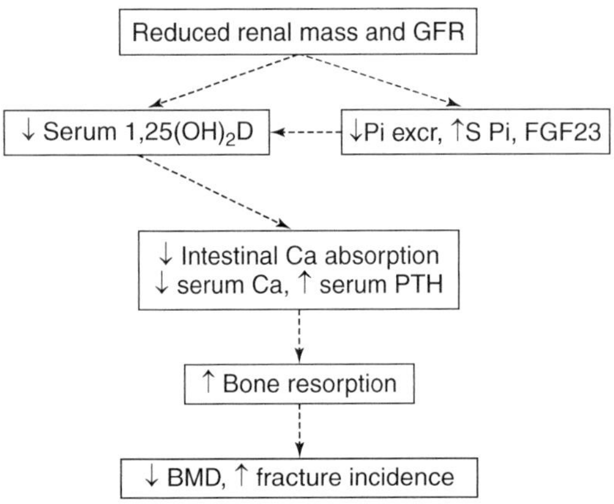

Fig. 18.4 Proposed mechanism by which changes in bone mineral density (BMD) and fractures may occur in patient's post-kidney donation

References

1. Alshayeb HM, Josephson MA, Sprague SM. CKD-mineral and bone disorder management in kidney transplant recipients. Am J Kidney Dis. 2013;61(2):310–25.
2. Rojas E, Carlini RG, Clesca P, Arminio A, Suniaga O, De Elguezabal K, et al. The pathogenesis of osteodystrophy after renal transplantation as detected by early alterations in bone remodeling. Kidney Int. 2003;63(5):1915–23.
3. Bonomini V, Bortolotti GC, Feletti C, Scolari MP. Serial histomorphometric and histochemical bone biopsy studies in dialysis and transplantation. J Urol Nephrol (Paris). 1975;81(12):941–50.
4. Bonomini V, Feletti C, Di Felice A, Buscaroli A. Bone remodelling after renal transplantation (RT). Adv Exp Med Biol. 1984;178:207–16.
5. Lehmann G, Ott U, Stein G, Steiner T, Wolf G. Renal osteodystrophy after successful renal transplantation: a histomorphometric analysis in 57 patients. Transplant Proc. 2007;39(10):3153–8.
6. Almond MK, Kwan JT, Evans K, Cunningham J. Loss of regional bone mineral density in the first 12 months following renal transplantation. Nephron. 1994;66(1):52–7.
7. Aroldi A, Ponticelli C. Skeletal complications after renal transplantation. Int J Artif Organs. 1998;21(5):251–4.
8. Blaslov K, Katalinic L, Kes P, Spasovski G, Smalcelj R, Basic-Jukic N. What is the impact of immunosuppressive treatment on the post-transplant renal osteopathy? Int Urol Nephrol. 2014;46(5):1019–24.
9. Brandenburg VM, Politt D, Ketteler M, Fassbender WJ, Heussen N, Westenfeld R, et al. Early rapid loss followed by long-term consolidation characterizes the development of lumbar bone mineral density after kidney transplantation. Transplantation. 2004;77(10):1566–71.
10. Haffner D, Schuler U. Metabolic bone disease after renal transplantation. Curr Opin Pediatr. 2014;26(2):198–206.
11. Harrington KD, Murray WR, Kountz SL, Belzer FO. Avascular necrosis of bone after renal transplantation. J Bone Joint Surg Am. 1971;53(2):203–15.
12. Nehme D, Rondeau E, Paillard F, Moreau JF, Nussaume O, Kanfer A, et al. Aseptic necrosis of bone following renal transplantation: relation with hyperparathyroidism. Nephrol Dial Transplant. 1989;4(2):123–8.
13. Rodino MA, Shane E. Osteoporosis after organ transplantation. Am J Med. 1998;104(5):459–69.
14. ter Meulen CG, Hilbrands LB, van den Bergh JP, Hermus AR, Hoitsma AJ. The influence of corticosteroids on quantitative ultrasound parameters of the calcaneus in the 1st year after renal transplantation. Osteoporos Int. 2005;16(3):255–62.
15. Ugur A, Guvener N, Isiklar I, Turan M, Erdal R, Haberal M. Osteoporosis after renal transplantation: single center experience. Transplantation. 2001;71(5):645–9.
16. van den Ham EC, Kooman JP, Christiaans ML, van Hooff JP. The influence of early steroid withdrawal on body composition and bone mineral density in renal transplantation patients. Transpl Int. 2003;16(2):82–7.
17. Aroldi A, Tarantino A, Montagnino G, Cesana B, Cocucci C, Ponticelli C. Effects of three immunosuppressive regimens on vertebral bone density in renal transplant recipients: a prospective study. Transplantation. 1997;63(3):380–6.
18. Briner VA, Landmann J, Brunner FP, Thiel G. Cyclosporin A-induced transient rise in plasma alkaline phosphatase in kidney transplant patients. Transpl Int. 1993;6(2):99–107.
19. Campistol JM, Holt DW, Epstein S, Gioud-Paquet M, Rutault K, Burke JT. Bone metabolism in renal transplant patients treated with cyclosporine or sirolimus. Transpl Int. 2005;18(9):1028–35.
20. Gaber AO, Matas AJ, Henry ML, Brennan DC, Stevens RB, Kapur S, et al. Antithymocyte globulin induction in living donor renal transplant recipients: final report of the TAILOR registry. Transplantation. 2012;94(4):331–7.
21. El-Faramawi M, Rohr N, Jespersen B. Steroid-free immunosuppression after renal transplantation-long-term experience from a single centre. Nephrol Dial Transplant. 2006;21(7):1966–73.
22. Webster AC, Pankhurst T, Rinaldi F, Chapman JR, Craig JC. Monoclonal and polyclonal antibody therapy for treating acute rejection in kidney transplant recipients: a systematic review of randomized trial data. Transplantation. 2006;81(7):953–65.
23. Calne R, Moffatt SD, Friend PJ, Jamieson NV, Bradley JA, Hale G, et al. Campath IH allows low-dose cyclosporine monotherapy in 31 cadaveric renal allograft recipients. Transplantation. 1999;68(10):1613–6.
24. Ciancio G, Burke GW, Gaynor JJ, Mattiazzi A, Roohipour R, Carreno MR, et al. The use of Campath-1H as induction therapy in renal

transplantation: preliminary results. Transplantation. 2004;78(3):426–33.
25. Kaufman DB, Leventhal JR, Axelrod D, Gallon LG, Parker MA, Stuart FP. Alemtuzumab induction and prednisone-free maintenance immunotherapy in kidney transplantation: comparison with basiliximab induction–long-term results. Am J Transplant. 2005;5(10):2539–48.
26. Shapiro R, Basu A, Tan H, Gray E, Kahn A, Randhawa P, et al. Kidney transplantation under minimal immunosuppression after pretransplant lymphoid depletion with thymoglobulin or campath. J Am Coll Surg. 2005;200(4):505–15; quiz A59-61.
27. Ciancio G, Burke GW, Gaynor JJ, Carreno MR, Cirocco RE, Mathew JM, et al. A randomized trial of three renal transplant induction antibodies: early comparison of tacrolimus, mycophenolate mofetil, and steroid dosing, and newer immune-monitoring. Transplantation. 2005;80(4):457–65.
28. (HHS) OUSDoHaHS. Organ Procurement and Transplantation Network; U.S. Department of Health and Human Services. 2015.
29. Horvat LD, Shariff SZ, Garg AX, Donor Nephrectomy Outcomes Research N. Global trends in the rates of living kidney donation. Kidney Int. 2009;75(10):1088–98.
30. USRDS. USRDS 2015 annual data report: atlas of chronic kidney disease and end-stage renal disease in the United States. In: NIH N, Bethesda: National Institutes of Health, editor. 2015.
31. Grams ME, Sang Y, Levey AS, Matsushita K, Ballew S, Chang AR, et al. Kidney-failure risk projection for the living kidney-donor candidate. N Engl J Med. 2016;374(5):411–21.
32. Muzaale AD, Massie AB, Wang MC, Montgomery RA, McBride MA, Wainright JL, et al. Risk of end-stage renal disease following live kidney donation. JAMA. 2014;311(6):579–86.
33. Mjoen G, Hallan S, Hartmann A, Foss A, Midtvedt K, Oyen O, et al. Long-term risks for kidney donors. Kidney Int. 2014;86(1):162–7.
34. Kasiske BL, Anderson-Haag T, Israni AK, Kalil RS, Kimmel PL, Kraus ES, et al. A prospective controlled study of living kidney donors: three-year follow-up. Am J Kidney Dis. 2015;66(1):114–24.
35. Kasiske BL, Kumar R, Kimmel PL, Pesavento TE, Kalil RS, Kraus ES, et al. Abnormalities in biomarkers of mineral and bone metabolism in kidney donors. Kidney Int. 2016;90(4):861–8.
36. Moe S, Drueke T, Cunningham J, Goodman W, Martin K, Olgaard K, et al. Definition, evaluation, and classification of renal osteodystrophy: a position statement from Kidney Disease: Improving Global Outcomes (KDIGO). Kidney Int. 2006;69(11):1945–53.
37. McCarthy JT, Kumar R. Behavior of the vitamin D endocrine system in the development of renal osteodystrophy. Semin Nephrol. 1986;6(1):21–30.
38. McCarthy JT, Kumar R. Renal osteodystrophy. Endocrinol Metab Clin N Am. 1990;19(1):65–93.
39. McCarthy JT, Rajiv K. Role of the vitamin D system in the pathogenesis of renal osteodystrophy. In: Kumar R, editor. Vitamin D: basic and clinical aspects. Dortrecht: Martinus Nijhoff Publishers; 1984. p. 611–40.
40. Ghanekar H, Welch BJ, Moe OW, Sakhaee K. Post-renal transplantation hypophosphatemia: a review and novel insights. Curr Opin Nephrol Hypertens. 2006;15(2):97–104.
41. Martin KJ, Olgaard K, Coburn JW, Coen GM, Fukagawa M, Langman C, et al. Diagnosis, assessment, and treatment of bone turnover abnormalities in renal osteodystrophy. Am J Kidney Dis. 2004;43(3):558–65.
42. Bricker NS, Slatopolsky E, Reiss E, Avioli LV. Caclium, phosphorus, and bone in renal disease and transplantation. Arch Intern Med. 1969;123(5):543–53.
43. London G, Coyne D, Hruska K, Malluche HH, Martin KJ. The new kidney disease: improving global outcomes (KDIGO) guidelines - expert clinical focus on bone and vascular calcification. Clin Nephrol. 2010;74(6):423–32.
44. Malluche HH. Bone disease in renal failure. Introduction. Miner Electrolyte Metab. 1991;17(4):209–10.
45. Malluche HH, Ritz E, Lange HP, Kutschera L, Hodgson M, Seiffert U, et al. Bone histology in incipient and advanced renal failure. Kidney Int. 1976;9(4):355–62.
46. Dempster DW, Compston JE, Drezner MK, Glorieux FH, Kanis JA, Malluche H, et al. Standardized nomenclature, symbols, and units for bone histomorphometry: a 2012 update of the report of the ASBMR Histomorphometry Nomenclature Committee. J Bone Miner Res. 2013;28(1):2–17.
47. Moore C, Yee J, Malluche H, Rao DS, Monier-Faugere MC, Adams E, et al. Relationship between bone histology and markers of bone and mineral metabolism in African-American hemodialysis patients. Clin J Am Soc Nephrol. 2009;4(9):1484–93.
48. Malluche HH, Mawad H, Monier-Faugere MC. Effects of treatment of renal osteodystrophy on bone histology. Clin J Am Soc Nephrol. 2008;3(Suppl 3):S157–63.
49. Malluche HH, Monier-Faugere MC. Renal osteodystrophy: what's in a name? Presentation of a clinically useful new model to interpret bone histologic findings. Clin Nephrol. 2006;65(4):235–42.
50. Qi Q, Monier-Faugere MC, Geng Z, Malluche HH. Predictive value of serum parathyroid hormone levels for bone turnover in patients on chronic maintenance dialysis. Am J Kidney Dis. 1995;26(4):622–31.
51. Malluche HH, Monier-Faugere MC. The role of bone biopsy in the management of patients with renal osteodystrophy. J Am Soc Nephrol. 1994;4(9):1631–42.
52. Malluche HH, Mawad HW, Monier-Faugere MC. Renal osteodystrophy in the first decade of the new millennium: analysis of 630 bone biopsies

in black and white patients. J Bone Miner Res. 2011;26(6):1368–76.
53. Reiss E, Canterbury JM, Kanter A. Circulating parathyroid hormone concentration in chronic renal insufficiency. Arch Intern Med. 1969;124(4):417–22.
54. Potts JT, Reita RE, Deftos LJ, Kaye MB, Richardson JA, Buckle RM, et al. Secondary hyperparathyroidism in chronic renal disease. Arch Intern Med. 1969;124(4):408–12.
55. Norman ME, Mazur AT, Borden S, Gruskin A, Anast C, Baron R, et al. Early diagnosis of juvenile renal osteodystrophy. J Pediatr. 1980;97(2):226–32.
56. Baron R, Mazur A, Norman M. Histomorphometric classification of juvenile renal osteodystrophy: prevalence of mineralizing defect. In: Norman AW, Schaefer K, Herrath DV, Grigoleit H-G, editors. Vitamin D: chemical, biochemical and clinical endocrinology of calcium metabolism. Berlin: Walter de Gruyter; 1982. p. 835–40.
57. Slatopolsky E, Brown A, Dusso A. Pathogenesis of secondary hyperparathyroidism. Kidney Int Suppl. 1999;73:S14–9.
58. Slatopolsky E. The intact nephron hypothesis: the concept and its implications for phosphate management in CKD-related mineral and bone disorder. Kidney Int Suppl. 2011;121:S3–8.
59. Slatopolsky E, Bricker NS. The role of phosphorus restriction in the prevention of secondary hyperparathyroidism in chronic renal disease. Kidney Int. 1973;4(2):141–5.
60. Slatopolsky E, Brown A, Dusso A. Role of phosphorus in the pathogenesis of secondary hyperparathyroidism. Am J Kidney Dis. 2001;37(1 Suppl 2):S54–7.
61. Martin DR, Ritter CS, Slatopolsky E, Brown AJ. Acute regulation of parathyroid hormone by dietary phosphate. Am J Physiol Endocrinol Metab. 2005;289(4):E729–34.
62. Slatopolsky E, Caglar S, Gradowska L, Canterbury J, Reiss E, Bricker NS. On the prevention of secondary hyperparathyroidism in experimental chronic renal disease using "proportional reduction" of dietary phosphorus intake. Kidney Int. 1972;2(3):147–51.
63. Slatopolsky E, Delmez JA. Pathogenesis of secondary hyperparathyroidism. Miner Electrolyte Metab. 1995;21(1–3):91–6.
64. McCarthy JT, Kumar R. Renal osteodystrophy. In: Jacobson HR, Striker GE, Klahr S, editors. The principles and practice of nephrology. St. Louis: Mosby-Year Book, Inc.; 1995. p. 1032–45.
65. DeLuca HF. The kidney as an endocrine organ involved in the function of vitamin D. Am J Med. 1975;58(1):39–47.
66. Eisman JA, Hamstra AJ, Kream BE, DeLuca HF. 1,25-Dihydroxyvitamin D in biological fluids: a simplified and sensitive assay. Science. 1976;193(4257):1021–3.
67. Hollis BW. Assay of circulating 1,25-dihydroxyvitamin D involving a novel single-cartridge extraction and purification procedure. Clin Chem. 1986;32(11):2060–3.
68. Ishimura E, Nishizawa Y, Inaba M, Matsumoto N, Emoto M, Kawagishi T, et al. Serum levels of 1,25-dihydroxyvitamin D, 24,25-dihydroxyvitamin D, and 25-hydroxyvitamin D in nondialyzed patients with chronic renal failure. Kidney Int. 1999;55(3):1019–27.
69. Mason RS, Lissner D, Wilkinson M, Posen S. Vitamin D metabolites and their relationship to azotaemic osteodystrophy. Clin Endocrinol. 1980;13(4):375–85.
70. Scharla S, Schmidt-Gayk H, Reichel H, Mayer E. A sensitive and simplified radioimmunoassay for 1,25-dihydroxyvitamin D3. Clin Chim Acta. 1984;142(3):325–38.
71. Yumita S, Suzuki M, Akiba T, Akizawa T, Seino Y, Kurokawa K. Levels of serum 1,25(OH)2D in patients with pre-dialysis chronic renal failure. Tohoku J Exp Med. 1996;180(1):45–56.
72. Coburn JW, Koppel MH, Brickman AS, Massry SG. Study of intestinal absorption of calcium in patients with renal failure. Kidney Int. 1973;3(4):264–72.
73. Juttmann JR, Hagenouw-Taal JC, Lameyer LD, Ruis AM, Birkenhager JC. Intestinal calcium absorption, serum phosphate, and parathyroid hormone in patients with chronic renal failure and osteodystrophy before and during hemodialysis. Calcif Tissue Res. 1978;26(2):119–26.
74. Chanard JM, Drueke T, Zingraff J, Man NK, Russo-Marie F, Funck-Brentano JL. Effects of haemodialysis on fractional intestinal absorption of calcium in uraemia. Eur J Clin Investig. 1976;6(3):261–4.
75. Recker RR, Saville PD. Calcium absorption in renal failure: its relationship to blood urea nitrogen, dietary calcium intake, time on dialysis, and other variables. J Lab Clin Med. 1971;78(3):380–8.
76. Faul C, Amaral AP, Oskouei B, Hu MC, Sloan A, Isakova T, et al. FGF23 induces left ventricular hypertrophy. J Clin Invest. 2011;121(11):4393–408.
77. Gutierrez O, Isakova T, Rhee E, Shah A, Holmes J, Collerone G, et al. Fibroblast growth factor-23 mitigates hyperphosphatemia but accentuates calcitriol deficiency in chronic kidney disease. J Am Soc Nephrol. 2005;16(7):2205–15.
78. Gutierrez OM, Januzzi JL, Isakova T, Laliberte K, Smith K, Collerone G, et al. Fibroblast growth factor 23 and left ventricular hypertrophy in chronic kidney disease. Circulation. 2009;119(19):2545–52.
79. Gutierrez OM, Mannstadt M, Isakova T, Rauh-Hain JA, Tamez H, Shah A, et al. Fibroblast growth factor 23 and mortality among patients undergoing hemodialysis. N Engl J Med. 2008;359(6):584–92.
80. Isakova T, Xie H, Yang W, Xie D, Anderson AH, Scialla J, et al. Fibroblast growth factor 23 and risks of mortality and end-stage renal disease in patients with chronic kidney disease. JAMA. 2011;305(23):2432–9.
81. Pande S, Ritter CS, Rothstein M, Wiesen K, Vassiliadis J, Kumar R, et al. FGF-23 and sFRP-4 in

chronic kidney disease and post-renal transplantation. Nephron Physiol. 2006;104(1):23–32.
82. Cunningham J, Fraher LJ, Clemens TL, Revell PA, Papapoulos SE. Chronic acidosis with metabolic bone disease. Effect of alkali on bone morphology and vitamin D metabolism. Am J Med. 1982;73(2):199–204.
83. Eiam-ong S, Kurtzman NA. Metabolic acidosis and bone disease. Miner Electrolyte Metab. 1994;20(1–2).72–80.
84. Marone CC, Wong NL, Sutton RA, Dirks JH. Acidosis and renal calcium excretion in experimental chronic renal failure. Nephron. 1981;28(6):294–6.
85. Seeman E, Wahner HW, Offord KP, Kumar R, Johnson WJ, Riggs BL. Differential effects of endocrine dysfunction on the axial and the appendicular skeleton. J Clin Invest. 1982;69(6):1302–9.
86. Bakr AM. Bone mineral density and bone turnover markers in children with chronic renal failure. Pediatr Nephrol. 2004;19(12):1390–3.
87. Cochat P, Braillon P, Feber J, Hadj-Aissa A, Dubourg L, Liponski I, et al. Body composition in children with renal disease: use of dual energy X-ray absorptiometry. Pediatr Nephrol. 1996;10(3):264–8.
88. Ersoy FF. Osteoporosis in the elderly with chronic kidney disease. Int Urol Nephrol. 2007;39(1):321–31.
89. Georgiou E, Virvidakis K, Douskas G, Lambrinoudaki I, Voudiklari S, Katsoudas S, et al. Body composition changes in chronic hemodialysis patients before and after hemodialysis as assessed by dual-energy x-ray absorptiometry. Metabolism. 1997;46(9):1059–62.
90. Johnson DW, McIntyre HD, Brown A, Freeman J, Rigby RJ. The role of DEXA bone densitometry in evaluating renal osteodystrophy in continuous ambulatory peritoneal dialysis patients. Perit Dial Int. 1996;16(1):34–40.
91. Atsumi K, Kushida K, Yamazaki K, Shimizu S, Ohmura A, Inoue T. Risk factors for vertebral fractures in renal osteodystrophy. Am J Kidney Dis. 1999;33(2):287–93.
92. Ensrud KE, Lui LY, Taylor BC, Ishani A, Shlipak MG, Stone KL, et al. Renal function and risk of hip and vertebral fractures in older women. Arch Intern Med. 2007;167(2):133–9.
93. Alem AM, Sherrard DJ, Gillen DL, Weiss NS, Beresford SA, Heckbert SR, et al. Increased risk of hip fracture among patients with end-stage renal disease. Kidney Int. 2000;58(1):396–9.
94. Ball AM, Gillen DL, Sherrard D, Weiss NS, Emerson SS, Seliger SL, et al. Risk of hip and renal fracture among dialysis transplant recipients. JAMA. 2002;288(23):3014–8.
95. Chen YJ, Kung PT, Wang YH, Huang CC, Hsu SC, Tsai WC, et al. Greater risk of hip fracture in hemodialysis than in peritoneal dialysis. Osteoporos Int. 2014;25(5):1513–8.
96. Coco M, Rush H. Increased incidence of hip fractures in dialysis patients with low serum parathyroid hormone. Am J Kidney Dis. 2000;36(6):1115–21.
97. Jadoul M, Albert JM, Akiba T, Akizawa T, Arab L, Bragg-Gresham JL, et al. Incidence and risk factors for hip or other bone fractures among hemodialysis patients in the Dialysis Outcomes and Practice Patterns Study. Kidney Int. 2006;70(7): 1358–66.
98. Mittalhenkle A, Gillen DL, Stehman-Breen CO. Increased risk of mortality associated with hip fracture in the dialysis population. Am J Kidney Dis. 2004;44(4):672–9.
99. Rudser KD, de Boer IH, Dooley A, Young B, Kestenbaum B. Fracture risk after parathyroidectomy among chronic hemodialysis patients. JASN. 2007;18(8):2401–7.
100. Stehman-Breen CO, Sherrard DJ, Alem AM, Gillen DL, Heckbert SR, Wong CS, et al. Risk factors for hip fracture among patients with end-stage renal disease. Kidney Int. 2000;58(5):2200–5.
101. Evenepoel P, Claes K, Kuypers D, Maes B, Bammens B, Vanrenterghem Y. Natural history of parathyroid function and calcium metabolism after kidney transplantation: a single-centre study. Nephrol Dial Transplant. 2004;19(5):1281–7.
102. Evenepoel P, Meijers BKI, de Jonge H, Naesens M, Bammens B, Claes K, et al. Recovery of hyperphosphatoninism and renal phosphorus wasting one year after successful renal transplantation. Clin J Am Soc Nephrol. 2008;3(6):1829–36.
103. Amer H, Griffin MD, Stegall MD, Cosio FG, Park WD, Kremers WK, et al. Oral paricalcitol reduces the prevalence of posttransplant hyperparathyroidism: results of an open label randomized trial. Am J Transplant. 2013;13(6):1576–85.
104. Carlini RG, Rojas E, Weisinger JR, Lopez M, Martinis R, Arminio A, et al. Bone disease in patients with long-term renal transplantation and normal renal function. Am J Kidney Dis. 2000;36(1):160–6.
105. Borchhardt K, Sulzbacher I, Benesch T, Fodinger M, Sunder-Plassmann G, Haas M. Low-turnover bone disease in hypercalcemic hyperparathyroidism after kidney transplantation. Am J Transplant. 2007;7(11):2515–21.
106. Monier-Faugere MC, Mawad H, Qi Q, Friedler RM, Malluche HH. High prevalence of low bone turnover and occurrence of osteomalacia after kidney transplantation. J Am Soc Nephrol. 2000;11(6):1093–9.
107. Boot AM, Nauta J, Hokken-Koelega AC, Pols HA, de Ridder MA, de Muinck Keizer-Schrama SM. Renal transplantation and osteoporosis. Arch Dis Child. 1995;72(6):502–6.
108. Brandenburg VM, Ketteler M, Heussen N, Politt D, Frank RD, Westenfeld R, et al. Lumbar bone mineral density in very long-term renal transplant recipients: impact of circulating sex hormones. Osteoporos Int. 2005;16(12):1611–20.
109. Brandenburg VM, Westenfeld R, Ketteler M. The fate of bone after renal transplantation. J Nephrol. 2004;17(2):190–204.
110. Bubenicek P, Sotornik I, Vitko S, Teplan V. Early bone mineral density loss after renal transplantation

and pre-transplant PTH: a prospective study. Kidney Blood Press Res. 2008;31(3):196–202.
111. Caglar M, Adeera L. Factors affecting bone mineral density in renal transplant patients. Ann Nucl Med. 1999;13(3):141–5.
112. Chao SH, Tsai KS, Chieng PU, Lee PH, Lee CJ, Lee CS. Bone mineral density profile in uremic and renal transplant patients. Transplant Proc. 1994;26(4):2009–11.
113. Cueto-Manzano AM, Konel S, Hutchison AJ, Crowley V, France MW, Freemont AJ, et al. Bone loss in long-term renal transplantation: histopathology and densitometry analysis. Kidney Int. 1999;55(5):2021–9.
114. Durieux S, Mercadal L, Orcel P, Dao H, Rioux C, Bernard M, et al. Bone mineral density and fracture prevalence in long-term kidney graft recipients. Transplantation. 2002;74(4):496–500.
115. Feber J, Cochat P, Braillon P, Castelo F, Martin X, Glastre C, et al. Bone mineral density after renal transplantation in children. J Pediatr. 1994;125(6 Pt 1):870–5.
116. Grotz WH, Mundinger FA, Gugel B, Exner V, Kirste G, Schollmeyer PJ. Bone-fracture and osteodensitometry with dual-energy X-ray absorptiometry in kidney-transplant recipients. Transplantation. 1994;58(8):912–5.
117. Grotz WH, Mundinger FA, Gugel B, Exner VM, Kirste G, Schollmeyer PJ. Bone mineral density after kidney transplantation. A cross-sectional study in 190 graft recipients up to 20 years after transplantation. Transplantation. 1995;59(7):982–6.
118. Gupta AK, Huang M, Prasad GV. Determinants of bone mineral density in stable kidney transplant recipients. J Nephrol. 2012;25(3):373–83.
119. Horber FF, Casez JP, Steiger U, Czerniak A, Montandon A, Jaeger P. Changes in bone mass early after kidney transplantation. J Bone Miner Res. 1994;9(1):1–9.
120. Kwan JT, Almond MK, Evans K, Cunningham J. Changes in total body bone mineral content and regional bone mineral density in renal patients following renal transplantation. Miner Electrolyte Metab. 1992;18(2–5):166–8.
121. Moreno A, Torregrosa JV, Pons F, Campistol JM, Martinez de Osaba MJ, Oppenheimer F. Bone mineral density after renal transplantation: long-term follow-up. Transplant Proc. 1999;31(6):2322–3.
122. Nielsen HE, Melsen F, Christensen MS. Bone lesions following renal transplantation. Bone mineral density and amount of trabecular bone. Scand J Urol Nephrol Suppl. 1977;42:127–9.
123. Weisinger JR, Carlini RG, Rojas E, Bellorin-Font E. Bone disease after renal transplantation. Clin J Am Soc Nephrol. 2006;1(6):1300–13.
124. Fan SL, Kumar S, Cunningham J. Long-term effects on bone mineral density of pamidronate given at the time of renal transplantation. Kidney Int. 2003;63(6):2275–9.
125. Giannini S, D'Angelo A, Carraro G, Antonello A, Di Landro D, Marchini F, et al. Persistently increased bone turnover and low bone density in long-term survivors to kidney transplantation. Clin Nephrol. 2001;56(5):353–63.
126. Jeffery JR, Leslie WD, Karpinski ME, Nickerson PW, Rush DN. Prevalence and treatment of decreased bone density in renal transplant recipients: a randomized prospective trial of calcitriol versus alendronate. Transplantation. 2003;76(10):1498–502.
127. Julian BA, Laskow DA, Dubovsky J, Dubovsky EV, Curtis JJ, Quarles LD. Rapid loss of vertebral mineral density after renal transplantation. N Engl J Med. 1991;325(8):544–50.
128. Coen G. Fracturing osteoporosis after kidney transplantation–what are the options? Nephrol Dial Transplant. 1996;11(4):567–9.
129. Davidson JK, Tsakiris D, Briggs JD, Junor BJ. Osteonecrosis and fractures following renal transplantation. Clin Radiol. 1985;36(1):27–35.
130. Elmstedt E, Svahn T. Skeletal complications following renal transplantation. Acta Orthop Scand. 1981;52(3):279–86.
131. Evarts CM, Phalen GS. Osseous avascular necrosis associated with renal transplantation. Clin Orthop. 1971;78:330–5.
132. Levine E, Erken EH, Price HI, Meyers AM, Solomon L. Osteonecrosis following renal transplantation. AJR Am J Roentgenol. 1977;128(6):985–91.
133. Ramsey-Goldman R, Dunn JE, Dunlop DD, Stuart FP, Abecassis MM, Kaufman DB, et al. Increased risk of fracture in patients receiving solid organ transplants. J Bone Miner Res. 1999;14(3):456–63.
134. O'Shaughnessy EA, Dahl DC, Smith CL, Kasiske BL. Risk factors for fractures in kidney transplantation. Transplantation. 2002;74(3):362–6.
135. Parker CR, Freemont AJ, Blackwell PJ, Grainge MJ, Hosking DJ. Cross-sectional analysis of renal transplantation osteoporosis. J Bone Miner Res. 1999;14(11):1943–51.
136. Patel S, Kwan JTC, McCloskey E, McGee G, Thomas G, Johnson D, et al. Prevalence and causes of low bone density and fractures in kidney transplant patients. J Bone Miner Res. 2001;16(10):1863–70.
137. Nam JH, Moon JI, Chung SS, Kim SI, Park KI, Song YD, et al. Prevalence and risk factors for vertebral fractures in renal transplants. Transplant Proc. 2000;32(7):1877.
138. Falkiewicz K, Bidzinska B, Demissie M, Boratynska M, Zmonarski SC, Tworowska K, et al. Influence of vitamin D receptor gene polymorphisms on secondary hyperparathyroidism and bone density after kidney transplantation. Transplant Proc. 2005;37(2):1023–5.
139. Kanaan N, Claes K, Devogelaer JP, Vanderschueren D, Depresseux G, Goffin E, et al. Fibroblast growth factor-23 and parathyroid hormone are associated with post-transplant bone mineral density loss. CJASN. 2010;5(10):1887–92.
140. Young A, Hodsman AB, Boudville N, Geddes C, Gill J, Goltzman D, et al. Bone and mineral metabolism

and fibroblast growth factor 23 levels after kidney donation. Am J Kidney Dis. 2012;59(6):761–9.
141. Gonzalez MT, Gonzalez C, Grino JM, Castelao AM, Marinoso ML, Serrano S, et al. Long-term evolution of renal osteodystrophy after kidney transplantation: comparative study between intact PTH levels and bone biopsy. Transplant Proc. 1990;22(4):1407–11.
142. Isaksson E, Sterner G. Early development of secondary hyperparathyroidism following renal transplantation.[Erratum appears in Nephron Clin Pract. 2012;121(3–4): c111]. Nephron. 2012;121(1–2):c68–72.
143. Kawarazaki H, Shibagaki Y, Fukumoto S, Kido R, Nakajima I, Fuchinoue S, et al. The relative role of fibroblast growth factor 23 and parathyroid hormone in predicting future hypophosphatemia and hypercalcemia after living donor kidney transplantation: a 1-year prospective observational study. Nephrol Dial Transplant. 2011;26(8):2691–5.
144. Kokado Y, Takahara S, Ichimaru N, Toki K, Kyo M, Permpongkosol S, et al. Factors influencing vertebral bone density after renal transplantation. Transpl Int. 2000;13(Suppl 1):S431–5.
145. Roe SD, Porter CJ, Godber IM, Hosking DJ, Cassidy MJ. Reduced bone mineral density in male renal transplant recipients: evidence for persisting hyperparathyroidism. Osteoporos Int. 2005;16(2):142–8.
146. Torres A, Rodriguez AP, Concepcion MT, Garcia S, Rufino M, Martin B, et al. Parathyroid function in long-term renal transplant patients: importance of pre-transplant PTH concentrations. Nephrol Dial Transplant. 1998;13:94–7.
147. Bozkaya G, Nart A, Uslu A, Onman T, Aykas A, Dogan M, et al. Impact of calcineurin inhibitors on bone metabolism in primary kidney transplant patients. Transplant Proc. 2008;40(1):151–5.
148. Stein E, Ebeling P, Shane E. Post-transplantation osteoporosis. Endocrinol Metab Clin North Am. 2007;36(4):937–63.
149. Westenfeld R, Schlieper G, Woltje M, Gawlik A, Brandenburg V, Rutkowski P, et al. Impact of sirolimus, tacrolimus and mycophenolate mofetil on osteoclastogenesis-implications for post-transplantation bone disease. Nephrol Dial Transplant. 2011;26(12):4115–23.
150. Zand MS. Immunosuppression and immune monitoring after renal transplantation. Semin Dial. 2005;18(6):511–9.
151. Vincenti F, Schena FP, Paraskevas S, Hauser IA, Walker RG, Grinyo J, et al. A randomized, multicenter study of steroid avoidance, early steroid withdrawal or standard steroid therapy in kidney transplant recipients. Am J Transplant. 2008;8(2):307–16.
152. Woodle ES, Peddi VR, Tomlanovich S, Mulgaonkar S, Kuo PC, Investigators TS. A prospective, randomized, multicenter study evaluating early corticosteroid withdrawal with thymoglobulin in living-donor kidney transplantation. Clin Transpl. 2010;24(1):73–83.
153. Walker JK, Alloway RR, Roy-Chaudhury P, Mogilishetty G, Cardi MA, Weimert NA, et al. A prospective trial of a steroid-free/calcineurin inhibitor minimization regimen in human leukocyte antigen (HLA)-identical live donor renal transplantation. Transplantation. 2009;87(3):408–14.
154. Woodle ES, Vincenti F, Lorber MI, Gritsch HA, Hricik D, Washburn K, et al. A multicenter pilot study of early (4-day) steroid cessation in renal transplant recipients under simulect, tacrolimus and sirolimus. Am J Transplant. 2005;5(1):157–66.
155. de Nijs RNJ, Jacobs JWG, Bijlsma JWJ, Lems WF, Laan R, Houben HHM, et al. Prevalence of vertebral deformities and symptomatic vertebral fractures in corticosteroid treated patients with rheumatoid arthritis. Rheumatology. 2001;40(12):1375–83.
156. Kalpakcioglu BB, Engelke K, Genant HK. Advanced imaging assessment of bone fragility in glucocorticoid-induced osteoporosis. Bone. 2011;48(6):1221–31.
157. Ebeling PR. Approach to the patient with transplantation-related bone loss. J Clin Endocrinol Metab. 2009;94(5):1483–90.
158. Loke YK, Cavallazzi R, Singh S. Risk of fractures with inhaled corticosteroids in COPD: systematic review and meta-analysis of randomised controlled trials and observational studies. Thorax. 2011;66(8):699–708.
159. Van Staa TP, Leufkens HGM, Abenhaim L, Zhang B, Cooper C. Use of oral corticosteroids and risk of fractures. J Bone Miner Res. 2000;15(6):993–1000.
160. Thierry A, Mourad G, Buchler M, Kamar N, Villemain F, Heng AE, et al. Steroid avoidance with early intensified dosing of enteric-coated mycophenolate sodium: a randomized multicentre trial in kidney transplant recipients. Nephrol Dial Transplant. 2012;27(9):3651–9.
161. Srinivas TR, Meier-Kriesche HU. Minimizing immunosuppression, an alternative approach to reducing side effects: objectives and interim result. Clin J Am Soc Nephrol. 2008;3(Suppl 2):S101–16.
162. Lee Y-J, Kim B, Lee JE, Kim Y-G, Kim DJ, Kim S-J, et al. Randomized trial of cyclosporine and tacrolimus therapy with steroid withdrawal in living-donor renal transplantation: 5-year follow-up. Transpl Int. 2010;23(2):147–54.
163. Mainra R, Elder G. Review article: managing bone complications after kidney transplantation. Nephrology (Carlton). 2009;14(4):437–42.
164. Palmer SC, Strippoli GF, McGregor DO. Interventions for preventing bone disease in kidney transplant recipients: a systematic review of randomized controlled trials. Am J Kidney Dis. 2005;45(4):638–49.
165. Nikkel LE, Mohan S, Zhang A, McMahon DJ, Boutroy S, Dube G, et al. Reduced fracture risk with early corticosteroid withdrawal after kidney transplant. Am J Transplant. 2012;12(3):649–59.
166. Kumar R. Glucocorticoid-induced osteoporosis. Curr Opin Nephrol Hypertens. 2001;10(5):589–95.

167. Compston JE. Osteoporosis after liver transplantation. Liver Transpl. 2003;9(4):321–30.
168. Jeon SH, Kim SJ, Kim JS, Kang HS. Immunosuppressant FK506 decreases the intracellular magnesium in the human osteoblast cell by inhibiting the ERK1/2 pathway. Life Sci. 2009;84(1–2):23–7.
169. Ponticelli C, Aroldi A. Osteoporosis after organ transplantation. Lancet. 2001;357(9268):1623.
170. Monegal A, Navasa M, Guanabens N, Peris P, Pons F, de Osaba MJM, et al. Bone disease after liver transplantation: a long-term prospective study of bone mass changes, hormonal status and histomorphometric characteristics. Osteoporos Int. 2001;12(6):484–92.
171. Collini A, De Bartolomeis C, Barni R, Ruggieri G, Bernini M, Carmellini M. Calcineurin-inhibitor induced pain syndrome after organ transplantation. Kidney Int. 2006;70(7):1367–70.
172. Villaverde V, Cantalejo M, Balsa A, Mola EM. Leg bone pain syndrome in a kidney transplant patient treated with tacrolimus (FK506). Ann Rheum Dis. 1999;58(10):653–4.
173. Naredo Sanchez E, Balsa Criado A, Sanz Guajardo A, Pantoja Zarza L, Martin Mola E, Gijon BJ. Leg bone pain syndrome due to cyclosporine in a renal transplant patient. Clin Exp Rheumatol. 1994;12(6):653–6.
174. Lan GB, Xie XB, Peng LK, Liu L, Song L, Dai HL. Current status of research on osteoporosis after solid organ transplantation: pathogenesis and management. Biomed Res Int. 2015;2015:413169.
175. Romero DF, Buchinsky FJ, Rucinski B, Cvetkovic M, Bryer HP, Liang XG, et al. Rapamycin - a bone-sparing immunosuppressant. J Bone Miner Res. 1995;10(5):760–8.
176. Alvarez-Garcia O, Carbajo-Perez E, Garcia E, Gil H, Molinos I, Rodriguez J, et al. Rapamycin retards growth and causes marked alterations in the growth plate of young rats. Pediatr Nephrol. 2007;22(7):954–61.
177. Charpentier B, Medina Pestana JO, Del CRM, Rostaing L, Grinyo J, Vanrenterghem Y, et al. Long-term exposure to belatacept in recipients of extended criteria donor kidneys. Am J Transplant. 2013;13(11):2884–91.
178. Dobbels F, Wong S, Min Y, Sam J, Kalsekar A. Beneficial effect of belatacept on health-related quality of life and perceived side effects: results from the BENEFIT and BENEFIT-EXT trials. Transplantation. 2014;98(9):960–8.
179. Durrbach A, Pestana JM, Pearson T, Vincenti F, Garcia VD, Campistol J, et al. A phase III study of belatacept versus cyclosporine in kidney transplants from extended criteria donors (BENEFIT-EXT study). Am J Transplant. 2010;10(3):547–57.
180. Pestana JO, Grinyo JM, Vanrenterghem Y, Becker T, Campistol JM, Florman S, et al. Three-year outcomes from BENEFIT-EXT: a phase III study of belatacept versus cyclosporine in recipients of extended criteria donor kidneys. Am J Transplant. 2012;12(3):630–9.
181. Rostaing L, Neumayer HH, Reyes-Acevedo R, Bresnahan B, Florman S, Vitko S, et al. Belatacept-versus cyclosporine-based immunosuppression in renal transplant recipients with pre-existing diabetes. Clin J Am Soc Nephrol. 2011;6(11):2696–704.
182. Rostaing L, Vincenti F, Grinyo J, Rice KM, Bresnahan B, Steinberg S, et al. Long-term belatacept exposure maintains efficacy and safety at 5 years: results from the long-term extension of the BENEFIT study. Am J Transplant. 2013;13(11):2875–83.
183. Vanrenterghem Y, Bresnahan B, Campistol J, Durrbach A, Grinyo J, Neumayer HH, et al. Belatacept-based regimens are associated with improved cardiovascular and metabolic risk factors compared with cyclosporine in kidney transplant recipients (BENEFIT and BENEFIT-EXT studies). Transplantation. 2011;91(9):976–83.
184. Boquist L, Bergdahl L, Andersson L. Hyperparathyroidism after renal transplantation and long-term hemodialysis. Scand J Urol Nephrol. 1971;5(3):243–50.
185. Evenepoel P. Recovery versus persistence of disordered mineral metabolism in kidney transplant recipients. Semin Nephrol. 2013;33(2):191–203.
186. Evenepoel P, Kuypers D, Maes B, Messiaen T, Vanrenterghem Y. Persistent hyperparathyroidism after kidney transplantation requiring parathyroidectomy. Acta Otorhinolaryngol Belg. 2001;55(2):177–86.
187. Fleseriu M, Licata AA. Failure of successful renal transplant to produce appropriate levels of 1,25-dihydroxyvitamin D. Osteoporos Int. 2007;18(3):363–8.
188. Blohme I, Eriksson A. Parathyroidectomy after renal transplantation. Scand J Urol Nephrol Suppl. 1977;42:134–6.
189. Brunt LM, Wells SA Jr. Surgical treatment of secondary hyperparathyroidism. Ann Chir Gynaecol. 1983;72(3):139–45.
190. Buck BA, Robertson RD. Indications for parathyroidectomy in advanced renal disease. Surg Gynecol Obstet. 1971;133(2):218–24.
191. Cerilli J, Limbert JG, Ferris TF, Tzagournis M. Subtotal parathyroidectomy for tertiary hyperparathyroidism thirty-two months after renal transplantation. Am J Surg. 1973;125(5):636–8.
192. Chou FF, Hsieh KC, Chen YT, Lee CT. Parathyroidectomy followed by kidney transplantation can improve bone mineral density in patients with secondary hyperparathyroidism. Transplantation. 2008;86(4):554–7.
193. Conzo G, Perna AF, Sinisi AA, Palazzo A, Stanzione F, Della Pietra C, et al. Total parathyroidectomy without autotransplantation in the surgical treatment of secondary hyperparathyroidism of chronic kidney disease. J Endocrinol Investig. 2012;35(1):8–13.
194. Copley JB, Wuthrich RP. Therapeutic management of post-kidney transplant hyperparathyroidism. Clin Transplant. 2011;25(1):24–39.

195. Cruzado JM, Moreno P, Torregrosa JV, Taco O, Mast R, Gomez-Vaquero C, et al. A randomized study comparing parathyroidectomy with Cinacalcet for treating hypercalcemia in kidney allograft recipients with hyperparathyroidism. J Am Soc Nephrol. 2016;27(8):2487–94.
196. Dewberry LK, Weber C, Sharma J. Near total parathyroidectomy is effective therapy for tertiary hyperparathyroidism. Am Surg. 2014;80(7):646–51.
197. Evenepoel P, Claes K, Kuypers DR, Debruyne F, Vanrenterghem Y. Parathyroidectomy after successful kidney transplantation: a single centre study. Nephrol Dial Transplant. 2007;22(6):1730–7.
198. Foley RN, Li S, Liu J, Gilbertson DT, Chen SC, Collins AJ. The fall and rise of parathyroidectomy in U.S. hemodialysis patients, 1992 to 2002. J Am Soc Nephrol. 2005;16(1):210–8.
199. Garcia A, Mazuecos A, Garcia T, Gonzalez P, Ceballos M, Rivero M. Effect of parathyroidectomy on renal graft function. Transplant Proc. 2005;37(3):1459–61.
200. Dahl E, Nordal KP, Halse J, Flatmark A. Pretransplant parathyroidectomy in renal failure: effects on bone histology and aluminum deposits during dialysis and after kidney transplantation. Scand J Urol Nephrol. 1992;26(3):283–8.
201. Callender GG, Malinowski J, Javid M, Zhang Y, Huang H, Quinn CE, et al. Parathyroidectomy prior to kidney transplant decreases graft failure. Surgery. 2017;161(1):44–50.
202. Lou I, Schneider DF, Leverson G, Foley D, Sippel R, Chen H. Parathyroidectomy is underused in patients with tertiary hyperparathyroidism after renal transplantation. Surgery. 2016;159(1):172–9.
203. Querings K, Girndt M, Geisel J, Georg T, Tilgen W, Reichrath J. 25-hydroxyvitamin D deficiency in renal transplant recipients. J Clin Endocrinol Metab. 2006;91(2):526–9.
204. Cozzolino M, Brancaccio D, Cannella G, Messa P, Gesualdo L, Marangella M, et al. VDRA therapy is associated with improved survival in dialysis patients with serum intact PTH <=150 pg/mL: results of the Italian FARO survey. Nephrol Dial Transplant. 2012;27(9):3588–94.
205. Trillini M, Cortinovis M, Ruggenenti P, Reyes Loaeza J, Courville K, Ferrer-Siles C, et al. Paricalcitol for secondary hyperparathyroidism in renal transplantation. J Am Soc Nephrol. 2015;26(5):1205–14.
206. Brown EM, Gamba G, Riccardi D, Lombardi M, Butters R, Kifor O, et al. Cloning and characterization of an extracellular Ca(2+)-sensing receptor from bovine parathyroid. Nature. 1993;366(6455):575–80.
207. Brown EM, Hebert SC. A cloned Ca(2+)-sensing receptor: a mediator of direct effects of extracellular Ca2+ on renal function? J Am Soc Nephrol. 1995;6(6):1530–40.
208. Brown EM, Hebert SC. A cloned extracellular Ca(2+)-sensing receptor: molecular mediator of the actions of extracellular Ca2+ on parathyroid and kidney cells? Kidney Int. 1996;49(4):1042–6.
209. Brown EM, MacLeod RJ. Extracellular calcium sensing and extracellular calcium signaling. Physiol Rev. 2001;81(1):239–97.
210. Chou YH, Pollak MR, Brandi ML, Toss G, Arnqvist H, Atkinson AB, et al. Mutations in the human Ca(2+)-sensing-receptor gene that cause familial hypocalciuric hypercalcemia. Am J Hum Genet. 1995;56(5):1075–9.
211. Quinn SJ, Ye CP, Diaz R, Kifor O, Bai M, Vassilev P, et al. The Ca2+−sensing receptor: a target for polyamines. Am J Phys. 1997;273(4 Pt 1):C1315–23.
212. Riccardi D, Park J, Lee WS, Gamba G, Brown EM, Hebert SC. Cloning and functional expression of a rat kidney extracellular calcium/polyvalent cation-sensing receptor. Proc Natl Acad Sci U S A. 1995;92(1):131–5.
213. Zhang C, Miller CL, Gorkhali R, Zou J, Huang K, Brown EM, et al. Molecular basis of the extracellular ligands mediated signaling by the calcium sensing receptor. Front Physiol. 2016;7:441.
214. Nemeth EF. Calcimimetic and calcilytic drugs: just for parathyroid cells? Cell Calcium. 2004;35(3):283–9.
215. Nemeth EF, Heaton WH, Miller M, Fox J, Balandrin MF, Van Wagenen BC, et al. Pharmacodynamics of the type II calcimimetic compound cinacalcet HCl. J Pharmacol Exp Ther. 2004;308(2):627–35.
216. Al-Moasseb Z, Aitken E. Natural history of serum calcium and parathyroid hormone following renal transplantation. Transplant Proc. 2016;48(10):3285–91.
217. Jeon HJ, Kim H, Yang J. Bone disease in post-transplant patients. Curr Opin Endocrinol Diabetes Obes. 2015;22(6):452–8.
218. Komaba H, Fukagawa M. Basic and clinical aspects of calcimimetics. Calcimimetics : a promising treatment for persistent hypercalcemia after kidney transplantation. Clin Calcium. 2008;18(1):60–6.
219. Leca N, Laftavi M, Gundroo A, Kohli R, Min I, Karam J, et al. Early and severe hyperparathyroidism associated with hypercalcemia after renal transplant treated with cinacalcet. Am J Transplant. 2006;6(10):2391–5.
220. Leonard N, Brown JH. Persistent and symptomatic post-transplant hyperparathyroidism: a dramatic response to cinacalcet. Nephrol Dial Transplant. 2006;21(6):1736.
221. Muirhead N, Zaltman JS, Gill JS, Churchill DN, Poulin-Costello M, Mann V, et al. Hypercalcemia in renal transplant patients: prevalence and management in Canadian transplant practice. Clin Transpl. 2014;28(2):161–5.
222. Sharma AK, Masterson R, Holt SG, Tan SJ, Hughes PD, Chu M, et al. Impact of cinacalcet pre-transplantation on mineral metabolism in renal transplant recipients. Nephrology (Carlton). 2016;21(1):46–54.
223. Torregrosa JV, Barros X. Management of hypercalcemia after renal transplantation. Nefrologia. 2013;33(6):751–7.

224. Apostolou T, Kollia K, Damianou L, Kaitsioti H, Kotsiev V, Dracopoulos S, et al. Hypercalcemia due to resistant hyperparathyroidism in renal transplant patients treated with the calcimimetic agent cinacalcet. Transplant Proc. 2006;38(10):3514–6.
225. Bahner U, Brandl M, Nies C, Schmidt-Gayk H. Use of cinacalcet HCl to achieve the recommended targets of bone metabolism in a patient with therapy-resistant renal hyperparathyroidism. J Ren Nutr. 2008;18(4):383–8.
226. Bergua C, Torregrosa JV, Cofan F, Oppenheimer F. Cinacalcet for the treatment of hypercalcemia in renal transplanted patients with secondary hyperparathyroidism. Transplant Proc. 2007;39(7):2254–5.
227. Bergua C, Torregrosa JV, Fuster D, Gutierrez-Dalmau A, Oppenheimer F, Campistol JM. Effect of cinacalcet on hypercalcemia and bone mineral density in renal transplanted patients with secondary hyperparathyroidism. Transplantation. 2008;86(3):413–7.
228. Borchhardt KA, Diarra D, Sulzbacher I, Benesch T, Haas M, Sunder-Plassmann G. Cinacalcet decreases bone formation rate in hypercalcemic hyperparathyroidism after kidney transplantation. Am J Nephrol. 2010;31(6):482–9.
229. Borchhardt KA, Heinzl H, Mayerwoger E, Horl WH, Haas M, Sunder-Plassmann G. Cinacalcet increases calcium excretion in hypercalcemic hyperparathyroidism after kidney transplantation. Transplantation. 2008;86(7):919–24.
230. Cho ME, Duan Z, Chamberlain CE, Reynolds JC, Ring MS, Mannon RB. Cinacalcet improves bone density in post-kidney transplant hyperparathyroidism. Transplant Proc. 2010;42(9):3554–8.
231. Cohen JB, Gordon CE, Balk EM, Francis JM. Cinacalcet for the treatment of hyperparathyroidism in kidney transplant recipients: a systematic review and meta-analysis. Transplantation. 2012;94(10):1041–8.
232. Copley JB, Germain M, Stern L, Pankewycz O, Katznelson S, Shah T, et al. Evaluation of cinacalcet HCl treatment after kidney transplantation. Transplant Proc. 2010;42(7):2503–8.
233. Coyne DW, Delos SR. Evaluating the safety and rationale for cinacalcet posttransplant hyperparathyroidism and hypercalcemia. Am J Transplant. 2014;14(11):2446–7.
234. de Francisco AL. New strategies for the treatment of hyperparathyroidism incorporating calcimimetics. Expert Opin Pharmacother. 2008;9(5):795–811.
235. Dong BJ. Cinacalcet: an oral calcimimetic agent for the management of hyperparathyroidism. Clin Ther. 2005;27(11):1725–51.
236. El-Amm JM, Doshi MD, Singh A, Migdal S, Morawski K, Sternbauer D, et al. Preliminary experience with cinacalcet use in persistent secondary hyperparathyroidism after kidney transplantation. Transplantation. 2007;83(5):546–9.
237. Evenepoel P, Cooper K, Holdaas H, Messa P, Mourad G, Olgaard K, et al. A randomized study evaluating cinacalcet to treat hypercalcemia in renal transplant recipients with persistent hyperparathyroidism. Am J Transplant. 2014;14(11):2545–55.
238. Gomez Marques G, Obrador Mulet A, Vilar Gimeno A, Pascual Felip MJ, Alarcon Zurita A, Molina Guasch M, et al. Treatment with cinacalcet of secondary hyperparathyroidism after renal transplantation. Transplant Proc. 2009;41(6):2139–43.
239. Guerra R, Auyanet I, Fernandez EJ, Perez MA, Bosch E, Ramirez A, et al. Hypercalcemia secondary to persistent hyperparathyroidism in kidney transplant patients: analysis after a year with cinacalcet. J Nephrol. 2011;24(1):78–82.
240. Henschkowski J, Bischoff-Ferrari HA, Wuthrich RP, Serra AL. Renal function in patients treated with cinacalcet for persistent hyperparathyroidism after kidney transplantation. Kidney Blood Press Res. 2011;34(2):97–103.
241. Kamar N, Gennero I, Spataru L, Esposito L, Guitard J, Lavayssiere L, et al. Pharmacodynamic effects of cinacalcet after kidney transplantation: once-versus twice-daily dose. Nephrol Dial Transplant. 2008;23(11):3720–6.
242. Ketteler M, Martin KJ, Cozzolino M, Goldsmith D, Sharma A, Khan S, et al. Paricalcitol versus cinacalcet plus low-dose vitamin D for the treatment of secondary hyperparathyroidism in patients receiving haemodialysis: study design and baseline characteristics of the IMPACT SHPT study. Nephrol Dial Transplant. 2012;27(5):1942–9.
243. Kruse AE, Eisenberger U, Frey FJ, Mohaupt MG. Effect of cinacalcet cessation in renal transplant recipients with persistent hyperparathyroidism. Nephrol Dial Transplant. 2007;22(8):2362–5.
244. Nakai K, Fujii H, Yoshikawa M, Kono K, Yonekura Y, Goto S, et al. Effect of cinacalcet cessation on hyperparathyroidism in kidney transcaplant patients after long-term dialysis therapy. Clin Exp Nephrol. 2015;19(6):1184–8.
245. Grotz W, Nagel C, Poeschel D, Cybulla M, Petersen KG, Uhl M, et al. Effect of ibandronate on bone loss and renal function after kidney transplantation. J Am Soc Nephrol. 2001;12(7):1530–7.
246. Haas M, Leko-Mohr Z, Roschger P, Kletzmayr J, Schwarz C, Mitterbauer C, et al. Zoledronic acid to prevent bone loss in the first 6 months after renal transplantation. Kidney Int. 2003;63(3):1130–6.
247. Coco M, Pullman J, Cohen HW, Lee S, Shapiro C, Solorzano C, et al. Effect of risedronate on bone in renal transplant recipients. J Am Soc Nephrol. 2012;23(8):1426–37.
248. El-Agroudy AE, El-Husseini AA, El-Sayed M, Mohsen T, Ghoneim MA. A prospective randomized study for prevention of postrenal transplantation bone loss. Kidney Int. 2005;67(5):2039–45.
249. Nowacka-Cieciura E, Cieciura T, Baczkowska T, Kozinska-Przybyl O, Tronina O, Chudzinski W, et al. Bisphosphonates are effective prophylactic of early bone loss after renal transplantation. Transplant Proc. 2006;38(1):165–7.

250. Torregrosa JV, Fuster D, Gentil MA, Marcen R, Guirado L, Zarraga S, et al. Open-label trial: effect of weekly risedronate immediately after transplantation in kidney recipients. Transplantation. 2010;89(12):1476–81.
251. Abediazar S, Nakhjavani MR. Effect of alendronate on early bone loss of renal transplant recipients. Transplant Proc. 2011;43(2):565–7.
252. Friedlander MA, Lemke JH, Horst RL. The effect of uninephrectomy on mineral metabolism in normal human kidney donors. Am J Kidney Dis. 1988;11(5):393–401.
253. Gossmann J, Wilhelm A, Kachel HG, Jordan J, Sann U, Geiger H, et al. Long-term consequences of live kidney donation follow-up in 93% of living kidney donors in a single transplant center. Am J Transplant. 2005;5(10):2417–24.
254. Westerberg PA, Ljunggren O, Larsson TE, Wadström J, Linde T. Fibroblast growth factor-23 and mineral metabolism after unilateral nephrectomy. Nephrol Dial Transplant. 2010;25(12):4068–71.
255. Ponte B, Trombetti A, Hadaya K, Ernandez T, Fumeaux D, Iselin C, et al. Acute and long term mineral metabolism adaptation in living kidney donors: a prospective study. Bone. 2014;62:36–42.
256. Huan Y, Kapoor S, Deloach S, Ommen E, Meyers K, Townsend RR. Changes in biomarkers associated with living kidney donation. Am J Nephrol. 2013;38(3):212–7.
257. Khosla S. Odanacatib: location and timing are everything. J Bone Miner Res. 2012;27(3):506–8.
258. Riggs BL, Melton LJ 3rd. Bone turnover matters: the raloxifene treatment paradox of dramatic decreases in vertebral fractures without commensurate increases in bone density. J Bone Miner Res. 2002;17(1):11–4.

Part VI

Obesity and Adipokines

19 Obesity in Kidney Disease

Peter Stenvinkel

Introduction

Considering that the global prevalence of obesity has more than doubled between 1980 and 2014 [1], nephrologists have to face and address a new clinical problem. In fact, whereas protein-energy wasting (PEW) may be less common than anticipated, obesity is today a frequent and emerging condition in dialysis cohorts around the world [2]. The global pandemic of obesity carries a markedly increased risk for comorbid complications, such as type 2 diabetes, cancer, dyslipidemia, hypertension, inflammation, osteoarthritis, dementia, cardiovascular disease (CVD), and sleep apnea [3]. Thus, it is disappointing that no major success stories to combat the obesity epidemic have been reported [4]. When the society has become serious about addressing obesity, it may take decades to reverse obesity rates to the levels reported before the epidemic started. The obesity spreading patterns seem predictable around the world, and emerging data show that low- and middle-income countries, such as China [5], India [6], and Brazil [7], are currently undergoing a similar transition from normal weight to overweight and obesity as industrialized countries already have encountered. Obesity increases the risk for chronic kidney disease (CKD) and its progression to end-stage renal disease (ESRD) [8]. In fact, a high body mass index (BMI) ranks as one of the strongest risk factors for new-onset CKD [9], and obese patients have a greater incidence of glomerulosclerosis [3]. The dimension of the obesity epidemic and the impact of this epidemic on the kidney call for efforts to understand the epidemiology and the mechanism(s) of CKD associated with obesity and set as a public health priority for the development of treatment policies to halt this growing problem.

Definition and Assessment of Obesity

Obesity is most commonly defined based on BMI, i.e., a person's weight (kg) divided by the square of his or her height (m); a BMI between 20 and 25 kg/m^2 is by the World Health Organization (WHO) considered as normal weight, a BMI between 25 and 30 kg/m^2 as overweight, and BMI >30 kg/m^2 as obese with increasing grading as BMI increases. The population norms of BMI are different based on ethnic and racial background [10]. Since BMI is so easy to calculate, this metric is often used in nutritional guidelines. However, BMI is a poor estimate of fat mass distribution, especially in ESRD patients defined by imbalance of hydration status

P. Stenvinkel
Division of Renal Medicine, Department of Clinical Science, Intervention and Technology, Karolinska Institute, Stockholm, Sweden

Karolinska University Hospital, Stockholm, Sweden
e-mail: peter.stenvinkel@ki.se

C. M. Rhee et al. (eds.), *Endocrine Disorders in Kidney Disease*,
https://doi.org/10.1007/978-3-319-97765-2_19

[11]. Since disease risk increase with a waist circumference (WC) and waist-hip ratio (WHR) of >88 cm and >0.8, respectively, for females and of >102 cm and 0.9, respectively, for males, this simple measure seems superior to BMI for the correct classification of obesity [12]. Compared to anthropometric measurements, fat determination by single-frequency bioimpedance is not better [13], and for routine use WHR and anthropometrics are recommended [12]. The conicity index (an easy anthropometric estimate using WC, height, and weight to model the relative accumulation of abdominal fat without requiring the hip circumference) could be useful to identify non-overweight CKD patients with an estimate of the wasting component [14]. The somewhat confusing overlap between PEW and obesity is termed "obese sarcopenia" and indicates a problem to correctly assess nutritional status [15].

Adiposity: A Consequence or Cause of Overeating?

Like most chronic diseases that affect a large proportion of the population, the pathophysiology of obesity is severely complex, including genetic predisposition, environmental changes, and individual preferences. More than 150 genetic loci are related with the development of obesity and type 2 diabetes [16]. Although much improvement in identifying genetic changes induced by obesity has already been made, studies are missing defining the liable key loci [17]. The remarkable growth of the prevalence of obesity in the world with a fixed genetic background [18] is partly explained by the strong link between a sedentary inactive lifestyle and obesity [19]. Studies of obesity require a deep perception of energy balance, i.e., increased adiposity results from the loss of the homeostatic control of caloric intake and energy expenditure. Since normal mitochondrial function associates with a healthier metabolic phenotype in obese children [20] and offsprings of type 2 diabetics display impaired mitochondrial function [21], oxidative capacity stimulation may be key for a lean phenotype. Moreover, since cold exposure and beta-adrenergic agonists can induce browning of white adipose tissue (increase energy expenditure and produce heat rousing), stimulation of brown fat depots may be a future treatment of obesity [22]. A recent study identified miR-378 as a key regulatory component underlying expansion and obesity resistance of brown adipose tissue and, thus, adds novel insights into the cross talk between brown and white adipose tissue [23].

It has been estimated that during our lifetime we will eat approximately 35 tons of food. Thus, the food we consume is the single most important and versatile environmental determinant of human health. Increased intake of energy-dense food and sodas are considered to be a major cause of obesity. However, although it is acknowledged that eating too little calories is not the cause, but a symptom of anorexia nervosa, it is still believed that consumption of fewer calories will lead to the solution of the obesity problem. Since eating disorders may be due to altered neurotransmitter system function, it has been suggested that overeating could be regarded as a symptom rather than the cause of obesity [24, 25]. The current paradigm that overeating of easy digestible carbohydrates and the resulting imbalance between "energy out and in" as the main cause of obesity has been confronted [26]. Instead it has been suggested that the host response to diverse nutrients commit to overeating and obesity. Thus, a much more complex sum of synchronized alterations, including neurocognitive factors [27], mutation of the uricase gene [28], psychosocial stress [29], changes in the epigenome [30], gut dysbiosis [31], adenovirus infection [32], and metabolic changes triggered by specific nutrients [26], may promote obesity. It is evident that whereas some nutrients promote insulin resistance and fat accumulation, other nutrients, such as anti-oxidants, plant food, probiotics and nuts, counteract the negative effects of a calorie-rich diet by beneficial effects on mitochondrial health [26]. Thus, invigoration of mitochondrial oxidative capacity could be the key for a slender phenotype. Plant phenols, a large group of metabolites that include tannins, flavonoids (anthocyanins and flavonols), and stilbenoids, may counter insulin resistance and fat buildup [26]. Polyphenols lower triglycerides and body weight by increasing energy expenditure, increase fat utilization, and balance glucose homeostasis. A high intake of total polyphenols, total flavonoids, and stilbenes is associated with a reduced risk of diabetes in elderly persons at risk of CVD [33]. As resveratrol has favorable effects on energy metabolism and mitochondrial oxidative capacity, this "caloric restriction mimetic" may be a future treatment for obese and insulin-resistant individuals. Berries also show anti-obesity effects as they not only blocked the metabolic effects [34] but also changed hepatic gene expression and DNA methylation patterns [35] of a high-fat diet. Although nuts are rich in fat and calories, they do not increase body weight and have favorable effects (especially walnuts) on the cardiometabolic profile. Since the nuclear factor (erythroid-derived 2)-like 2 (Nrf2) is a transcription factor and key activator of antioxidant genes, it can be conjectured that depressed intake of nutrients rich in Nrf2 stimulators, such as polyphenols, resveratrol, allicins, lycopene, and caffeine, increases risk of obesity [36]. It was recently reported that a high-quality diet pattern, i.e., greater intake of fruits, vegetables, whole grains, seeds/nuts, and yogurt intake, was associated with decreased adiposity, while red/processed meats were associated with greater regional adiposity [37]. Since fish eaters have lower BMI than meat eaters [38], the impact of marine lipids on insulin resistance and fat buildup deserves further attention.

Does Increased Intake of Fructose Cause Obesity?

Sugar or other fructose-containing composites in fruits and vegetables, in sucrose, and in high-fructose corn syrup (HFCS) have hitherto been considered as empty calories. In contrast to glucose, fructose is not important for biochemical reactions and humans operate well without it. Since fructose intake does not evoke an increase in glucose and insulin levels, its potential for weight gain has been regarded as minimal. However, in the USA the marked increase in fructose intake with the introduction of HFCS in the early 1970s has paralleled the rise in BMI [39]. Indeed, the establishment of HFCS in soft drinks may have added not only to the obesity epidemic [40] but also, via stimulation of uric acid, to hypertension, type 2 diabetes, and CKD [41]. As lowering of uric acid has beneficial effects on the metabolic syndrome, studies that examine if low-fructose and low-purine diets reduce weight and decrease cardiovascular risk should be supported. High intake of fructose induces appearances of the metabolic syndrome and boosts leptin resistance [42], causes intracellular ATP depletion [43], blocks satiety signals [44], and reduces resting energy expenditure [45]. Fructose metabolites also drive excessive food consumption by stimulation of dopamine and affecting the reward system in the brain. In fact, in many ways fructose mimes the effect of its metabolic cousin ethanol, another nonessential energy source [46]. Moreover, since fructose triggers vasopressin [47] and enhances urinary sodium reabsorption [48], this may indirectly promote overweight status. Because vasopressin stimulates fat accumulation [49], blocks fat oxidation [50], and induces insulin resistance and fatty liver accumulation [51], this ties hyperosmolarity to obesity. Indeed, water loading reduces hepatic fat content [51], and high salt intake with low water intake diminishes insulin sensitivity [52] and forecasts obesity and diabetes [53, 54]. Thus, promotion of more water intake could be a novel strategy to reduce energy consumption [55].

Gut Microbiota: An Emerging Player in Obesity and Kidney Disease

The nutritional value of the approximately 35 tons of food we ingest during our lifetime is shaped by the gut microbiota, an environmental factor that influences whole-body metabolism by affecting energy balance. Gut microbiota affect gut permeability, metabolic endotoxemia, and the production of short-chain fatty acids, which protect against diet-induced obesity [56]. The switch from a low-fat, plant polysaccharide-rich diet to a high-sucrose and high-fat diet leads to a rapid transformation in the mice microbiota [57]. As a study in twins discordant for obesity reported that fat mass and obesity-associated metabolic phenotype were transmissible to mice with fecal cultures [58], it signifies a central role of the gut microflora for fat buildup. In accordance, a study in wild hibernating bears showed that transplantation of summer (but not winter) bear microbiota to germ-free mice promoted adiposity without impairing glucose tolerance. Thus, seasonal variation in the microbiota contributes to host energy metabolism in hibernating brown bears [59]. Recent insights show that specific personal and microbiome features enable accurate glucose response prediction [60], which may lead to the opportunity for a personalized modulation of the microbiome by nutritional and pre- and probiotic intervention [61]. Also fecal transplantation [62] and probiotics [63] carry therapeutic potential for imminent treatment of obesity. Moreover, since noncaloric artificial sweeteners, such as saccharin, sucralose, and aspartame, induce glucose intolerance by changing the gut microbiota toward a composition known to associate with metabolic disease [64], patients should be discouraged to use artificial sweeteners. Since antibiotics may alter gut microbiota, especially if frequently prescribed to children, antibiotic-induced gut microbiota dysbiosis may contribute to the obesity epidemic [65]. Taken together, dietary interventions that take into consideration the specific metabolic effects of nutrients may have a better chance to decrease weight instead of only focusing on traditional hypocaloric diets in the treatment of obesity. It is fascinating that the rapid spread of obesity around the world resembles pandemics of infectious origin. As human adenovirus 36 stimulates enzymes and transcription factors that accumulate triglycerides and differentiate pre-adipocytes into mature adipocytes, virus infections may be a cause of obesity [66]. Indeed, a recent meta-analysis showed that human adenovirus 36 infection increased the risk of weight gain in adults but not in children [67]. Since Ad-36 antibodies associate with lower triglycerides [68], adenovirus infections may relate to a "healthy obesity" phenotype (vide infra).

Gross Obesity but Not Overweight Status Increases the Risk for Death and Comorbidity

Obesity is associated with disparate comorbid conditions including CVD, type 2 diabetes, metabolic syndrome, dyslipidemia, hypertension, various cancers, gallbladder disease, obstructive sleep apnea, nonalcoholic steatohepatitis, hypovitaminosis D, osteoarthritis, and psychosocial problems. Obesity is also associated with a significantly worse outcome for many cancers [69] and is related to persistent inflammation in both the general population [70] and in CKD [71]. In the general population, gross obesity increases death risk [72]. However, whereas gross obesity (BMI >35 kg/m^2) was associated with higher all-cause mortality in the general population, a meta-analysis showed that being obese in the range between 30 and 35 kg/m^2 was not associated with higher mortality and being overweight (BMI 25–30 kg/m^2) was actually associated with lower all-cause mortality [73]. Thus, BMI shows a U-shaped association with clinical outcomes, with the best fallout in overweight and mildly obese CKD patients [74]. This implies that fat mass accumulation may also have favorable effects. In accordance with results in the general population, a study in 54,506 CKD stage 3 patients showed that in comparison with patients with BMI of 18.5–24.9 kg/m^2, overweight patients and patients with obesity class 1–2 have lower risk for cardiovascular and malignancy-related death [75]. It should be noted that about 30% of obese patients seem to be protected against obesity-related metabolic complications [76]. Individuals with "healthy obesity" are characterized by relatively low visceral fat mass, normal adipose tissue function, low macrophage infiltration, and normal insulin sensitivity [76].

Obesity: An Independent Risk Factor for CKD

Obesity is an autonomous risk factor for development of CKD in the general population [8, 77, 78]. Hsu et al. [79] showed that higher baseline

BMI remained an independent predictor for ESRD also following adjustments for diabetes mellitus and hypertension. Moreover, data from 2585 individuals followed for 19 years showed that BMI independently predicted new-onset CKD [80]. European data showed that obesity increased the risk of microalbuminuria [81] and loss of residual renal function after start of dialysis [82]. Moreover, CKD is strongly associated with components of the metabolic syndrome [83]. Besides indirect effects on kidney disease incidence and its progression (via diabetes, atherosclerosis, and hypertension), adiposity has effects that may directly affect kidney function [84]. Since obesity as measured by WC is associated with higher risk for ESRD even after adjustment for BMI [85], distribution of fat mass likely has an impact on the risk for kidney dysfunction. Hyperinsulinemia, which commonly accompanies obesity, promotes mesangial expansion, glomerular hyperfiltration, glomerular hypertrophy, and increased filtration fraction. These alterations may promote glomerulosclerosis [86] and segmental glomerulosclerosis [87]. In addition, obesity-associated hyperleptinemia promotes renal fibrosis and oxidative stress and activates the sympathetic nervous system [88], factors that increase risk of kidney dysfunction.

Treatment of Obesity in CKD

Unfortunately, despite the magnitude of the obesity problem, treatment modalities for obesity are not well developed. Since obesity may in some cases be countered through lower calorie consumption and increased physical activity, adherence to a healthy lifestyle should always be the primary aim when nephrologists handle obese CKD patients. Indeed, differences in lifestyle and body composition are associated with reductions in insulin sensitivity in moderate-severe CKD [89]. Unfortunately, since only minor and short-duration studies have been conducted, sketchy data exist on the effects of intentional weight loss in CKD [90]. The development of anti-obesity drugs has been full of calamities, and at present nephrologists do not really have efficient pharmacological treatment to offer this vulnerable patient group. Only small studies have been conducted [91], and cases of impaired renal function associated with the use of the anti-obesity drugs have been reported [92]. Bariatric surgery has become the standard for effective intervention in the general population, and a more than 50% weight loss [93] and lower incidence of cardiovascular events at long-term follow-up [94] have been reported. Bariatric surgery was also more efficient in the prevention of type 2 diabetes than usual care. Several reports in limited numbers of patients indicate a significant improvement in renal parameters after bariatric surgery [95–99]. It is remarkable that diabetic nephropathy resolved in 58% of 52 obese type 2 diabetic patients that underwent bariatric surgery [100]. Although higher complication rates were reported in CKD patients after bariatric surgery, the incidence of complications remained <10% [101]. Thus, since dialysis patients have excellent medium-term weight loss and an acceptable (but increased) risk-benefit ratio [102], dialysis should not be considered as a contraindication to bariatric surgery.

The Obesity Paradox: Should Weight Gain Be Promoted in Dialysis Patients?

The observation that elevated BMI confers a survival advantage to ESRD patients was first reported in 1999 [103] and subsequently confirmed in most, but not all [104], studies based on North American [105, 106], European [107, 108], and Asian [109] dialysis cohorts. Furthermore, a study of 123,383 hemodialysis patients showed that higher BMI was associated with lower mortality across all dialysis vintage and age groups [110]. However, the obesity paradox has not been confirmed in a group of nondiabetic patients with mild-moderate CKD [111]. There may be many reasons why obesity is associated with a survival advantage. Whereas residual confounding by PEW, inflammation, and competing mortality risk factors may in part explain the "obesity paradox" phenomenon, other factors doubtlessly contribute. Because an increase in BMI may reflect more lean body mass, the association between increased BMI and better outcome does not automatically imply that fat mass is protective. Indeed, the protection observed with high BMI is likely to be connected to high muscle mass [112, 113]. A retrospective study of 119,099 Japanese hemodialysis patients reported that the "obesity paradox" only existed when obesity was defined by BMI and lower levels of serum creatinine were associated with poor outcomes in all BMI groups [114]. It is also likely that high BMI is a reflection of preserved appetite and energy stores. Because good appetite is associated with better outcomes in dialysis patients [115] and obese patients are more likely to expend extra calories, this may indirectly explain the alliance between high BMI and better outcomes. Besides indicating well-preserved energy stores, the larger amount of fat mass may be associated with improved hemodynamic tolerance, better stem cell mobilization, less stress response as a result of neurohormonal alterations, and more competent disposal of lipophilic uremic toxins [3]. The observations of the "obesity paradox" have led some to argue that weight gain should be encouraged in dialysis patients regardless of its body compartment, i.e., fat or muscle mass. However, obesity has not been shown to have any advantageous effects on self-rated health status and physical function in analogy to normal weight or moderately overweight hemodialysis patients [106].

Although overweight status and obesity are associated with several complications of peritoneal dialysis (PD), such as increased risk of peritonitis, PD catheter loss and technique failure, and a more rapid decline of residual renal function [116–118], the impact of overweight status on outcome in PD patients is less clear. Whereas the mortality of obese PD patients was reported to be worse in comparison with normal body weight [119], Snyder et al. [120] reported a survival benefit for overweight and obese PD patients. Weight gain and accumulation of fat mass is a common metabolic complication of PD that may lead to significant clinical problems.

High BMI has been associated with a "paradoxically" better outcome in many other chronic debilitating disorders, such as congestive heart failure, rheumatoid arthritis, dementia, coronary heart disease, and cancer. It is striking that a high BMI is associated with a survival advantage in the very same chronic debilitating diseases that obesity is a risk factor for. As persistent low-grade inflammation is a common feature in all the chronic diseases in which the "obesity paradox" has been proclaimed, the impact of persistent inflammation on the association between BMI and outcome needs examination. It was lately studied if the documented association between high BMI and better outcome would be affected by the presence of systemic inflammation in about 6000 European hemodialysis patients [108]. Whereas the study confirmed that lower BMI was associated with higher mortality, it also revealed that when inflammation was taken into consideration, a major catalyzing effect of inflammation was evident [121]. Whereas high BMI had a protective action and was linked to longer survival rates for chronically inflamed dialysis patients, no protective effect of high BMI was found in non-inflamed dialysis patients. The observed correlation persisted even after controlling for a large number of non-modifiable and modifiable factors, such as hospitalization, catheter use, Kt/V, blood flow, and blood pressure that can influence survival rates. Thus, the implications of obesity in dialysis patients carry differential prognostic information in those who are inflamed or not inflamed. Thus, dialysis patients who are overweight and show signs of chronic inflammation should not be endorsed to lose weight. Treatment of inflamed patients, regardless of whether they are over- or underweight, should focus on resolving the inflammatory process and treating the underlying causes.

Obesity and Kidney Transplantation

Since the prevalence of obesity in US patients awaiting a kidney transplant increased from around 12% to 25% between 1987 and 2001 [122], nephrologists need to be aware of the potential risks of obesity on renal graft function and magnitude of postoperative complications. In a retrospective study, obesity was an independent risk factor for graft loss and death in recipients of kidney transplant [123]. Another retrospective study revealed recipient BMI and dialysis vintage as independent risk factors for delayed graft function [124]. Pretransplant overweight status or obesity was also associated with an incrementally higher risk of delayed graft function in other studies [125, 126]. A recent meta-analysis showed that obese (BMI >30 kg/m^2) transplant recipients only had a slightly increased risk of graft loss and do experience a similar survival as recipients with normal BMI [127]. Since there is a higher risk for postoperative complications and delayed graft function after renal transplantation, there is a controversy regarding which BMI cutoff level should be used [128]. A recent debate concluded that with the exception of morbid obesity (BMI >40 kg/m^2), outcomes of obese patients undergoing transplantation are better than in dialysis patients who are not undergoing renal transplantation [128]. As BMI is a poor measure of body fat composition in ESRD patients, further research should be carried out to define the optimal cutoff using more clear-cut fat assessment methods. Indeed, WC is an independent risk factor for new-onset diabetes after renal transplantation (NODAT) [129], a condition associated with poor graft function, higher rates of cardiovascular complications, and poor prognosis.

Summary and Conclusion

Increased fat mass increases the risk of CKD both by direct renal effects and indirectly via hypertension, atherosclerosis, and diabetes. Nephrologists should master methods to assess fat mass distribution and know how to manage the obese CKD patient. The treatment of obesity requires a varied approach including, but not limited to, weight-reduction and physical exercise programs. Nephrologists should aim for interventions that increase muscle mass and decrease visceral fat mass. This should be achieved in a multidisciplinary approach including dietitians and physiotherapists.

References

1. Rokholm B, Baker JL, Sørensen TI. The levelling off of the obesity epidemic since the year 1999 – a review of evidence and perspectives. Obes Rev. 2010;11:835–46.
2. Koefoed M, Kromann CB, Juliussen SR, Hvidtfeldt D, Ekelund B, Frandsen NE, et al. Nutritional status of maintenance Dialysis patients: low lean body mass index and obesity are common, protein-energy wasting is uncommon. PLoS One. 2016;11:e0150012.
3. Stenvinkel P, Zoccali C, Ikizler TA. Obesity in CKD – what should nephrologists know? J Am Soc Nephrol. 2013;24:1727–36.
4. Ng M, Fleming T, Robinson M, Thomson B, Graetz N, Margono C, et al. Global, regional, and national prevalence of overweight and obesity in children and adults during 1980–2013: a systematic analysis for the Global Burden of Disease Study 2013. Lancet. 2014;384:766–81.
5. Yu Z, Han S, Chu J, Zhu C, Guo X. Trends in overweight and obesity among children and adolescents in China from 1981 to 2010: a meta-analysis. PLoS One. 2012;7:e51949.
6. Gupta R, Sharma KK, Gupta A, Agrawal A, Mohan I, Gupta VP, et al. Persistent high prevalence of cardiovascular risk factors in the urban middle class in India: Jaipur Heart Watch-5. J Assoc Physicians India. 2012;60:11–6.
7. Schmitt AC, Cardoso MR, Lopes H, Pereira WM, Pereira EC, de Rezende DA, et al. Prevalence of metabolic syndrome and associated factors in women aged 35 to 65 years who were enrolled in a family health program in Brazil. Menopause. 2013;20:470–6.
8. Kramer HJ, Saranathan A, Luke A, Durazo-Arvizu R, Guichan C, Hou S, et al. Increasing body mass index and obesity in the incident ESRD population. J Am Soc Nephrol. 2006;17:1453–9.
9. Obermayr RP, Temml C, Knechtelsdorfer M, Gutjahr G, Kletzmayr J, Heiss S, et al. Predictors of new-onset decline in kidney function in a general middle-european population. Nephrol Dial Transplant. 2008;23:1265–73.
10. WHO Expert Consultation. Appropriate body-mass index for Asian populations and its implications for policy and intervention strategies. Lancet. 2004;363:157–63.
11. Rodrigues J, Santin F, Barbosa Brito FS, Carrero JJ, Lindholm B, Cuppari L, et al. Sensitivity and specificity of body mass index as a marker of obesity in elderly patients on hemodialysis. J Ren Nutr. 2016;26:65–71.
12. Zoccali C, Torino C, Tripepi G, Mallamaci F. Assessment of obesity in chronic kidney disease: what is the best measure? Curr Opin Nephrol Hypertens. 2012;21:641–6.
13. Silva M, Vale B, Lemos C, Torres M, Bregman R. Body adiposity index assess body fat with high

accuracy in nondialyzed chronic kidney disease patients. Obesity. 2012;21:546–52.
14. Cordeiro AC, Qureshi AR, Stenvinkel P, Heimbürger O, Axelsson J, Bárány P, et al. Abdominal fat deposition is associated with increased inflammation, protein-energy wasting and worse outcome in patients undergoing haemodialysis. Nephrol Dial Transpl. 2010;25:562–8.
15. Honda H, Qureshi AR, Axelsson J, Heimburger O, Suliman ME, Barany P, et al. Obese sarcopenia in end-stage renal disease patients is associated with inflammation and increased mortality. Am J Clin Nutr. 2007;86:633–8.
16. Drong AW, Lindgren CM, McCarthy MI. The genetic and epigenetic basis of type 2 diabetes and obesity. Clin Pharmacol Ther. 2012;92:707–15.
17. Youngson NA, Morris MJ. What obesity research tells us about epigenetic mechanisms. Philos Trans R Soc Lond Ser B Biol Sci. 2013;368:20110337.
18. Christakis NA, Fowler JH. The spread of obesity in a large social network over 32 years. N Engl J Med. 2007;357:370–9.
19. Knight JA. Physical inactivity: associated diseases and disorders. Ann Clin Lab Sci. 2012;42:320–37.
20. Fleischman A, Kron M, Systrom DM, Hrovat M, Grinspoon SK. Mitochondrial function and insulin resistance in overweight and normal-weight children. J Clin Endocrinol Metab. 2009;94:4923–30.
21. Morino K, Petersen KF, Dufour S, Befroy D, Frattini J, Shatzkes N, et al. Reduced mitochondrial density and increased IRS-1 serine phosphorylation in muscle of insulin-resistant offspring of type 2 diabetic parents. J Clin Invest. 2005;115:3587–93.
22. Kim SH, Plutsky J. Brown fat and browning for the treatment of obesity and related metabolic disorders. Diabetes Metab J. 2016;40:12–21.
23. Pan D, Mao C, Quattrochi B, Friedline RH, Zhu LJ, Jung DY, et al. MicroRNA-378 controls classical brown fat expansion to counteract obesity. Nat Commun. 2014;5:4725.
24. Taube G. Treat obesity as physiology, not physics. Nature. 2012;492:155.
25. Ludwig DS, Friedman M. Increasing adiposity: consequence or cause of overeating? JAMA. 2014;311:2167–8.
26. Stenvinkel P. Obesity a a disease with many etiologies disguised in the same oversized phenotype: has the overeating thery failed? Nephrol Dial Transpl. 2015;30:1656–64.
27. Milanski M, Degasperi G, Coope A, Morari J, Denis R, Cintra DE, et al. Saturated fatty acids produce an inflammatory response predominantly through the activation of TLR4 signaling in hypothalamus: implications for the pathogenesis of obesity. J Neurosci. 2009;29:359–70.
28. Johnson RJ, Stenvinkel P, Martin SL, Jani A, Sanchez-Lozada LG, Hill JO, et al. Redefining metabolic syndrome as a fat storage condition based on studies of comparative physiology. Obesity. 2013;21:659–64.
29. Karasu SR. Of mind and matter: psychological dimensions in obesity. Am J Psychother. 2012;66:111–28.
30. Bays H, Scinta W. Adiposopathy and epigenetics: an introduction to obesity as a transgenerational disease. Curr Med Res Opin. 2015;31:2059–69.
31. Festi D, Schiumerini R, Birtolo C, Marzi L, Montrone L, Scaioli E, et al. Gut microbiota and its pathophysiology in disease paradigms. Dig Dis. 2011;29:518–24.
32. Mitra AK, Clarke K. Viral obesity: fact or fiction? Obesity. 2010;11:289–96.
33. Tresserra-Rimbau A, Guasch-Ferré M, Salas-Salvadó J, Toledo E, Corella D, Castañer O, et al. Intake of total polyphenols and some classes of Polyphenols is inversely associated with diabetes in elderly people at high cardiovascular disease risk. J Nutr. 2016;146:767–77.
34. Heyman L, Axling U, Blanco N, Sterner O, Holm C, Berger K. Evaluation of beneficial metabolic effects of berries in high-fat fed C57BL/6J mice. J Nutr Metab. 2014;2014:403041.
35. Heyman-Lindén L, Seki Y, Storm P, Jones HA, Charron MJ, Berger K, et al. Berry intake changes hepatic gene expression and DNA methylation patterns associated with high-fat diet. J Nutr Biochem. 2016;27:79–95.
36. Cardozo LF, Pedruzzi LM, Stenvinkel P, Stockler-Pinto MB, Daleprane JB, Leite M, et al. Nutritional strategies to modulate inflammation and oxidative stress pathways via activation of the master antioxidant switch Nrf2. Biochimie. 2013;95:1525–33.
37. Shah RV, Murthy VL, Allison MA, Ding J, Budoff M, Frazier-Wood AC, et al. Diet and adipose tissue distributions: the multi-ethnic study of atherosclerosis. Nutr Metab Cardiovasc Dis. 2016;26:185–93.
38. Spencer EA, Appleby PN, Davey GK, Key TJ. Diet and body mass index in 38000 EPIC-Oxford meat-eaters, fish-eaters, vegetarians and vegans. Int J Obes Relat Metab Disord. 2003;27:728–34.
39. Johnson RJ, Segal MS, Sautin Y, Nakagawa T, Feig DI, Kang DH, et al. Potential role of sugar (fructose) in the epidemic of hypertension, obesity and the metabolic syndrome, diabetes, kidney disease, and cardiovascular disease. Am J Clin Nutr. 2007;86:899–906.
40. Perez-Pozo SE, Schold J, Nakagawa T, Sánchez-Lozada LG, Johnson RJ, Lillo JL. Excessive fructose intake induces the features of metabolic syndrome in healthy adult men: role of uric acid in the hypertensive response. Int J Obes. 2010;34:454–61.
41. Johnson RJ, Sanchez-Lozada LG, Nakagawa T. The effect of fructose on renal biology and disease. J Am Soc Nephrol. 2012;21:2036–9.
42. Shapiro A, Mu W, Roncal C, Cheng KY, Johnson R, Scarpace PJ. Fructose-induced leptin resistance exacerbates weight gain in response to subsequent high-fat feeding. Am J Physiol Regul Integr Comp Physiol. 2008;295:R1370–5.

43. Friedman MI, Harris RB, Ramirez I, Tordoff MG. Fatty acid oxidation affects food intake by altering hepatic energy status. Am J Physiol Regul Integr Comp Physiol. 1999;276:R1046–53.
44. Lane MD, Cha SH. Effect of glucose and fructose on food intake via malonyl-CoA signaling in the brain. Biochem Biophys Res Commun. 2009;382:1–5.
45. Cox CL, Stanhope KL, Schwarz JM, Graham JL, Hatcher B, Griffen SC, et al. Consumption of fructose-sweetened beverages for 10 weeks reduces net fat oxidation and energy expenditure in overweight/obese men and women. Eur J Clin Nutr. 2012;66:201–8.
46. Lustig RH. Fructose: It's "alcohol without the buzz". Adv Nutr. 2013;4:226–35.
47. Wolf JP, Nguyen NU, Dumoulin G, Berthelay S. Influence of hypertonic monosaccharide infusions on the release of plasma arginine vasopressin in normal humans. Horm Metab Res. 1992;24:379–83.
48. Cabral PD, Hong NJ, Hye Khan MA, Ortiz PA, Beierwaltes WHI, Mig JD, et al. Fructose stimulates Na/H exchange activity and sensitizes the proximal tubule to angiotensin II. Hypertension. 2014;63:e68–73.
49. Johnson RJ, Nakagawa T, Sanchez-Lozada LG, Shafiu M, Sundaram S, Le M, et al. Sugar, uric acid, and the etiology of diabetes and obesity. Diabetes. 2013;62:3307–15.
50. Rofe AM, Williamson DH. Metabolic effects of vasopressin infusion in the starved rat. Reversal of ketonemia. Biochem J. 1983;212:231–9.
51. Taveau C, Chollet C, Waeckel L, Desposito D, Bicket DG, Arthus MF, et al. Vasopressin and hydration play a major role in the development of glucose intolerance and hepatic steatosis in obese rats. Diabetologia. 2015;58:1081–90.
52. Donovan DS, Soloman CG, Seely EW, Williams GH, Simonson DC. Effect of sodium intake on insulin sensitivity. Am J Phys. 1993;264:E730–4.
53. Larsen SC, Ängquist L, Sørensen TI, Heitmann BL. 24h urinary sodium excretion and subsequent change in weight, waist circumference and body composition. PlosOne. 2013;8:e69689.
54. Libuda L, Kersting M, Alexy U. Consumption of dietary salt measured by urinary sodium excretion and its association with body weight status in healthy children and adolescents. Public Health Nutr. 2012;15:433–41.
55. An R, McCaffrey J. Plain water consumption in relation to energy intake and diet quality among US adults, 2005–2012. J Hum Nutr Diet. 2016;29(5):624–32.
56. Lin HV, Frassetto A, Kowalik EJ, Nawrocki AR, Lu MM, Kosinski JR, et al. Butyrate and propionate protect against diet-induced obesity and regulate gut hormones via free fatty acid receptor 3-independent mechanisms. PlosOne. 2012;7:e35240.
57. Turnbaugh PJ, Ridaura VK, Faith JJ, Rey FE, Knight R, Gordon JI. The effect of diet on the human gut microbiome: a metagenomic analysis in humanized gnotobiotic mice. Sci Transl Med. 2009;1:6ra14.
58. Ridaura VK, Faith JJ, Rey FE, Cheng J, Duncan AE, Kau AL, et al. Gut microbiota from twins discordant for obesity modulate metabolism in mice. Science. 2013;341:1241214.
59. Sommer F, Ståhlman MI, Lkayeva O, Arnemo JM, Kindberg J, Josefsson J, et al. The gut microbiota modulates energy metabolism in the hibernating Brown bear Ursus arctos. Cell Rep. 2016;14:1655–61.
60. Zeevi D, Korem T, Zmora N, Israeli D, Rothschild D, Weinberger A, et al. Personalized nutrition by prediction of glycemic responses. Cell Rep. 2015;163:1079–94.
61. Zmora N, Zeevi D, Korem T, Segal E, Elinav E. Taking it personally: personalized utilization of the human microbiome in health and disease. Cell Host Microbe. 2016;19:12–20.
62. Gupta A, Allen-Vercoe E, Petrof EO. Fecal microbiota transplantation: in perspective. Therap Adv Gastroenterol. 2016;9:229–39.
63. Kobyliak N, Conte C, Cammarota G, Haley AP, Styriak I, Gaspar L, et al. Probiotics in prevention and treatment of obesity: a critical view. Nutr Metab (Lond). 2016;13:14.
64. Suez J, Korem T, Zeevi D, Zilberman-Schapira G, Thaiss CA, Maza O, et al. Artificial sweeteners induce glucose intolerance by altering the gut microbiota. Nature. 2014;514:181–6.
65. Principi N, Esposito S. Antibiotic administration and the development of obesity in children. Int J Antimicrob Agents. 2016;47(3):171–7.
66. Atkinson RL. Could viruses contribute to the worldwide epidemic of obesity? In t J Pediatr Obes. 2008;3(Suppl 1):37–43.
67. Xy MY, Cao B, Wang DF, Guo JH, Chen KL, Shi M, et al. Human adenovirus 36 infection increased the risk of obesity: a meta-analysis update. Medicine (Baltimore). 2015;94:e2357.
68. Atkinson RL, Dhurandhar NV, Allison DB, Bowen RL, Israel BA, Albu JB, et al. Human adenovirus-36 is associated with increased body weight and paradoxical reduction of serum lipids. Int J Obes. 2005;29:281–6.
69. Gilbert CA, Slingerland JM. Cytokines, obesity, and cancer: new insights on mechanisms linking obesity to cancer risk and progression. Annu Rev Med. 2013;64:45–57.
70. You T, Nicklas BJ. Chronic inflammation: role of adipose tissue and modulation by weight loss. Curr Diabetes Rev. 2006;2:29–37.
71. Axelsson J, Qureshi AR, Suliman ME, Honda H, Pecoits-Filho R, Heimbürger O, et al. Truncal fat mass as a contributor to inflammation in end-stage renal disease. Am J Clin Nutr. 2004;80:1222–9.
72. Greenberg JA. Obesity and early mortality in the U.S. Obesity (Silver Spring). 2013;21:405–12.
73. Flegal KM, Kit BK, Orpana H, Graubard BI. Association of all-cause mortality with overweight and obesity using standard body mass index categories: a systematic review and meta-analysis. JAMA. 2013;309:71–82.

74. Lu JL, Kalantar-ZAdeh K, Ma JZ, Quarles LD, Kovesdy CP. Association of body mass index with outcomes in patients with CKD. J Am Soc Nephrol. 2014;25:2088–96.
75. Navaneethan SD, Schold JD, Arrigain S, Kirwan JP, Nally JV. Body mass index and causes of death in chronic kidney disease. Kidney Int. 2016;89:675–82.
76. Blüher M. Are there still healthy obese patients? Curr Opin Endocrinol Diabetes Obes. 2012;19:341–6.
77. Chertow GM, Hsu C-Y, Johansen KL. The enlarging body of evidence: obesity and chronic kidney disease. J Am Soc Nephrol. 2006;17:1501–2.
78. Ejerblad E, Fored CM, Lindblad P, Fryzek J, McLaughlin JK, Nyrén O. Obesity and risk for chronic renal failure. J Am Soc Nephrol. 2006;17:1695–702.
79. Hsu CY, McCulloch CE, Iribarren C, Darbinian J, Go AS. Body mass index and risk for end-stage renal disease. Ann Intern Med. 2006;144:21–8.
80. Fox CS, Larson MG, Leip EP, Culleton B, Wilson PW, Levy D. Predictors of new-onset kidney disease in a community-based population. JAMA. 2004;291:844–50.
81. Pinto-Sietsma SJ, Navis G, Janssen WM, de Zeeuw D, Gans RO, de Jong PE, et al. A central body fat distribution is related to renal function impairment, even in lean subjects. Am J Kidney Dis. 2003;41:733–41.
82. Drechsler C, de Mutsert R, Grootendorst DC, Boeschoten EW, Krediet RT, le Cessie S, et al. Association of body mass index with decline in residual kidney function after initiation of dialysis. Am J Kidney Dis. 2009;53:1014–23.
83. Chen J, Muntner P, Hamm LL, Jones DW, Batuman V, Fonseca V, et al. The metabolic syndrome and chronic kidney disease in U.S. adults. Ann Intern Med. 2004;140:167–74.
84. Wickman C, Kramer H. Obesity and kidney disease: potential mechanisms. Semin Nephrol. 2013;33:14–22.
85. Kramer H, Gutiérrez OM, Judd SE, Muntner P, Warnock DG, Tanner RM, et al. Waist circumference, body mass index, and ESRD in the REGARDS (Reasons for Geographic and Racial Differences in Stroke) study. Am J Kidney Dis. 2016;67:62–9.
86. Brenner BM. Hemodynamically mediated glomerular injury and the progressive nature of kidney disease. Kidney Int. 1983;23:647–55.
87. Warnke RA, Kempson RL. The nephrotic syndrome in massive obesity: a study by light, immunofluorescence, and electron microscopy. Arch Pathol Lab Med. 1978;102:431–8.
88. Wolf G, Ziyadeh FN. Leptin and renal fibrosis. Contrib Nephrol. 2006;151:175–83.
89. de Boer IH, Zelnick L, Afkarian M, Ayers E, Curtin L, Himmelfarb J, Ikizler TA, et al. Impaired glucose and insulin homeostasis in moderate-severe CKD. J Am Soc Nephrol. 2016;27(9):2861–71.
90. Navaneethan SD, Yehnert H, Moustarah F, Schreiber MJ, Schauer PR, Beddhu S. Weight loss interventions in chronic kidney disease: a systematic review and meta-analysis. Clin J Am Soc Nephrol. 2009;4:1565–74.
91. Tong PC, Lee ZS, Sea MM, Chow CC, Ko GT, Chan WB, et al. The effect of orlistat-induced weight loss, without concomitant hypocaloric diet, on cardiovascular risk factors and insulin sensitivity in young obese Chinese subjects with or without type 2 diabetes. Arch Intern Med. 2002;162:2428–35.
92. Coutinho AK, Glancey GR. Orlistat, an under-recognised cause of progressive renal impairment. Nephrol Dial Transplant. 2013;(Suppl 4):iv172–4.
93. Buchwald H, Avidor Y, Braunwald E, Jensen MD, Pories W, Fahrbach K, et al. Bariatric surgery: a systematic review and meta-analysis. JAMA. 2004;292:1724–37.
94. Sjöström L, Peltonen M, Jacobson P, Sjöström CD, Karason K, Wedel H, et al. Bariatric surgery and long-term cardiovascular events. JAMA. 2012;307:56–65.
95. Kiortis DN, Christou MA. Management of obesity-induced kidney disease: a critical review of the literature. Obes Facts. 2012;5:821–32.
96. Alexander JW, Goodman HR, Hawver LR, Cardi MA. Improvement and stabilization of chronic kidney disease after gastric bypass. Surg Obes Relat Dis. 2009;5:237–41.
97. Hou CC, Shyu RS, Lee WJ, Ser KH, Lee YC, Chen SC. Improved renal function 12 months after bariatric surgery. Surg Obes Relat Dis. 2012;9:202–6.
98. Bueter M, Dubb SS, Gill A, Joannou L, Ahmed A, Frankel AH, et al. Renal cytokines improve early after bariatric surgery. Br J Surg. 2010;97:1838–44.
99. Amor A, Jiménez A, Moizé V, Ibarzabal A, Flores L, Lacy AM, et al. Weight loss independently predicts urinary albumin excretion normalization in morbidly obese type 2 diabetic patients undergoing bariatric surgery. Surg Endosc. 2013;27:2046–51.
100. Heneghan HM, Cetin D, Navaneethan SD, Orzech N, Brethauer SA, Schauer PR. Effects of bariatric surgery on diabetic nephropathy after 5 years of follow-up. Surg Obes Relat Dis. 2013;9:7–14.
101. Turgeon NA, Perez S, Mondestin M, Davis SS, Lin E, Tata S, et al. The impact of renal function on outcomes of bariatric surgery. J Am Soc Nephrol. 2012;23:885–94.
102. Jamal MH, Corcelles R, Daigle CR, Rogula T, Korh M, Schauer PR, et al. Safety and effectiveness of bariatric surgery in dialysis patients and kidney transplantation candidates. Surg Obes Relat Dis. 2015;11:419–23.
103. Fleischmann E, Teal N, Dudley J, May W, Bower JD, Salahudeen AK. Influence of excess weight on mortality and hospital stay in 1346 hemodialysis patients. Kidney Int. 1999;55:1560–7.
104. de Mutsert R, Snijder MB, van der Sman-de Beer F, Seidell JC, Boeschoten EW, Krediet RT, et al. Association between body mass index and mortality is similar in the hemodialysis population and the

general population at high age and equal duration of follow-up. J Am Soc Nephrol. 2007;18:967–74.
105. Kalantar-Zadeh K, Kopple JD, Kilpatrick RD, McAllister CJ, Shinaberger CS, Gjertson DW, et al. Association of morbid obesity and weight change over time with cardiovascular survival in hemodialysis patients. Am J Kidney Dis. 2005;46:489–500.
106. Johansen KL, Kutner NG, Young B, Chertow GM. Association of body size with health status in patients beginning dialysis. Am J Clin Nutr. 2006;83:543–9.
107. Chazot C, Gassia JP, Di Benedetto A, Cesare S, Ponce P, Marcelli D. Is there any survival advantage of obesity in southern European haemodialysis patients? Nephrol Dial Transpl. 2009;24:2871–6.
108. Stenvinkel P, Gillespie IA, Tunks J, Addison J, Kronenberg F, Drueke TB, et al. Inflammation modifies the paradoxical association between body mass index and mortality in hemodialysis patients. J Am Soc Nephrol. 2016;27(5):1479–86.
109. Park J, Jin DC, Molnar MZ, Dukkipati R, Kim YL, Jing J, et al. Mortality predictability of body size and muscle mass surrogates in Asian vs white and African American hemodialysis patients. Mayo Clin Proc. 2013;88:479–86.
110. Vashistha T, Mehrotra R, Park J, Streja E, Dukkipati R, Nissenson AR, et al. Effect of age and dialysis vintage on obesity paradox in long-term hemodialysis patients. Am J Kidney Dis. 2014;63:612–22.
111. Madero M, Sarnak MJ, Wang X, Castaneda Sceppa C, Greene T, Beck GJ, et al. Body mass index and mortality in CKD. Am J Kidney Dis. 2007;50:404–11.
112. Noori N, Kopple JD, Kovesdy CP, Feroze U, Sim JJ, Murali SB, et al. Mid-arm muscle circumference and quality of life and survival in maintenance hemodialysis patients. Clin J Am Soc Nephrol. 2010;5:2258–68.
113. Beddhu S, Pappas LM, Ramkumar N, Samore MH. Effects of body size and body composition on survival in hemodialysis patients. J Am Soc Nephrol. 2003;14:2366–72.
114. Sakao Y, Ojima T, Yasuda H, Hashimoto S, Hasegawa T, Iseki K, et al. Serum creatinine modifies associations between body mass index and mortality and morbidity in prevalent hemodialysis patients. PlosOne. 2016;11:e0150003.
115. Carrero JJ, Qureshi AR, Axelsson J, Avesani CM, Suliman ME, Kato S, et al. Comparison of nutritional and inflammatory markers in dialysis patients with reduced appetite. Am J Clin Nutr. 2007;85:695–70.
116. Piraino B, Bernardini J, Centa PK, Johnston JR, Sorkin MI, Piraino B, Bernardini J, et al. The effect of body weight on CAPD related infections and catheter loss. Perit Dial Int. 1991;11(1):64–8.
117. Grzegorzewska AE, Mariak I. Differences in clinical and laboratory data of peritoneal dialysis patients selected according to body mass index. Adv Perit Dial. 2003;19:222–6.
118. McDonald SP, Collins JF, Rumpsfeld M, Johnson DW. Obesity is a risk factor for peritonitis in the Australian and New Zealand peritoneal dialysis patient populations. Perit Dial Int. 2004;24:340–6.
119. McDonald SP, Collins JF, Johnson DW. Obesity is associated with worse peritoneal dialysis outcomes in the Australia and New Zealand patient populations. J Am Soc Nephrol. 2003;14:1894–901.
120. Snyder JJ, Foley RN, Gilbertson DT, Vonesh EF, Collins AJ. Body size and outcomes on peritoneal dialysis in the United States. Kidney Int. 2003;64:1838–44.
121. Carrero JJ, Stenvinkel P. Of persistent inflammation as a catalyst for other risk factors in chronic kidney disease; a hypothesis proposal. Clin J Am Soc Nephrol. 2009;4(Suppl1):S49–55.
122. Friedman AN, Miskulin DC, Rosenberg IH, Levey AS. Demographics and trends in overweight and obesity in patients at time of kidney transplantation. Am J Kidney Dis. 2003;41:480–7.
123. Grosso G, Corona D, Mistretta A, Zerbo D, Sinagra N, Giaquinta A, et al. The role of obesity in kidney transplantation outcome. Transplant Proc. 2012;44:1864–8.
124. Weissenbacher A, Jara M, Ulmer H, Biebl M, Bösmüller C, Schneeberger S, et al. Recipient and donor body mass index as important risk factors for delayed kidney graft function. Transplantation. 2012;93:524–9.
125. Molnar MZ, Kovesdy CP, Mucsi I, Bunnapradist S, Streja E, Krishnan M, et al. Higher recipient body mass index is associated with post-transplant delayed kidney graft function. Kidney Int. 2011;80:218–24.
126. Hatamizadeh P, Molnar MZ, Streja E, Lertdumrongluk P, Krishnan M, Kovesdy CP, et al. Recipient-related predictors of kidney transplantation outcomes in the elderly. Clin Transpl. 2013;27:436–43.
127. Hill CJ, Courtney AE, Cardwell CR, Maxwell AP, Lucarelli G, Veroux M, et al. Recipient obesity and outcomes after kidney transplantation: a systematic review and meta-analysis. Nephrol Dial Transpl. 2015;30:1403–11.
128. Sever MS, Zoccali C. Moderator's view: Pretransplant weight loss in dialysis patients: cum Grano salis. Nephrol Dial Transpl. 2015;30:1810–3.
129. Dedinska I, Laca L, Miklusica J, Rosenberger J, Zilinska Z, Galajda P, et al. Waist circumference as an independent risk factor for NODAT. Ann Transplant. 2015;20:154–9.

20 Adiponectin and Leptin in Kidney Disease Patients

Jerry Zhong Yu, Kamyar Kalantar-Zadeh,
and Connie M. Rhee

Introduction

Adiponectin is a type of adipokine, namely, a hormonally active molecule secreted by adipose tissue with pervasive effects on multiple organ systems. In the general population, adiponectin has demonstrated anti-inflammatory and cardio-protective properties, and a number of studies have shown that higher levels are associated with favorable cardiovascular outcomes and survival (Table 20.1). However, in patients with non-dialysis-dependent (NDD) and dialysis-dependent chronic kidney disease (CKD), higher adiponectin levels have been paradoxically associated with adverse cardiovascular outcomes and higher mortality risk (Table 20.2). Similarly, leptin is an adipokine which has been identified as having an important role in the regulation of inflammation and energy metabolism. In the general population, high serum leptin has been associated with adverse cardiovascular outcomes, but these observations are in contradistinction to findings observed in patients with end-stage renal disease (ESRD). The objective of this chapter is to review and discuss the existing body of evidence examining the interrelationships of adiponectin and leptin and outcomes in the general population as well as in those with varying degrees of impaired kidney function.

J. Z. Yu (✉)
Nephrology Associates Medical Group, Riverside, CA, USA

K. Kalantar-Zadeh
Division of Nephrology and Hypertension, Departments of Medicine, Pediatrics, Public Health, and Nursing Sciences, University of California Irvine School of Medicine, Orange, CA, USA

C. M. Rhee
Division of Nephrology and Hypertension, Departments of Medicine and Public Health, University of California Irvine School of Medicine, Orange, CA, USA

Adiponectin

Background Physiology

Adiponectin is a 240-amino acid hormone produced exclusively by adipose tissue, and it is encoded by the APM1 gene located on chromosome 3q27 as the most abundantly transcribed gene in adipocytes [17]. Adiponectin circulates in high concentrations ranging from 5 to 30 μg/mL, and it accounts for 0.01% of total serum proteins [18]. Adiponectin is synthesized as a monomer of 28–30 kDa, and it is assembled into trimer, hexamer (low molecular weight [LMW]), and high molecular weight (HMW) forms, with LMW adiponectin as the predominant isoform in circulation. HMW adiponectin levels as well as the ratio of HMW adiponectin to total adiponectin have been found to be strong predictors of insulin sensitivity in comparison with adiponectin monomers alone [19, 20].

C. M. Rhee et al. (eds.), *Endocrine Disorders in Kidney Disease*,
https://doi.org/10.1007/978-3-319-97765-2_20

Table 20.1 Studies of adiponectin and cardiovascular disease in the general population

Study	Study population	Adiponectin	*N*	Age (years)	Study type	Follow-up	Primary outcome	Results	Conclusion
Matsuda et al. [1]	CAD risk factors undergoing CT coronary	Serum adiponectin	298	67 ± 10.3	Cross-sectional	–	Multivessel coronary disease by CT coronary	ADPN in addition to risk factors predictive of CAD (AUC 0.72; 95%CI 0.66–0.77)	APDN is risk factor for multivessel CAD
Kawagoe et al. [2]	Known CAD undergoing PCI for LAD lesion	Intracoronary adiponectin	48	65 ± 11, 69 ± 11	Prospective	66 mos	Cardiovascular event occurrence	OR 5.25 for CV event in ADPN negative group	ADPN protective against CV events
Yoon et al. [3]	CAD risk factors	Serum adiponectin	1033	57.17 ± 7.16 55.40 ± 7.29	Cross-sectional	–	Carotid intima-media thickness	OR for CIMT thickening 0.42 in men; 0.47 in women	ADPN protective against atherosclerosis
Yamashita et al. [4]	Non-DM undergoing cardiac catheterization	Serum adiponectin	97	66.2 ± 8.4	Cross-sectional	–	CAD	Low ADPN HR 3.47 (1.27–9.89) for CAD	Low ADPN increases risk for CAD severity
Komura et al. [5]	Known CAD ± DM	Total ADPN, HMW ADPN	186	64.2 ± 0.9 non-DM; 63.2 ± 1.1 DM	Cross-sectional	–	Risk factors for CAD	HMW ADPN correlates to HDL	ADPN correlates to CAD risk factors
Pischon et al. [6]	Health Professionals Follow-up study with MI during follow-up	Serum adiponectin	266	65.2	Nested case control	6 yrs	Fatal and nonfatal MI and coronary heart disease	Highest quintile ADPN lowest risk for MI (RR 0.56; 95% CI 0.32–0.99)	ADPN protective against CVD

Abbreviations: *CAD* coronary artery disease, *CT* computed tomography, *ADPN* adiponectin, *PCI* percutaneous coronary intervention, *LAD* left anterior descending, *mos* months, *CV* cardiovascular, *CIMT* carotid intima-media thickness, *DM* diabetes, *HMW* high molecular weight, *MI* myocardial infarction, *yrs* years

Table 20.2 Studies of adiponectin, cardiovascular disease, and survival in non-dialysis-dependent chronic kidney disease, dialysis, and kidney transplant recipient populations

Study	Study population	*N*	Age (years)	ADPN measurements	Follow-up	Primary outcome	All-cause mortality HR (95% CI)	Total CVD HR (95% CI)	Conclusion
Imawashi et al. [7]	NDD-CKD	150	67.7 ± 0.8	Baseline	31.9 ± 1.5 mos	CVD	–	0.86 (0.75–0.96)	Low adiponectin predictor of CVD
Menon et al. [8]	NDD-CKD	585	52 ± 12	Baseline	10 yrs	All-cause mortality, CVD	1.03 (1.01–1.05)	1.06 (1.03–1.09)	High adiponectin associated with increased mortality
Jorsal et al. [9]	NDD-CKD	438	42.3 ± 10.4	Baseline	8.1 yrs	All-cause mortality, CVD	1.75 (1.47–2.10)	1.50 (1.26–1.78)	High adiponectin associated with increased all-cause and CV mortality
Zoccali et al. [10]	HD	227	59.9 ± 15.0	Baseline	31 ± 13 mos	All-cause mortality, CVD	–	0.97 (0.93–0.99)	High adiponectin associated with decreased CV events
Diez et al. [11]	HD + PD	184	67.8 ± 11.7 52.1 ± 16.9	Baseline +12 months	33.9 ± 15.7 mos	All-cause mortality, CVD	0.68 (0.49–0.95)	0.43 (0.21–0.86)	High adiponectin associated with decreased all-cause and CV mortality
Takemoto et al. [12]	HD	68	58.8 ± 13.6, 61.0 ± 8.2	Baseline	8 yrs	All-cause mortality, CVD	–	Men: 0.74 (0.57–0.97) women: 0.79 (0.67–0.94)	High adiponectin associated with decreased CV events but not overall mortality
Abdallah et al. [13]	HD	133	54.6 ± 17.3	Baseline	24 ± 9 mos	All-cause mortality, CVD	1.17 (1.08–1.28)	1.23 (1.11–1.32)	Low adiponectin associated with increased CV events
Drechsler et al. [14]	HD	1255	65.7 ± 8.3	Baseline +182 day follow- up	3.96 yrs	All-cause mortality, CVD	1.09 (1.06–1.57)	1.33 (1.05–1.69)	Rising adiponectin associated with increased risk for mortality, CVA, MI
Rao et al. [15]	HD	176	62.2 ± 12.3	Baseline + yearly	3.96 yrs	All-cause mortality, CVD	1.08 (1.00–1.17) for baseline; 1.04 (1.01–1.07) for time dependent	–	Lower baseline adiponectin associated with prevalent CV disease. Non-linear association of adiponectin with mortality and CV outcomes.
Alam et al. [16]	Posttransplant	987	51 ± 12.8	Baseline	51 mos	All-cause mortality, graft failure	1.44 (1.13–1.85)	–	High adiponectin associated with increased all-cause mortality and graft failure

Abbreviations: *ADPN* adiponectin, *CVD* cardiovascular disease, *NDD-CKD* non-dialysis-dependent chronic kidney disease, *HD* hemodialysis, *CV* cardiovascular, *PD* peritoneal dialysis, *CVA* stroke, *MI* myocardial infarction

Adiponectin mediates its intracellular effects through the adenosine monophosphate-activated protein kinase (AMPK) pathway. Adiponectin exhibits its intracellular effects via two receptors, namely, ADIPOR1 and ADIPOR2, each of which contain seven transmembrane domains and are transmembrane G-protein receptors. ADIPOR1 has a high affinity for HMW adiponectin, while AdipoR2 has intermediate affinity for all adiponectin isoforms. ADIPOR1 is expressed primarily in the skeletal muscle, while ADIPOR2 is expressed in the liver [21]. ADIPOR1 induces extracellular calcium influx that allows for the activation of calmodulin-dependent protein kinase kinase (CaMKK) and AMPK which are further involved in the control of energy metabolism. AdipoR2 activates and increases expression of peroxisome proliferator-activated receptor α (PPAR-α) ligands and increases energy consumption [21]. Single nucleotide polymorphisms have been identified in the promoter region of both ADIPOR1 and ADIPOR2 adiponectin receptors, and homozygous individuals have been observed to have overall greater abdominal obesity versus non-homozygous individuals.

Interaction Between Adiponectin and the Kidney

ADIPOR1 and AMPK are expressed in the kidney, and adiponectin is renally excreted in healthy individuals [21]. Animal data suggest that adiponectin may have an anti-inflammatory and reno-protective role. In vitro studies using animal models showed that ADIPOR1 is expressed in glomerular endothelial cells, podocytes, mesangial cells, and Bowman's capsule epithelial cells within the glomerulus which are exposed to urinary adiponectin. Exposure of these cells to HMW adiponectin resulted in increased phosphorylation of AMPK confirming the functionality of ADIPOR1 within the glomerulus [22]. Studies of adiponectin gene knockout mice show that adiponectin accumulates in renal tissue in the setting of kidney damage. Absence of adiponectin is associated with impaired kidney function, fibrosis, albuminuria, and inflammatory response, which may be ameliorated with adiponectin repletion [23].

In human studies, cross-sectional data in type 2 diabetic patients show that urinary adiponectin concentrations are positively correlated with microalbuminuria and higher mean brachial-ankle pulse velocity, suggesting that urine adiponectin may be associated with microvascular and macrovascular disease [24]. Longitudinal studies in type 1 diabetic patients have shown that urinary adiponectin is positively correlated with albuminuria, blood pressure, and glycated hemoglobin (HbA1c) and negatively correlated with kidney function. Moreover, changes in urinary adiponectin exceeded increases in serum adiponectin suggesting a role in renal injury independent of increased glomerular filtration [25]. However, in a study of patients with CKD due to type 2 diabetes, increasing urinary HMW adiponectin levels were associated with impaired kidney function but were not associated with albuminuria [26].

Adiponectin and Cardiovascular Risk Factors

Adiponectin and Obesity

A study of Pima Indians has shown that plasma adiponectin concentrations are in fact lower in obesity [27] and are negatively correlated with body mass index (BMI), body fat percentage, waist-to-thigh ratio, fasting plasma insulin levels, and 2-hour plasma glucose concentrations [28]. Obese patients with type 2 diabetes have been shown to have decreased APM1 gene expression and mRNA transcription in adipose tissue compared to nonobese patients [29]. In contrast, weight loss leads to elevation of plasma adiponectin levels in both diabetic and nondiabetic patients [10–12, 30].

Adiponectin and Type 2 Diabetes Mellitus

Numerous studies have established an association between higher adiponectin levels and enhanced insulin sensitivity. For example, in animal studies, adiponectin has been shown to reverse insulin resistance in lipoatrophic mice, presumed to be due to the reduction of triglyceride content in muscle and liver and subsequent increase in molecules that augment fatty acid utilization in muscle [31]. A systematic review and meta-analysis of 13 prospective studies have also examined the relationship between adiponectin and the risk of developing type 2 diabetes. In analyses that accounted for obesity, every 1-μg/mL increment in the log of adiponectin levels was associated with a 28% lower risk of developing type 2 diabetes (adjusted relative risk [aRR] 0.72 [95% CI] 0.67–0.78; $p < 0.001$), supporting the hypothesis that adiponectin increases insulin sensitivity in humans as well [32].

Adiponectin and Type 1 Diabetes Mellitus

A number of studies have observed that type 1 diabetic patients have higher adiponectin concentrations. In a substudy of the Coronary Artery Calcification in Type 1 Diabetes (CACTI) prospective cohort, 86 type 1 diabetic patients underwent hyperinsulinemic-euglycemic clamp testing in order to investigate the role of adiponectin in insulin sensitization. Results showed that type 1 diabetic patients had higher mean total adiponectin levels (12.3 ± 5.8 vs. 9.6 ± 5.5 μl/ml, respectively; p=0.03) and higher mean HMW adiponectin levels than their nondiabetic controls (6.5 ± 4.6 vs. 4.4 ± 3.5 μl/ml, respectively; p= 0.02) and that for any given level of adiponectin, type 1 diabetic patients had decreased insulin sensitivity compared to their nondiabetic controls as manifested by a lower glucose infusion rate [33].

Observational studies suggest that higher adiponectin levels in type 1 diabetic patients are associated with higher risk of microvascular complications including retinopathy [34] and progression of diabetic nephropathy [35]. It is unclear if these complications are directly related to adiponectin or are a marker of greater insulin resistance. Nevertheless, these observations challenge the cardioprotective role of adiponectin in patients with type 1 diabetes mellitus.

Adiponectin and Cardiovascular Disease

A number of studies have sought to examine the relationship between adiponectin and cardiovascular disease (Table 20.1). Existing data strongly suggest that adiponectin has anti-atherogenic and anti-inflammatory roles. In cellular and vascular injury, serum adiponectin levels are elevated and directly linked to vascular intima specific collagen [36]. Human studies have shown that diabetic patients with underlying coronary disease have lower adiponectin levels compared to the general population and diabetics without coronary disease [30]. Adiponectin also increases COX-2 in endothelial cells [37]. In addition, adiponectin levels were observed to inhibit expression of cell adhesion molecules suggesting a role in downregulation of inflammatory response [38]. In vitro studies suggest that adiponectin has a central role in vasodilation via its effect on nitric oxide (NO). Adiponectin has enzymatic regulation of endothelial nitric oxide synthase (eNOS) via a host of different mechanisms including increasing mRNA stability, increasing Ser1179 phosphorylation, and associating with scaffolding proteins [39].

In response to in vitro studies that suggest that adiponectin serves a cardioprotective function, population-based studies have examined adiponectin's impact on the development of coronary vascular disease. For example, in a cross-sectional study of 298 patients, Matsuda et al. looked at multivessel coronary disease on CT coronary angiography (CTCA) in relationship to adiponectin levels [1]. In this study, low adiponectin, along with four other traditional risk factors for coronary artery disease including age, sex, high triglyceride levels, and diabetes mellitus, were noted to have predictive values for multivessel disease found on CTCA (ROC analysis, AUC 0.72; 95% CI, 0.67–0.78). In addition, low adiponectin was noted to be associated with multivessel disease independent of the other risk factors. However, when low HDL and abdominal obesity were accounted for, the AUC decreased and was deemed to not be predictive for coronary artery disease in this study. However, further cross-sectional studies suggest that HMW adiponectin directly correlates to serum HDL levels [5].

In another study, Yoon et al. attempted to correlate adiponectin to carotid intima-media thickness as a surrogate for atherosclerosis [3]. This cross-sectional study of 1033 Korean participants showed that at the highest quartile of adiponectin (defined as >9.90 mg/L in men and > 13.4 mg/L in women), adiponectin was associated with reduced subclinical atherosclerosis (OR 0.42 [95% CI] 0.25–0.77 and 0.47 [95% CI] 0.29–0.75, respectively). In addition, when adiponectin was added to the risk prediction model, AUC of the ROC analysis was observed to increase by 0.025 and 0.022 in men and women, respectively, demonstrating its predictive value for carotid intima-media thickness.

Kawagoe et al., based on an earlier study suggesting that local intracoronary adiponectin influences coronary perfusion, examined intracoronary adiponectin's impact as a predictor of adverse coronary events including unstable angina, heart failure, and myocardial infarction [2]. In this study, 48 patients with left anterior descending artery stenosis requiring percutaneous coronary intervention were divided into high vs. low adiponectin groups (greater or less than 0 μg/mL at the left coronary artery, respectively). Coronary adiponectin was calculated as the plasma adiponectin level at the great cardiac vein minus the level at the orifice of the left coronary artery. Retrospective examination of patient records over a period of 66 months demonstrated a higher incidence of adverse coronary events in the low adiponectin group as compared with the high adiponectin group (7 events among 11 patients vs. 9 events among 37 patients, respectively; $p = 0.02$).

Coronary artery disease as measured directly by coronary artery angiogram in relationship to baseline adiponectin levels and metabolic syndrome was the subject of a cross-sectional study by Yamashita et al. [4]. In this analysis, 97 patients without diabetes mellitus undergoing elective coronary angiography participated in this study. In multivariate analyses, low adiponectin levels (defined as <4.5 μg/mL) were found to be a predictor of multivessel disease (OR 3.47 [95% CI] 1.27–9.89). Combination of low adiponectin with additional components of metabolic syndrome was not associated with increased incidence of multivessel coronary artery disease, but the combination of adiponectin levels >4.5 μg/mL and <3 components of metabolic syndrome were associated with decreased prevalence of multivessel coronary artery disease (OR 0.23 [95% CI] 0.09–0.56).

To further quantify the role of adiponectin in diabetes mellitus, Wu et al. conducted the first systematic review and meta-analysis of five prospective studies and one nested case-control study that examined the relationship between serum adiponectin levels and cardiovascular disease in patients with type 1 and 2 diabetes mellitus [40]. Data in type 1 diabetics showed that adiponectin was inversely related to risk of coronary heart disease, whereas studies in type 2 diabetic patients showed mixed associations between serum adiponectin concentrations and type 2 diabetes.

Adiponectin and Mortality Risk

General Population

Pischon et al. conducted a nested case-control study among 18,225 male participants from the Health Professionals Follow-Up Study that examined the association of baseline adiponectin levels with the primary outcome of the incidence of fatal and nonfatal coronary heart disease over a total duration of 6 years [6]. In this study, higher adiponectin levels showed associations with higher HDL cholesterol levels and lower triglyceride, C-reactive protein, HbA1c, and BMI levels. In multivariable analyses, adiponectin was inversely associated with the risk of myocardial infarction, such that the highest quintile of adiponectin demonstrated a RR of 0.56 (95% CI) 0.32–0.99. Adiponectin was therefore observed to be favorably associated with cardiovascular risk factors and decreased risk of fatal and nonfatal coronary disease.

Non-dialysis-Dependent Chronic Kidney Disease

Multiple observational studies have shown that adiponectin levels are increased in patients with kidney disease and that the degree of adiponectin elevation corresponds to the extent of renal dysfunction (Table 20.2). In the NDD-CKD population, it is currently unclear whether adiponectin serves as a cardiovascular protective agent or as an indicator of increased mortality risk.

An early prospective study conducted by Becker et al. examined a population of 227 non-diabetic patients with NDD-CKD (average GFR 63 ml/min/1.73m^2) [41]. Baseline adiponectin, insulin, and insulin resistance were measured, and patients had a follow-up period that averaged 54 months. Despite the varying stages of CKD, mean baseline adiponectin levels in this population did not show any statistically significant differences according to CKD status (6.6 ± 2.8 μg/ml vs. 6.1 ± 4.2 μg/ml for controls vs. CKD patients, respectively). However, higher fasting insulin levels and greater insulin resistance were observed in the CKD group as compared with age, sex, and BMI-matched controls. Ten patients during the follow-up period experienced non-cardiovascular events; these patients were noted to have lower adiponectin levels at baseline compared to patients who did not experience cardiovascular events (3.0 ± 1.3 vs. 6.5 ± 4.5 μg/ml, respectively). In addition, they were noted to have increased fasting insulin and serum glucose levels, as well as greater insulin resistance. This study suggests that in NDD-CKD patients, adiponectin serves as a vasoprotective agent and that hypoadiponectinemia may be a cardiovascular risk factor.

The hypothesis that adiponectin may serve a cardioprotective role in CKD has been further supported by subsequent studies. Included among these studies is a prospective analysis by Imawashi et al. that followed a group of 150 Japanese NDD-CKD patients with the goal of determining adiponectin's association with cardiovascular morbidity and mortality, including death secondary to cardiovascular disease [7]. Unlike the Becker et al. study, patients with diabetes and diabetic nephropathy were included in this trial. Baseline adiponectin levels were directly linked with increasing CKD stage. During an average follow-up period over 31.9 ± 1.5 months, patients who developed de novo cardiovascular events, including cardiovascular death, were noted to have lower adiponectin levels at baseline as compared with those who did not (5.0 ± 1.3 vs. 8.4 ± 0.7 μg/ml, respectively). Recurrent ischemic heart disease was also noted to be associated with lower adiponectin levels. When adjusted for pre-existing ischemic heart disease, smoking, and CKD stage, each 1 μg/ml increment in adiponectin level was associated with a HR of 0.86 (95% CI) 0.75–0.96; $p = 0.004$) for cardiovascular events and mortality. Therefore, the authors concluded that higher adiponectin levels may have a cardioprotective function independent of the elevations ensuing from kidney dysfunction.

Not all studies have corroborated a cardioprotective role of adiponectin; however, Jorsal et al. studied a cohort of 438 patients with type 1 diabetes mellitus with NDD diabetic nephropathy as defined by the presence of macroalbuminuria [25]. This group had a mean ± SD eGFR of 66 ± 28 ml/min/1.73 m^2. They were followed for an average of 8.1 years and matched with 440 patients with type 1 diabetes without macroalbuminuria. Baseline characteristics showed that patients with diabetic nephropathy had higher adiponectin levels compared to those without nephropathy. Upon follow-up, it was observed that baseline adiponectin levels were an independent predictor of all-cause mortality when adjusted for covariates that included age, sex, presence of nephropathy, blood pressure, HbA1c, creatinine, cholesterol, and antihypertensive treatment. Associations with fatal and nonfatal cardiovascular events did not reach statistical significance. In addition, adjusted analyses showed that baseline adiponectin levels predicted progression to ESRD with a HR of 2.72 (95% CI) 1.27–5.84; $p = 0.10$.

Menon et al. conducted a secondary analysis of the Modification of Diet in Renal Disease (MDRD) study to examine the association of adiponectin with cardiovascular outcomes and mortality risk [8]. Unlike the aforementioned studies which largely focused upon stage 1–2 CKD patients, this study focused on 820 patients with stage 3–4 CKD (mean ± SD eGFR of the cohort was 33 ± 12 ml/min/1.73m^2) with an average follow-up of 10 years. Results of fully adjusted Cox regression models showed that each 1 µg/ml increase in adiponectin was associated with a 3% higher risk of all-cause mortality after adjustment for cardiovascular risk factors: HR 1.03 (95% CI) 1.00–1.07; $p = 0.05$. Adiponectin was also found to be associated with higher cardiovascular mortality: HR 1.07 (95% CI) 1.03–1.11; $p = 0.001$.

Dialysis-Dependent End-Stage Renal Disease

Serum adiponectin level has been observed to be approximately 2.5-fold higher in ESRD patients than in average healthy subjects [10]. Among studies of ESRD patients, the evidence is mixed with respect to associations of adiponectin with mortality risk (Table 20.2). However, multiple studies suggest that higher adiponectin levels may have a protective role in this population.

In one of the seminal studies conducted to date, Zoccali et al. conducted a prospective study following 227 Caucasian ESRD patients on hemodialysis who had no symptoms of heart failure with a mean ± SD follow-up of 31 ± 13 months. Adiponectin levels were collected at baseline, and the primary endpoints of the study were cardiovascular events and all-cause mortality risk. Baseline adiponectin levels were found to directly correlate with HDL while inversely correlating with triglyceride, insulin, and BMI levels. Results showed that the lowest tertile of adiponectin was associated with higher risk of adverse cardiovascular events (ref: highest tertile): RR 1.56 (95% CI) 1.12–1.99. After adjustment for Framingham cardiovascular risk factors, C-reactive protein, homocysteine, as well as hemoglobin, albumin, calcium, phosphate, and duration of hemodialysis, each 1 µg/mL increment in adiponectin level was associated with a 3% reduction in fatal and nonfatal cardiovascular events: HR 0.97 (95% CI) 0.93–0.99; $p = 0.04$. Hence, this study suggested a cardioprotective role for adiponectin in ESRD patients.

Subsequent studies have suggested that adiponectin's relationship with mortality may be dependent upon obesity status. In a prospective cohort study of 537 hemodialysis patients, Zoccali et al. examined whether the association between adiponectin and mortality is modified by waist circumference (WC) as a proxy of visceral body fat [42]. Investigators observed that WC negatively correlated with C-reactive protein. In survival analyses, higher adiponectin levels were associated with lower all-cause mortality among patients in the lowest tertile of WC but were associated with higher mortality among patients in the highest tertile of WC.

There have been numerous corollary studies following the trial conducted by Zoccali et al. For example, Takemoto et al. conducted a prospective cohort study of 68 Japanese hemodialysis patients [12]. This trial was distinguished by an exceptionally long follow-up period of 8 years following measurement of baseline adiponectin levels. Primary outcomes included coronary heart disease as defined by angina pectoris and fatal or nonfatal myocardial infarction. Baseline adiponectin levels were much higher in females than in male patients (15.70 ± 7.10 vs. 9.34 ± 4.28 µg/mL, respectively). Data analyses showed that plasma adiponectin was positively correlated with serum HDL cholesterol levels ($R = 0.043$; $p = 0.009$) and inversely correlated with waist circumference ($R = -0.48$; $p = 0.002$) and serum creatinine ($R = -0.39$; $p = 0.02$) which were independent parameters that influence plasma adiponectin concentrations. In Cox regression analyses, higher plasma adiponectin levels were associated with lower risk of coronary heart disease: HR 0.74 (95% CI) 0.57–0.97 in men and HR 0.79 (95% CI) 0.67–0.94 in women. However, significant associations were not observed with all-cause mortality: HR 1.03 (95% CK) 0.91–1.17 in men and HR 0.98 (95% CI) 0.91–1.06 in women.

Diez et al. conducted a retrospective study of 164 hemodialysis and peritoneal dialysis patients that examined longitudinal adiponectin levels collected at baseline and 12 months with a mean ± SD follow-up of 33.9 ± 15.7 months [11]. Results showed that compared to peritoneal dialysis patients, those receiving hemodialysis had lower baseline adiponectin levels. In multivariate adjusted Cox regression analyses, baseline, 1 year, and mean adiponectin levels were shown to be associated with lower all-cause mortality risk. The same pattern of findings was observed for cardiovascular mortality and nonfatal cardiovascular events. However, these associations did not persist when restricted to hemodialysis patients only.

However, not all studies have corroborated a potential cardioprotective role of adiponectin. Drechsler et al. examined the data from 1255 participants from the German *Die Deutsche Diabetes Dialyse* (4D) study who underwent baseline and 6-month adiponectin measurements [14]. Primary endpoints included sudden death, stroke, myocardial infarction, combined cardiovascular events, and all-cause mortality. In crude analyses, baseline adiponectin levels were associated with higher risk of sudden death, stroke, and combined cardiovascular events (HRs 1.26, 1.40, and 1.66, respectively). However, in multivariate analyses, associations with stroke did not persist, and baseline adiponectin was associated with a higher risk of combined cardiovascular events (HR 1.27 [95% CI] 1.05–1.52) and sudden death (HR 1.39 [95% CI] 1.02–1.89). Baseline adiponectin levels were not associated with higher risk of all-cause death risk in crude or multivariate analyses. The highest tertile of baseline adiponectin levels were associated with higher incidence of cardiovascular events and stroke (HR 1.33 [95% CI] 1.03–1.72 and HR 2.39 [95% CI] 1.28–4.48, respectively). No associations were observed between the highest tertile of adiponectin and all-cause death. Rising adiponectin levels defined as an increase of levels 12.3% above baseline were associated with higher risk of adverse events. Increasing adiponectin levels showed positive correlations with rise in NT-pro-BNP and inverse correlations with change in BMI. In crude analyses, patients with rising adiponectin levels were observed to have higher rates of sudden death, myocardial infarction, and all-cause mortality: HR 1.51 (95% CI) 1.02–2.25, HR 1.66 (95% CI) 1.15–2.39, and HR 1.29 (95% CI) 1.06–1.57, respectively. However, these associations did not persist after multivariate adjustment.

Rao et al. conducted a secondary analysis of 182 hemodialysis-dependent patients from the HEMO study that measured baseline and yearly adiponectin levels over an average of 3.96 years of follow-up [15]. The primary outcome was defined as all-cause mortality, and secondary outcomes consisted of first hospitalization for cardiac causes and death from cardiac causes. Higher adiponectin levels were found to be associated with a lower risk for vascular disease with ORs of 0.70 (95% CI) 0.51–0.95. The relationship between baseline plasma adiponectin and all-cause mortality as well as cardiovascular hospitalization risk was nonlinear and best described with a quadratic transformation, but even this did not reach statistical significance. In unadjusted Cox analyses, changes in adiponectin levels from baseline did not show a statistically significant association with all-cause mortality nor cardiovascular disease outcomes. Upon adjustment for covariates which included C-reactive protein and IL-6, statistically significant associations were observed. However, subsequent adjustment for various covariates showed mixed findings, with unclear conclusions drawn from these analyses.

Kidney Transplantation Recipients

ESRD patients who undergo kidney transplantation have been observed to have lower serum adiponectin levels compared to pretransplant patients but remain higher relative to that of non-ESRD populations [43, 44]. With respect to outcomes in this population (Table 20.2), Alam et al. examined 987 Hungarian ESRD patients who underwent kidney transplantation and were followed for median duration of 51 months with a primary outcome of all-cause mortality and graft failure [16]. This study showed that adiponectin was independently associated with all-cause mortality with a HR of 1.44 (95% CI) 1.13–1.85. Compared to those in the lowest tertile, patients in the highest tertile of baseline adiponectin levels had an adjusted mortality HR of 1.80 (95% CI) 1.09–2.96. In addition, higher adiponectin levels were predictive of graft failure with a HR of 1.83 (95% CI) 1.48–2.26, but these associations became nonsignificant in fully adjusted models.

Leptin

Leptin is a 16-kDa adipocytokine composed of a 167-amino-acid protein that is expressed primarily by adipose tissue. It functions via receptors in the hypothalamus and regulates neuroendocrine functions, energy intake, and inflammation [45]. Leptin has a broad and important role in regulating the physiology of energy metabolism, inflammatory response, and energy storage [46–48]. It is known that leptin levels directly correlate with BMI and body fat composition and are inversely associated with malnutrition markers [49–51]. In the general population, leptin has been associated with higher risk of cerebral vascular disease, carotid intimal hyperplasia, and cardiovascular disease and is thought to be potently pro-atherogenic and pro-inflammatory [52–55]. Notably, in comparison with the general population, ESRD patients have been found to have significantly higher leptin levels, and this is hypothesized to be a result of increased production rather than decreased renal clearance [56].

Leptin, Cardiovascular Disease, and Mortality

There are very few studies which have investigated leptin's association with cardiovascular risk and mortality in the ESRD population, although small prospective and cross-sectional analyses have suggested a potentially cardioprotective role for leptin (Table 20.3). A small prospective observational study in a cohort of 53 Chinese hemodialysis patients has shown that leptin levels above the median value were associated with lower cardiovascular and all-cause mortality [59]. However, small cross-sectional studies have failed to show an association between leptin and vascular disease [58], left ventricular hypertrophy [62], and anemia [60] in the ESRD population. Further investigations are necessary to elucidate the role in leptin in the ESRD population.

Conclusion

Adiponectin and leptin are important adipokines that act on multiple organ systems. Serum adiponectin levels are strongly affected by obesity and insulin sensitivity. In studies of the general population, higher serum adiponectin levels have been suggested to have cardioprotective functions, whereas lower levels have been associated with higher risk of morbidity. In patients with kidney dysfunction, higher levels of adiponectin have been observed. However, the impact of higher adiponectin levels upon the cardiovascular morbidity and mortality of NDD-CKD and ESRD populations remains in dispute. It is unclear if higher adiponectin levels are a marker of the inflammatory state in ESRD or rather reflect general nutritional deficiency rather than a physiological response to renal failure. In the general population, high leptin levels are associated with pro-inflammatory and atherogenic responses, as well as a higher risk of cardiovascular disease. However, these associations have not been observed in the ESRD population, and small studies suggest high leptin levels may be associated with improved cardiovascular outcome. Further trials are needed to categorically qualify the role of adiponectin and leptin upon the cardiovascular health and survival of kidney disease patients.

Table 20.3 Studies of leptin, cardiovascular risk factors, cardiovascular disease, and survival in dialysis populations

Study	Study population	Study type	*N*	Age	Follow-up time	Primary outcome	All-cause mortality HR (95% CI)	CVD mortality HR (95% CI)	Conclusion
Diez et al. [57]	ESRD on PD and HD	Cross-sectional	82 (38 HD)	54.4	–	Association with vascular disease	–	–	No association between leptin and vascular disease
Diez et al. [58]	ESRD on HD	Prospective observational	118	65.1	24.7 mos	Association with CVD and all-cause mortality	No association	No association	No association between leptin and leptin/BMI ratio with CVD or all-cause mortality
Bian et al. [59]	ESRD on HD	Prospective observational	53	66	5 yrs	Association with all-cause mortality	HR 0.21 (0.06 to 0.72)	–	Low leptin associated with increased all-cause mortality
Nasri et al. [60]	ESRD on HD	Cross-sectional	36	47	–	Association with hemoglobin	–	–	Serum leptin correlated with hemoglobin; serum leptin correlated with BMI
Nasri et al. [60]	ESRD on HD	Cross-sectional	41	46	–	Association with left ventricular hypertrophy	–	–	No association between serum leptin and left ventricular hypertrophy
Park et al. [61]	ESRD on PD	Prospective observational	131	50.8	5 years	Association with all-cause mortality	Higher L/A RR 1.17 (1.07–1.27) for all-cause mortality	–	Higher leptin, lower ADPN, and higher L/A associated with increased risk of mortality

Abbreviations: *CVD* cardiovascular disease, *ESRD* end-stage renal disease, *PD* peritoneal dialysis, *HD* hemodialysis, *ADPN* adiponectin, *L/A* leptin to adiponectin ratio

References

1. Matsuda M, Tamura R, Kishida N, et al. Predictive value of adiponectin in patients with multivessel coronary atherosclerosis detected on computed tomography angiography. J Atheroscler Thromb. 2013;20:767–76.
2. Kawagoe J, Ishikawa T, Iwakiri H, Date H, Imamura T, Kitamura K. Association between adiponectin production in coronary circulation and future cardiovascular events in patients with coronary artery disease. Int Heart J. 2014;55:239–43.
3. Yoon JH, Kim SK, Choi HJ, et al. Adiponectin provides additional information to conventional cardiovascular risk factors for assessing the risk of atherosclerosis in both genders. PLoS One. 2013;8:e75535.
4. Yamashita T, Matsuda M, Nishimoto O, et al. Combination of serum adiponectin level and metabolic syndrome is closely associated with coronary artery disease in Japanese subjects with good glycemic control. Intern Med. 2010;49:721–7.
5. Komura N, Kihara S, Sonoda M, et al. Clinical significance of high-molecular weight form of adiponectin in male patients with coronary artery disease. Circ J. 2008;72:23–8.
6. Pischon T, Girman CJ, Hotamisligil GS, Rifai N, Hu FB, Rimm EB. Plasma adiponectin levels and risk of myocardial infarction in men. JAMA. 2004;291:1730–7.
7. Iwashima Y, Horio T, Kumada M, et al. Adiponectin and renal function, and implication as a risk of cardiovascular disease. Am J Cardiol. 2006;98:1603–8.
8. Menon V, Li L, Wang X, et al. Adiponectin and mortality in patients with chronic kidney disease. J Am Soc Nephrol. 2006;17:2599–606.
9. Jorsal A, Tarnow L, Frystyk J, et al. Serum adiponectin predicts all-cause mortality and end stage renal disease in patients with type I diabetes and diabetic nephropathy. Kidney Int. 2008;74:649–54.
10. Zoccali C, Mallamaci F, Tripepi G, et al. Adiponectin, metabolic risk factors, and cardiovascular events among patients with end-stage renal disease. J Am Soc Nephrol. 2002;13:134–41.
11. Diez JJ, Estrada P, Bajo MA, et al. High stable serum adiponectin levels are associated with a better outcome in prevalent dialysis patients. Am J Nephrol. 2009;30:244–52.
12. Takemoto F, Katori H, Sawa N, et al. Plasma adiponectin: a predictor of coronary heart disease in hemodialysis patients--a Japanese prospective eight-year study. Nephron Clin Pract. 2009;111:c12–20.
13. Abdallah E, Waked E, Nabil M, El-Bendary O. Adiponectin and cardiovascular outcomes among hemodialysis patients. Kidney Blood Press Res. 2012;35:247–53.
14. Drechsler C, Krane V, Winkler K, Dekker FW, Wanner C. Changes in adiponectin and the risk of sudden death, stroke, myocardial infarction, and mortality in hemodialysis patients. Kidney Int. 2009;76:567–75.
15. Rao M, Li L, Tighiouart H, et al. Plasma adiponectin levels and clinical outcomes among haemodialysis patients. Nephrol Dial Transplant. 2008;23:2619–28.
16. Alam A, Molnar MZ, Czira ME, et al. Serum adiponectin levels and mortality after kidney transplantation. Clin J Am Soc Nephrol. 2013;8:460–7.
17. Maeda K, Okubo K, Shimomura I, Funahashi T, Matsuzawa Y, Matsubara K. cDNA cloning and expression of a novel adipose specific collagen-like factor, apM1 (adipose most abundant gene transcript 1). 1996. Biochem Biophys Res Commun. 2012;425:556–9.
18. Nigro E, Scudiero O, Monaco ML, et al. New insight into adiponectin role in obesity and obesity-related diseases. Biomed Res Int. 2014;2014:658913.
19. Pajvani UB, Hawkins M, Combs TP, et al. Complex distribution, not absolute amount of adiponectin, correlates with thiazolidinedione-mediated improvement in insulin sensitivity. J Biol Chem. 2004;279:12152–62.
20. Arner P. The adipocyte in insulin resistance: key molecules and the impact of the thiazolidinediones. Trends Endocrinol Metab. 2003;14:137–45.
21. Yamauchi T, Iwabu M, Okada-Iwabu M, Kadowaki T. Adiponectin receptors: a review of their structure, function and how they work. Best Pract Res Clin Endocrinol Metab. 2014;28:15–23.
22. Cammisotto PG, Bendayan M. Adiponectin stimulates phosphorylation of AMP-activated protein kinase alpha in renal glomeruli. J Mol Histol. 2008;39:579–84.
23. Ohashi K, Iwatani H, Kihara S, et al. Exacerbation of albuminuria and renal fibrosis in subtotal renal ablation model of adiponectin-knockout mice. Arterioscler Thromb Vasc Biol. 2007;27:1910–7.
24. Jeon WS, Park JW, Lee N, et al. Urinary adiponectin concentration is positively associated with micro- and macro-vascular complications. Cardiovasc Diabetol. 2013;12:137.
25. Jorsal A, Petersen EH, Tarnow L, et al. Urinary adiponectin excretion rises with increasing albuminuria in type 1 diabetes. J Diabetes Complicat. 2013;27:604–8.
26. Kopf S, Oikonomou D, von Eynatten M, et al. Urinary excretion of high molecular weight adiponectin is an independent predictor of decline of renal function in type 2 diabetes. Acta Diabetol. 2014;51:479–89.
27. Arita Y, Kihara S, Ouchi N, et al. Paradoxical decrease of an adipose-specific protein, adiponectin, in obesity. Biochem Biophys Res Commun. 1999;257:79–83.
28. Weyer C, Funahashi T, Tanaka S, et al. Hypoadiponectinemia in obesity and type 2 diabetes: close association with insulin resistance and hyperinsulinemia. J Clin Endocrinol Metab. 2001;86:1930–5.
29. Statnick MA, Beavers LS, Conner LJ, et al. Decreased expression of apM1 in omental and subcutaneous adipose tissue of humans with type 2 diabetes. Int J Exp Diabetes Res. 2000;1:81–8.
30. Hotta K, Funahashi T, Arita Y, et al. Plasma concentrations of a novel, adipose-specific protein, adiponectin,

in type 2 diabetic patients. Arterioscler Thromb Vasc Biol. 2000;20:1595–9.
31. Yamauchi T, Kamon J, Waki H, et al. The fat-derived hormone adiponectin reverses insulin resistance associated with both lipoatrophy and obesity. Nat Med. 2001;7:941–6.
32. Li S, Shin HJ, Ding EL, van Dam RM. Adiponectin levels and risk of type 2 diabetes: a systematic review and meta-analysis. JAMA. 2009;302:179–88.
33. Pereira RI, Snell-Bergeon JK, Erickson C, et al. Adiponectin dysregulation and insulin resistance in type 1 diabetes. J Clin Endocrinol Metab. 2012;97:E642–7.
34. Hadjadj S, Aubert R, Fumeron F, et al. Increased plasma adiponectin concentrations are associated with microangiopathy in type 1 diabetic subjects. Diabetologia. 2005;48:1088–92.
35. Sarahcimo M, Forsblom C, Thorn L, et al. Serum adiponectin and progression of diabetic nephropathy in patients with type 1 diabetes. Diabetes Care. 2008;31:1165–9.
36. Okamoto Y, Arita Y, Nishida M, et al. An adipocyte-derived plasma protein, adiponectin, adheres to injured vascular walls. Horm Metab Res. 2000;32:47–50.
37. Lee FP, Jen CY, Chang CC, et al. Mechanisms of adiponectin-mediated COX-2 induction and protection against iron injury in mouse hepatocytes. J Cell Physiol. 2010;224:837–47.
38. Ouchi N, Kihara S, Arita Y, et al. Novel modulator for endothelial adhesion molecules: adipocyte-derived plasma protein adiponectin. Circulation. 1999;100:2473–6.
39. Cheng KK, Lam KS, Wang Y, et al. Erratum. Adiponectin-induced endothelial nitric oxide synthase activation and nitric oxide production are mediated by APPL1 in endothelial cells. Diabetes. 2007;56:1387–94. Diabetes 2016;65:3218.
40. Wu Z, Cheng Y, Aung LH, Li B. Association between adiponectin concentrations and cardiovascular disease in diabetic patients: a systematic review and meta-analysis. PLoS One. 2013;8:e78485.
41. Becker B, Kronenberg F, Kielstein JT, et al. Renal insulin resistance syndrome, adiponectin and cardiovascular events in patients with kidney disease: the mild and moderate kidney disease study. J Am Soc Nephrol. 2005;16:1091–8.
42. Zoccali C, Postorino M, Marino C, et al. Waist circumference modifies the relationship between the adipose tissue cytokines leptin and adiponectin and all-cause and cardiovascular mortality in haemodialysis patients. J Intern Med. 2011;269:172–81.
43. Chudek J, Adamczak M, Karkoszka H, et al. Plasma adiponectin concentration before and after successful kidney transplantation. Transplant Proc. 2003;35:2186–9.
44. Adamczak M, Szotowska M, Chudek J, Karkoszka H, Cierpka L, Wiecek A. Plasma adiponectin concentration in patients after successful kidney transplantation – a single-center, observational study. Clin Nephrol. 2007;67:381–90.
45. Mantzoros CS. The role of leptin in human obesity and disease: a review of current evidence. Ann Intern Med. 1999;130:671–80.
46. Hukshorn CJ, Lindeman JH, Toet KH, et al. Leptin and the proinflammatory state associated with human obesity. J Clin Endocrinol Metab. 2004;89:1773–8.
47. Dervisoglu E, Eraldemir C, Kalender B, Kir HM, Caglayan C. Adipocytokines leptin and adiponectin, and measures of malnutrition-inflammation in chronic renal failure: is there a relationship? J Ren Nutr. 2008;18:332–7.
48. Fantuzzi G. Adipose tissue, adipokines, and inflammation. J Allergy Clin Immunol. 2005;115:911–9. quiz 20
49. Heimburger O, Lonnqvist F, Danielsson A, Nordenstrom J, Stenvinkel P. Serum immunoreactive leptin concentration and its relation to the body fat content in chronic renal failure. J Am Soc Nephrol. 1997;8:1423–30.
50. Johansen KL, Mulligan K, Tai V, Schambelan M. Leptin, body composition, and indices of malnutrition in patients on dialysis. J Am Soc Nephrol. 1998;9:1080–4.
51. Nishizawa Y, Shoji T, Tanaka S, et al. Plasma leptin level and its relationship with body composition in hemodialysis patients. Am J Kidney Dis. 1998;31:655–61.
52. Lieb W, Sullivan LM, Harris TB, et al. Plasma leptin levels and incidence of heart failure, cardiovascular disease, and total mortality in elderly individuals. Diabetes Care. 2009;32:612–6.
53. Vavruch C, Lanne T, Fredrikson M, Lindstrom T, Ostgren CJ, Nystrom FH. Serum leptin levels are independently related to the incidence of ischemic heart disease in a prospective study of patients with type 2 diabetes. Cardiovasc Diabetol. 2015; 14:62.
54. Batsis JA, Sahakyan KR, Singh P, Bartels SJ, Somers VK, Lopez-Jimenez F. Leptin, adiposity, and mortality: results from the National Health and nutrition examination survey III, 1988 to 1994. Mayo Clin Proc. 2015;90:481–91.
55. Adya R, Tan BK, Randeva HS. Differential effects of leptin and adiponectin in endothelial angiogenesis. J Diabetes Res. 2015;2015:648239.
56. Merabet E, Dagogo-Jack S, Coyne DW, et al. Increased plasma leptin concentration in end-stage renal disease. J Clin Endocrinol Metab. 1997;82:847–50.
57. Diez JJ, Iglesias P, Fernandez-Reyes MJ, et al. Serum concentrations of leptin, adiponectin and resistin, and their relationship with cardiovascular disease in patients with end-stage renal disease. Clin Endocrinol. 2005;62:242–9.
58. Diez JJ, Bossola M, Fernandez-Reyes MJ, et al. Relationship between leptin and all-cause and cardiovascular mortality in chronic hemodialysis patients. Nefrologia. 2011;31:206–12.
59. Bian X, Liu N, Bai Y, et al. Association of leptin with mortality in patients on maintenance hemodialysis: a prospective study. Iran J Kidney Dis. 2014;8:314–20.

60. Nasri H. Association of serum leptin with anemia in maintenance hemodialysis patients. Saudi J Kidney Dis Transpl. 2006;17:521–5.
61. Park JT, Yoo TH, Kim JK, et al. Leptin/adiponectin ratio is an independent predictor of mortality in nondiabetic peritoneal dialysis patients. Perit Dial Int. 2013;33:67–74.
62. Nasri H. Serum leptin concentration and left ventricular hypertrophy and function in maintenance hemodialysis patients. Minerva Urol Nefrol. 2006;58:189–93.

Part VII

Other Pituitary Disorders

21 Growth Hormone Disorders and Abnormal Stature in Kidney Disease

Amira Al-Uzri, Annabelle N. Chua, and Bradley A. Warady

Prevalence of Short Stature in CKD

Severe short stature, a frequent complication experienced by children with chronic kidney disease (CKD), is defined as a height standard deviation score (SDS) of −1.88 or worse, equivalent to ≤ third percentile for age and sex. The reported prevalence varies from 12 to 50% based on the era of reporting (being higher in older reports) and also by the level of kidney function (being more pronounced at lower levels of kidney function) [1–4]. Two important studies from North America have revealed different prevalence data. The Chronic Kidney Disease in Children (CKiD) study, an observational longitudinal study that was initiated in 2006 and that includes children with CKD stages 2–4, has reported the prevalence of short stature to be 12% in their cohort of 799 children [2]. In comparison, the North American Pediatric Renal Trials and Collaborative Studies (NAPRTCS), a voluntary registry that has collected data on children with CKD stages 2–4 since 1994, has reported a 35.5% prevalence of short stature in children with CKD at the time of registry entry [5]. A greater height deficit was noted for younger patients with growth failure, being documented in 58% of patients <1 year of age as compared to 22% of those >12 years of age.

In contrast to those with mild to moderate CKD, there is a higher prevalence of severe short stature in children on dialysis with over 40% of children having a height SDS of −1.88 or worse, which tends to improve in the youngest patients following kidney transplantation [6–8].

The Impact of Growth Retardation in Children with CKD

Emerging evidence suggests that short stature in children with CKD is not merely a cosmetic issue for children and parents but rather a complication of CKD that is associated with higher morbidity and mortality, as well as lower health-related quality of life (HRQoL).

Early work by Furth et al. revealed that short stature in children on dialysis was associated with higher rates of hospitalization and mortality when compared to those with normal heights [9–12].

A. Al-Uzri
Division of Pediatric Kidney Services and Hypertension, Department of Pediatrics, Oregon Health and Science University, Portland, OR, USA

A. N. Chua
Department of Pediatrics, Duke University School of Medicine, Durham, NC, USA

B. A. Warady (✉)
University of Missouri—Kansas City School of Medicine, Kansas City, MO, USA

Division of Pediatric Nephrology, Department of Pediatrics, Children's Mercy Hospital, Kansas City, MO, USA
e-mail: bwarady@cmh.edu

C. M. Rhee et al. (eds.), *Endocrine Disorders in Kidney Disease*,
https://doi.org/10.1007/978-3-319-97765-2_21

Most recently, the CKiD study has shown that children with CKD stages 2–4 have a lower overall HRQoL compared to healthy children [13], and one of the factors that may influence that outcome is height. In a CKiD analysis of patient and parent data derived from the Pediatric Quality of Life Inventory (PedsQL; Version 4.0) and its four domains (e.g., physical, emotional, social, and school), investigators reported statistically significant associations between improvement in height SDS and better HRQoL scores in the physical functioning and social functioning domains by parent proxy reports, implying that parents of children with short stature believe that physical and social functioning domains are impacted by growth [1].

Factors Related to Growth in CKD

The etiology of growth retardation in children with CKD is undoubtedly multifactorial in origin. Factors that influence the development of growth failure include age at onset of CKD and abnormal birth history, protein and calorie malnutrition, metabolic acidosis, primary renal disorder and severity of renal impairment, chronic kidney disease-mineral bone disorders, alterations of the growth hormone/insulin-like growth factor I (GH/IGF-I) axis, and pubertal delay.

Infants with CKD pose a unique challenge in terms of overall management and are particularly vulnerable to growth failure in the first two years of life, a period in which approximately one-third of the final height is attained in healthy children [14, 15]. Studies by Betts et al. revealed that more than half of the children who developed renal insufficiency during infancy were at or below the third percentile for height in later years, whereas those who developed renal insufficiency later during childhood were closer to normal in height. In addition, a seminal finding was that reduced growth velocity occurred when the energy intake fell below 80% of the recommended dietary allowance (RDA) [15].

Infants and children with CKD and end-stage renal disease (ESRD) oftentimes have inadequate nutritional intake with the mean caloric intake reported to range from 62–85% of dietary reference intake (DRI), emphasizing the importance of periodic assessment of the nutritional status [16–19]. The assessment frequency should be greatest in the youngest patients and in those with advanced stages of CKD. Improving the caloric intake to meet at least 100% of the DRI has been shown to result in an improved linear growth rate, particularly in infants [20–22]. In turn, if the voluntary intake is not sufficient to meet 100% of the DRI for calories, supplemental enteral feeds either orally or via nasogastric/gastrostomy tube may be required [20, 23]. In addition, the provision of a low protein diet to infants with CKD has resulted in diminished linear growth; therefore, current recommendations are that the dietary protein intake for infants and children with CKD should provide 100% of the DRI, using proteins of high biologic value [18, 24].

The impact of abnormal birth parameters on the growth of infants and children with CKD was explored by Greenbaum et al. in a report from the CKiD study [25]. In that analysis of 426 children, low birth weight (LBW) (<2500 g) and SGA (birth weight < 10th percentile for gestational age) were noted to be present in 17% and 14% of the cohort, respectively. A negative effect of LBW (-0.43 ± 0.14; $P < 0.01$) and SGA (-0.29 ± 0.16; $P = 0.07$) on height SDS highlighted both LBW and SGA as risk factors for short stature in children with CKD [25]. Another large study by Franke et al., of 435 children with CKD stages 3–5, documented the high frequency of abnormal birth exposures in that 31.8% of children with CKD had a history of prematurity and 27.8% had a history of SGA compared to only 8.0% and 8.1%, respectively, in 61 children in the reference group [26]. In a subsequent longitudinal follow-up study of 509 children in which poor growth was defined as height SDS <2, Frank et al. observed that the rate of prematurity and SGA was significantly higher in children who grew poorly (43.2% and 36.8%), compared to those with good growth (25.6% and 18.9%) ($P < 0.001$) [27].

The influence that the primary renal disorder has on linear growth and attainment of final adult height is evident when comparing those children born with non-glomerular disorders versus acquired glomerular disease. For example, children born with aplastic/dysplastic/hypoplastic kidneys and CKD have more severe growth impairment relative to children with glomerular diseases, reflecting the longer burden of CKD that starts at birth [2, 5, 28]. In addition, many children with early-onset CKD have renal tubular injury which results in urinary losses of salt and base which can predispose to poor growth if adequate salt supplementation or sodium bicarbonate is not provided [2, 29].

Indeed, metabolic acidosis has been demonstrated to contribute to poor growth as evidenced by impaired growth in children with untreated renal tubular acidosis (RTA) and in those with CKD [30]. Metabolic acidosis may contribute to poor growth for a variety of reasons, including its association with resistance to the anabolic actions of growth hormone [14, 18, 31]. In addition, metabolic acidosis suppresses albumin synthesis, promotes calcium efflux from bone, and promotes protein degradation.

The relationship between the level of kidney function and growth was clearly demonstrated in a NAPRTCS analysis in which children were divided into three cohorts at the time of registry entry based upon their creatinine clearance. Patients with observed mean height SDS values of −1.92, −1.48, and −0.8 had mean creatinine clearance values of 10–25, 26–50, and >50 mL/min/1.73 m^2 [5]. In a more recent longitudinal analysis from the CKiD study, a decrease in height SDS of 0.14 was noted for each 10/mL min/1.73 m^2 decrease in glomerular filtration rate (GFR) [2].

Finally, CKD-associated mineral and bone disorders range from high-turnover lesions of secondary hyperparathyroidism to low-turnover lesions of osteomalacia and adynamic bone disease, both of which can contribute to growth failure [32]. Secondary hyperparathyroidism may lead to poor linear growth as it influences the expression of key regulators of endochondral bone formation thereby altering the normal architecture of the growth plate cartilage [18]. Adynamic bone disease has been shown to lead to growth failure in children undergoing chronic peritoneal dialysis in association with high-dose pulse calcitriol therapy [33].

Disturbances of the Growth Hormone-IGF Axis in CKD

Growth hormone is freely filtered by the glomerulus; in turn, plasma levels rise as renal function declines, resulting in normal or high serum levels of growth hormone in children with CKD [6]. Recognition of the normal or high fasting serum levels of growth hormone in children with CKD or ESRD and growth impairment has led to the concept of growth hormone insensitivity or resistance in uremia. Several mechanisms contribute to growth hormone resistance and likely involve the growth hormone receptor (GHR), growth hormone signal transduction, and insulin-like growth factor I (IGF-I) which is the mediator of most actions of growth hormone. In addition to the effect of uremia on the development of growth hormone resistance, the growth hormone-IGF-I axis is sensitive to nutritional deficiencies, inflammation, and acidosis, all of which are common complications of CKD [34].

One mechanism of growth hormone resistance in CKD is the reduced density of growth hormone receptors in target organs, which is reflected by a decreased serum growth hormone-binding protein (GHBP) concentration. The GHBP concentration has been used as a surrogate marker of GHR number given that GHBP is a cleaved product of the growth hormone receptor with release of the extracellular domain into the circulation. The GHBP concentration has been found to be low in children with CKD and is proportionate to the degree of renal dysfunction [35]. Another mechanism to explain growth hormone resistance is a defect in the post-receptor growth hormone-activated Janus kinase/signal transducer and activator of transcription (JAK/STAT) signaling, both of which must be intact for growth hormone-stimulated IGF-I gene expression to occur. Activation of JAK2 occurs after binding of growth hormone to its receptor. JAK2 then self-phosphorylates, followed by phosphorylation of the GHR and subsequently STAT 1a, STAT 3, STAT 5a, and STAT 5b, which are members of a larger family of cytoplasmic transcription factors. These phosphorylated STATs form dimers which then enter the nucleus where they bind specific deoxyribonucleic acid sequences to activate or repress their target genes, including IGF-I and some suppressors of cytokine signaling (SOCS). Impaired phosphorylation of JAK2 and STAT proteins, as well as the nuclear levels of phosphorylated STAT proteins, occurs in CKD thereby leading to impaired IGF-I gene expression [36].

Decreased bioactivity of IGF-I due to an excess of circulating IGF-binding proteins (IGFBPs) is yet another explanation for growth hormone resistance in CKD. IGFBPs are normally cleared through the kidney; therefore, accumulation of IGFBPs occurs in CKD in relation to the degree of kidney dysfunction. Serum IGFBP-1, IGFBP-2, IGFBP-4, and IGFBP-6 levels and immunoreactive low molecular fragments of IGFBP-3 are elevated and form high-affinity complexes with IGF-I and insulin-like growth factor 2 (IGF-2), thereby reducing bioavailability (Fig. 21.1) [14, 37]. In addition, increased IGFBP-1 mRNA and IGFBP-2 mRNA have been noted in liver tissue in experimental uremic states which suggests that hepatic production of IGFBP-1 and IGFBP-2 also contributes to elevated IGFBPs in CKD [38].

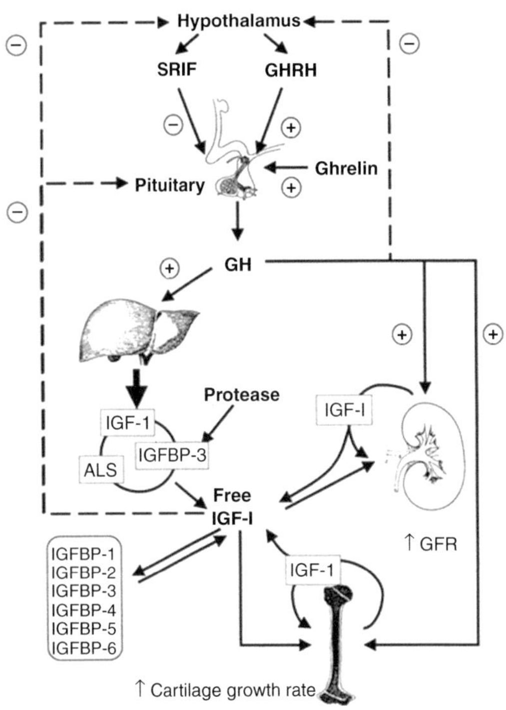

Fig. 21.1 Deranged somatotropic axis in chronic renal failure. The reduced effectiveness of endogenous IGF-I likely is due to decreased levels of free, bioactive IGF-I as levels of circulating inhibitory IGFBP are increased. In addition, less IGF-I is circulating in the complex with ALS and IGFBP-3 as a result of increased proteolysis of IGFBP-3 (From Mahan and Warady [14], Fig. 1B, with permission of Springer)

Delayed Puberty in Children with CKD

Pulsatile secretion of growth hormone increases at puberty and the growth hormone system is modified by gonadarche. Estrogens potentiate growth hormone release in response to growth hormone-releasing peptide or growing hormone-releasing hormone. Appropriate growth is achieved only in the presence of gonadarche [39, 40]. As such, children with CKD oftentimes experience delayed puberty, lagging approximately two years behind their peers in the onset and progression of gonadarche [41]. In addition, the minimal prespurt height velocity in children with CKD has been noted to be reduced by 50%, the peak height velocity is reduced by 50%, and the duration of the pubertal growth spurt is shortened by one year [42]. The mechanism for the pubertal delay is at least in part related to the fact that the presence of CKD can interfere with the neurohypophyseal reproductive axis at every level [43]. Children with CKD exhibit disturbances in the gonadotropic hormone axis with elevated gonadotropin levels due to decreased renal clearance and reduction of the pituitary secretion of bioactive luteinizing hormone (LH) as compared to healthy adolescents. Schaefer et al. observed a three- to fourfold increase in the estimated plasma half-life of LH, a marked reduction in the pulsatile LH secretory rate, and a relative increase in the apparent basal secretion of immunoreactive LH in uremic patients compared to healthy controls [44]. In the renal transplant recipients, none of the LH secretory and clearance characteristics were significantly different from controls, suggesting reversibility of the changes observed in uremic patients after recovery of renal function. In fact, they demonstrated an inverse relationship between the plasma half-life of bioactive LH and GFR. In pubertal females with CKD, the altered secretory pattern of LH may perturb the emergence of the physiological periodical changes in LH pulsatility which is required for regular ovarian cycles, thereby leading to delayed menarche, reduced fertility, and menstrual disorders [44].

Plasma testosterone concentrations are also decreased in CKD, and free testosterone levels are further decreased due to a rise in sex hormone-binding globulins, thereby resulting in suboptimal pubertal growth and development [45]. Other abnormalities that contribute to pubertal delay include suppression of pulsatile gonadotropin-releasing hormone (GnRH) secretion due to elevations of prolactin levels, as well as elevated levels of inhibin which is a negative regulator of pituitary function produced by the Sertoli cell [43, 46].

Finally, many children with CKD and post-renal transplant are treated with steroids. Steroids reduce growth hormone pulsatility which is important during the peripubertal years. In the setting of steroid therapy, the normal physiological increase in growth hormone secretion that occurs during puberty is reduced, and the association between sex steroid plasma concentrations and growth hormone release observed in healthy adolescents is blunted, resulting in delayed, attenuated growth [6, 47, 48].

Growth in Infants with CKD

The first two years of life is a period of very rapid growth with high calorie and protein requirements. Growth in early infancy is principally dependent on nutrition rather than growth hormone, with the rate of growth as high as 1.5 cm per month in the first six months of life [49]. Infants with CKD, however, commonly experience feeding difficulties, vomiting, and infections which can lead to inadequate nutritional intake, thereby resulting in the loss of as much as 2 height SD scores [50–52]. In addition, salt depletion, which is known to limit growth, may occur in infants born with salt-wasting renal disorders [29]. As such, enteral feeding by nasogastric or gastrostomy tube is considered an essential tool to optimize nutrition and growth, as well as to provide necessary medications and supplements in young infants [53]. An increase or maintenance of length SDS has been reported to be greater in infants with CKD who received gastrostomy feeding as compared to nasogastric tube or on demand feeding, likely as a result of the decreased propensity for emesis with use of a gastrostomy [52]. Aggressive nutritional support may not always be sufficient, however, to achieve normal or catch-up growth rates, and in many of those cases, the introduction of recombinant human growth hormone (rhGH) therapy may be indicated [50, 54, 55].

Growth in Children on Dialysis

As with growth failure in CKD, growth failure in children on dialysis is multifactorial in origin, being influenced by nutritional, metabolic, and hormonal alterations [52, 56]. In addition, patients with congenital renal disease and inherited metabolic disorders who experience impaired kidney function from birth regularly achieve a significantly smaller final adult height as compared to patients with disorders typically first manifesting in later childhood. While still suboptimal, the growth of pediatric ESRD patients has demonstrated improvement over the past few decades, which suggests overall improvement in the management of these patients, with greater attention to the modifiable factors which influence growth outcomes [28, 29, 57–59]. One such factor is dialysis adequacy. While the achievement of standard dialysis adequacy targets has not routinely been associated with catch-up growth in dialysis patients, the provision of daily hemodiafiltration to a small number of children has been associated with exceptional growth, likely the result of "optimal" solute clearance and enhanced nutritional intake [60]. Further evaluation of this treatment approach and the resultant impact on growth should be encouraged.

In peritoneal dialysis (PD) patients in particular, contributors to growth failure include poor nutritional intake and significant protein losses in the PD effluent, the latter often occurring in the setting of high transport characteristics of the peritoneal membrane [19, 56, 57]. Adequate nutritional intake is particularly difficult to achieve in infants on PD as they are prone to gastroesophageal reflux and vomiting due to uremia, raised intra-abdominal pressure due to the presence of dialysate, and the need to concentrate feeds and minimize volume for oliguric/anuric infants [61]. As such, enteral feeding via nasogastric tube feeding or gastrostomy tube is often essential, with slightly improved preservation of growth noted in infants on PD fed via gastrostomy tube, as noted above [52]. Finally, rhGH usage has been associated with improved height velocity in the PD population [62].

Growth in Children Following Renal Transplantation

Renal transplantation results in an improved GFR and tubular function; however, spontaneous catch-up growth oftentimes is suboptimal to compensate for the height deficit acquired pretransplant. The main factors which contribute to longitudinal growth retardation following renal transplantation include corticosteroid treatment, chronological age at time of transplant, pretransplant growth deficit, and level of GFR [63, 64]. As noted previously, corticosteroids affect growth hormone pulsatility, which is particularly important during the peripubertal years. Corticosteroid therapy also decreases growth hormone receptor and IGF-I expression and increases plasma levels of IGF-inhibiting IGFBPs, thereby limiting the bioavailability of IGF [65, 66]. Glucocorticoid treatment additionally has a direct effect on growth plate function by suppressing chondrocyte proliferation, reducing bone formation, and altering endochondral ossification [67, 68]. Strategies to decrease or eliminate corticosteroid exposure with low-dose and alternate-day regimens or complete steroid avoidance have been associated with improvement in growth parameters post-renal transplant [69–72].

Not unexpectedly, given the relationship between renal insufficiency and growth, an estimated GFR (eGFR) 30 days after transplant has been shown to be predictive of the impact of transplantation on long-term height *Z* score, with those recipients with an eGFR <60 mL/min/1.73 m^2 experiencing a reduced height *Z* score [73].

Factors that may result in better catch-up/accelerated growth in the posttransplant period include living-donor transplant (independent of GFR) and preemptive transplantation [64, 74, 75]. While the etiology of the improved growth noted following living-related donor renal transplantation as compared to deceased donor transplantation is not entirely clear, it has been speculated that patterns of cytokines and other mediator molecules may change in the period of death and in association with prolonged cold ischemia time for deceased donor kidneys [74]. Preemptive renal transplantation may improve final height by avoiding the decreased growth velocity that has been associated with a prolonged period of time on dialysis.

Growth Hormone Treatment in Children with CKD

As noted previously, disturbances of the growth hormone-IGF-I axis which leads to insufficient levels of bioactive IGF-I and a state of growth hormone insensitivity have been well described in children with CKD. The rationale for the use of pharmacologic doses of rhGH in the setting of CKD is, in turn, to tilt the balance toward a greater availability of bioactive IGF-I [6]. At present, recommendations within both the KDOQI nutrition guidelines and the KDIGO bone guidelines are that rhGH treatment should be considered for children with CKD stages 2–5 and those on dialysis with short stature (height SDS ≤ 1.88 or height for age ≤ third percentile) and with potential for linear growth [19, 76]. A three-month observation period is proposed prior to starting rhGH treatment to correct nutritional and metabolic abnormalities and to monitor the impact of these interventions [19, 76]. Close monitoring of the nutritional status of children with CKD is always mandatory, and correction of metabolic acidosis to a serum bicarbonate level of at least 22 mEq/L is important to promote growth and enhance protein energy metabolism [77, 78].

The initial short-term studies that were conducted to address the use of rhGH treatment in children with CKD clearly demonstrated a positive effect of rhGH on height velocity and height SDS [79, 80]. Longer follow-up studies of children with CKD who received five years of rhGH treatment have demonstrated continued improved growth, and the treatment has permitted a substantial percentage of children to reach a normal final adult height [59].

The recommended dose of rhGH for children with CKD is 0.35 mg/kg/week (or 28–33 IU/m^2/week) divided into daily subcutaneous injections [6, 81]. The identical starting dose is recommended for patients with CKD and receiving conservative management, dialysis patients, and transplant recipients. The dose should be reevaluated and potentially modified every 3–4 months to account for changes in patient weight that may have occurred in the interim. Whereas the first rhGH product that was approved by the FDA for the treatment of short stature in children with CKD was Nutropin® in the early 1990s, over time, other brands of rhGH therapy became available with comparable efficacy and safety. In turn, these products have been used by pediatric endocrinologists/nephrologists for the treatment of short stature in CKD, with the specific product used often based on insurance preferences [82, 83]. Trials using long-acting and PEGylated rhGH which can ease the burden of daily injections for children are currently underway [84, 85].

The anticipated growth response to rhGH treatment in children with CKD is influenced by a variety of factors; some of the factors are potentially modifiable such as nutrition, bone metabolism, medication adherence, and the length of treatment with rhGH, whereas others are non-modifiable such as age, pubertal growth, level of kidney function, and genetic factors [86]. To maximize the efficiency of rhGH treatment, the healthcare provider should take into consideration the interplay of the above factors so as to optimize growth management on an individualized basis.

For example, the total length of treatment with rhGH is a determinant of the overall growth response, and it should be anticipated that growth velocity will be highest during the first year of treatment compared to subsequent years. Fine reported a deceleration in height velocity of a CKD cohort from 4.2 cm/year in the first year of rhGH treatment to 2.3 cm in the second year of therapy [87].

Haffner et al. demonstrated a relationship between the efficacy of rhGH therapy and the degree of renal impairment when he revealed first and second year growth responses of 9.3 and 7.1 cm/year, respectively, in 74 CKD patients versus 7.2 and 5.4 cm/year, respectively, in 29 children on dialysis [88]. Similar findings have been published by Nissel et al. based on data from the Pfizer International Growth Database (KIGS) which revealed a higher cumulative increase in mean height SDS and near-final height SDS in patients on conservative management (+1.5 and −1.7) compared to patients on dialysis (1.1 and −3.0) and after kidney transplantation (+1.1 and −2.4) (each $P < 0.05$), respectively [62]. The NAPRTCS has also reported a positive impact of rhGH therapy on the growth of the transplant population [89].

The preference for the early initiation of therapy in terms of patient age is based on the finding that younger children with short stature and CKD on rhGH therapy experience the highest annual growth rates [62]. Franke et al. reported an accelerated change in height SDS from −2.4 at four years of age to −1.55 at eight years of age among 384 children on renal replacement therapy who were treated with rhGH [90]. It is worth mentioning that children ≤5 years of age comprised 42% of the total cohort.

In contrast and as part of a review of the KIGS registry, Nissel et al. reviewed the effect of puberty on attaining near-final height in 240 children on rhGH treatment [62]. In this large cohort, 38% of the cohort were prepubertal, 47% were early Tanner II/III, and 15% were Tanner IV/V. The authors reported that near-final height SDS was positively associated with the duration of rhGH therapy and negatively associated with delayed puberty. Furthermore, the increment in height SDS during the first year of rhGH treatment was higher in prepubertal patients with normal onset of puberty and late pubertal patients (each +0.5), compared with prepubertal patients with delayed onset of puberty (+0.2) and early pubertal patients.

Predictive models for an individual's response to rhGH therapy have been proposed with the hope of optimizing the growth potential for every patient. Mehls et al. published a mathematical equation to predict the individual growth response to rhGH therapy taking into account age, etiology of renal failure, rhGH dose, and GFR. Interestingly, the derived equation explained only 37% of the overall variability of the growth response during the first and second years of rhGH therapy [91].

Mahan et al. [92] derived growth prediction curves based on the height velocity responses documented during the first year of rhGH treatment in 270 prepubertal children with CKD enrolled in the Genentech National Cooperative Growth Study. As the height velocity at any age in patients who were treated with rhGH therapy was higher than the pretreatment height velocity (Fig. 21.2), the authors proposed to use a height velocity below −1 SD for age as an indicator of inadequate response to rhGH therapy. This finding would signal the treating provider of the need to evaluate for other factors that may lower the response to rhGH treatment, such as metabolic abnormalities or medication nonadherence [92].

The use of an IGF-I generation test to measure the amount of IGF generated after seven doses of rhGH to predict the height velocity over the next 12 months has been promoted by some, but failed to show a correlation with growth velocity in 16 children with CKD [93].

Complications of Growth Hormone Therapy

Reports on the adverse effects of rhGH treatment in children with CKD are scant and reflect the excellent safety profile associated with its use in the CKD population. A meta-analysis by the Cochrane group addressed the reported adverse effects associated with rhGH treatment in 16 publications (809 children enrolled) [81]. Adverse effects reported to be related to rhGH use were described in 13 studies (677 children). Reported side effects included asthma/wheezing, elevated fasting glucose, papilledema, granuloma formation, lymph node swelling, claudication, hypertension, and worsening of preexisting idiopathic scoliosis. More targeted adverse events associated with rhGH usage were reported by Fine et al. from the NAPRTCS registry in a study which assessed the incidence of slipped capital femoral epiphysis, avascular necrosis, intracranial hypertension, and malignancies [94]. No statistically significant differences in the incidence of any of these complications were noted among those treated with rhGH and a control group over a 6.5-year interval.

A later study based on data in the NAPRTCS registry confirmed the safety of rhGH in renal transplant recipients with respect to the issue of malignancy. The study evaluated the five-year follow-up of 513 rhGH-treated kidney transplant recipients compared to 2263 controls and revealed that the percentages of patients who developed a malignancy in the two groups were similar at approximately 1.9% [89]. However, a more

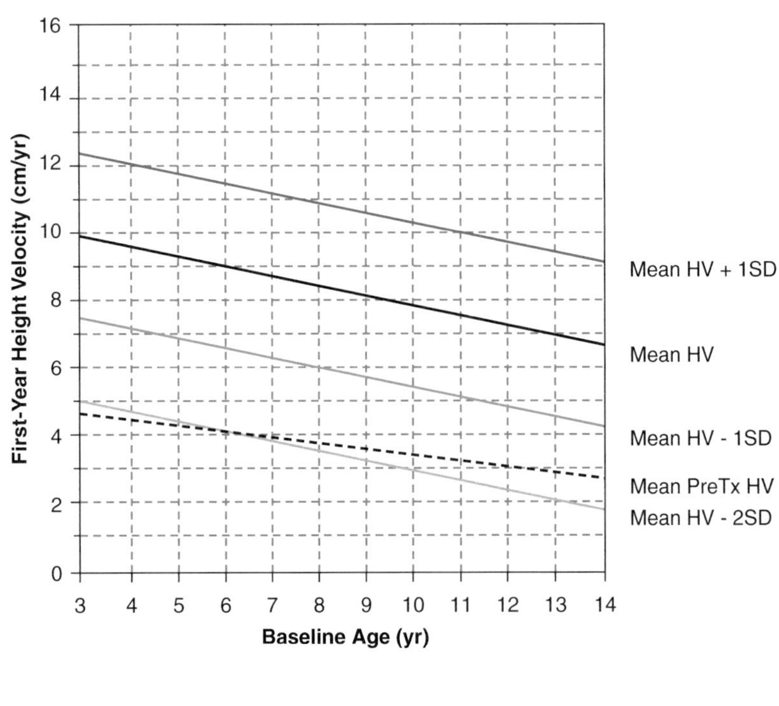

Fig. 21.2 First year fitted curves by age expressed as height velocity (HV) for prepubertal children with CKD during rhGH treatment compared to pretreatment (PreTx) height velocity (From Mahan et al. [92], with permission of Springer)

recent analysis of the NAPRTCS registry showed a slight increase in the rate of posttransplant lymphoproliferative disease (PTLD) in those children with CKD who received rhGH and went on to receive a kidney transplant (18/407 or 4.4%) compared to those who never used rhGH (23/1240 or 1.9%) ($P = 0.009$) [95]. Continued monitoring of this issue is clearly of utmost importance.

Effect of rhGH Therapy on the Progression of CKD

Growth hormone therapy increases renal plasma flow and GFR and reduces renal vascular resistance through the action of IGF-I [96, 97]. In turn, a sustained increase in renal plasma flow may have a deleterious effect on kidney function as a result of hyperfiltration injury and subsequent nephron loss. Thankfully, this effect has not been demonstrated in children with short stature and CKD receiving long-term rhGH therapy. A five-year follow-up study compared changes in GFR in two cohorts of children with CKD stages 2–4: one from the European KIGS registry of patients who received rhGH therapy and one from the ESCAPE study of subjects who did not receive rhGH therapy. No statistically significant differences in the rate of GFR decline for the two cohorts were demonstrated [98].

Utilization of rhGH for Patients with CKD

Data pertaining to the safety and efficacy of rhGH therapy support its use in children with CKD and on renal replacement therapy (including dialysis patients and transplant recipients) who experience severe short stature/poor height velocity after addressing any nutritional or metabolic abnormalities that could compromise growth [19, 76, 81]. Despite this, the percentage of children with short stature and CKD who meet the criteria for rhGH treatment in the United States but fail to receive the treatment remains substantial at 70–75% [1, 2, 8]. Low utilization of rhGH in children with severe short stature has also been reported in Europe by the ESPN/ERA-EDTA registry based on data from 20 countries. Severe short stature was reported in 42.6% of 1612 children followed between 1990 and 2011, yet only 20% of the population reported the use of rhGH [28]. Whereas the low utilization may be partially related to the strict rhGH approval process that exists in Europe, the fact that utilization is also low in those European countries in which rhGH is reimbursed suggests that the attitudes of physicians and patients regarding the therapy are influential as well [99].

In a study designed to help explain the low utilization of rhGH based on medical record review, Greenbaum et al. found that of 110/307 children with CKD who fell below the fifth percentile for height, only 49% of them had been prescribed rhGH. The most common reasons reported for the somewhat low utilization of rhGH were family refusal, secondary hyperparathyroidism and poor control of renal osteodystrophy, and a history of noncompliance. Delays of drug availability related to insurance company approval were another contributing factor [100]. Interestingly, in a substantial percentage of cases, no apparent reason for the lack of rhGH utilization was included in the medical record.

Other proposed causes for poor rhGH utilization include challenges associated with the need for daily injections and presumed rapid referral for kidney transplantation and the opportunity for catch-up/or better growth, particularly when using steroid-avoidance protocols [71].

Finally, despite its efficacy in the transplant population, the use of rhGH in children with short stature in this patient cohort may also be low because of concern related to the risk of graft rejection. A meta-analysis by Wu et al. reported that a higher percentage (35/205) of transplant recipients who were receiving rhGH experienced a rejection episode compared to those who were not receiving rhGH therapy (19/185) with a risk ratio of 1.56 (95%, CI 0.97–2.53) [101]. However, it appears that the higher rejection rate in transplant recipients who receive rhGH is limited to those with a history of two or more prior rejection episodes [7, 81, 102]. Therefore, with vigilant follow-up, the majority of children with short stature post-kidney transplant can safely be treated with rhGH.

Evolution of Short Stature in Children with CKD

As noted above, although final adult height remains suboptimal for children with CKD/ESRD, improvement in the height SDS of these children has been observed over the past two decades, likely as a result of the provision of optimal nutrition, improved metabolic bone management, correction of acid-base abnormalities, and the use of rhGH.

Improvement in the growth of the CKD population might be best reflected by the significant improvement in the height SDS score of children at the time of kidney transplantation. The NAPRTCS has revealed an improvement in the height SDS from −2.4 in 1987 to −1.7 in 2013 (Fig. 21.3) [103]. The same is reflected by data from the European Society for Pediatric Nephrology/European Renal Association and European Dialysis and Transplant Association registry on more than 1600 patients who received renal replacement therapy [28]. The percentage of patients who reached a final adult height within the normal range increased from 50% for those who reached adulthood between 1990 and 1995 to 63% who reached adulthood from 2006 to 2011. Most importantly, however, the height SDS did not change significantly between onset of renal replacement therapy and final adult height, all of which suggests that the height gains experienced were likely due to improved pre-ESRD care.

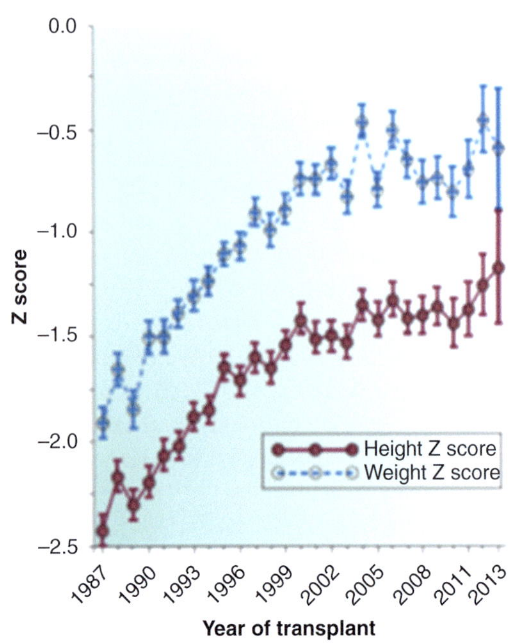

Fig. 21.3 Height and weight *Z* score at the time of kidney transplantation in the NAPRTCS registry between 1987 and 2013 (From Bertram et al. [104], with permission of Springer)

Improvement in the final adult height SDS of children on renal replacement therapy has also been documented over time. The mean height SDS was observed to improve from −3.03 to −1.80 ($p < 0.001$) when comparing growth data of 732 patients collected by the European Dialysis and Transplant Association registry (blue bars) in 1985–1988, with data from 384 patients collected in a German registry (red bars) from 1998 to 2009 (Fig. 21.4) [90]. Eighty-eight percent and 78%, respectively, of the two cohorts were comprised of transplant recipients. In a study by Fine et al. in which the outcome of over 10,000 transplant recipients in the NAPRTCS registry was reviewed, marked improvement in the final adult height SDS was noted in all age groups, most notably in children above 12 years of age in whom the mean height SDS improved from −1.75 to −0.92 from 1991 to 2002 [73].

Summary

Short stature is common among children with CKD and those requiring renal replacement therapy and is associated with an increase in the rates of hospitalization and mortality and a lower HRQoL. Correction of the metabolic abnormalities associated with CKD such as metabolic acidosis, bone disease, and salt depletion, along with the provision of adequate nutrition particularly in the first 2 years of life, usually improves growth in children. If not, the use of rhGH for treatment of short stature in CKD is safe and efficacious, and its early use should be encouraged with a goal of achieving a normal final adult height. The underutilization of rhGH mandates continued attention to those factors that currently preclude its use in children with CKD and poor growth.

Fig. 21.4 Comparison of mean height SDS for children in European Dialysis and Transplant Association (EDTA) registry (blue bars) from 1985 to 1988 and the German registry (red bars) from 1998 to 2009 revealed an improvement in height SDS from −3.03 to −1.80 ($p < 0.001$) (From Franke et al. [90], with permission of Springer)

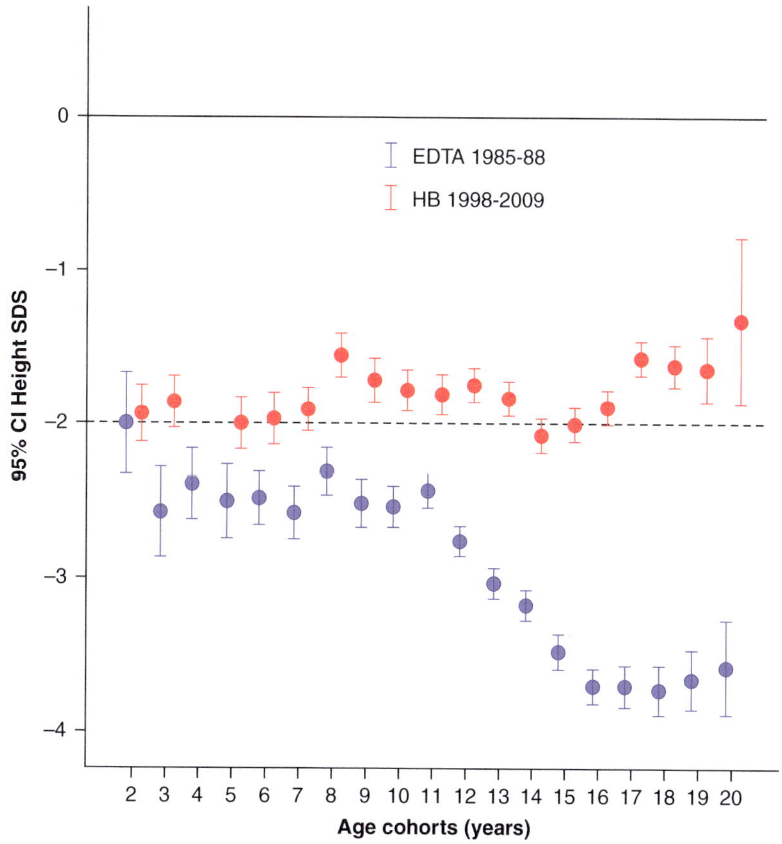

References

1. Al-Uzri A, Matheson M, Gipson DS, Mendley SR, Hooper SR, Yadin O, et al. The impact of short stature on health-related quality of life in children with chronic kidney disease. J Pediatr. 2013;163(3):736–41.e1.
2. Rodig NM, McDermott KC, Schneider MF, Hotchkiss HM, Yadin O, Seikaly MG, et al. Growth in children with chronic kidney disease: a report from the Chronic Kidney Disease in Children Study. Pediatr Nephrol. 2014;29(10):1987–95.
3. Salevic P, Radovic P, Milic N, Bogdanovic R, Paripovic D, Paripovic A, et al. Growth in children with chronic kidney disease: 13 years follow up study. J Nephrol. 2014;27(5):537–44.
4. Seikaly MG, Ho PL, Emmett L, Fine RN, Tejani A. Chronic renal insufficiency in children: the 2001 Annual Report of the NAPRTCS. Pediatr Nephrol. 2003;18(8):796–804.
5. Seikaly MG, Salhab N, Gipson D, Yiu V, Stablein D. Stature in children with chronic kidney disease: analysis of NAPRTCS database. Pediatr Nephrol. 2006;21(6):793–9.
6. Rees L. Growth hormone therapy in children with CKD after more than two decades of practice. Pediatr Nephrol. 2016;31(9):1421–35.
7. Mehls O, Fine RN. Growth hormone treatment after renal transplantation: a promising but underused chance to improve growth. Pediatr Nephrol. 2013;28(1):1–4.
8. Seikaly MG, Salhab N, Warady BA, Stablein D. Use of rhGH in children with chronic kidney disease: lessons from NAPRTCS. Pediatr Nephrol. 2007;22(8):1195–204.
9. Furth SL, Hwang W, Yang C, Neu AM, Fivush BA, Powe NR. Growth failure, risk of hospitalization and death for children with end-stage renal disease. Pediatr Nephrol. 2002;17(6):450–5.
10. Furth SL, Stablein D, Fine RN, Powe NR, Fivush BA. Adverse clinical outcomes associated with short stature at dialysis initiation: a report of the North American Pediatric Renal Transplant Cooperative Study. Pediatrics. 2002;109(5):909–13.
11. Furth SLAD, Hwang W, Neu AM, Powe NR, FIvush PA. Does poor growth predict morbidity and mortality in children with chronic renal failure and on dialysis? Semin Nephrol. 2001;21:463–9.
12. Wong CS, Gipson DS, Gillen DL, Emerson S, Koepsell T, Sherrard DJ, et al. Anthropometric measures and risk of death in children with end-stage renal disease. Am J Kidney Dis. 2000;36(4):811–9.
13. Gerson AC, Wentz A, Abraham AG, Mendley SR, Hooper SR, Butler RW, et al. Health-related qual-

ity of life of children with mild to moderate chronic kidney disease. Pediatrics. 2010;125(2):e349–57.
14. Mahan JD, Warady BA, Consensus C. Assessment and treatment of short stature in pediatric patients with chronic kidney disease: a consensus statement. Pediatr Nephrol. 2006;21(7):917–30.
15. Betts PR, Magrath G. Growth pattern and dietary intake of children with chronic renal insufficiency. Br Med J. 1974;2(5912):189–93.
16. Simmons JM, Wilson CJ, Potter DE, Holliday MA. Relation of calorie deficiency to growth failure in children on hemodialysis and the growth response to calorie supplementation. N Engl J Med. 1971;285(12):653–6.
17. Norman LJ, Coleman JE, Macdonald IA, Tomsett AM, Watson AR. Nutrition and growth in relation to severity of renal disease in children. Pediatr Nephrol. 2000;15(3–4):259–65.
18. Kuizon BD, Salusky IB. Growth retardation in children with chronic renal failure. J Bone Miner Res. 1999;14(10):1680–90.
19. KDOQI Work Group. KDOQI Clinical Practice Guideline for Nutrition in Children with CKD: 2008 update. Executive summary. Am J Kidney Dis. 2009;53(3 Suppl 2):S11–104.
20. Ledermann SE, Shaw V, Trompeter RS. Long-term enteral nutrition in infants and young children with chronic renal failure. Pediatr Nephrol. 1999;13:870–5.
21. Kari JA, Gonzalez C, Ledermann SE, Shaw V, Rees L. Outcome and growth in infants with severe chronic renal failure. Kidney Int. 2000;57:1681–7.
22. Arnold WC, Danford D, Holliday MA, Arnold WC. Effects of caloric supplementation on growth in children with uremia. Kidney Int. 1983;24(2):205–9.
23. Kuizon BD, Nelson PA, Salusky IB. Tube feeding in children with end-stage renal disease. Miner Electrolyte Metab. 1997;23(3–6):306–10.
24. Uauy RD, Hogg RJ, Brewer ED, Reisch JS, Cunningham C, Holliday MA. Dietary protein and growth in infants with chronic renal insufficiency: a report from the Southwest Pediatric Nephrology Study Group and the University of California, San Francisco. Pediatr Nephrol. 1994;8(1):45–50.
25. Greenbaum LA, Munoz A, Schneider MF, Kaskel FJ, Askenazi DJ, Jenkins R, et al. The association between abnormal birth history and growth in children with CKD. Clin J Am Soc Nephrol. 2011;6(1):14–21.
26. Franke D, Volker S, Haase S, Pavicic L, Querfeld U, Ehrich JH, et al. Prematurity, small for gestational age and perinatal parameters in children with congenital, hereditary and acquired chronic kidney disease. Nephrol Dial Transplant. 2010;25(12):3918–24.
27. Franke D, Alakan H, Pavicic L, Gellermann J, Muller D, Querfeld U, et al. Birth parameters and parental height predict growth outcome in children with chronic kidney disease. Pediatr Nephrol. 2013;28(12):2335–41.
28. Harambat J, Bonthuis M, van Stralen KJ, Ariceta G, Battelino N, Bjerre A, et al. Adult height in patients with advanced CKD requiring renal replacement therapy during childhood. Clin J Am Soc Nephrol. 2014;9(1):92–9.
29. Parekh RS, Flynn JT, Smoyer WE, Milne JL, Kershaw DB, Bunchman TE, et al. Improved growth in young children with severe chronic renal insufficiency who use specified nutritional therapy. J Am Soc Nephrol. 2001;12(11):2418–26.
30. Caldas A, Broyer M, Dechaux M, Kleinknecht C. Primary distal tubular acidosis in childhood: clinical study and long-term follow-up of 28 patients. J Pediatr. 1992;121(2):233–41.
31. Maniar S, Kleinknecht C, Zhou X, Motel V, Yvert JP, Dechaux M. Growth hormone action is blunted by acidosis in experimental uremia or acid load. Clin Nephrol. 1996;46(1):72–6.
32. Salusky IB, Goodman WG. Growth hormone and calcitriol as modifiers of bone formation in renal osteodystrophy. Kidney Int. 1995;48(3):657–65.
33. Kuizon BD, Goodman WG, Juppner H, Boechat I, Nelson P, Gales B, et al. Diminished linear growth during intermittent calcitriol therapy in children undergoing CCPD. Kidney Int. 1998;53(1):205–11.
34. Rabkin R, Sun DF, Chen Y, Tan J, Schaefer F. Growth hormone resistance in uremia, a role for impaired JAK/STAT signaling. Pediatr Nephrol. 2005;20(3):313–8.
35. Tonshoff B, Cronin MJ, Reichert M, Haffner D, Wingen AM, Blum WF, et al. Reduced concentration of serum growth hormone (GH)-binding protein in children with chronic renal failure: correlation with GH insensitivity. The European Study Group for Nutritional Treatment of Chronic Renal Failure in Childhood. The German Study Group for Growth Hormone Treatment in Chronic Renal Failure. J Clin Endocrinol Metab. 1997;82(4):1007–13.
36. Schaefer F, Chen Y, Tsao T, Nouri P, Rabkin R. Impaired JAK-STAT signal transduction contributes to growth hormone resistance in chronic uremia. J Clin Invest. 2001;108(3):467–75.
37. Powell DR, Liu F, Baker BK, Hinzt RL, Kale A, Suwanichkul A, et al. Effect of chronic renal failure and growth hormone therapy on the insulin-like growth factors and their binding proteins. Pediatr Nephrol. 2000;14(7):579–83.
38. Tonshoff B, Powell DR, Zhao D, Durham SK, Coleman ME, Domene HM, et al. Decreased hepatic insulin-like growth factor (IGF)-I and increased IGF binding protein-1 and -2 gene expression in experimental uremia. Endocrinology. 1997;138(3):938–46.
39. Styne DM. The regulation of pubertal growth. Horm Res. 2003;60(Suppl 1):22–6.
40. Lane PH. Puberty and chronic kidney disease. Adv Chronic Kidney Dis. 2005;12(4):372–7.
41. Hokken-Koelega AC, Saenger P, Cappa M, Greggio N. Unresolved problems concerning optimal therapy of puberty in children with chronic renal diseases. J Pediatr Endocrinol Metab. 2001;14(Suppl 2):945–52.
42. Schaefer F, Seidel C, Binding A, Gasser T, Largo RH, Prader A, et al. Pubertal growth in chronic renal failure. Pediatr Res. 1990;28(1):5–10.

43. Holley JL. The hypothalamic-pituitary axis in men and women with chronic kidney disease. Adv Chronic Kidney Dis. 2004;11(4):337–41.
44. Schaefer F, Veldhuis JD, Robertson WR, Dunger D, Scharer K. Immunoreactive and bioactive luteinizing hormone in pubertal patients with chronic renal failure. Cooperative Study Group on Pubertal Development in Chronic Renal Failure. Kidney Int. 1994;45(5):1465–76.
45. Belgorosky A, Ferraris JR, Ramirez JA, Jasper H, Rivarola MA. Serum sex hormone-binding globulin and serum nonsex hormone-binding globulin-bound testosterone fractions in prepubertal boys with chronic renal failure. J Clin Endocrinol Metab. 1991;73(1):107–10.
46. Mitchell R, Schaefer F, Morris ID, Scharer K, Sun JG, Robertson WR. Elevated serum immunoreactive inhibin levels in peripubertal boys with chronic renal failure. Cooperative Study Group on Pubertal Development in Chronic Renal Failure (CSPCRF). Clin Endocrinol. 1993;39(1):27–33.
47. Schaefer F, Hamill G, Stanhope R, Preece MA, Scharer K. Pulsatile growth hormone secretion in peripubertal patients with chronic renal failure. Cooperative Study Group on Pubertal Development in Chronic Renal Failure. J Pediatr. 1991;119(4):568–77.
48. Rees L, Greene SA, Adlard P, Jones J, Haycock GB, Rigden SP, et al. Growth and endocrine function after renal transplantation. Arch Dis Child. 1988;63(11):1326–32.
49. Rees L. Management of the infant with end-stage renal failure. Nephrol Dial Transplant. 2002;17(9):1564–7.
50. Abitbol CL, Zilleruelo G, Montane B, Strauss J. Growth of uremic infants on forced feeding regimens. Pediatr Nephrol. 1993;7(2):173–7.
51. Karlberg J, Schaefer F, Hennicke M, Wingen AM, Rigden S, Mehls O. Early age-dependent growth impairment in chronic renal failure. European Study Group for Nutritional Treatment of Chronic Renal Failure in Childhood. Pediatr Nephrol. 1996;10(3):283–7.
52. Rees L, Azocar M, Borzych D, Watson AR, Buscher A, Edefonti A, et al. Growth in very young children undergoing chronic peritoneal dialysis. J Am Soc Nephrol. 2011;22(12):2303–12.
53. Rees L, Brandt ML. Tube feeding in children with chronic kidney disease: technical and practical issues. Pediatr Nephrol. 2010;25(4):699–704.
54. Fine RN, Attie KM, Kuntze J, Brown DF, Kohaut EC. Recombinant human growth hormone in infants and young children with chronic renal insufficiency. Genentech Collaborative Study Group. Pediatr Nephrol. 1995;9(4):451–7.
55. van Stralen KJ, Borzych-Duzalka D, Hataya H, Kennedy SE, Jager KJ, Verrina E, et al. Survival and clinical outcomes of children starting renal replacement therapy in the neonatal period. Kidney Int. 2014;86(1):168–74.
56. Schaefer F, Klaus G, Mehls O. Peritoneal transport properties and dialysis dose affect growth and nutritional status in children on chronic peritoneal dialysis. Mid-European Pediatric Peritoneal Dialysis Study Group. J Am Soc Nephrol. 1999;10(8):1786–92.
57. Rees L, Shaw V. Nutrition in children with CRF and on dialysis. Pediatr Nephrol. 2007;22(10):1689–702.
58. Bacchetta J, Harambat J, Cochat P, Salusky IB, Wesseling-Perry K. The consequences of chronic kidney disease on bone metabolism and growth in children. Nephrol Dial Transplant. 2012;27(8):3063–71.
59. Haffner D, Schaefer F, Nissel R, Wuhl E, Tonshoff B, Mehls O. Effect of growth hormone treatment on the adult height of children with chronic renal failure. German Study Group for Growth Hormone Treatment in Chronic Renal Failure. N Engl J Med. 2000;343(13):923–30.
60. Fischbach M, Terzic J, Menouer S, Dheu C, Seuge L, Zalosczic A. Daily on line haemodiafiltration promotes catch-up growth in children on chronic dialysis. Nephrol Dial Transplant. 2010;25(3):867–73.
61. Fischbach M, Warady BA. Peritoneal dialysis prescription in children: bedside principles for optimal practice. Pediatr Nephrol. 2009;24(9):1633–42. quiz 40, 42.
62. Nissel R, Lindberg A, Mehls O, Haffner D. Factors predicting the near-final height in growth hormone-treated children and adolescents with chronic kidney disease. J Clin Endocrinol Metab. 2008;93(4):1359–65.
63. Ulinski T, Cochat P. Longitudinal growth in children following kidney transplantation: from conservative to pharmacological strategies. Pediatr Nephrol. 2006;21(7):903–9.
64. Harambat J, Cochat P. Growth after renal transplantation. Pediatr Nephrol. 2009;24:1297.
65. Jux C, Leiber K, Hugel U, Blum W, Ohlsson C, Klaus G, et al. Dexamethasone impairs growth hormone (GH)-stimulated growth by suppression of local insulin-like growth factor (IGF)-I production and expression of GH- and IGF-I-receptor in cultured rat chondrocytes. Endocrinology. 1998;139(7):3296–305.
66. Koedam JA, Hoogerbrugge CM, Van Buul-Offers SC. Differential regulation of IGF-binding proteins in rabbit costal chondrocytes by IGF-I and dexamethasone. J Endocrinol. 2000;165(3):557–67.
67. Smink JJ, Buchholz IM, Hamers N, van Tilburg CM, Christis C, Sakkers RJ, et al. Short-term glucocorticoid treatment of piglets causes changes in growth plate morphology and angiogenesis. Osteoarthritis Cartilage. 2003;11(12):864–71.
68. Chrysis D, Ritzen EM, Savendahl L. Growth retardation induced by dexamethasone is associated with increased apoptosis of the growth plate chondrocytes. J Endocrinol. 2003;176(3):331–7.
69. Broyer M, Guest G, Gagnadoux MF. Growth rate in children receiving alternate-day corticosteroid treatment after kidney transplantation. J Pediatr. 1992;120(5):721–5.
70. Shapiro R, Scantlebury VP, Jordan ML, Vivas C, Ellis D, Lombardozzi-Lane S, et al. Pediatric renal transplantation under tacrolimus-based immunosuppression. Transplantation. 1999;67(2):299–303.

71. Sarwal MM, Yorgin PD, Alexander S, Millan MT, Belson A, Belanger N, et al. Promising early outcomes with a novel, complete steroid avoidance immunosuppression protocol in pediatric renal transplantation. Transplantation. 2001;72(1):13–21.
72. Jabs K, Sullivan EK, Avner ED, Harmon WE. Alternate-day steroid dosing improves growth without adversely affecting graft survival or long-term graft function. A report of the North American Pediatric Renal Transplant Cooperative Study. Transplantation. 1996;61(1):31–6.
73. Fine RN, Martz K, Stablein D. What have 20 years of data from the North American Pediatric Renal Transplant Cooperative Study taught us about growth following renal transplantation in infants, children, and adolescents with end-stage renal disease? Pediatr Nephrol. 2010;25(4):739–46.
74. Pape L, Ehrich JH, Zivicnjak M, Offner G. Living related kidney donation as an advantage for growth of children independent of glomerular filtration rate. Transplant Proc. 2006;38(3):685–7.
75. Pape L, Ehrich JH, Zivicnjak M, Offner G. Growth in children after kidney transplantation with living related donor graft or cadaveric graft. Lancet. 2005;366(9480):151–3.
76. Kidney Disease: Improving Global Outcomes (KDIGO) CKD-MBD Work Group. KDIGO clinical practice guideline for the diagnosis, evaluation, prevention, and treatment of Chronic Kidney Disease-Mineral and Bone Disorder (CKD-MBD). Kidney Int Suppl. 2009;(113):S1–S130.
77. Bergstrom J, Wang T, Lindholm B. Factors contributing to catabolism in end-stage renal disease patients. Miner Electrolyte Metab. 1998;24(1):92–101.
78. Sharma AP, Singh RN, Yang C, Sharma RK, Kapoor R, Filler G. Bicarbonate therapy improves growth in children with incomplete distal renal tubular acidosis. Pediatr Nephrol. 2009;24(8):1509–16.
79. Fine RN, Yadin O, Moulton L, Nelson PA, Boechat MI, Lippe BM. Five years experience with recombinant human growth hormone treatment of children with chronic renal failure. J Pediatr Endocrinol. 1994;7(1):1–12.
80. Mehls O, Tonshoff B, Haffner D, Wuhl E, Schaefer F. The use of recombinant human growth hormone in short children with chronic renal failure. J Pediatr Endocrinol. 1994;7(2):107–13.
81. Hodson EM, Willis NS, Craig JC. Growth hormone for children with chronic kidney disease. Cochrane Database Syst Rev. 2012;2:CD003264.
82. Hokken-Koelega A, Mulder P, De Jong R, Lilien M, Donckerwolcke R, Groothof J. Long-term effects of growth hormone treatment on growth and puberty in patients with chronic renal insufficiency. Pediatr Nephrol. 2000;14(7):701–6.
83. Schwarz HP, Walczak M, Birkholz-Walerzak D, Szalecki M, Nanu M, Woehling H, et al. Two-year data from a long-term phase IV study of recombinant human growth hormone in short children born small for gestational age. Adv Ther. 2016;33:423.
84. Hou L, Chen ZH, Liu D, Cheng YG, Luo XP. Comparative pharmacokinetics and pharmacodynamics of a PEGylated recombinant human growth hormone and daily recombinant human growth hormone in growth hormone-deficient children. Drug Design Dev Ther. 2016;10:13–21.
85. Saenger PH, Mejia-Corletto J. Long-acting growth hormone: an update. Endocr Dev. 2016;30:79–97.
86. Akchurin OM, Melamed ML, Hashim BL, Kaskel FJ, Del Rio M. Medication adherence in the transition of adolescent kidney transplant recipients to the adult care. Pediatr Transplant. 2014;18(5):538–48.
87. Fine RN, Kohaut EC, Brown D, Perlman AJ. Growth after recombinant human growth hormone treatment in children with chronic renal failure: report of a multicenter randomized double-blind placebo-controlled study. Genentech Cooperative Study Group. J Pediatr. 1994;124(3):374–82.
88. Haffner D, Wuhl E, Schaefer F, Nissel R, Tonshoff B, Mehls O. Factors predictive of the short- and long-term efficacy of growth hormone treatment in prepubertal children with chronic renal failure. The German Study Group for Growth Hormone Treatment in Chronic Renal Failure. J Am Soc Nephrol. 1998;9(10):1899–907.
89. Fine RN, Stablein D. Long-term use of recombinant human growth hormone in pediatric allograft recipients: a report of the NAPRTCS Transplant Registry. Pediatr Nephrol. 2005;20(3):404–8.
90. Franke D, Winkel S, Gellermann J, Querfeld U, Pape L, Ehrich JH, et al. Growth and maturation improvement in children on renal replacement therapy over the past 20 years. Pediatr Nephrol. 2013;28(10):2043–51.
91. Mehls O, Lindberg A, Nissel R, Haffner D, Hokken-Koelega A, Ranke MB. Predicting the response to growth hormone treatment in short children with chronic kidney disease. J Clin Endocrinol Metab. 2010;95(2):686–92.
92. Mahan JD, Warady BA, Frane J, Rosenfeld RG, Swinford RD, Lippe B, et al. First-year response to rhGH therapy in children with CKD: a National Cooperative Growth Study Report. Pediatr Nephrol. 2010;25(6):1125–30.
93. Al-Uzri A, Swinford RD, Nguyen T, Jenkins R, Gunsul A, Kachan-Liu SS, et al. The utility of the IGF-I generation test in children with chronic kidney disease. Pediatr Nephrol. 2013;28(12):2323–33.
94. Fine RN, Ho M, Tejani A, Blethen S. Adverse events with rhGH treatment of patients with chronic renal insufficiency and end-stage renal disease. J Pediatr. 2003;142(5):539–45.
95. Dharnidharka VR, Talley LI, Martz KL, Stablein DM, Fine RN. Recombinant growth hormone use pretransplant and risk for post-transplant lymphoproliferative disease – a report of the NAPRTCS. Pediatr Transplant. 2008;12(6):689–95.
96. Guler HP, Eckardt KU, Zapf J, Bauer C, Froesch ER. Insulin-like growth factor I increase glomeru-

lar filtration rate and renal plasma flow in man. Acta Endocrinol. 1989;121(1):101–6.
97. Kopple JD, Hirschberg R. Physiological effects of growth hormone and insulin-like growth factor I on the kidney. Miner Electrolyte Metab. 1990;16(1):82–8.
98. Mehls O, Lindberg A, Haffner D, Schaefer F, Wuhl E. Long-term growth hormone treatment in short children with CKD does not accelerate decline of renal function: results from the KIGS registry and ESCAPE trial. Pediatr Nephrol. 2015;30:2145.
99. van Huis M, Bonthuis M, Sahpazova E, Mencarelli F, Spasojević B, Reusz G, et al. Considerable variations in growth hormone policy and prescription in paediatric end-stage renal disease across European countries—a report from the ESPN/ERA-EDTA registry. Nephrol Dial Transplant. 2016;31(4):609–19.
100. Greenbaum LA, Hidalgo G, Chand D, Chiang M, Dell K, Kump T, et al. Obstacles to the prescribing of growth hormone in children with chronic kidney disease. Pediatr Nephrol. 2008;23(9):1531–5.
101. Wu Y, Cheng W, Yang XD, Xiang B. Growth hormone improves growth in pediatric renal transplant recipients – a systemic review and meta-analysis of randomized controlled trials. Pediatr Nephrol. 2013;28(1):129–33.
102. Broyer M. Results and side-effects of treating children with growth hormone after kidney transplantation – a preliminary report. Pharmacia & Upjohn Study Group. Acta Paediatr Suppl. 1996;417:76–9.
103. North American Pediatric Renal Trials and Cooperative Studies (NAPRTCS) 2014 Annual Transplant Report. https://web.emmes.com/study/ped/annlrept/annualrept2014.pdf. 2014.
104. Bertram JF, Goldstein SL, Pape L, et al. Kidney disease in children: latest advances and remaining challenges. Nat Rev Nephrol. 2016;12:182–91.

Other Pituitary Disorders and Kidney Disease

22

Wenyu Huang and Mark E. Molitch

Prolactin and Kidney Disease

Prolactin (PRL) is synthesized and secreted from the lactotrophs in the anterior pituitary [1]. Hypothalamic dopamine exerts tonic inhibition on PRL secretion [2], while several hypothalamic factors, including vasoactive intestinal polypeptide (VIP) and thyrotropin-releasing hormone (TRH), stimulate PRL secretion [3, 4]. In addition, the lactotrophs are also directly stimulated by estrogen [5–7], which explains the elevated PRL levels during pregnancy [8]. Following delivery, PRL increases with each suckling episode, stimulating milk production. In addition, circulating levels of PRL display a strong circadian rhythm, in which PRL levels peak during the first half of the sleep period followed by a gradual decrease to lower levels during daytime [9].

In patients with chronic kidney disease (CKD), there is an increase in PRL levels. The prevalence of hyperprolactinemia ranges from 18.3% in mild renal insufficiency [10, 11] to more than 70% in patients on hemodialysis (HD) and peritoneal dialysis (PD) [12, 13]. In patients with CKD who are also taking medications known to interfere with dopamine, PRL levels up to 2000 μg/L have been reported, which is a level usually associated with PRL-producing pituitary macroadenomas [10].

Pathophysiology

Multiple mechanisms exist to explain the elevation of PRL in CKD. One main mechanism is decreased renal clearance of PRL molecules [12]. In one study, the metabolic clearance rate of PRL was reported to be decreased by about 33% in patients with CKD [12]. Additionally, the secretion of PRL is also enhanced in CKD. Compared to that in normal subjects, the PRL secretion rate increases by about three- to fourfold in patients with CKD [12]. The mechanism underlying the increase in PRL release in CKD is believed to be resistance of PRL secretion to dopaminergic suppression [14]. Interestingly, resistance of PRL secretion to regulatory signals also exists for TRH, VIP, and chlorpromazine [14, 15], but not for metoclopramide [16], suggesting that several hypothalamic mechanisms regulating PRL secretion are differentially affected in CKD. PRL molecules are not removed by HD or PD [17]. Not surprisingly, after kidney transplant, hyperprolactinemia usually corrects or significantly improves, even within days [18].

W. Huang · M. E. Molitch (✉)
Division of Endocrinology, Metabolism and Molecular Medicine, Northwestern University Feinberg School of Medicine, Chicago, IL, USA
e-mail: molitch@northwestern.edu

C. M. Rhee et al. (eds.), *Endocrine Disorders in Kidney Disease*,
https://doi.org/10.1007/978-3-319-97765-2_22

Diagnosis of Hyperprolactinemia

PRL is commonly measured by two-site immunometric assays. It should be emphasized that breast and nipple manipulations can transiently increase PRL secretion, so PRL levels should not be checked shortly after a breast exam. Three distinct molecular forms of PRL have been identified, with corresponding molecular weights of 23 (monomeric), 50–60 (big PRL), and >100 kDA (big big PRL or macroprolactin). The high molecular forms are thought to result from dimerization or binding of PRL to IgG. Polyethylene glycol is commonly used to precipitate macroprolactin molecules before measuring PRL monomers in the supernatant to calculate the percentage of PRL recovery and has been shown to correlate well with the gold standard for measuring monomeric PRL, i.e., gel filtration chromatography [19]. A PRL recovery ≤40% is suggested as the cutoff for diagnosis of macroprolactinemia, while a recovery >50% makes the diagnosis of macroprolactinemia unlikely [19].

In normal individuals, the monomeric form of PRL accounts for 85–95% of PRL in circulation [20]. In CKD, an increase in PRL immunoreactivity exceeds that of PRL bioactivity [21]. While some studies found monomeric PRL to be the predominant form of PRL contributing to the hyperprolactinemia in patients with CKD [22] and on HD and PD [23], a recent study demonstrated that macroprolactin levels are positively correlated with a decline in renal function, suggesting that macroprolactin may also contribute to the hyperprolactinemia observed in CKD patients [24].

During evaluation for hyperprolactinemia, it is important to carefully check the medications that a patient is taking, as some medications have been shown to increase PRL levels [25] and that stopping of PRL-raising medications can significantly lower PRL levels, even in patients with CKD [10]. Normally, an MRI is not needed in the assessment of hyperprolactinemia in patients with CKD. However, if there is a concern that hyperprolactinemia may be caused by sellar or suprasellar lesion in patients with CKD, for example, patients presenting with headache, vision change, or defective visual field suggesting compression of optic chiasm, a pituitary MRI can be performed. However, given the potential severe complications associated with intravenous MRI contrast use in patients with CKD, the MRI should be performed either without contrast in patients with CKD but not on dialysis or, if medically necessary, with contrast in patients on HD who then require additional dialysis sessions to clear the contrast.

Clinical Manifestation of Hyperprolactinemia

Clinically, hyperprolactinemia can cause galactorrhea and hypogonadism (manifested as amenorrhea or oligomenorrhea, low libido, erectile dysfunction, gynecomastia, infertility, etc.). Galactorrhea is usually bilateral, multi-ductal, and milky. The color can range from clear to yellow, green, or brown [25, 26]. On the other hand, nipple discharge that is from a single duct, bloody or serosanguinous, or associated with palpable or radiologically evident breast mass, will need further evaluation for breast tumors [27]. A Sudan IV staining for fat droplets in the nipple discharge can confirm the diagnosis of milk [25]. While hyperprolactinemia generally causes hypogonadotropic hypogonadism, hypergonadotropic hypogonadism is also commonly seen in patients with CKD [28], suggesting different mechanisms leading to hypogonadism in CKD. Recently, it has been suggested that PRL levels are directly associated with endothelial dysfunction and with increased risk of cardiovascular events and mortality in CKD patients [29]. However, the direct relationship of hyperprolactinemia and increased cardiovascular risk is not firmly established, and there are no studies showing cardiovascular benefit from lowering PRL levels in such patients.

Treatment of Hyperprolactinemia

Indications for the treatment of hyperprolactinemia in patients with CKD include bothersome galactorrhea and hypogonadism. As most hyperprolactinemia in CKD is related to decreased kidney function, dopamine agonists can be considered for lowering PRL levels in these patients. It should be noted that there are very limited data available on the efficacy and safety of dopamine agonists in patients with

Table 22.1 Medications or substances that cause hyperprolactinemia

Antipsychotics
Gastrointestinal motility medications: e.g., metoclopramide (Reglan®)
Antidepressants: rare
Antihypertensive medications: verapamil, methyldopa, reserpine
Antinausea agents: chlorpromazine
Others: opioids, cocaine

CKD or on dialysis [30, 31]. Moreover, PRL secretion is resistant to dopaminergic suppression in CKD, so higher doses of dopamine agonists may be needed [14, 32].

Additionally, for patients with hyperprolactinemia possibly caused or exacerbated by medications, the offending medication(s) ideally should be considered for discontinuation. If the underlying condition warrants continuation of such medications, switching to another medication in the same class that has lower or no potential to cause hyperprolactinemia would be the most appropriate management. It is very important to work closely with the prescriber to address the adjustment of such medication [33, 34]. Below is a list of medications that commonly cause hyperprolactinemia (Table 22.1).

If the major concern is decreased reproductive hormone production, they can then be replaced judiciously. Estrogen replacement using oral contraceptives will not restore ovulation, and referral to a reproductive endocrinologist will usually be necessary if fertility is desired. Likewise, in male patients, replacement of testosterone will not usually help with spermatogenesis. The use of injectable follicle-stimulating hormone (FSH) and luteinizing hormone (LH) to stimulate spermatogenesis in patients with CKD has not been studied.

For patients who do not meet indications and who choose no intervention, it is reasonable to reassure the patient and monitor [35, 36].

Hypothalamic-Pituitary-Adrenal Axis and Kidney Disease

In CKD, many aspects of the physiology of the hypothalamic-pituitary-adrenal (HPA) axis are altered. Accordingly, diagnosis and treatment of disorders involving the HPA axis are affected by CKD.

Pathophysiology

Circulating Levels of Adrenocorticotropic Hormone (ACTH) and Cortisol

In patients with CKD, ACTH levels are usually found to be elevated [37–39], but there are conflicting data regarding the level of cortisol. While a number of studies have shown that morning and afternoon levels of plasma cortisol are similar in patients with CKD as compared to normal subjects [37, 38, 40], other studies have demonstrated that the mean morning plasma total and free cortisol levels and the mean 24-h plasma total cortisol levels were elevated in patients with CKD on chronic HD [39, 41, 42].

Circadian Rhythms of ACTH and Cortisol

In healthy individuals with normal sleep patterns, there is a strong circadian rhythm of ACTH and cortisol secretion. After reaching their nadir around midnight, ACTH and cortisol levels start to rise and reach their peaks in the morning after waking up, which is then followed by a decline throughout the day before reaching their nadir again at midnight.

Although circadian rhythms of plasma and salivary cortisol are largely preserved in patients with CKD [41, 43], patients with advanced CKD on chronic dialysis, compared to normal subjects, have higher trough levels of plasma and salivary cortisol at midnight [43], likely explained by higher levels of ACTH at that time point [44, 45].

Altered Metabolism of Endogenous Cortisol

Cortisol has a strong affinity to and is able to activate mineralocorticoid receptors. Normally, cortisol is converted to biologically inactive cortisone by 11-beta-hydroxysteroid dehydrogenase 2 (11-beta-HSD2) at mineralocorticoid target tissues, including the kidney, pancreas, and colon [46]. As a result, circulating cortisol does not normally activate mineralocorticoid receptors. In patients with CKD, it has been reported that there is ineffective deactivation of cortisol by 11-beta-HSD2 [47, 48], which may lead to exaggerated activation of the mineralocorticoid receptors and eventually hypertension [49].

Altered Metabolism of Exogenous Glucocorticoids

In addition to changes in metabolism of endogenous glucocorticoids in patients with CKD, there is prolongation of the half-life with reduced metabolic clearance rate of hydrocortisone and prednisolone, but a shortened half-life and increased metabolic clearance rate of dexamethasone, highlighting the distinct metabolism of exogenous steroids in CKD [50]. Moreover, it has also been demonstrated that orally administered dexamethasone has a lower absorption rate in patients with CKD as compared to normal subjects [40], which may explain why oral dexamethasone fails to suppress endogenous cortisol in some patients (see the following section under "Cushing's disease" for more discussion). Furthermore, there are also altered responses of cortisol to exogenous stimulators or suppressors, which are discussed below.

Adrenal Insufficiency in CKD

Diagnosis of Adrenal Insufficiency in CKD

Cosyntropin Stimulation Test

Patients with secondary or tertiary adrenal insufficiency, i.e., deficiency of cortisol due to inadequate ACTH or corticotropin-releasing hormone (CRH), respectively, are commonly diagnosed with cosyntropin (1 μg or 250 μg – the latter is the standard dose) stimulation tests. In the cosyntropin stimulation test, adrenally insufficient patients fail to mount an increase in cortisol levels to 18 μg/dL (some authors prefer 20 μg/mL) at 30 or 60 minutes after cosyntropin administration. It should be remembered in testing that an ACTH level should always be drawn with the baseline cortisol before administering the cosyntropin.

In one study, patients with CKD on HD or continuous ambulatory PD (CAPD) mount increases in cortisol levels after 1 μg, 5 μg, and 250 μg cosyntropin stimulation similar to those seen in healthy subjects [38]. In the same study, baseline cortisol levels were similar between the controls and dialysis patients, whereas baseline ACTH levels were higher in the patients on dialysis [38], consistent with other studies [37, 39, 40].

Metyrapone Stimulation Test

Metyrapone inhibits 11-beta-hydroxylase, a key enzyme in adrenal steroidogenesis, and results in suppression of cortisol production, which in turn stimulates secretion of ACTH and immediate precursors of cortisol, i.e., 11-deoxycortisol [51]. Therefore, the metyrapone stimulation test is able to assess the response of the whole HPA axis. However, it is less commonly used due to the limited availability of metyrapone and the possibility of inducing adrenal crisis in patients with adrenal insufficiency. In CKD patients, there appears to be a preserved response to metyrapone (30 mg/kg), as manifested by similar decreases in cortisol and increases in ACTH and 11-deoxycortisol after overnight oral metyrapone as in control subjects [40].

Insulin Tolerance Test (ITT)

Like the metyrapone stimulation test, the ITT also tests the integrity of the whole HPA axis. In the ITT, transient hypoglycemia induced by an exogenous intravenous insulin bolus (0.1 U/kg) leads to activation of the HPA axis and an increase in ACTH and cortisol levels. Although considered the gold standard for the diagnosis of adrenal insufficiency, the ITT is also not commonly recommended due to its inconvenience, complexity, and safety concerns [52]. Similarly to what was observed in the metyrapone stimulation test, patients on CAPD or chronic HD have normal cortisol responses in the ITT [40, 53], suggestive of the validity of both tests in diagnosing adrenal insufficiency.

The CRH Stimulation Test

The CRH stimulation test has been used to differentiate secondary and tertiary adrenal insufficiency, in which exogenous CRH generates higher ACTH levels in patients with tertiary, but not secondary, adrenal insufficiency [54]. In CKD patients on chronic dialysis, after correction of anemia by erythropoietin, the cortisol response to exogenous CRH was prolonged [55]. Furthermore, compared to ESRD patients not on dialysis and those on HD, patients on CAPD demonstrated a more normal response to CRH stimulation [56].

Etiology of Adrenal Insufficiency in CKD

It is likely that the most common cause of adrenal insufficiency in patients with CKD is prior treatment with exogenous steroids, as it is for those without CKD. It should be remembered that the HPA axis can be suppressed for more than 1 year with such steroid use and 10–15% of patients never recover their axis [57]. Autoimmune disease is the most common cause otherwise in the USA, but infections with tuberculosis and fungal diseases are relatively common causes in those coming from other countries. Anticoagulation with hemorrhage into both adrenal glands is another frequently overlooked cause.

Clinical Manifestation of Adrenal Insufficiency in CKD

Symptoms of adrenal insufficiency in CKD patients are similar to those in patients without CKD. The common presentations are fatigue, gastrointestinal symptoms including nausea, diarrhea and abdominal pain, hypotension, hyponatremia, etc. However, in patients with advanced CKD, such symptoms are relatively nonspecific. Additionally, patients with adrenal insufficiency can manifest as hypercalcemia in patients on dialysis [58, 59]. Indeed, the prevalence of hypercalcemia in CKD is around 1.3% [58].

Treatment of Adrenal Insufficiency in CKD

The mainstay of the treatment of secondary or tertiary adrenal insufficiency in CKD patients is similar to that in patients with normal renal function, i.e., replacement of glucocorticoids. The clinician should consider the altered metabolism of exogenous glucocorticoids, especially those commonly used in adrenal insufficiency including hydrocortisone, prednisone, etc. Usual hydrocortisone replacement doses are in the 15–25 mg/day range, given in divided doses. Adjustment of glucocorticoid doses should be mainly based on symptoms of the patients. Similar sick-day rules and use of stress dose glucocorticoids during extreme stress, e.g., surgery, should also apply; thus, 50–75 mg is usually given parenterally every 8 h [52, 60].

Cushing's Disease in CKD

Diagnosis of Cushing's Syndrome in CKD

Cushing's syndrome may be caused by exogenous steroids (the most common cause), excessive ACTH production by a pituitary tumor (Cushing's disease) or an ectopic tumor, or autonomous production of steroids by an adrenal adenoma/carcinoma with suppression of ACTH levels. The diagnosis of Cushing's syndrome relies on demonstrating cortisol levels that cannot be suppressed fully with dexamethasone and findings of elevated 24-h urine-free cortisol (UFC) levels and midnight salivary cortisol levels [61].

While higher cortisol levels were associated with higher mortality in patients on chronic HD [62], the diagnosis of Cushing's syndrome also appears to be altered in patients with CKD, as detailed below.

Dexamethasone Suppression Test

While most studies show that 1 mg of dexamethasone overnight does not adequately suppress the cortisol secretion in patients with CKD [41, 63, 64], one study showed normal suppression of cortisol by 1 mg oral dexamethasone in patients with various degrees of CKD including ESRD on HD [37]. Interestingly, despite seemingly inadequate suppression by the 1 mg dexamethasone overnight test in most studies, the regular two-day low-dose [63] and 3 mg overnight [40] dexamethasone tests are able to fully inhibit cortisol levels as in normal subjects. Conflicting results exist as to the metabolism of 1 mg dexamethasone administered orally. While one study shows that the metabolism of dexamethasone is similar in both CKD patients and normal subjects [63], another study suggested that there is inadequate absorption of 1 mg dexamethasone following oral administration, which may account for the insufficient suppression of cortisol by 1 mg, but not 3 mg, of dexamethasone [40]. Additionally, there seems to be some resistance of the HPA axis to exogenous steroids in CKD since 1 mg of IV dexamethasone in CKD patients does not suppress cortisol to the level seen in normal subjects after the same dose of IV dexamethasone [65]. When doing dexamethasone suppression tests, it is important to measure dexamethasone levels at the same time as cortisol levels to be sure an adequate amount of dexamethasone was taken.

Midnight Salivary Cortisol Test

An elevated midnight salivary cortisol level has an excellent ability to indicate the presence of Cushing's syndrome in subjects without CKD [66]. The validity of the midnight salivary cortisol test in the diagnosis of Cushing's syndrome in CKD is lacking. However, given the previous report that ESRD patients have higher nadir levels of salivary cortisol [43] in a 24-h period, the normal levels used in the current diagnostic criteria may result in more false-positive tests; therefore, this test will warrant further investigation.

24-Hour UFC Test

The utility of the 24-h UFC in diagnosing Cushing's syndrome is uncertain as it has been reported that patients with Cushing's disease complicated by CKD have either lower [67] or undetectable levels of UFC [68].

Because elevated levels of UFC can be found in non-Cushing's patients with CKD and that those with Cushing's and CKD may not have elevated levels, the measurement of UFC in this setting may be inaccurate and not useful.

Inferior Petrosal Sinus Sampling (IPSS)

Inferior petrosal sinus sampling (IPSS) is recommended)for confirming the pituitary source of ACTH-dependent Cushing's syndrome, which is most commonly due to a pituitary adenoma. There are no reports of the use of IPSS in the setting of CKD perhaps due to the known toxicity of radiocontrast media in CKD. Based on the understanding of Cushing's disease and the effects of CKD on the HPA axis, it is expected that there is still a pituitary-to-peripheral gradient of ACTH in patients with Cushing's disease complicated with CKD, as revealed by IPSS (Table 22.2).

Table 22.2 Dynamic tests for diagnosis of hypercortisolism in chronic kidney disease

1 mg overnight dexamethasone suppression test	Less suppression of cortisol, may cause false-positive results
Two-day, low-dose (0.5 mg every 6 h) dexamethasone suppression test	Similar response as in normal renal function
High-dose (3 mg) overnight dexamethasone suppression test	Similar response as in normal renal function
Midnight salivary cortisol test	Higher nadir level of cortisol, may cause false-positive results
24-h urine-free cortisol	Not useful

Clinical Manifestation of Cushing's Disease in CKD

Patients with Cushing's disease normally present with symptoms of hypercortisolism. Since cortisol affects almost every organ system, symptoms and signs of hypercortisolism are broad. The symptoms, in the order of prevalence, include weight gain, menstrual irregularity, hirsutism, psychiatric dysfunction, backache, muscle weakness, fractures, and loss of scalp hair. The clinical signs of hypercortisolism include truncal or generalized obesity, plethora, moon facies, hypertension, bruising, red-purple striae, muscle weakness, ankle edema, and skin hyperpigmentation [69].

Treatment of Cushing's Syndrome in CKD

Due to the absence of strong clinical evidence, there are no guidelines for treating Cushing's syndrome in CKD patients. As in patients with normal renal function, the principal treatment of Cushing syndrome in CKD should be surgical removal of the pituitary or adrenal tumor, followed by subsequent treatment(s) with radiotherapy and/or medications if necessary. Medical treatment of Cushing's syndrome includes pasireotide (a somatostatin analog), cabergoline (a dopamine agonist), adrenal enzyme inhibitors such as ketoconazole, and mifepristone (a glucocorticoid receptor antagonist). These agents can be considered in individual patients who do not attain control after surgical intervention [70, 71].

Arginine Vasopressin (AVP) and Kidney Disease

Pathophysiology

AVP, also called antidiuretic hormone (ADH), is secreted by magnocellular neurons in the supraoptic (SON) and paraventricular nuclei (PVN) of the hypothalamus. The AVP molecule is first synthesized as a pre-pro-vasopressin precursor in the cytoplasm of these neurons. The precursor then undergoes proteolytic cleavage into AVP, neurophysin II, and copeptin (also known as C-terminal pro-arginine vasopressin, CT-proAVP) during axonal transport from the cytosol to neuronal terminals at the posterior pituitary gland (neurohypophysis), where these molecules are stored in secretory vesicles. The peptide content in the secretory vesicles accounts for the typical bright signal observed on the T1-weighted MR images of the posterior pituitary. Upon stimulation by a variety of signals, including an increase in serum osmolarity, a decrease in intravascular volume, stress, nausea, etc., the SON and PVN neurons are activated, and their action potentials travel down the axons and eventually lead to fusion of the granular secretory vesicles with synaptic membranes at the axonal terminals and exocytosis of AVP and copeptin in equimolar amounts.

Upon its release into systemic circulation, AVP exerts its action at multiple tissues through activation of its various receptors, primarily vasopressin receptor 1a (V1a), receptor 1b (V1b), and receptor 2 (V2R). V1a receptors are mainly found in smooth muscles of the arterioles. Activation of V1a receptors results in constriction of the arterioles, leading to an increase in the systemic circulatory resistance and eventually an increase in blood pressure. V1b receptors are located in the anterior pituitary and are responsible for the stimulatory effect of AVP on ACTH secretion. Distinct from V1a and V1b receptors, V2Rs are mostly present in the principal cells of the distal convoluted tubes and the collecting ducts of the kidney. Binding of AVP to V2R activates the cyclic AMP signaling pathway, insertion of aquaporin 2 molecules (water channels) into the apical membrane of the principal cells, and subsequently absorption of water from the glomerular filtrate and urinary concentration. V2Rs are also found in extrarenal tissues, including the vascular endothelial cells in which activation of the V2Rs causes release of coagulation factor VIII and von Willebrand factor (vWF) and tissue plasminogen (t-PA) [72].

In patients on HD, AVP levels are found to be elevated owing to a variety of mechanisms, including decreased metabolic clearance rate [73–75] and impermeability of AVP molecules of the dialysis membranes [73, 76]. Since copeptin is co-secreted in equimolar amounts with AVP and that AVP has a short half-life in circulation, copeptin has been proposed as a surrogate marker of AVP secretion [77]. Indeed, similar to AVP, copeptin levels are also elevated in patients with CKD or on chronic HD [77, 78]. However, the rise in copeptin in CKD is much faster than that of AVP, suggesting differential metabolism of each molecule [77]. Interestingly, despite an increase in AVP levels, the ability of AVP to concentrate urine is diminished in CKD, highlighting an impaired signaling pathway of AVP in renal tubules [74, 79] which is at least partially due to a downregulation of V2R mRNA expression [80]. Moreover, there appears to be a defect in the response of AVP secretion to its stimulatory signals, at least in patients on HD [75]. Even though AVP levels do respond to the stimulation of very high osmolarity, e.g., hypertonic saline infusion during HD [81], AVP levels do not increase right after HD sessions which is contrary to the expected rise as a result of decreased intravascular volume during HD [76]. Accordingly, a recent study showed that plasma concentrations of copeptin decreased significantly after HD sessions if a high-flux membrane, but not a low-flux membrane, was used [78]. Taken together, these studies suggest that hypotension observed during an HD session is not fully compensated with sufficient increase in

AVP secretion, which may contribute to persistent hypotension during HD [82–84]. A recent study demonstrated that treatment with vasopressin during HD improves cardiovascular stability and allows for increased removal of excess extracellular fluid [85].

Central Diabetes Insipidus (DI) in CKD

Central DI is caused by deficiency or insufficiency of AVP, which is commonly a result of injury to the hypothalamus, pituitary stalk, or hypophysis. It is recognized that AVP resistance exists in patients with advanced CKD, manifested as hypotonic urine compared to plasma despite supramaximal doses of vasopressin [86], suggesting that higher doses of vasopressin may be needed in treating central DI in CKD. In contrast, a few studies have reported that central DI can be masked in advanced CKD until kidney transplantation. These findings likely result from the significant increase in AVP levels in CKD, which are subsequently corrected by renal transplantation [87, 88]. Taken together, the above contrasting observations highlight the balance between increased AVP and coexisting AVP resistance in CKD.

Syndrome of Inappropriate ADH Secretion (SIADH) in CKD

SIADH is a common cause of hyponatremia in which the action of AVP (ADH) is enhanced, which is therefore deemed inappropriate for the low serum sodium levels. In about one third of hyponatremic patients, AVP levels are found to be elevated, while AVP levels are either suppressed or even undetectable in the rest of the patients [89]. Importantly, in mild and moderate CKD, the ability of the kidney to dilute and concentrate urine is usually well preserved, so normonatremia is commonly maintained [90]. Therefore, diagnosis of SIADH can still be reliably made in these patients. However, in advanced renal failure, there is a decline in the ability of the kidney to dilute and concentrate the urine, with the diluting ability preserved longer than the concentrating ability. Eventually the urine osmolarity is fixed around 300 mOsm/L in end-stage renal disease [90]. Therefore, an impairment in free water excretion along with an increase in solute excretion can result in hyponatremia in advanced CKD [90]. Importantly, in contrast to the elevated AVP levels commonly found in CKD, patients with advanced CKD and hyponatremia tend to have low AVP levels [86], making it difficult to differentiate from SIADH.

AVP and Autosomal Dominant Polycystic Kidney Disease (ADPKD)

Recently, the AVP signaling pathway, especially activation of the V2Rs, has been implicated in the pathogenesis of kidney diseases, especially ADPKD [91]. In early stages, ADPKD is associated with a blunted osmolarity-regulated release of AVP and impaired sensitivity of peripheral tissues to AVP [92]. In a cohort of 241 patients with ADPKD and preserved renal function, copeptin levels are independently associated with disease progression, but not plasma osmolality [93]. Additionally, urine copeptin concentrations have been demonstrated to be a good surrogate marker for prediction of renal prognosis in ADPKD [94]. A possible pathogenic mechanism proposes that abnormal AVP signaling may result in the development of ADPKD. In this hypothesis, increased sensitivity of tubular cells to AVP leads to disruption of calcium signaling pathways initiated by aberrant signaling of polycystin-1 or polycystin-2, which eventually causes formation, development, and growth of renal cysts [95]. Therefore, it is likely that in ADPKD patients, there are both central and nephrogenic defects in osmoregulation and copeptin balance, and copeptin may serve as a marker to identify patients who could benefit from an intervention targeted at AVP signaling pathway by using the V2R antagonist vaptans [91, 96–98]. In a recent large-scale clinical trial, tolvaptan, a V2R antagonist, was shown to result in less renal volume expansion, slower worsening of kidney function, and less kidney pain over three years. However, there were higher discontinuation rates in the tolvaptan group due to aquaresis (excretion of electrolyte-free water) and hepatic adverse events [99].

References

1. Kleinberg DL, Noel GL, Frantz AG. Galactorrhea: a study of 235 cases, including 48 with pituitary tumors. N Engl J Med. 1977;296(11):589–600. https://doi.org/10.1056/NEJM197703172961103.
2. Freeman ME, Kanyicska B, Lerant A, Nagy G. Prolactin: structure, function, and regulation of secretion. Physiol Rev. 2000;80(4):1523–631.
3. Martinez de la Escalera G, Weiner RI. Dissociation of dopamine from its receptor as a signal in the pleiotropic hypothalamic regulation of prolactin secretion. Endocr Rev. 1992;13(2):241–55.
4. van den Pol AN. Excitatory neuromodulator reduces dopamine release, enhancing prolactin secretion. Neuron. 2010;65(2):147–9. https://doi.org/10.1016/j.neuron.2010.01.013.
5. Morel GR, Caron RW, Console GM, Soaje M, Sosa YE, Rodriguez SS, et al. Estrogen inhibits tuberoinfundibular dopaminergic neurons but does not cause irreversible damage. Brain Res Bull. 2009;80(6):347–52. https://doi.org/10.1016/j.brainresbull.2009.08.026.
6. DeMaria JE, Livingstone JD, Freeman ME. Ovarian steroids influence the activity of neuroendocrine dopaminergic neurons. Brain Res. 2000;879(1–2):139–47. doi:S0006-8993(00)02763-3 [pii].
7. Livingstone JD, Lerant A, Freeman ME. Ovarian steroids modulate responsiveness to dopamine and expression of G-proteins in lactotropes. Neuroendocrinology. 1998;68(3):172–9. doi:nen68172 [pii].
8. Molitch ME. Pituitary disorders during pregnancy. Endocrinol Metab Clin N Am. 2006;35(1):99–116., vi. https://doi.org/10.1016/j.ecl.2005.09.011.
9. Salvador J, Dieguez C, Scanlon MF. The circadian rhythms of thyrotrophin and prolactin secretion. Chronobiol Int. 1988;5(1):85–93.
10. Hou SH, Grossman S, Molitch ME. Hyperprolactinemia in patients with renal insufficiency and chronic renal failure requiring hemodialysis or chronic ambulatory peritoneal dialysis. Am J Kidney Dis. 1985;6(4):245–9. doi:S0272638685000981 [pii].
11. Travaglini P, Moriondo P, Togni E, Venegoni P, Bochicchio D, Conti A, et al. Effect of oral zinc administration on prolactin and thymulin circulating levels in patients with chronic renal failure. J Clin Endocrinol Metab. 1989;68(1):186–90.
12. Sievertsen GD, Lim VS, Nakawatase C, Frohman LA. Metabolic clearance and secretion rates of human prolactin in normal subjects and in patients with chronic renal failure. J Clin Endocrinol Metab. 1980;50(5):846–52. https://doi.org/10.1210/jcem-50-5-846.
13. Hagen C, Olgaard K, McNeilly AS, Fisher R. Prolactin and the pituitary-gonadal axis in male uraemic patients on regular dialysis. Acta Endocrinol. 1976;82(1):29–38.
14. Ramirez G, O'Neill WM Jr, Bloomer HA, Jubiz W. Abnormalities in the regulation of prolactin in patients with chronic renal failure. J Clin Endocrinol Metab. 1977;45(4):658–61. https://doi.org/10.1210/jcem-45-4-658.
15. Arnaout MA, Hamzeh YS, Ajlouni KM. Prolactin responses to vasoactive intestinal polypeptide and thyrotropin releasing hormone in chronic renal failure. Acta Endocrinol. 1991;125(6):651–6.
16. Leroith D, Danovitz G, Trestan S, Spitz IM. Dissociation of prolactin response to thyrotropin-releasing hormone and metoclopramide in chronic renal failure. J Clin Endocrinol Metab. 1979;49(6):815–7. https://doi.org/10.1210/jcem-49-6-815.
17. Olgaard K, Hagen C, McNeilly AS. Pituitary hormones in women with chronic renal failure: the effect of chronic intermittent haemo- and peritoneal dialysis. Acta Endocrinol. 1975;80(2):237–46.
18. Saha MT, Saha HH, Niskanen LK, Salmela KT, Pasternack AI. Time course of serum prolactin and sex hormones following successful renal transplantation. Nephron. 2002;92(3):735–7. doi:nef92735 [pii].
19. Olukoga AO, Kane JW. Macroprolactinaemia: validation and application of the polyethylene glycol precipitation test and clinical characterization of the condition. Clin Endocrinol. 1999;51(1):119–26.
20. Smith TP, Kavanagh L, Healy ML, McKenna TJ. Technology insight: measuring prolactin in clinical samples. Nat Clin Pract Endocrinol Metab. 2007;3(3):279–89. https://doi.org/10.1038/ncpendmet0447.
21. Mooradian AD, Morley JE, Korchik WP, Ma KW, Hartfel MA, Parsons JA. Comparison between bioactivity and immunoreactivity of serum prolactin in uraemia. Clin Endocrinol. 1985;22(3):241–7.
22. Rodriguez-Puyol D, Martin-Oar JE, Cachofeiro MV, del Pino D, Lopez-Novoa JM, Hernando L. Molecular heterogeneity of circulating prolactin in chronic uremic men and renal transplant recipients. J Clin Endocrinol Metab. 1986;62(2):352–6. https://doi.org/10.1210/jcem-62-2-352.
23. Yavuz D, Topcu G, Ozener C, Akalin S, Sirikci O. Macroprolactin does not contribute to elevated levels of prolactin in patients on renal replacement therapy. Clin Endocrinol. 2005;63(5):520–4. https://doi.org/10.1111/j.1365-2265.2005.02375.x.
24. Sari F, Sari R, Ozdem S, Sarikaya M, Cetinkaya R. Serum prolactin and macroprolactin levels in diabetic nephropathy. Clin Nephrol. 2012;78(1):33–9.
25. Huang W, Molitch ME. Evaluation and management of galactorrhea. Am Fam Physician. 2012;85(11):1073–80.
26. Santen RJ, Mansel R. Benign breast disorders. N Engl J Med. 2005;353(3):275–85. https://doi.org/10.1056/NEJMra035692.

27. Vaidyanathan L, Barnard K, Elnicki DM. Benign breast disease: when to treat, when to reassure, when to refer. Cleve Clin J Med. 2002;69(5):425–32.
28. Dhindsa S, Reddy A, Karam JS, Bilkis S, Chaurasia A, Mehta A, et al. Prevalence of subnormal testosterone concentrations in men with type 2 diabetes and chronic kidney disease. Eur J Endocrinol. 2015;173(3):359–66. https://doi.org/10.1530/eje-15-0359.
29. Carrero JJ, Kyriazis J, Sonmez A, Tzanakis I, Qureshi AR, Stenvinkel P, et al. Prolactin levels, endothelial dysfunction, and the risk of cardiovascular events and mortality in patients with CKD. Clin J Am Soc Nephrol. 2012;7(2):207–15. https://doi.org/10.2215/cjn.06840711.
30. Muir JW, Besser GM, Edwards CR, Rees LH, Cattell WR, Ackrill P, et al. Bromocriptine improves reduced libido and potency in men receiving maintenance hemodialysis. Clin Nephrol. 1983;20(6):308–14.
31. Vircburger MI, Prelevic GM, Peric LA, Knezevic J, Djukanovic L. Testosterone levels after bromocriptine treatment in patients undergoing long-term hemodialysis. J Androl. 1985;6(2):113–6.
32. Peces R, Horcajada C, Lopez-Novoa JM, Frutos MA, Casado S, Hernando L. Hyperprolactinemia in chronic renal failure: impaired responsiveness to stimulation and suppression. Normalization after transplantation. Nephron. 1981;28(1):11–6.
33. Molitch ME. Medication-induced hyperprolactinemia. Mayo Clin Proc. 2005;80(8):1050–7.
34. Molitch ME. Drugs and prolactin. Pituitary. 2008;11(2):209–18. https://doi.org/10.1007/s11102-008-0106-6.
35. Pena KS, Rosenfeld JA. Evaluation and treatment of galactorrhea. Am Fam Physician. 2001;63(9):1763–70.
36. Leung AK, Pacaud D. Diagnosis and management of galactorrhea. Am Fam Physician. 2004;70(3):543–50.
37. Oguz Y, Oktenli C, Ozata M, Ozgurtas T, Sanisoglu Y, Yenicesu M, et al. The midnight-to-morning urinary cortisol increment method is not reliable for the assessment of hypothalamic-pituitary-adrenal insufficiency in patients with end-stage kidney disease. J Endocrinol Investig. 2003;26(7):609–15. https://doi.org/10.1007/bf03347016.
38. Clodi M, Riedl M, Schmaldienst S, Vychytil A, Kotzmann H, Kaider A, et al. Adrenal function in patients with chronic renal failure. Am J Kidney Dis. 1998;32(1):52–5. https://doi.org/10.1053/ajkd.1998.v32.pm9669424.
39. McDonald WJ, Golper TA, Mass RD, Kendall JW, Porter GA, Girard DE, et al. Adrenocorticotropin-cortisol axis abnormalities in hemodialysis patients. J Clin Endocrinol Metab. 1979;48(1):92–5. https://doi.org/10.1210/jcem-48-1-92.
40. Ramirez G, Gomez-Sanchez C, Meikle WA, Jubiz W. Evaluation of the hypothalamic hypophyseal adrenal axis in patients receiving long-term hemodialysis. Arch Intern Med. 1982;142(8):1448–52.
41. Wallace EZ, Rosman P, Toshav N, Sacerdote A, Balthazar A. Pituitary-adrenocortical function in chronic renal failure: studies of episodic secretion of cortisol and dexamethasone suppressibility. J Clin Endocrinol Metab. 1980;50(1):46–51. https://doi.org/10.1210/jcem-50-1-46.
42. Kleeman CR, Levi J, Better O. Kidney and adrenocortical hormones. Nephron. 1975;15(3–5):261–78.
43. Raff H, Trivedi H. Circadian rhythm of salivary cortisol, plasma cortisol, and plasma ACTH in end-stage renal disease. Endocr Connect. 2013;2(1):23–31. https://doi.org/10.1530/ec-12-0058.
44. Deshmukh S, Phillips BG, O'Dorisio T, Flanigan MJ, Lim VS. Hormonal responses to fasting and refeeding in chronic renal failure patients. Am J Physiol Endocrinol Metab. 2005;288(1):E47–55. https://doi.org/10.1152/ajpendo.00163.2004.
45. Russcher M, Chaves I, Lech K, Koch BC, Nagtegaal JE, Dorsman KF, et al. An observational study on disturbed peripheral circadian rhythms in hemodialysis patients. Chronobiol Int. 2015;32(6):848–57. https://doi.org/10.3109/07420528.2015.1048868.
46. Albiston AL, Obeyesekere VR, Smith RE, Krozowski ZS. Cloning and tissue distribution of the human 11 beta-hydroxysteroid dehydrogenase type 2 enzyme. Mol Cell Endocrinol. 1994;105(2):R11–7.
47. Mongia A, Vecker R, George M, Pandey A, Tawadrous H, Schoeneman M, et al. Role of 11betaHSD type 2 enzyme activity in essential hypertension and children with chronic kidney disease (CKD). J Clin Endocrinol Metab. 2012;97(10):3622–9. https://doi.org/10.1210/jc.2012-1411.
48. N'Gankam V, Uehlinger D, Dick B, Frey BM, Frey FJ. Increased cortisol metabolites and reduced activity of 11beta-hydroxysteroid dehydrogenase in patients on hemodialysis. Kidney Int. 2002;61(5):1859–66. https://doi.org/10.1046/j.1523-1755.2002.00308.x.
49. Homma M, Tanaka A, Hino K, Takamura H, Hirano T, Oka K, et al. Assessing systemic 11beta-hydroxysteroid dehydrogenase with serum cortisone/cortisol ratios in healthy subjects and patients with diabetes mellitus and chronic renal failure. Metab Clin Exp. 2001;50(7):801–4. https://doi.org/10.1053/meta.2001.24213.
50. Kawai S, Ichikawa Y, Homma M. Differences in metabolic properties among cortisol, prednisolone, and dexamethasone in liver and renal diseases: accelerated metabolism of dexamethasone in renal failure. J Clin Endocrinol Metab. 1985;60(5):848–54. https://doi.org/10.1210/jcem-60-5-848.
51. Soule S, Van Zyl SC, Parolis G, Attenborough S, Peter D, Kinvig S, et al. The low dose ACTH stimulation test is less sensitive than the overnight metyrapone test for the diagnosis of secondary hypoadrenalism. Clin Endocrinol. 2000;53(2):221–7.
52. Charmandari E, Nicolaides NC, Chrousos GP. Adrenal insufficiency. Lancet. 2014;383(9935):2152–67. https://doi.org/10.1016/s0140-6736(13)61684-0.
53. Rodger RS, Dewar JH, Turner SJ, Watson MJ, Ward MK. Anterior pituitary dysfunction in patients with chronic renal failure treated by hemodialysis or continuous ambulatory peritoneal dialysis. Nephron. 1986;43(3):169–72.

54. Schmidt IL, Lahner H, Mann K, Petersenn S. Diagnosis of adrenal insufficiency: evaluation of the corticotropin-releasing hormone test and basal serum cortisol in comparison to the insulin tolerance test in patients with hypothalamic-pituitary-adrenal disease. J Clin Endocrinol Metab. 2003;88(9):4193–8. https://doi.org/10.1210/jc.2002-021897.
55. Ramirez G, Bittle PA, Sanders H, Rabb HA, Bercu BB. The effects of corticotropin and growth hormone releasing hormones on their respective secretory axes in chronic hemodialysis patients before and after correction of anemia with recombinant human erythropoietin. J Clin Endocrinol Metab. 1994;78(1):63–9. https://doi.org/10.1210/jcem.78.1.8288716.
56. Siamopoulos KC, Dardamanis M, Kyriaki D, Pappas M, Sferopoulos G, Alevisou V. Pituitary adrenal responsiveness to corticotropin-releasing hormone in chronic uremic patients. Perit Dial Int. 1990;10(2):153–6.
57. Crowley RK, Argese N, Tomlinson JW, Stewart PM. Central hypoadrenalism. J Clin Endocrinol Metab. 2014;99(11):4027–36. https://doi.org/10.1210/jc.2014-2476.
58. Sakao Y, Sugiura T, Tsuji T, Ohashi N, Yasuda H, Fujigaki Y, et al. Clinical manifestation of hypercalcemia caused by adrenal insufficiency in hemodialysis patients: a case-series study. Intern Med. 2014;53(14):1485–90.
59. Kato A, Shinozaki S, Goga T, Hishida A. Isolated adrenocorticotropic hormone deficiency presenting with hypercalcemia in a patient on long-term hemodialysis. Am J Kidney Dis. 2003;42(2):E32–6.
60. Bancos I, Hahner S, Tomlinson J, Arlt W. Diagnosis and management of adrenal insufficiency. Lancet Diabetes Endocrinol. 2015;3(3):216–26. https://doi.org/10.1016/s2213-8587(14)70142-1.
61. Nieman LK, Biller BM, Findling JW, Newell-Price J, Savage MO, Stewart PM, et al. The diagnosis of Cushing's syndrome: an Endocrine Society Clinical Practice Guideline. J Clin Endocrinol Metab. 2008;93(5):1526–40. https://doi.org/10.1210/jc.2008-0125.
62. Gracia-Iguacel C, Gonzalez-Parra E, Egido J, Lindholm B, Mahillo I, Carrero JJ, et al. Cortisol levels are associated with mortality risk in hemodialysis patients. Clin Nephrol. 2014;82(4):247–56.
63. Workman RJ, Vaughn WK, Stone WJ. Dexamethasone suppression testing in chronic renal failure: pharmacokinetics of dexamethasone and demonstration of a normal hypothalamic-pituitary-adrenal axis. J Clin Endocrinol Metab. 1986;63(3):741–6. https://doi.org/10.1210/jcem-63-3-741.
64. Olsen H, Mjoman M. Moderately impaired renal function increases morning cortisol and cortisol levels at dexamethasone suppression test in patients with incidentally detected adrenal adenomas. Clin Endocrinol. 2015;83:762. https://doi.org/10.1111/cen.12823.
65. Rosman PM, Farag A, Peckham R, Benn R, Tito J, Bacci V, et al. Pituitary-adrenocortical function in chronic renal failure: blunted suppression and early escape of plasma cortisol levels after intravenous dexamethasone. J Clin Endocrinol Metab. 1982;54(3):528–33. https://doi.org/10.1210/jcem-54-3-528.
66. Lindsay JR, Nieman LK. Differential diagnosis and imaging in Cushing's syndrome. Endocrinol Metab Clin N Am. 2005;34(2):403–21., x. https://doi.org/10.1016/j.ecl.2005.01.009.
67. Chan KC, Lit LC, Law EL, Tai MH, Yung CU, Chan MH, et al. Diminished urinary free cortisol excretion in patients with moderate and severe renal impairment. Clin Chem. 2004;50(4):757–9. https://doi.org/10.1373/clinchem.2003.029934.
68. Issa BG, Page MD, Read G, John R, Douglas-Jones A, Scanlon MF. Undetectable urinary free cortisol concentrations in a case of Cushing's disease. Eur J Endocrinol. 1999;140(2):148–51.
69. Stewart PM. The adrenal cortex. In: Kronenberg HM, Melmed S, Polonsky KS, Larsen PR, editors. Williams textbook of endocrinology. 11th ed. Philadelphia: Saunders Elsevier; 2008.
70. Molitch ME. Current approaches to the pharmacological management of Cushing's disease. Mol Cell Endocrinol. 2015;408:185–9. https://doi.org/10.1016/j.mce.2014.09.021.
71. Nieman LK, Biller BM, Findling JW, Murad MH, Newell-Price J, Savage MO, et al. Treatment of Cushing;s syndrome: an Endocrine Society Clinical Practice Guideline. J Clin Endocrinol Metab. 2015;100(8):2807–31. https://doi.org/10.1210/jc.2015-1818.
72. Juul KV, Bichet DG, Nielsen S, Norgaard JP. The physiological and pathophysiological functions of renal and extrarenal vasopressin V2 receptors. Am J Physiol Renal Physiol. 2014;306(9):F931–40. https://doi.org/10.1152/ajprenal.00604.2013.
73. Iitake K, Kimura T, Matsui K, Ota K, Shoji M, Inoue M, et al. Effect of haemodialysis on plasma ADH levels, plasma renin activity and plasma aldosterone levels in patients with end-stage renal disease. Acta Endocrinol. 1985;110(2):207–13.
74. Argent NB, Wilkinson R, Baylis PH. Metabolic clearance rate of arginine vasopressin in severe chronic renal failure. Clin Sci. 1992;83(5):583–7.
75. Shimamoto K, Watarai I, Miyahara M. A study of plasma vasopressin in patients undergoing chronic hemodialysis. J Clin Endocrinol Metab. 1977;45(4):714–20. https://doi.org/10.1210/jcem-45-4-714.
76. Ettema EM, Zittema D, Kuipers J, Gansevoort RT, Vart P, de Jong PE, et al. Dialysis hypotension: a role for inadequate increase in arginine vasopressin levels? A systematic literature review and meta-analysis. Am J Nephrol. 2014;39(2):100–9. https://doi.org/10.1159/000358203.
77. Roussel R, Fezeu L, Marre M, Velho G, Fumeron F, Jungers P, et al. Comparison between copeptin and vasopressin in a population from the community and in people with chronic kidney disease. J Clin Endocrinol Metab. 2014;99(12):4656–63. https://doi.org/10.1210/jc.2014-2295.

78. Mueller T, Gegenhuber A, Kronabethleitner G, Leitner I, Haltmayer M, Dieplinger B. Plasma concentrations of novel cardiac biomarkers before and after hemodialysis session. Clin Biochem. 2015;48(16–17):1163–6. https://doi.org/10.1016/j.clinbiochem.2015.07.031.
79. Pedersen EB, Thomsen IM, Lauridsen TG. Abnormal function of the vasopressin-cyclic-AMP-aquaporin2 axis during urine concentrating and diluting in patients with reduced renal function. A case control study. BMC Nephrol. 2010;11:26. https://doi.org/10.1186/1471-2369-11-26.
80. Teitelbaum I, McGuinness S. Vasopressin resistance in chronic renal failure. Evidence for the role of decreased V2 receptor mRNA. J Clin Invest. 1995;96(1):378–85. https://doi.org/10.1172/jci118044.
81. Rosansky SJ, Rhinehart R, Shade R. Effect of osmolar changes on plasma arginine vasopressin (PAVP) in dialysis patients. Clin Nephrol. 1991;35(4):158–64.
82. Thompson AM, Oliver JA. Endogenous and exogenous vasopressin during hemodialysis. Semin Dial. 2009;22(5):472–5. https://doi.org/10.1111/j.1525-139X.2009.00615.x.
83. Hegbrant J, Thysell H, Martensson L, Ekman R, Boberg U. Changes in plasma levels of vasoactive peptides during standard bicarbonate hemodialysis. Nephron. 1993;63(3):303–8.
84. Rho M, Perazella MA, Parikh CR, Peixoto AJ, Brewster UC. Serum vasopressin response in patients with intradialytic hypotension: a pilot study. Clin J Am Soc Nephrol. 2008;3(3):729–35. https://doi.org/10.2215/cjn.05341107.
85. van der Zee S, Thompson A, Zimmerman R, Lin J, Huan Y, Braskett M, et al. Vasopressin administration facilitates fluid removal during hemodialysis. Kidney Int. 2007;71(4):318–24. https://doi.org/10.1038/sj.ki.5001885.
86. Tannen RL, Regal EM, Dunn MJ, Schrier RW. Vasopressin-resistant hyposthenuria in advanced chronic renal disease. N Engl J Med. 1969;280(21):1135–41. https://doi.org/10.1056/nejm196905222802101.
87. Kim KM, Kim SM, Lee J, Lee SY, Kwon SK, Kim HY. Newly developed central diabetes insipidus following kidney transplantation: a case report. Transplant Proc. 2013;45(7):2804–6. https://doi.org/10.1016/j.transproceed.2013.02.141.
88. Kim DD, Holdaway IM. Unmasking of undiagnosed pre-existing central diabetes insipidus after renal transplantation. Pituitary. 2012;15(1):106–9. https://doi.org/10.1007/s11102-010-0259-y.
89. Ellison DH, Berl T. Clinical practice. The syndrome of inappropriate antidiuresis. N Engl J Med. 2007;356(20):2064–72. https://doi.org/10.1056/NEJMcp066837.
90. Kovesdy CP. Significance of hypo- and hypernatremia in chronic kidney disease. Nephrol Dial Transplant. 2012;27(3):891–8. https://doi.org/10.1093/ndt/gfs038.
91. Bankir L, Bouby N, Ritz E. Vasopressin: a novel target for the prevention and retardation of kidney disease? Nat Rev Nephrol. 2013;9(4):223–39. https://doi.org/10.1038/nrneph.2013.22.
92. Ho TA, Godefroid N, Gruzon D, Haymann JP, Marechal C, Wang X, et al. Autosomal dominant polycystic kidney disease is associated with central and nephrogenic defects in osmoregulation. Kidney Int. 2012;82(10):1121–9. https://doi.org/10.1038/ki.2012.225.
93. Boertien WE, Meijer E, Li J, Bost JE, Struck J, Flessner MF, et al. Relationship of copeptin, a surrogate marker for arginine vasopressin, with change in total kidney volume and GFR decline in autosomal dominant polycystic kidney disease: results from the CRISP cohort. Am J Kidney Dis. 2013;61(3):420–9. https://doi.org/10.1053/j.ajkd.2012.08.038.
94. Nakajima A, Lu Y, Kawano H, Horie S, Muto S. Association of arginine vasopressin surrogate marker urinary copeptin with severity of autosomal dominant polycystic kidney disease (ADPKD). Clin Exp Nephrol. 2015;19:1199. https://doi.org/10.1007/s10157-015-1101-7.
95. Chebib FT, Sussman CR, Wang X, Harris PC, Torres VE. Vasopressin and disruption of calcium signalling in polycystic kidney disease. Nat Rev Nephrol. 2015;11(8):451–64. https://doi.org/10.1038/nrneph.2015.39.
96. Bolignano D, Cabassi A, Fiaccadori E, Ghigo E, Pasquali R, Peracino A, et al. Copeptin (CTproAVP), a new tool for understanding the role of vasopressin in pathophysiology. Clin Chem Lab Med. 2014;52(10):1447–56. https://doi.org/10.1515/cclm-2014-0379.
97. Baur BP, Meaney CJ. Review of tolvaptan for autosomal dominant polycystic kidney disease. Pharmacotherapy. 2014;34(6):605–16. https://doi.org/10.1002/phar.1421.
98. Torres VE. Vasopressin antagonists in polycystic kidney disease. Kidney Int. 2005;68(5):2405–18. https://doi.org/10.1111/j.1523-1755.2005.00703.x.
99. Torres VE, Chapman AB, Devuyst O, Gansevoort RT, Grantham JJ, Higashihara E, et al. Tolvaptan in patients with autosomal dominant polycystic kidney disease. N Engl J Med. 2012;367(25):2407–18. https://doi.org/10.1056/NEJMoa1205511.

Endocrine System in Acute Kidney Injury

23

Alice Sabatino, Graziano Ceresini, Michela Marina, and Enrico Fiaccadori

Introduction

Acute kidney injury (AKI) is frequent among hospitalized patients, especially in the intensive care unit (ICU) setting (incidence rates of 20–30%), with 2–5% of cases requiring renal replacement therapy (RRT) [1]. The average mortality risk associated with AKI still remains very high, though highly variable (16–49%) according to severity of illness, clinical setting, and comorbidities [2]. In critically ill patients, AKI seldom occurs as an isolated organ failure and more often represents a key component of the multiple organ failure syndrome. Thus, the implications of the syndrome might go beyond the already complex role of the organ in fluid, electrolyte/acid-base homeostasis, blood pressure control, and waste product excretion. The physiologic role of the kidney extends in fact to multiple endocrine functions. The occurrence of endocrine abnormalities during AKI may be expected for several reasons: (a) several hormones are synthesized or activated in the kidney (erythropoietin, angiotensins I and II, vitamin D, etc.); (b) the organ is very important for metabolism and excretion of hormones; (c) the kidney is a target organ for several hormones involved in the regulation of its excretory and endocrine functions; and (d) AKI is a heterogeneous syndrome caused by different etiological factors and mechanisms and is characterized by profound derangements of the internal milieu, influencing the secretion, transport, transformation, degradation, and action of hormones.

The present chapter is aimed at focusing on some of the main renal-endocrine pathways involved in AKI, focusing on the most severe forms of AKI, and with special regard to the ICU setting. To this end, glucose homeostasis derangements and insulin resistance, the hypothalamus-pituitary-thyroid axis, calcium-phosphorus metabolism and vitamin D, as well as erythropoietin will be reviewed.

Glucose Homeostasis and Insulin Resistance

Glucose homeostasis is severely deranged in patients with AKI, and both hyper- and hypoglycemia can be commonly observed in this clinical setting since both altered insulin metabolism and insulin resistance may coexist [3], the latter also representing an independent predictor for worse outcomes. Loss of kidney metabolic function and critical illness-associated hyperglycemia (CIAH) may contribute to insulin resistance in AKI, as well as uremia in and of itself may play a role by

A. Sabatino (✉) · E. Fiaccadori
Renal Failure Unit, Parma University Medical School, Parma, PR, Italy

G. Ceresini · M. Marina
Endocrinology of the Development and Aging Unit, Parma University Medical School, Parma, PR, Italy

C. M. Rhee et al. (eds.), *Endocrine Disorders in Kidney Disease*,
https://doi.org/10.1007/978-3-319-97765-2_23

reducing peripheral and hepatic glucose uptake. Glycemic control in patients with AKI is made more complicated by the provision of calories from nutrients under the form of enteral/parenteral nutrition and from carbohydrate and carbohydrate-like energy substrates administered to the patients under the form of citrate, glucose, and lactate in the solutions commonly used in the dialysis/hemofiltration procedures (dialysate and replacement fluids) (Table 23.1). In fact, when standard modalities of continuous or prolonged intermittent RRT with citrate, glucose, and eventually lactate solutions are employed, an estimated 300–1200 Kcal/day may be given to the patient, with large differences due to the different operational characteristics of the RRT modalities themselves [3]. In general, in the critically ill, the risk of hypoglycemia increases up to four to eight times as compared to conventional insulin treatments when intensive insulin treatment (IIT) protocols are applied (i.e., aimed at glycemic values in the normal range of 80–110 mg/dL [4.44–6.11 mmol/L]) [4]. Insufficient caloric supply may further negatively affect the relationship between IIT protocols and incidence of hypoglycemia [5, 6]. Among trauma patients on IIT aimed at serum glucose values of 70–149 mg/dL (3.9–8.3 mmol/L), hypoglycemia (<60 mg/dl [<3.3 mmol/L]) was observed in 76% of cases with coexisting AKI or end-stage renal disease (ESRD), as compared to 35% in patients with normal renal function [7]. In parallel, glycemic variability was greatly increased [7]. Percentages were, respectively, 29% and 0% when only severe hypoglycemia episodes (<40 mg/dl [<2.2 mmol/L]) were considered [7]. For this reason, in patients with AKI, targeting higher glycemic values could reduce the incidence of hypoglycemia.

Table 23.1 Calorie equivalent of carbohydrate metabolism substrates in dialysis/hemofiltration fluids

Substrate	Molecular weight	Kcal/mmol	Kj/mmol
Glucose	198[a]	0.73	3.06
Citrate	192[b]	0.59	3.07
Lactate	89	0.33	1.37

[a]As glucose monohydrate
[b]As citrate anion

The key role of the kidney in insulin metabolism and glucose regulation sets the stage for the association between reduced kidney function and the increased risk for hypoglycemia in AKI [3]. In fact, insulin is, for a large extent, metabolized by the kidneys (50% of its clearance), and renal gluconeogenesis contributes to about 30% to glucose systemic appearance [3, 8].

Higher glycemic values are currently suggested as targets as compared with earlier recommendations (Table 23.2) [9–14]: up to 180 mg/dL [10 mmol/L] vs. 110 mg/dL [6.11 mmol/L] in the Sepsis Survival Campaign recommendations [9], 144–180 mg/dL [8–10 mmol/L] in the case of the American Diabetes Association guidelines [14], and 140–180 mg/dL [7.8–10 mmol/L] in the ASPEN guidelines [10]. In the specific case of patients with AKI, it seems prudent to aim for higher blood glucose concentrations as suggested in the 2012 Kidney Disease Improving Global Outcomes (KDIGO) guidelines (110–149 mg/dl)

Table 23.2 Guideline recommendations on glycemic control in critically ill patients in the ICU and in patients with AKI [9–14]

Guidelines	Patients	Glycemic control range
Sepsis Survival Campaign *Intensive Care Med* 2013; 39:165–228	Critically ill patients with sepsis	<180 mg/dl
American Diabetes Association *Diabetes Care.* 2010;33(suppl 1):S11–S61	Critically ill patients	144–180 mg/dl
ASPEN *JPEN* 2013;37:23–36	Critically ill patients	140–180 mg/dl
KDIGO *Kidney Int* 2012;29(suppl):1–138	AKI in the ICU	110–149 mg/dl
European Best Practice Guidelines *NDT* 2012;27:4263–4272	AKI in the ICU	110–180 mg/dl
KDOQI on KDIGO 2012 *AJKD* 2013;61:649–672	AKI in the ICU	110–149 mg/dl

AKI acute kidney injury, *ASPEN* American Society of Parenteral and Enteral Nutrition, *ICU* intensive care unit, *KDIGO* Kidney Disease Improving Global Outcomes

[11] and in the European Renal Best Practice (ERBP) comments to the KDIGO guidelines (140–180 mg/dl) [12], albeit with limited evidence.

Hypothalamic-Pituitary-Thyroid Axis in AKI

The synthesis of thyroid hormones is controlled by the hypothalamus, which releases thyrotropin-releasing hormone (TRH) and stimulates the thyrotropic cells in the pituitary to synthesize and secrete thyroid-stimulating hormone (TSH). TSH stimulates the thyroid gland to synthesize and secrete thyroid hormones, and its synthesis is regulated by a negative feedback mechanism operated by circulating levels of thyroid hormones. The thyroid gland predominantly secretes the inactive thyroid hormone thyroxine (T4), which is converted to the active thyroid hormone triiodothyronine (T3) in the peripheral target organs. Different types of deiodinases (D1–D3) are responsible for the peripheral conversion of T4 to T3 or to the biologically inactive reverse T3 (rT3). Thyroid hormones are essential for the regulation of energy metabolism and have profound effects on differentiation and growth.

Critical illness is often associated with alterations in thyroid hormone concentrations in patients with no previous thyroid disease (euthyroid sick syndrome, ESS) (Table 23.3) [15]. In the course of acute illness or severe physical stress, a rapid decline of circulating T3 levels is usually observed, whereas rT3 levels are upregulated. A decrease in D1 activity and an increase in D3 activity are responsible for the observed changes in thyroid hormone homeostasis [16]. Circulating T4 levels may rise only transiently, although T4 levels may also decrease during prolonged ICU stays in the more severely ill [17]. In critically ill patients, changes in the markers of thyroid function are very common and are often associated with alterations in other endocrine axes [18]. Thus, the ESS should not be viewed as an isolated abnormal event but as part of a generalized systemic endocrine response to illness. The decrease in circulating T3 and T4 during the first 24 h after the insult reflects the severity of illness and correlates with mortality risk [19]. Whether or not these changes reflect a beneficial and adaptive response to the severity of illness or rather contribute to adverse outcome remains currently unclear, and the mechanisms behind the observed changes are still not fully understood. Inflammatory markers such as cytokines have been demonstrated to affect deiodinase activity and are able to mimic the acute stress response of the thyroid axis [20]. However, cytokine antagonists failed to restore normal thyroid function after endotoxemic challenge [21]. Other potential factors of the ESS include low concentrations of thyroid hormone-binding proteins, reduced thyroid hormone uptake, and metabolism by elevated levels of free fatty acids and bilirubin [22]. Patients who need prolonged intensive care and enter a more chronic phase of illness display low levels of circulating T3 and T4. Despite low circulating thyroid hormone levels and thus reduced negative feedback, pulsatile TSH and hypothalamic TRH expression are low, pointing to a central suppression of the thyroid axis in which an important role is played by cytokines [23]. Patients with prolonged critical illness that present with this clinical picture (lower TSH, T4 and T3, and higher rT3 levels) have a higher mortality rate as compared with those surviving prolonged critical illness [24]. In particular, the reduced T4 level has been shown to relate to the severity of illness [25].

Table 23.3 Alterations in thyroid hormones during critical illness

Critical illness	T3	T4	TSH
Acute phase	↓	↑	Normal
Chronic phase	↓	↓	No change/↓

Several mechanisms contribute to the inhibition of deiodinase 1 and therefore to the low serum T3 concentrations in critically ill patients with ESS: (a) exogenous glucocorticoid therapy; (b) circulating inhibitors of deiodinase activity, such as free (nonesterified) fatty acids; (c) treatment with drugs that inhibit deiodinase 1 activity, such as amiodarone and high doses of propranolol; and (d) cytokines (such as tumor necrosis factor, interferon alpha, NF-kB, and interleukin-6) [20, 26]. Peripheral changes in thyroid hormone metabolism occur quite early in the process of critical illness and are present in all forms of acute stress. Furthermore, such changes are very similar to the changes evoked by short-term fasting and likely partly brought about by the lack of normal nutritional intake during acute illness. The immediate fall in circulating T3 during starvation has been interpreted as an attempt of the body to reduce its energy expenditure and prevent protein wasting. Hence, the rapid changes during the acute phase of illness could be considered beneficial and an adaptive response that does not warrant intervention. During the prolonged phase of illness, a hypothalamic suppression also occurs, suggesting that patients in this situation could benefit from treatment. From the current literature, however, it remains controversial whether administration of thyroid hormone to critically ill patients is beneficial or harmful [27].

The interactions between the kidney and thyroid hormones (TH) are well known. Thyroid hormones contribute to growth and development of the kidney and to water and electrolyte homeostasis. Thyroid hormones are known to influence renal function by both indirect (prerenal) and direct (renal) effects. As a matter of fact, on one hand, the effects of thyroid hormones on the cardiovascular system and the renal blood flow (RBF) mediate prerenal effects, while direct renal effects are mediated by the action of thyroid hormones on glomerular filtration rate, tubular secretory and reabsorptive processes, as well as the hormonal influences on renal tubular physiology [28] (Fig. 23.1).Renal function is significantly influenced by thyroid dysfunction. Congenital hypothyroidism is associated with increased prevalence of congenital renal anomalies [29], this very fact supporting a key role of TH in early embryogenesis [29]. Both hypo- and hyperthyroidisms affect glomerular filtration rate, renal blood flow, tubular function, and electrolyte and water metabolism [29–31]. The kidney not only contributes to the metabolism of TH but is also an important target organ for these hormones [30, 32].

TH participate in the control of tubular transport of sodium, by their effects on the sodium-potassium ATP pump (Na/K ATPase) and permeability of the proximal tubule membrane to potassium [33]. Both in the adult [34] and the pediatric [35] settings, primary hypothyroidism is associated with a reversible increase in serum creatinine. More than half of adult patients with hypothyroidism have reduced glomerular filtra-

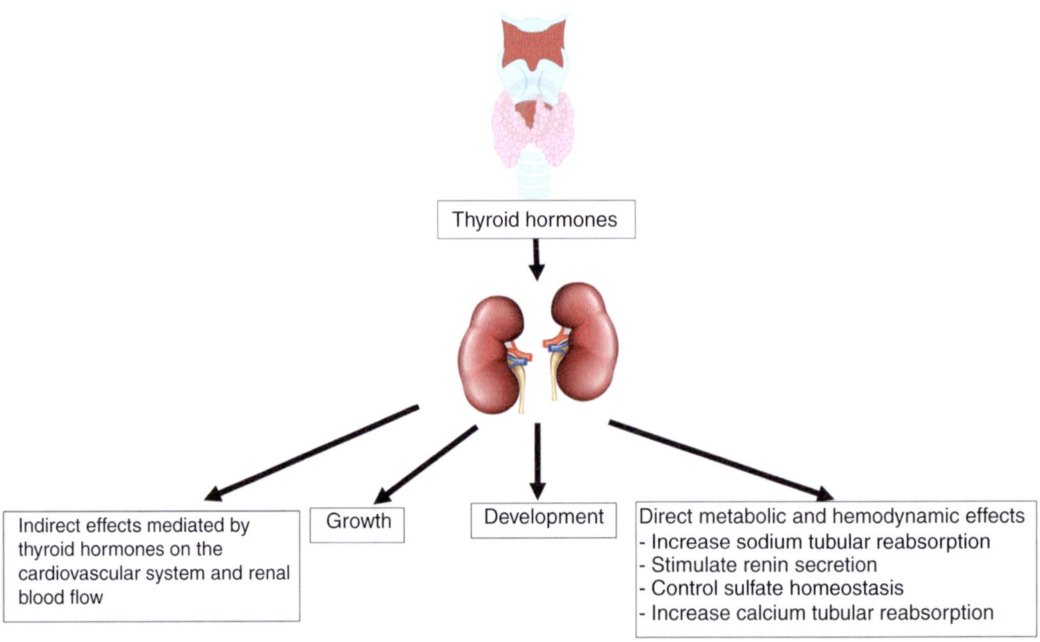

Fig. 23.1 Direct and indirect effects of thyroid hormones in the kidney

tion rate (GFR) and renal plasma flow values that are normalized following levothyroxine administration [32]. On the other hand, hyperthyroidism is characterized by an increase in renal plasma flow and GFR [36]. Total body water and exchangeable potassium are decreased in hyperthyroidism, and the amount of exchangeable sodium is increased, while serum electrolyte concentrations are usually normal. These alterations are typical of endogenous hyperthyroidism and exogenous thyrotoxicosis. Renal function modifications in hyperthyroidism are at least in part due to hemodynamic changes such as increased systolic volume, heart rate, and cardiac output and reduced peripheral vascular resistance [37].

In patients with CKD, serum T3 correlates with many markers of inflammation, nutrition, and endothelial activation [38]. In addition, low T3 levels are independent predictors for all-cause and cardiovascular disease mortality in euthyroid patients with end-stage renal disease, probably due, at least in part, to an intimate association with inflammation and malnutrition [38]. The effect of AKI on thyroid function and TH has not been studied in detail. AKI is associated with alterations in thyroid function similar to those found in other forms of ESS in critically ill patients. A recent study of 35 AKI patients found a high prevalence of altered thyroid function tests (~80%) [39]. The most common derangement was the presence of ESS with low T3 only (~65%). Other small cross-sectional studies reported low T4 and T3 and normal levels of rT3 [40].

Low levels of T3 are explained not only by a reduction in the tissue 5′-monodeiodinase activity but also by changes in the amount of thyroid hormone that is bound to serum proteins, as found in other forms of ESS [40, 41]. No differences between anuric/oliguric and polyuric patients have been documented, suggesting that alterations in thyroid function during AKI are nonspecific [39]. Although the administration of TH in toxic and ischemic AKI animal models has been shown to be effective in promoting recovery [42–44], recent data have suggested that thyroid hormone therapy was associated with worse outcomes in patients with AKI, in particular mortality risk as well as need for dialysis or transplant [45].

Vitamin D and Calcium-Phosphorus Metabolism

Dysregulated mineral metabolism, including derangements in calcium and phosphate levels, is relatively well characterized in CKD, and correction of hypocalcemia, vitamin D deficiency, and hyperphosphatemia in CKD patients now represent standard of care [46–48]. These alterations are all associated with an increased risk of death and negative cardiovascular outcomes in patients with CKD and end-stage renal disease [49, 50]. Interestingly enough, although hypocalcemia and hyperphosphatemia are commonly observed in patients with AKI, the literature on mineral metabolism in this patient population is relatively limited.

AKI causes a rapid dysregulation of minerals normally handled by the kidneys. Specifically, vitamin D levels are reduced [51], and ionized calcium levels frequently decrease in patients with AKI. Serum albumin is also reduced in critically ill patients as a consequence of inflammation, stress, and sepsis, contributing to total calcium decrease. Interestingly, while both 25OH vitamin D (25(OH)D) and 1,25(OH)2 vitamin D (1,25(OH)2D) levels are decreased in patients with AKI, only the bioavailable fraction of 25(OH)D, calculated as the sum of the albumin-bound and free fractions, correlated with severity of sepsis and risk of death [52]. Ionized serum calcium can be further reduced by renal replacement itself, especially when citrate is utilized as anticoagulant in citrate-based protocols aimed at regional anticoagulation. Citrate in fact chelates ionized calcium, which is the main cofactor in the coagulation cascade, causing ionized hypocalcemia and impaired thrombin generation [53]. In a study on 116 patients undergoing a total of 807 citrate-based sustained low-efficiency dialysis (SLED) sessions [54], patients' ionized calcium values were only slightly reduced during SLED, 1.06 mmol/L ± 0.11 mmol/L (before) versus 0.99 [±0.09] mmol/L), and systemic intravenous calcium administration was needed only in 28 of 807 sessions (3.5%) [54]. However, during regional citrate anticoagulation for RRT, systemic hypocalcemia, and therefore systemic anticoagulation, is prevented both by partial removal of citrate by RRT itself (65–75%) and by metabolism of citrate-calcium complexes in the liver, kidney, and muscles to form bicarbonate [53].

Serum phosphate levels are variable in renal failure, according to the clinical setting (acute vs. chronic) and the coexistence of critical illness. Hypophosphatemia is a frequent finding in critically ill patients with AKI requiring renal replacement therapy (e.g., CRRT) [55, 56]. Low serum phosphorus levels are associated with failure to wean from the ventilator, increased in-hospital mortality, subsequent development of CKD, and long-term mortality [57, 58]. The pathophysiology of phosphate disturbances in patients with AKI is multifactorial and may reflect both comorbid conditions and severity of illness as well as the acute reduction in renal clearance due to AKI itself or an increase in phosphorus clearance by RRT [58]. The use of dialysis/hemofiltration fluids enriched with phosphate may reduce the incidence of hypophosphatemia during RRT [55, 56].

Vitamin D is a fat-soluble vitamin that is produced endogenously and has a key role in bone metabolism and calcium homeostasis. Its synthesis is triggered by ultraviolet rays from sunlight striking the skin and uses cholesterol as substrate (Fig. 23.2). The inactive vitamin D produced in the skin (cholecalciferol or vitamin D3) must undergo two hydroxylations for activation. The first one occurs in the liver and produces 25-hydroxyvitamin D (25(OH)D) or calcidiol. The second occurs primarily in the kidney and produces the physiologically active 1,25-dihydroxyvitamin D (1,25(OH)2D), also known as calcitriol, through the action of the enzyme 1α-hydroxylase (Fig. 23.2) [59]. Extrarenal synthesis also has been described in vascular cells, parathyroid gland, macrophages, and some cancer cells [60]. In CKD, 1,25(OH)2D levels start to decline in stage 2 and continue to decrease as GFR falls [61]. The majority of ESRD patients initiating hemodialysis have low 1,25(OH)2D levels, and the lowest levels correlate with significantly higher mortality during the first 90 days of dialysis [62]. There are limited data on 1,25(OH)2D levels in patients with AKI, and the relationship of 1,25(OH)2D levels to clinical outcomes in patients with AKI has not been elucidated. A recent pilot study found lower levels of 25(OH)D and 1,25(OH)2D in critically ill patients with AKI in comparison to healthy controls [59]. In a prospective study with 60 patients, 1,25(OH)2D levels were significantly decreased in patients with AKI compared to hos-

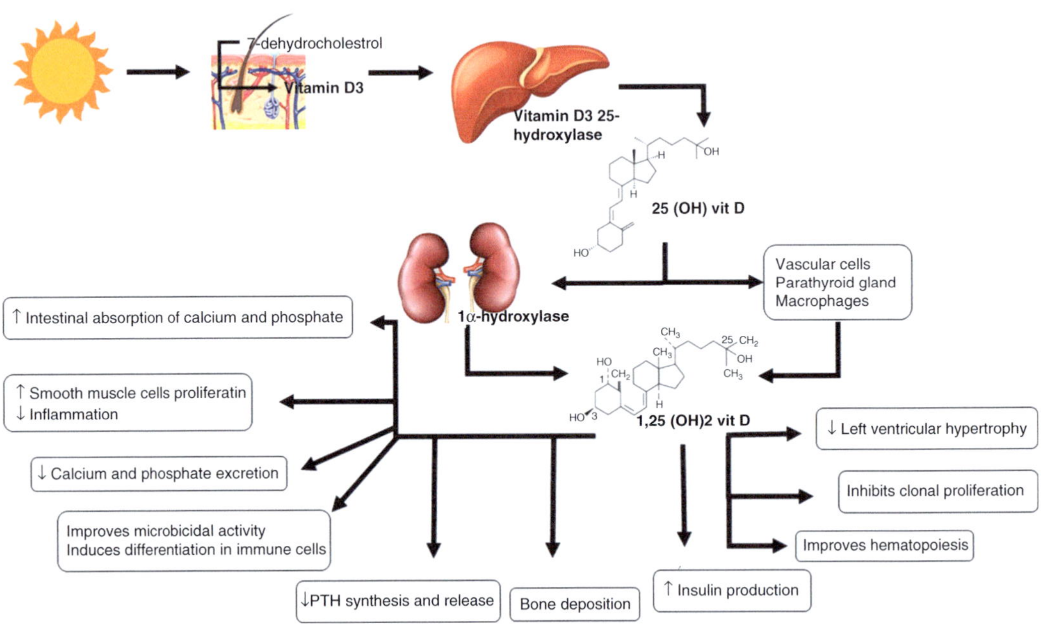

Fig. 23.2 Synthesis and function of vitamin D. Vitamin D synthesis starts in the skin, is triggered by ultraviolet radiation, and uses cholesterol as a substrate

pitalized patients without AKI [63]. However, the available evidence doesn't show any correlation between levels of 1,25(OH)2D and mortality in AKI patients [59, 63, 64]. Fibroblast growth factor-23 (FGF-23) normally inhibits the production of 1,25(OH)2D by downregulating the renal 1α-hydroxylase, and levels of these hormones are inversely correlated [65, 66]. FGF-23 levels were significantly higher in patients with AKI compared with control patients (1471 vs. 263 RU/mL) and were associated with death and need for RRT [63]. FGF-23 levels at enrollment (or within 48 h of AKI) were better predictors of the need for RRT than serum creatinine or any other mineral metabolism parameters examined. However, measures of FGF-23 were obtained after AKI diagnosis, and the mechanisms behind its increase could not be elucidated. A recent animal model study demonstrated that FGF-23 levels do increase one hour after induction of AKI, even before the rise of creatinine levels, suggesting that FGF-23 could be an early marker of AKI [65]. The mechanism responsible for its increase is likely to be independent from the classic regulators of FGF-23 (PTH, vitamin D, and phosphate) and, however, is related to increased production, not decreased clearance [65]. The animal study results were also validated in humans undergoing cardiac surgery [65]. Another more recent study of 250 patients undergoing cardiac surgery also reported an early increase in FGF-23 and a positive correlation with the severity of AKI or death [66]; they also confirmed that the elevations in FGF-23 among patients with AKI occurred independent of any alterations in PTH, phosphate, or vitamin D metabolites [66].

Erythropoietin

Erythropoietin (EPO) is a complex molecule, which regulates red blood cell production in the bone marrow. Approximately 90% of systemic EPO in adults is produced by peritubular interstitial fibroblasts in the renal cortex and outer medulla of the kidney (Fig. 23.3). A feedback mechanism involving the level of oxygen in the tissues appears to regulate EPO production. Hypoxia-inducible factor (HIF) regulates transcription of the EPO gene in the kidney, which

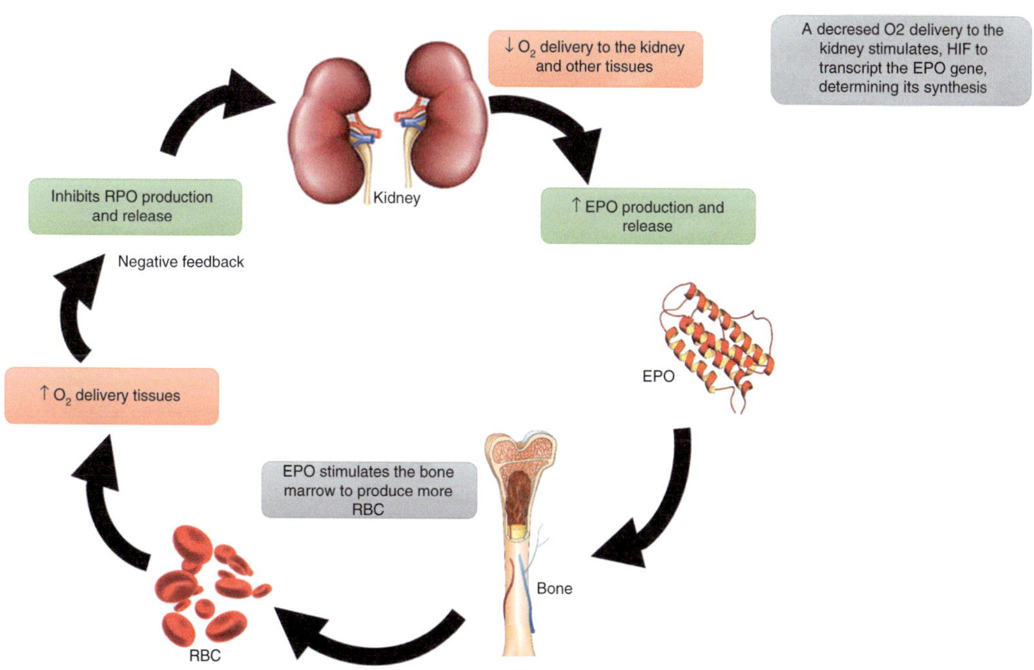

Fig. 23.3 Erythropoietin production and control. EPO production is regulated by a feedback mechanism involving the level of oxygen in the tissues and the hypoxia-inducible factor (HIF). EPO erythropoietin, HIF hypoxia-inducible factor, RBC red blood cells

determines EPO synthesis. This process is dependent on local oxygen tension. HIF is quickly destroyed in well-oxygenated cells through the ubiquitin-proteasome pathway by the tumor suppressor protein VHL, but when oxygen delivery decreases, VHL ceases its proteolysis of HIF, allowing it to go to the nucleus and increase EPO production [67].

The principal physiological function of EPO is red blood cell production in the bone marrow. However, some effects regarding tissue protection of EPO in the kidney have been demonstrated in some animals and clinical studies. Experimental studies have shown that EPO administration protects kidney tissue from damage, may improve renal function in ischemia-reperfusion (IR) and contrast-induced injury models of AKI, and exerts a renoprotective anti-inflammatory action [68–70], and its effect in the clinical setting has not been definitely demonstrated [71]. EPO activates endothelial nitric oxide synthase, and this effect on the endothelium may be critical for the renal tissue protective effects of EPO. EPO is an extremely potent stimulator of endothelial progenitor cells, whose function is partly dependent on nitric oxide bioavailability. Endothelial progenitor cells appear to be involved in endothelial recovery after injury. EPO limits AKI in part by stimulating vascular repair and by mobilizing endothelial progenitor cells and increasing tubular cell proliferation. These findings suggest that EPO may exert a protective effect via an interaction with the microvasculature.

Angiogenesis and EPO's renoprotective effects may be influenced by vascular endothelial growth factor (VEGF). The vascular EPO/EPO receptor system promoted postischemic angiogenesis by upregulating the VEGF/VEGF receptor system, both directly by promoting neovascularization and indirectly by mobilizing endothelial progenitor cells and bone marrow-derived proangiogenic cells [72]. It appears that angiogenesis is impaired and blood vessels are less responsive to VEGF in the absence of EPO receptors.

Little is known about EPO production during AKI. In a recent cohort study on 98 patients, plasma EPO concentration was higher in AKI patients when compared to non-AKI patients and correlated to hospital length of stay [73]. Interestingly, in AKI patients, the levels of plasma EPO did not correlate with hemoglobin concentration, low arterial oxygen tension, and inflammation markers but with insulin-like growth factor binding protein-1 (IGFBP-1), a marker of insulin resistance and systemic stress [73], suggesting that plasma EPO concentration in AKI patients may reflect systemic stress rather than low arterial oxygen tension and inflammation [73]. Data on the possible positive effects of EPO administration in clinical AKI have been mainly obtained in the heart surgery setting [74–79], with controversial results. A recent meta-analysis [80] has suggested that EPO administration before surgery in patients not at high risk of AKI could effectively decrease its incidence and ICU and hospital length of stay; however, no advantage was demonstrated in high-risk patients. In addition, EPO could only protect against injury resulting from ischemia but not inflammation. Consistently, patients with high-risk factors for AKI usually present with some inflammation-associated diseases.

References

1. Mehta RL, Cerdá J, Burdmann EA, et al. International Society of Nephrology's 0by25 initiative for acute kidney injury (zero preventable deaths by 2025): a human rights case for nephrology. Lancet. 2015;385:2616–43.
2. Susantitaphong P, Cruz DN, Cerda J, et al. World incidence of AKI: a meta-analysis. Clin J Am Soc Nephrol. 2013;8:1482–93.
3. Fiaccadori E, Sabatino A, Morabito S, et al. Hyper/hypoglycemia and acute kidney injury in critically ill patients. Clin Nutr. 2016;35:317–21.
4. Van den Berghe G, Wilmer A, Hermans G, et al. Intensive insulin therapy in the medical ICU. N Engl J Med. 2006;354:449–61.
5. Van den Berghe G. What's new in glucose control in the ICU? Int Care Med. 2013;39:823–5.
6. Preiser GC. Glycemic control and nutrition. J Parent Ent Nutr. 2011;35:671–2.
7. Stamou SC, Nussbaum M, Carew JD, et al. Hypoglycemia with intensive insulin therapy after cardiac surgery: predisposing factors and association with mortality. J Thorac Cardiovasc Surgery. 2011;142:166–73.

8. Meyer C, Dostou JM, Gerich JE. Role of the human kidney in glucose counterregulation. Diabetes. 1999;48:943–8.
9. Dellinger RP, Levy MM, Rhodes A, et al. Surviving sepsis campaign: international guidelines for management of severe sepsis and septic shock, 2012. Intensive Care Med. 2013;39:165–228.
10. McMahon MM, Nystrom E, Braunschweig C, et al. A.S.P.E.N. Clinical guidelines: nutrition support of adult patients with hyperglycemia. J Parenter Enter Nutr. 2013;37:23–36.
11. KDIGO. Clinical practice guidelines for acute kidney injury. Kidney Int. 2012;(suppl. 2):1–138.
12. Ad-hoc working group of ERBP, Fliser D, Laville M, et al. A European renal best practice (ERBP) position statement on the Kidney Disease Improving Global Outcomes (KDIGO) clinical practice guidelines on acute kidney injury: part 1: definitions, conservative management and contrast-induced nephropathy. Nephrol Dial Transplant. 2012;27:4263–72.
13. Palevsky PM, Liu KD, Brophy PD, et al. KDOQI US commentary on the 2012 KDIGO clinical practice guideline for acute kidney injury. AJKD. 2013;61:649–72.
14. American Diabetes Association. Standards of medical care in diabetes-2010. Diabetes Care. 2010;33:S11–61.
15. Adler SM, Wartofsky L. The nonthyroidal illness syndrome. Endocrinol Metab Clin N Am. 2007;36:657–72.
16. Peeters RP, Wouters PJ, Kaptein E, van Toor H, Visser TJ, Van den Berghe G. Reduced activation and increased inactivation of thyroid hormone in tissues of critically ill patients. J Clin Endocrinol Metab. 2003;88:3202–11.
17. den Berghe V, Baxter RC, Weekers F, Wouters P, Bowers CY, Veldhuis JD. A paradoxical gender dissociation within the growth hormone/insulin-like growth factor I axis during protracted critical illness. J Clin Endocrinol Metab. 2000;85:183–92.
18. Brierre S, Kumari R, Deboisblanc BP. The endocrine system during sepsis. Am J Med Sci. 2004;328:238–47.
19. Ray DC, Macduff A, Drummond GB, et al. Endocrine measurements in survivors and non-survivors from critical illness. Intensive Care Med. 2002;28:1301–8.
20. Van der Poll T, Romijn JA, Wiersinga WM, Sauerwein HP. Tumor necrosis factor: a putative mediator of the sick euthyroid syndrome in man. J Clin Endocrinol Metab. 1990;71:1567–72.
21. van der Poll T, Endert E, Coyle SM, Agosti JM, Lowry SF. Neutralization of TNF does not influence endotoxininduced changes in thyroid hormone metabolism in humans. Am J Phys. 1999;276:R357–62.
22. Mebis L, Van den Berghe G. Thyroid axis function and dysfunction in critical illness. Best Pract Res Clin Endocrinol Metab. 2011;25:745–57.
23. Mebis L, Debaveye Y, Ellger B, et al. Changes in the central component of the hypothalamus-pituitary-thyroid axis in a rabbit model of prolonged critical illness. Crit Care. 2009;13:R147.
24. Peeters RP, Wouters PJ, van Toor H, Kaptein E, Visser TJ, Van den Berghe G. Serum 3,3′,5′-triiodothyronine (rT3) and 3,5,3′-triiodothyronine/rT3 are prognostic markers in critically ill patients and are associated with postmortem tissue deiodinase activities. J Clin Endocrinol Metab. 2005;90:4559–65.
25. Maldonado LS, Murata GH, Hershman JM, Braunstein GD. Do thyroid function tests independently predict survival in the critically ill? Thyroid. 1992;2:119–23.
26. Stouthard JM, van der Poll T, Endert E, et al. Effects of acute and chronic interleukin-6 administration on thyroid hormone metabolism in humans. J Clin Endocrinol Metab. 1994;79:1342–6.
27. Langouche L, Van den Berghe G. Hypothalamic–pituitary hormones during critical illness: a dynamic neuroendocrine response. In: Fliers E, Korbonits M, Romijn JA, editors. Handbook of clinical neurology, Clinical Neuroendocrinology, vol. 124 (3rd series): Elsevier BV; 2014. p. 116–26.
28. Basu G, Mohapatra A. Interactions between thyroid disorders and kidney disease. Indian J Endocrinol Metab. 2012;16:204–13.
29. Kumar J, Gordillo R, Kaskel FJ, Druschel CM, Woroniecki RP. Increased prevalence of renal and urinary tract anomalies in children with congenital hypothyroidism. J Pediatr. 2009;154:263–6.
30. Kaptein EM. Thyroid function in renal failure. Contrib Nephrol. 1986;50:64–72.
31. Kaptein EM, Quion-Verde H, Chooljian CJ, et al. The thyroid in end-stage renal disease. Medicine. 1988;67:187–97.
32. den Hollander JG, Wulkan RW, Mantel MJ, Berghout A. Correlation between severity of thyroid dysfunction and renal function. Clin Endocrinol. 2005;62:423–7.
33. Lin HH, Tang MJ. Thyroid hormone upregulates Na,K-ATPase alpha and beta mRNA in primary cultures of proximal tubule cells. Life Sci. 1997;60:375–82.
34. Karanikas G, Schütz M, Szabo M, et al. Isotopic renal function studies in severe hypothyroidism and after thyroid hormone replacement therapy. Am J Nephrol. 2004;24:41–5.
35. del-Rio Camacho G, Tapia Ceballos L, Picazo Angelín B, Ruiz Moreno JA, Hortas Nieto ML, Romero González J. Renal failure and acquired hypothyroidism. Pediatr Nephrol. 2003;18:290–2.
36. Vargas F, Moreno JM, Rodríguez-Gómez I, et al. Vascular and renal function in experimental thyroid disorders. Eur J Endocrinol. 2006;154:197–212.
37. Woeber KA. Thyrotoxicosis and the heart. N Engl J Med. 1992;327:94–9889. Enia G, Panuccio V, Cutrupi S et al. Subclinical hypothyroidism is linked to micro-inflammation and predicts death in continuous ambulatory peritoneal dialysis. Nephrol Dial Transplant. 2007; 22: 538–544.
38. Carrero JJ, Qureshi AR, Axelsson J, et al. Clinical and biochemical implications of low thyroid hormone levels (total and free forms) in euthyroid

patients with chronic kidney disease. J Intern Med. 2007;262:690–701.
39. Iglesias P, Olea T, Vega-Cabrera C, et al. Thyroid function tests in acute kidney injury. J Nephrol. 2013;26:164–72.
40. Chen WL, Huang WS, Lin YF, Shieh SD. Changes in thyroid hormone metabolism in exertional heat stroke with or without acute renal failure. J Clin Endocrinol Metab. 1996;81:625–9.
41. Bello G, Ceaichisciuc I, Silva S, Antonelli M. The role of thyroid dysfunction in the critically ill: a review of the literature. Minerva Anestesiol. 2010;76:919–28.
42. Siegel NJ, Gaudio KM, Katz LA, et al. Beneficial effect of thyroxin on recovery from toxic acute renal failure. Kidney Int. 1984;25:906–11.
43. Cronin RE, Brown DM, Simonsen R. Protection by thyroxine in nephrotoxic acute renal failure. Am J Phys. 1986;251:F408–16.
44. Sutter PM, Thulin G, Stromski M, et al. Beneficial effect of thyroxin in the treatment of ischemic acute renal failure. Pediatr Nephrol. 1988;2:1–7.
45. Nigwekar SU, Strippoli GFM, Navaneethan SD. Thyroid hormones for acute kidney injury. Cochrane Database Syst Rev. 2013;(1):CD006740.
46. National Kidney Foundation. K/DOQI clinical practice guidelines for bone metabolism and disease in chronic kidney disease. Am J Kidney Dis. 2003;42:S1–S201.
47. Kidney Disease: Improving Global Outcomes (KDIGO) CKD-MBD Work Group. KDIGO clinical practice guideline for the diagnosis, evaluation, prevention, and treatment of Chronic Kidney Disease-Mineral and Bone Disorder (CKD-MBD). Kidney Int Suppl. 2009;113:S1–S130.
48. Uhlig K, Berns JS, Kestenbaum B, et al. KDOQI US commentary on the 2009 KDIGO clinical practice guideline for the diagnosis, evaluation, and treatment of CKD-mineral and bone disorder (CKD-MBD). Am J Kidney Dis. 2010(55):773–99.
49. Block GA, Klassen PS, Lazarus JM, Ofsthun N, Lowrie EG, Chertow GM. Mineral metabolism, mortality, and morbidity in maintenance hemodialysis. J Am Soc Nephrol. 2004;15:2208–18.
50. Ravani P, Malberti F, Tripepi G, et al. Vitamin D levels and patient outcome in chronic kidney disease. Kidney Int. 2009;75:88–95.
51. Druml W, Schwarzenhofer M, Apsner R, Hörl WH. Fat-soluble vitamins in patients with acute renal failure. Miner Electrolyte Metab. 1998;24:220–6.
52. Leaf DE, Waikar SS, Wolf M, Cremers S, Bhan I, Stern L. Dysregulated mineral metabolism in patients with acute kidney injury and risk of adverse outcomes. Clin Endocrinol (Oxf). 2013;79:491–8.
53. Morabito S, Pistolesi V, Tritapepe L, Fiaccadori E. Regional citrate anticoagulation for RRTs in critically ill patients with AKI. Clin J Am Soc Nephrol. 2014;9:2173–88.
54. Fiaccadori E, Regolisti G, Cademartiri C, et al. Efficacy and safety of a citrate-based protocol for sustained low-efficiency dialysis in AKI using standard dialysis equipment. Clin J Am Soc Nephrol. 2013;8:1670–8.
55. Morabito S, Pistolesi V, Tritapepe L, et al. Continuous veno-venous hemofiltration using a phosphate-containing replacement fluid in the setting of regional citrate anticoagulation. Int J Artif Organs. 2013;36:845–52.
56. Morabito S, Pistolesi V, Tritapepe L, et al. Continuous venovenous hemodiafiltration with a low citrate dose regional anticoagulation protocol and a phosphate-containing solution: effects on acid-base status and phosphate supplementation needs. BMC Nephrol. 2013;14:232.
57. Demirjian S, Teo BW, Guzman JA, et al. Hypophosphatemia during continuous hemodialysis is associated with prolonged respiratory failure in patients with acute kidney injury. Nephrol Dial Transplant. 2011;26:3508–14.
58. Schiffl H, Lang SM. Severe acute hypophosphatemia during renal replacement therapy adversely affects outcome of critically ill patients with acute kidney injury. Int Urol Nephrol. 2013;45:191–7.
59. Vijayan A, Li T, Dusso A, Jain S, Coyne DW. Relationship of 1,25 dihydroxy Vitamin D Levels to Clinical Outcomes in Critically Ill Patients with Acute Kidney Injury. J Nephrol Ther. 2015;5(1):190. [Epub ahead of print].
60. Valdivielso JM, Cannata-Andía J, Coll B, Fernández E. A new role for vitamin D receptor activation in chronic kidney disease. Am J Physiol Renal Physiol. 2009;297:F1502–9.
61. Levin A, Bakris GL, Molitch M, et al. Prevalence of abnormal serum vitamin D, PTH, calcium, and phosphorus in patients with chronic kidney disease: results of the study to evaluate early kidney disease. Kidney Int. 2007;71:31–8.
62. Wolf M, Shah A, Gutierrez O, et al. Vitamin D levels and early mortality among incident hemodialysis patients. Kidney Int. 2007;72:1004–13.
63. Leaf DE, Wolf M, Waikar SS, et al. FGF-23 levels in patients with AKI and risk of adverse outcomes. Clin J Am Soc Nephrol. 2012;7:1217–23.
64. Lai L, Qian J, Yang Y, et al. Is the serum vitamin D level at the time of hospital-acquired acute kidney injury diagnosis associated with prognosis? PLoS One. 2013;8:e64964.
65. Christov M, Waikar S, Pereira R, et al. Plasma FGF23 levels increase rapidly after acute kidney injury. Kidney Int. 2013;84:776–85.
66. Leaf DE, Christov M, Jüppner H, et al. Fibroblast growth factor 23 levels are elevated and associated with severe acute kidney injury and death following cardiac surgery. Kidney Int. 2016;89:939–48.
67. Diskin CJ, Stokes TJ, Dansby LM, Radcliff L, Carter TB. Beyond anemia: the clinical impact of the physiologic effects of erythropoietin. Semin Dial. 2008;21:447–54.
68. Tögel FE, Ahlstrom JD, Yang Y, Hu Z, Zhang P, Westenfelder C. Carbamylated erythropoietin outperforms erythropoietin in the treatment of AKI-on-CKD

and other AKI models. J Am Soc Nephrol.2016; pii: ASN.2015091059. [Epub ahead of print].

69. Gardner DS, Welham SJ, Dunford LJ, McCulloch TA, Hodi Z, Sleeman P, O'Sullivan S, Devonald MA. Remote conditioning or erythropoietin before surgery primes kidneys to clear ischemia-reperfusion-damaged cells: a renoprotective mechanism? Am J Physiol Renal Physiol. 2014;306:F873–84.
70. Coldewey SM, Khan AI, Kapoor A, Collino M, Rogazzo M, Brines M, Cerami A, Hall P, Sheaff M, Kieswich JE, Yaqoob MM, Patel NS, Thiemermann C. Erythropoietin attenuates acute kidney dysfunction in murine experimental sepsis by activationof the β-common receptor. Kidney Int. 2013;84:482–90.
71. Zhao C, Lin Z, Luo Q, Xia X, Yu X, Huang F. Efficacy and safety of erythropoietin to prevent acute kidney injury in patients with critical illness or perioperative care: a systematic review and meta analysis of randomized controlled trials. J Cardiovasc Pharmacol. 2015;65:593–600.
72. Nakano M, Satoh K, Fukumoto Y, et al. Important role of erythropoietin receptor to promote VEGF expression and angiogenesis in peripheral ischemia in mice. Circ Res. 2007;100:662–9.
73. Yamashita T, Noiri E, Hamasaki Y, et al. Erythropoietin concentration in acute kidney injury is associated with insulin-like growth factor-binding protein-1. Nephrology (Carlton). 2015; https://doi.org/10.1111/nep.12656. [Epub ahead of print].
74. de Seigneux S, Ponte B, Weiss L, Pugin J, Romand JA, Martin PY, et al. Epoetin administrated after cardiac surgery: effects on renal function and inflammation in a randomized controlled study. BMC Nephrol. 2012;13:132.
75. Kim JH, Shim JK, Song JW, Song Y, Kim HB, Kwak YL. Effect of erythropoietin on the incidence of acute kidney injury following complex valvular heart surgery: a double blind, randomized clinical trial of efficacy and safety. Crit Care. 2013;17:R254.
76. Oh SW, Chin HJ, Chae DW, Na KY. Erythropoietin improves long-term outcomes in patients with acute kidney injury after coronary artery bypass grafting. J Korean Med Sci. 2012;27:506–11.
77. Song YR, Lee T, You SJ, Chin HJ, Chae DW, Lim C, et al. Prevention of acute kidney injury by erythropoietin in patients undergoing coronary artery bypass grafting: a pilot study. Am J Nephrol. 2009;30:253–60.
78. Tasanarong A, Duangchana S, Sumransurp S, Homvises B, Satdhabudha O. Prophylaxis with erythropoietin versus placebo reduces acute kidney injury and neutrophil gelatinase-associated lipocalin in patients undergoing cardiac surgery: a randomized, double-blind controlled trial. BMC Nephrol. 2013;14:136.
79. Yoo YC, Shim JK, Kim JC, Jo YY, Lee JH, Kwak YL. Effect of single recombinant human erythropoietin injection on transfusion requirements in preoperatively anemic patients undergoing valvular heart surgery. Anesthesiology. 2011;115:929–37.
80. Tie HT, Luo MZ, Lin D, Zhang M, Wan JY, Wu QC. Erythropoietin administration for prevention of cardiac surgery-associated acute kidney injury: a meta-analysis of randomized controlled trials. Eur J Cardiothorac Surg. 2015;48:32–9.

24 Nutrition and Endocrine Disorders in Kidney Disease

Anuja Shah and Joel Kopple

Introduction

Advancement in chronic kidney failure is often marked by a progressive increase in the frequency and severity of markers of protein energy wasting (PEW), such as, hypoalbuminemia, low lean body mass, and increased net protein degradation. Hypoalbuminemia and reduced lean body mass are associated with increased morbidity and mortality in patients with chronic kidney disease (CKD) [1, 2] Although PEW is less common in non-dialyzed CKD patients especially in the earlier stages of CKD where the prevalence of PEW is lowest, it occurs in approximately 40% of maintenance hemodialysis (MHD) patients [3]. Many hormonal disturbances affect protein-energy status in CKD. These can be broadly divided into those altering nutrient intake, those causing impaired anabolism, and those increasing net protein and fat degradation. Abnormal nutrient intake may also alter hormonal pathways. The kidney is both an endocrine target organ and a synthesizer of certain hormones. The kidney also degrades many peptide hormones, some steroid hormones, and, in proteinuric patients, it may excrete substantial amounts of vitamin D.

In previous chapters, the actions of various hormones in CKD patients are discussed in detail. In this chapter, we will limit our review to the interactions between hormonal activity and protein-energy status of patients.

Parathyroid Hormone

Parathyroid hormone (PTH) causes protein degradation and negative nitrogen balance. Abnormal muscle physiology is a common feature of primary hyperparathyroidism and secondary hyperparathyroidism and in cancer-related increases in parathyroid hormone-related peptide. In primary hyperparathyroidism, muscle wasting, weakness, and myalgias are common symptoms [4]. Confounding the isolated effects of parathyroid hormone, the hypercalcemia in this disorder can itself lead to anorexia, constipation, and nausea, along with neuromuscular and neuropsychiatric symptoms [5]. Elevated serum PTH is almost universal in advanced renal failure. Its association with muscle wasting in uremia has been noted for many years [6]. Garber demonstrated in rats that PTH stimulates the synthesis and release of alanine and glutamine from skeletal muscle proteins [7]. By administering parathyroid hormone or its N-terminal fragments to rats for four days, Baczynski et al. showed that PTH decreased

A. Shah (✉)
Division of Nephrology and Hypertension, Harbor-UCLA Medical Center, Torrance, CA, USA

J. Kopple
Division of Nephrology, Department of Medicine, Harbor-UCLA Medical Center, Torrance, CA, USA

C. M. Rhee et al. (eds.), *Endocrine Disorders in Kidney Disease*, https://doi.org/10.1007/978-3-319-97765-2_24

energy production, transfer, and utilization in skeletal muscle. The calcium channel blocker verapamil blocked the observed effects [8]. Massry et al. demonstrated another mechanism of impaired energy utilization by PTH: the inhibition of long chain fatty acid oxidation with PTH injections. Activity of carnitine palmitoyl transferase, creatine phosphate, and adenosine triphosphate also were reduced following injection [9].

Studies by Kir et al. in cancer-associated cachexia have shown that PTH-related peptide increases the amount of brown adipose tissue which promotes both fat and muscle wasting [10]. This same group studied 5/6 nephrectomized rats and showed that PTH and PTH-related peptide mediate muscle and fat wasting through a common mechanism involving the PTH receptor. 5/6 nephrectomized rats had increased energy expenditure, heat production, and weight loss accompanied by an increase in thermogenic gene expression of *Ucp1*, *Dio2, Cidea*, and *Pgc1a*, and an induction of muscle wasting-related gene increases *urf-1*, *Atrogin-1*, and *Myostatin*. There was also a decrease in IGF-1 levels. In a knockout model of the PTH receptor in adipocytes, the weight loss and increased energy expenditure in these 5/6 nephrectomized rats was greatly attenuated. Induction of atrophy-related genes *Murf-1*, *Atrogin-1*, and *Myostatin* was also inhibited in these knockout CKD rats. In other experiments, these authors showed that PTH stimulated mRNA levels of the thermogenic *Ucp1*, *Dio2*, and *Pgc1a* in inguinal fat cells [11]. Taken together, these studies suggest multiple mechanisms by which PTH may induce a catabolic state. Hence, aggressive management of the bone-mineral axis in CKD patients should be considered important in maintaining nutritional status in these patients.

Many clinical studies in CKD patients have confirmed the catabolic effects seen in animal models. Cuppari et al. showed that MHD patients with secondary hyperparathyroidism had higher resting energy expenditure and that the resting energy expenditure decreased six months post parathyroidectomy in the patients that had follow-up measurements [12]. PTH is also directly correlated with the net protein degradation rate in MHD patients [13]. In a study of 32 Chinese MHD patients of whom 16 underwent parathyroidectomy, serum albumin was significantly increased by three months post surgery, and by six months serum albumin was statistically greater than in the nonoperative group. Body mass index and skinfold thickness were significantly increased by six months post surgery in the parathyroidectomy group [14]. Another study also reported an increase in serum albumin after parathyroidectomy [15]. However, differences in nutritional status due to PTH levels in end-stage kidney disease (ESKD) patients have not been seen consistent. Cuppari et al. compared nutritional parameters between 16 ESKD patients with a serum PTH level over 420 pg/ml and 16 ESKD patients with a parathyroid hormone level less than 290 pg/ml. Although serum urea nitrogen levels were greater in the higher serum PTH group and there was a trend toward higher net protein degradation rate in the higher PTH group ($p = 0.08$), no differences were observed between serum albumin, skinfold thickness, and weight between these two groups [16].

Nutritional management can also affect PTH levels. Low phosphorus intake and vitamin D supplements are a cornerstone of the management of secondary hyperparathyroidism. Multiple studies of ketoacid/essential amino acid (KA/EAA) supplemented very low-protein diets (SVLPDs) have shown a decrease in serum PTH levels with the diets [17, 18]. The high calcium in the KA/EAA supplements and the low phosphorus content of the SVLPDs may have contributed to lower serum PTH levels with these diets. The lower acid load from the lower protein intake may engender less acidosis and also attenuate some of the deleterious effects of secondary hyperparathyroidism on the bone. However, in one study, four days on a low-protein diet induced secondary hyperparathyroidism, possibly from decreased calcium absorption [19]. Nutrient intake can have a complex interplay with serum PTH levels, and during nutritional management of CKD, serum PTH levels should be monitored.

Vitamin D

The mineral bone axis in CKD is described in detail in Chaps. 14, 15, 16, 17, and 18. Therefore, this chapter will focus on the relation of vitamin D compounds to protein-energy status. Serum levels of both 25 hydroxycholecalciferol (25(OH)vitamin D3) and 1,25-dihydroxycholecalciferol (calcitriol, 1,25(OH)2 vitamin D3) are often low in CKD. Cholecalciferol is produced in the skin and its production is stimulated by sunlight. Cholecalciferol is also found in some foods. Cholecalciferol is transported to the liver where it is hydroxylated in the 25 position to form 25(OH) vitamin D3. 25(OH) vitamin D3 is transported to the kidney where it is hydroxylated in the 5 position to form calcitriol. Ergocalciferol (vitamin D2), which is primarily derived from fungi and some plants, undergoes conversion in the body to vitamin D3. The many contributing factors to vitamin D deficiency in CKD patients include the increasing age of CKD patients (which is associated with decreased cutaneous synthesis of cholecalciferol in response to sunlight), decreased exposure to sun due to fewer people working out of doors, clothing and increased sunscreen use which also limits sunshine exposure, and losses of vitamin D into urine in proteinuric patients. Serum calcitriol levels are also low due to the decreased enzymatic apparatus in the kidney for vitamin D synthesis due to kidney disease, the decreased availability of the 25 (OH) vitamin D substrate for calcitriol synthesis, inhibition of calcitriol synthesis by FGF-23, and the treatment of hyperparathyroidism which decreases stimulation of 1,25 production [20].

Severe 1,25 (OH)2D3 deficiency can lead to a myopathy that features type II fiber atrophy, internal myonuclei, and derangement of the intermyofibrillar network. Vitamin D, through its actions on the vitamin D receptor (VDR) in skeletal muscle, increases gene expression of contractile proteins and myogenic proteins [21, 22]. It also has nongenomic effects on calcium signaling in skeletal muscle, affecting mitochondrial function, and muscle contractility, and by modulating insulin signaling [23]. In vitro studies indicate that vitamin D inhibits myostatin, a protein that inhibits muscle growth [24]. In one study 25 (OH) D3, but not 1,25 (OH)2D3, reduced protein degradation but not protein synthesis in skeletal muscle from partially nephrectomized rats [25]. This suggests that there may be independent functions of 25(OH) D in muscle. The substantial physiological effects of vitamin D on muscle and the common occurrence of vitamin D deficiency in CKD patients have made vitamin D an attractive therapeutic agent for myopathy in advanced CKD patients and PEW.

The available data for the benefits on protein-energy status and decreasing fall risk and increasing muscle strength have been less robust in CKD than in other populations [20]. Two cross-sectional studies show an association between vitamin D status and muscle strength in CKD patients. Gordon. et al. observed a relationship between serum 1,25(OH)2 D levels and gait speed and sit-to-stand time in stage 3–4 CKD patients [26]. Zahed et al. observed that lower serum 25(OH) D levels were associated with lower muscle force in MHD patients [27]. 50,000 IU/week of ergocalciferol given for six months to MHD patients improved the equilibrated net protein catabolic rate from 0.91 ± 0.23 to 0.98 ± 0.32 ($P = 0.01$) [28]. However, in a study of 276 MHD patients randomized to ergocalciferol or placebo treatment, there was no difference in fall risk after six months of therapy [29]. On the other hand, case studies of advanced CKD patients have observed improvement in myopathy which can be marked with calcitriol or 25 (OH)D3 treatment (JDK unpublished observations) [30].

Testosterone

Testosterone's anabolic actions are mediated through a number of different pathways. As early as the 1960s, it was known that steroids could modulate ribosomal function skeletal muscle [31]. Since then several mechanisms of testosterone action on skeletal muscle growth and function have been elucidated. Testosterone also stimulates insulin-like growth factor 1 (IGF-1) expression which has downstream anabolic effects as well, which will be reviewed later in this chapter [31].

Testosterone induces hypertrophy of both type 1 and type 2 muscle fibers but more so in type 1 muscle fibers [32]. Fernando et al. observed that injection of testosterone in muscle increased net protein synthesis without any effect on breakdown; it increased re-utilization of intracellular amino acids without increasing transport of amino acids [33]. Adult myofibrils contain hundreds of myonuclei. Hypertrophy of the myofibrils over 26% is accompanied by an increase in the number of myonuclei; this is thought to happen to enhance protein synthesis [32]. Anabolic steroids increase the number of myonuclei in the skeletal muscle of athletes but more in type 1 fibers [32, 34]. Additionally there is evidence that testosterone can increase the density of centrally located myonuclei in skeletal muscle myofibrils in both type 1 and type 2 fibers in steroid using athletes whereas in no steroid use. It is though that these myofibrils are primed for muscle regeneration and fusion with new myotubes [35]. Testosterone also plays a role in the function of satellite cells, the local stem cells of skeletal muscle. These cells are an important source of new myonuclei for hypertrophying muscle [36]. In myoblast culture systems, testosterone can stimulate mitosis of satellite cells, and the number of satellite cells was observed to be higher in men receiving testosterone treatment for 20 weeks [37]. This may be mediated through Notch, a transmembrane receptor that can regulate cell differentiation; activated Notch expression increased in older men treated with testosterone [38]. In addition to local stem cells, androgens can also induce commitment of mesenchymal pluripotent stem cells to a myogenic lineage [39]. Androgen receptors are also transcription regulators. There are androgen receptors on skeletal muscle cells [32] and satellite cells [40]. Testosterone treatment for 1 month has been shown to increase androgen receptor activity but with longer-term treatment (six months) decreased back to pretreatment levels [41].

In addition to its effects on muscle, testosterone also affects adipose tissue. It inhibits lipid uptake and lipoprotein lipase activity [42]. Testosterone inhibits adipocyte precursor cell differentiation. Testosterone also increases beta-adrenergic receptors on adipocytes, stimulating lipolysis [43]. However, these effects may be different in visceral vs. subcutaneous fat [44].

There is a negative correlation between testosterone levels and renal function with an approximate prevalence of testosterone deficiency of 44% in CKD 5D [45]. Low testosterone levels are independently associated with lower muscle strength and decreased fat-free mass in men with CKD [46]. Increased visceral adiposity is also independently associated with hypogonadism in men with predialysis CKD [47]. Nutrient intake can also affect testosterone levels. During caloric restriction, testosterone levels decreased by 11% in 32 non-obese men restricted to 50% of their needs [48]. In one study of CKD 3–4 patients, lower testosterone levels were even associated with increased mortality [49]. The association with mortality has also been shown in male dialysis patients [50]. Johansen et al. showed that intramuscular androgen supplementation can also improve lean body mass and muscle strength in nonhypogonadal men and women on MHD. When combined with exercise therapy, this group observed a 3.1 ± 2.2 kg increase in lean body mass in men and women MHD patients after 12 weeks of therapy. Women received half the dose of men (100 vs. 200 mg of nandrolone decanoate) [51]. Macdonald et al. evaluated dose responsiveness of appendicular lean mass in CKD 5 men and women to nandrolone. A dose-response increase in appendicular lean body mass was observed, but tolerability of the high doses was limited in women due to virilization [52]. Lean body mass (LBM) is also increased in predialysis patients treated with nandrolone decanoate [53].

Glucocorticoids

Serum cortisone concentrations are generally normal in patients with advanced CKD and ESKD unless a specific illness is present that increases or decreases serum levels. Cortisol is a catabolic agent and glucocorticoids are often used in the treatment of inflammatory disease in patients with CKD. Glucocorticoids also antagonize the effects of insulin. Endogenous glucocorticoids also contribute to muscle wasting by the suppression of the phosphorylation of Akt by activation of the glucocorticoid receptor. The decrease in p-Akt upregulates proteolytic pathways [54]. Glucocorticoids increase muscle protein catabolism through the ubiquitin-proteasome pathway in a tissue-specific manner [55]. In CKD patients treated with glucocorticoids, effort should be paid to prevent or minimize PEW. Since glucocorticoids also promote mobilization of the bone, patients receiving large doses of glucocorticoids, for example, for the treatment of vasculitis or transplant rejection reactions, can develop negative calcium balance [56]. Treatment with growth hormone may mitigate some adverse effects of glucocorticoids [57].

Growth Hormone and Insulin-Like Growth Factors 1 and 2

Growth hormone (GH) has extensive metabolic effects including stimulation of protein anabolism, bone growth, calcium retention, bone mineralization, and lipolysis [58]. Adipose tissue often decreases with GH treatment. These characteristics of GH have made it an attractive target for clinical trials for the treatment of PEW in advanced CKD and MHD and peritoneal dialysis patients. GH is the key endocrine regulator of postnatal growth. Excess GH leads to acromegaly while GH deficiency in growing children leads to dwarfism [58]. Most of the effects of growth hormone on anabolism are mediated through insulin-like growth factor-1 (IGF-1) [59], but GH also has direct, IGF-1-independent effects on gluconeogenesis and lipolysis [60, 61]. GH mediates the release of IGF-1 primarily from the liver but also from the bone, muscle, and kidney as well as other organs [62]. The IGF system includes IGF-1 and IGF-2, various receptors, and six IGF-binding proteins. IGF-2 is thought to function independently of GH but in concert with IGF-1 to regulate growth and metabolism [63, 64]. The mechanisms of action of GH are discussed in Chap. 21 and will not be reviewed further here.

ESKD is a GH- and IGF-1-resistant state. Despite having normal or increased serum GH levels, children with CKD have blunted growth and blunted metabolic responses to GH [65, 66]. About 50% of GH and 99% of IGF-1 are bound to proteins in plasma; the increased levels of some IGF-binding proteins in serum of CKD patients, in part from both decreased filtration of some low molecular weight IGFBP-3 fragments and increased hepatic production of IGFBP-1 and IGFBP-2, contribute to the resistance to GH and IGF [67, 68]. A decrease in GH receptor expression and abnormalities in post-receptor signaling contribute to GH resistance in experimental kidney failure [66, 69]. GH mediates some of its effect through the JAK/SAT pathway, which may be impaired in uremia [70]. Abnormalities in nutrient intake may also affect GH activity in CKD. In starvation, GH increases while IGF-levels fall, and low energy intake is a common occurrence in advanced non-dialyzed CKD patients [71, 72].

Multiple short-term studies have shown improvement in markers of PEW in chronic dialysis patients [73–77], although even with improvement, most of these patients continue to display evidence for PEW [78]. Using full nitrogen balance studies conducted in MHD patients with PEW for several weeks per patient, Kopple et al. confirmed that GH treatment induced positive protein balance [79]. After six months of therapy, Hansen et al. demonstrated an increase in lean body mass and decrease in fat mass in MHD patients; the dosages used led to levels of GH seen in acromegaly but without significant side effects, suggesting again a GH-resistant state in CKD [80]. Also, after a six-month trial of GH therapy in 139 hemodialysis patients with varying doses of recombinant growth hormone therapy, Feldt-Rasmussen et al. demonstrated increased lean body mass and health-related quality of life and a trend toward increased albumin [81]. The largest trial of GH in MHD patients, the OPPORTUNITY trial, was terminated early but showed a decrease in total body fat and weight and high-sensitivity C-reactive protein and an increase in high-density lipoprotein cholesterol. There was no effect on mortality or other nutritional parameters, probably at least partly due to the short duration of the trial [82].

Thus, GH therapy appears to improve some markers of nutritional status, but long-term potential effects on morbidity and mortality in dialysis patients are still unknown. Similarly, human IGF-1, when administered to continuous ambulatory peritoneal dialysis (CAPD) patients, led to markedly positive nitrogen balance [83], and low serum levels of IGF-1 are associated with an increased risk of death in MHD patients. However, MHD patients with higher serum albumin levels and low serum IGF-I do not have an increased mortality risk possibly indicating that the association between low serum IGF-1 and mortality is less due to malnutrition and more closely associated within inflammatory illness or oxidant stress [84]. More long-term epidemiological studies and controlled interventional trials are needed to resolve these questions.

Insulin

Chapters 1, 2, 3, 4, 5, and 6 of this book review insulin effects in CKD in detail. Only a brief discussion will be provided here. Insulin resistance, which reflects the body's ability to utilize and dispose of glucose, and CKD are strongly related. Diabetes can affect PEW by decreasing gastric motility and impairing nutrient intake. Diabetic ESKD patients are reported to be especially prone to PEW, presumably due to insulinopenia or insulin resistance [85].

Clamp studies also show that advanced CKD is an insulin-resistant state, meaning that there is a decrease in glucose uptake for a given level of glucose and insulin [86]. Metabolic acidemia, hyperparathyroidism, inflammation and oxidative stress, and, most likely, abnormal adipokine production contribute to insulin resistance in CKD [87]. Obesity is also linked to insulin resistance and is of growing importance in the prevalence of CKD [88, 89]. Insulin resistance is associated with accelerated protein catabolism and skeletal muscle breakdown [90]. Insulin prevents protein degradation through the Class I phosphatidylinositol 3-kinase (PI3K)/Akt pathway [91]. In advanced CKD, signaling through this pathway is suppressed; the suppression may be partially attenuated by improvement in acidemia [92]. Abnormal insulin signaling likely enhances muscle breakdown by three pathways: ubiquitin-mediated proteasome activation, lysosomal protein degradation, and caspase-3-mediated muscle atrophy [92]. The result of abnormal insulin function in advanced CKD is a tendency toward muscle loss of muscle in these patients.

Stomach-Derived Hormones Ghrelin and Obestatin

Inadequate nutrient intake is one of the most important factors causing PEW in CKD patients [93]. Stomach-derived hormones play a role in appetite or anorexia regulation and may play a role in the nutritional status of CKD patients. Preproghrelin is the precursor for both ghrelin and obestatin. Cleavage and modification produce these hormones.

Ghrelin is a stomach-derived circulating hormone secreted by the oxyntic glands in the fundus of the stomach that stimulates food intake [94, 95]. Ghrelin secretion is increased by low energy intake and is decreased by food intake, glucose load, insulin, and somatostatin [96–99]. Ghrelin levels are negatively correlated with body mass index, proportion of fat mass, and fasting levels of insulin and leptin in normal individuals [99–101]. Ghrelin stimulates growth hormone, prolactin, and adrenocorticotropic hormone, providing feedback loop from the stomach to the hypothalamic-pituitary axis [102, 103]. Acyl ghrelin is its orexigenic form, while des-acyl ghrelin may be anorexigenic [104]. Total ghrelin levels (acyl and des-acyl ghrelin) are elevated in those with CKD and PEW. Differences degradation and excretion likely contribute to these increased levels [105]. However levels of both acyl ghrelin and des-acyl ghrelin are not consistently elevated across the spectrum of CKD and ESKD and not across pediatric and adult CKD [106, 107]. Peritoneal dialysis patients have lower ghrelin levels than hemodialysis or predialysis patients, which may be evidence of peritoneal glucose absorption suppressing ghrelin [99, 108]. Total and acyl ghrelin are also removed by hemodialysis [109]. Ghrelin levels may play a role in insulin sensitivity in CKD, and preserved insulin sensitivity is associated with increased ghrelin levels in nondiabetic CKD patients [110]. In animal models, ghrelin administration reduced the loss of muscle mass in nephrectomized rats [111]. Administration of acyl ghrelin acutely increased energy intake during one meal but only nonsignificantly increased energy intake over 24 h in maintenance peritoneal dialysis patients [112]. However, ghrelin levels do not correlate well with appetite levels in CKD [107].

Obestatin antagonizes the effects of ghrelin. In rats, it has been shown to inhibit food intake, cause jejunal contraction, and cause weight loss [113]. When obestatin and ghrelin are administered together, food intake does not change [113]. It has also been reported that obestatin partially inhibits ghrelin-stimulated GH secretion [114]. Non-dialysis patients have consistently been found to have lower levels than healthy volunteers, but reported levels in hemodialysis patients and the interaction between BMI and obestatin levels are inconsistent [107, 115]. Borges et al. examined the association between ghrelin and obestatin levels and nutritional parameters in patients with CKD. Higher levels were seen in ESKD than CKD, but no association between obestatin levels and nutritional status was identified [107].

Adipokines

Chapter 20 on adipokines discusses their effects in detail. Therefore we will not delve into an extensive discussion here. Adipokines are fat cell-derived cytokines with endocrine functions. Leptin and adiponectin are adipokines that have known effect on nutritional status in normal human physiology and likely play a role in nutritional status in CKD.

Leptin suppresses appetite in healthy humans, increases satiety, and is directly correlated with body fat in non-CKD individuals [116]. In one study of MHD patients, leptin levels correlate positively with C-reactive protein, but these findings are not consistent across multiple studies [117, 118]. High leptin levels are associated with a higher BMI, skinfold thickness, and albumin in MHD patients [117]. Hyperleptinemia is also associated visceral adiposity and lower testosterone levels in non-dialyzed CKD patients [47]. Overall it is still unclear if leptin is protective or not in CKD and therapeutic targets to affect PEW in leptin activity remain to be elucidated.

In normal physiology, adiponectin's functions include anti-atherogenesis, anti-inflammation, and insulin sensitization [119]. In obesity, decreased levels are associated with insulin resistance and obesity related complications [120]. In CKD plasma levels are elevated and directly correlated with ESKD [121]. In predialysis CKD, higher adiponectin levels are positively associated with PEW [122]. The reasons why adiponectin seems to be anti-inflammatory and provides cardiovascular protection in normal individuals and associated with PEW in CKD may be part of the phenomenon of reverse epidemiology in kidney disease [123]. Overall, the effects of adiponectin on nutrition and CKD are still unclear.

Thyroid Hormone

Thyroid hormone is discussed in detail in Chaps. 7 and 8. We will provide a very limited discussion here. Thyroid hormone regulates many aspects of metabolism and the basal metabolic rate. Tissue-specific receptor isoforms, transporters, and cofactors mediate the various effects of thyroid hormone. Thyroid hormone mainly exhibits effects through the nuclear receptors thyroid hormone receptor alpha and beta (TRα and TRβ) [124]. Hyperthyroidism is associated with higher metabolism, increased lipolysis, weight loss, and decreased serum cholesterol levels. Hypothyroidism is associated with lower metabolism, decreased lipolysis, weight gain, reduced cholesterol clearance, and elevated serum cholesterol [125]. With low energy intake or fasting, the hypothalamic thyroid axis is downregulated, thereby conserving energy [126]. Brown adipose tissue has both TRα and TRβ. The generation of heat in response to cold by brown adipose tissue requires both adrenergic and thyroid axis stimulation [127]. Thyroid hormone affects both peripheral and central adrenergic signaling [128]. Thyroid hormone increases hepatic gluconeogenesis, increases glucose transporter GLUT4 expression in skeletal muscle, and reduces insulin levels. [129] Thyroid hormone regulates fat metabolism; it stimulates both lipolysis and lipogenesis and can decrease low-density lipoprotein levels [125].

There is a high prevalence of subclinical hypothyroidism in CKD. In a study of non-dialyzed CKD patients in Japan, the prevalence of primary hypothyroidism (TSH $\geq$ 4.83 mU/L) in CKD stage 1 + 2, CKD stage 3 + 4, and CKD stage 5 was 9%, 20%, and 56%, respectively ($p < 0.05$). The serum TSH and thyroglobulin levels decreased, without replacement therapy, after the initiation of hemodialysis and iodine restriction. This study suggests an impairment of urinary excretion of iodine may be one cause of hypothyroidism in CKD [130]. Metabolic acidosis may also play a role; oral bicarbonate therapy may improve thyroid function in CKD [131]. Clearly, the hypothalamic thyroid axis plays an important role in nutritional status in humans, and abnormal nutritional status is an important aspect of CKD. Large clinical trials on the effects of alteration of the thyroid hormone axis on nutritional status in CKD are lacking. The association of thyroid dysfunction with adverse outcomes implores further study into possible therapeutic targets in the thyroid hormone axis [132].

References

1. Beddhu S, Pappas LM, Ramkumar N, Samore M. Effects of body size and body composition on survival in hemodialysis patients. J Am Soc Nephrol. 2003;14(9):2366–72.
2. Kalantar-Zadeh K, Block G, McAllister CJ, Humphreys MH, Kopple JD. Appetite and inflammation, nutrition, anemia, and clinical outcome in hemodialysis patients. Am J Clin Nutr. 2004;80(2):299–307.
3. Mehrotra R, Kopple JD. Causes of protein-energy malnutrition in chronic renal failure. Baltimore: Lippincott Williams & Wilkins; 2012.
4. Patten BM, Bilezikian JP, Mallette LE, Prince A, Engel WK, Aurbach GD. Neuromuscular disease in primary hyperparathyroidism. Ann Intern Med. 1974;80(2):182–93.
5. Weiner M, Epstein FH. Signs and symptoms of electrolyte disorders. Yale J Biol Med. 1970;43(2):76–109.
6. Floyd M, Ayyar DR, Barwick DD, Hudgson P, Weightman D. Myopathy in chronic renal failure. Q J Med. 1974;43(172):509–24.
7. Garber AJ. Effects of parathyroid hormone on skeletal muscle protein and amino acid metabolism in the rat. J Clin Invest. 1983;71(6):1806–21.
8. Baczynski R, Massry SG, Magott M, el-Belbessi S, Kohan R, Brautbar N. Effect of parathyroid hormone on energy metabolism of skeletal muscle. Kidney Int. 1985;28(5):722–7.
9. Smogorzewski M, Piskorska G, Borum PR, Massry SG. Chronic renal failure, parathyroid hormone and fatty acids oxidation in skeletal muscle. Kidney Int. 1988;33(2):555–60.
10. Kir S, White JP, Kleiner S, Kazak L, Cohen P, Baracos VE, Spiegelman BM. Tumour-derived PTH-related protein triggers adipose tissue browning and cancer cachexia. Nature. 2014;513(7516):100–4. https://doi.org/10.1038/nature13528.
11. Kir S, Komaba H, Garcia AP, Economopoulos KP, Liu W, Lanske B, Hodin RA, Spiegelman BM. PTH/PTHrP receptor mediates cachexia in models of kidney failure and cancer. Cell Metab. 2016;23(2):315–23. https://doi.org/10.1016/j.cmet.2015.11.003.
12. Cuppari L, de Carvalho AB, Avesani CM, Kamimura MA, Dos Santos Lobao RR, Draibe SA. Increased resting energy expenditure in hemodialysis patients with severe hyperparathyroidism. J Am Soc Nephrol. 2004;15(11):2933–9. https://doi.org/10.1097/01.ASN.0000141961.49723.BC.
13. Rezende LT, Cuppari L, Carvalho AB, Canziani ME, Manfredi SR, Cendoroglo M, Sigulem DM, Draibe SA. Nutritional status of hemodialysis patients with secondary hyperparathyroidism. Braz J Med Biol Res. 2000;33(11):1305–11.
14. Chen C, Wu H, Zhong L, Wang X, Xing ZJ, Gao BH. Impacts of parathyroidectomy on renal anemia and nutritional status of hemodialysis patients with secondary hyperparathyroidism. Int J Clin Exp Med. 2015;8(6):9830–8.
15. Yasunaga C, Nakamoto M, Matsuo K, Nishihara G, Yoshida T, Goya T. Effects of a parathyroidectomy on the immune system and nutritional condition in chronic dialysis patients with secondary hyperparathyroidism. Am J Surg. 1999;178(4):332–6.
16. Campos SR, Gusmao MH, Almeida AF, Pereira LJ, Sampaio LR, Medeiros JM. Nutritional status and food intake of continuous peritoneal dialysis patients with and without secondary hyperparathyroidism. J Bras Nefrol. 2012;34(2):170–7.
17. Di Iorio BR, Minutolo R, De Nicola L, Bellizzi V, Catapano F, Iodice C, Rubino R, Conte G. Supplemented very low protein diet ameliorates responsiveness to erythropoietin in chronic renal failure. Kidney Int. 2003;64(5):1822–8. https://doi.org/10.1046/j.1523-1755.2003.00282.x.
18. Malvy D, Maingourd C, Pengloan J, Bagros P, Nivet H. Effects of severe protein restriction with ketoanalogues in advanced renal failure. J Am Coll Nutr. 1999;18(5):481–6.
19. Kerstetter JE, O'Brien KO, Insogna KL. Low protein intake: the impact on calcium and bone homeostasis in humans. J Nutr. 2003;133(3):855S–61S.
20. Molina P, Carrero JJ, Bover J, Chauveau P, Mazzaferro S, Torres PU. Vitamin D, a modulator

of musculoskeletal health in chronic kidney disease. J Cachexia Sarcopenia Muscle. 2017;8:686. https://doi.org/10.1002/jcsm.12218.

21. Girgis CM, Mokbel N, Cha KM, Houweling PJ, Abboud M, Fraser DR, Mason RS, Clifton-Bligh RJ, Gunton JE. The vitamin D receptor (VDR) is expressed in skeletal muscle of male mice and modulates 25-hydroxyvitamin D (25OHD) uptake in myofibers. Endocrinology. 2014;155(9):3227–37. https://doi.org/10.1210/en.2014-1016.
22. Ceglia L, Harris SS. Vitamin D and its role in skeletal muscle. Calcif Tissue Int. 2013;92(2):151–62. https://doi.org/10.1007/s00223-012-9645-y.
23. Sinha A, Hollingsworth KG, Ball S, Cheetham T. Improving the vitamin D status of vitamin D deficient adults is associated with improved mitochondrial oxidative function in skeletal muscle. J Clin Endocrinol Metab. 2013;98(3):E509–13. https://doi.org/10.1210/jc.2012-3592.
24. Garcia LA, King KK, Ferrini MG, Norris KC, Artaza JN. 1,25(OH)2vitamin D3 stimulates myogenic differentiation by inhibiting cell proliferation and modulating the expression of promyogenic growth factors and myostatin in C2C12 skeletal muscle cells. Endocrinology. 2011;152(8):2976–86. https://doi.org/10.1210/en.2011-0159.
25. Harter HR, Birge SJ, Martin KJ, Klahr S, Karl IE. Effects of vitamin D metabolites on protein catabolism of muscle from uremic rats. Kidney Int. 1983;23(3):465–72.
26. Gordon PL, Doyle JW, Johansen KL. Association of 1,25-dihydroxyvitamin D levels with physical performance and thigh muscle cross-sectional area in chronic kidney disease stage 3 and 4. J Ren Nutr. 2012;22(4):423–33. https://doi.org/10.1053/j.jrn.2011.10.006.
27. Zahed N, Chehrazi S, Falaknasi K. The evaluation of relationship between vitamin D and muscle power by micro manual muscle tester in end-stage renal disease patients. Saudi J Kidney Dis Transpl. 2014;25(5):998–1003.
28. Blair D, Byham-Gray L, Lewis E, McCaffrey S. Prevalence of vitamin D [25(OH)D] deficiency and effects of supplementation with ergocalciferol (vitamin D2) in stage 5 chronic kidney disease patients. J Ren Nutr. 2008;18(4):375–82. https://doi.org/10.1053/j.jrn.2008.04.008.
29. Miskulin DC, Majchrzak K, Tighiouart H, Muther RS, Kapoian T, Johnson DS, Weiner DE. Ergocalciferol supplementation in hemodialysis patients with vitamin D deficiency: a randomized clinical trial. J Am Soc Nephrol. 2016;27(6):1801–10. https://doi.org/10.1681/ASN.2015040468.
30. Schoenfeld PJ MJ, Barnes B, Teitelbaum SL. Amelioration of myopathy with 25-hydroxyvitamin D3 therapy [25(OH)D3] in patients on chronic hemodialysis. Abstracts Third Workshop on Vitamin D, Asilomar, 1977. p. 160.
31. Breuer CB, Florini JR. Amino acid incorporation into protein by cell-free systems from rat skeletal muscle. IV. Effects of animal age, androgens, and anabolic agents on activity of muscle ribosomes. Biochemistry. 1965;4(8):1544–50.
32. Kadi F. Adaptation of human skeletal muscle to training and anabolic steroids. Acta Physiol Scand Suppl. 2000;646:1–52.
33. Ferrando AA, Tipton KD, Doyle D, Phillips SM, Cortiella J, Wolfe RR. Testosterone injection stimulates net protein synthesis but not tissue amino acid transport. Am J Phys. 1998;275(5 Pt 1):E864–71.
34. Sinha-Hikim I, Artaza J, Woodhouse L, Gonzalez-Cadavid N, Singh AB, Lee MI, Storer TW, Casaburi R, Shen R, Bhasin S. Testosterone-induced increase in muscle size in healthy young men is associated with muscle fiber hypertrophy. Am J Phys Endocrinol Metab. 2002;283(1):E154–64. https://doi.org/10.1152/ajpendo.00502.2001.
35. Kadi F. Cellular and molecular mechanisms responsible for the action of testosterone on human skeletal muscle. A basis for illegal performance enhancement. Br J Pharmacol. 2008;154(3):522–8. https://doi.org/10.1038/bjp.2008.118.
36. Moss FP, Leblond CP. Satellite cells as the source of nuclei in muscles of growing rats. Anat Rec. 1971;170(4):421–35. https://doi.org/10.1002/ar.1091700405.
37. Sinha-Hikim I, Roth SM, Lee MI, Bhasin S. Testosterone-induced muscle hypertrophy is associated with an increase in satellite cell number in healthy, young men. Am J Phys Endocrinol Metab. 2003;285(1):E197–205. https://doi.org/10.1152/ajpendo.00370.2002.
38. Sinha-Hikim I, Cornford M, Gaytan H, Lee ML, Bhasin S. Effects of testosterone supplementation on skeletal muscle fiber hypertrophy and satellite cells in community-dwelling older men. J Clin Endocrinol Metab. 2006;91(8):3024–33. https://doi.org/10.1210/jc.2006-0357.
39. Bhasin S, Taylor WE, Singh R, Artaza J, Sinha-Hikim I, Jasuja R, Choi H, Gonzalez-Cadavid NF. The mechanisms of androgen effects on body composition: mesenchymal pluripotent cell as the target of androgen action. J Gerontol A Biol Sci Med Sci. 2003;58(12):M1103–10.
40. Doumit ME, Cook DR, Merkel RA. Testosterone up-regulates androgen receptors and decreases differentiation of porcine myogenic satellite cells in vitro. Endocrinology. 1996;137(4):1385–94. https://doi.org/10.1210/endo.137.4.8625915.
41. Ferrando AA, Sheffield-Moore M, Yeckel CW, Gilkison C, Jiang J, Achacosa A, Lieberman SA, Tipton K, Wolfe RR, Urban RJ. Testosterone administration to older men improves muscle function: molecular and physiological mechanisms. Am J Phys Endocrinol Metab. 2002;282(3):E601–7. https://doi.org/10.1152/ajpendo.00362.2001.
42. De Pergola G. The adipose tissue metabolism: role of testosterone and dehydroepiandrosterone. Int J Obes Relat Metab Disord. 2000;24(Suppl 2):S59–63.
43. Xu X, De Pergola G, Eriksson PS, Fu L, Carlsson B, Yang S, Eden S, Bjorntorp P. Postreceptor events involved in the up-regulation of beta-adrenergic receptor mediated lipolysis by testosterone in rat white adipocytes. Endocrinology. 1993;132(4):1651–7. https://doi.org/10.1210/endo.132.4.8384992.

44. Arner P. Differences in lipolysis between human subcutaneous and omental adipose tissues. Ann Med. 1995;27(4):435–8.
45. Carrero JJ, Qureshi AR, Nakashima A, Arver S, Parini P, Lindholm B, Barany P, Heimburger O, Stenvinkel P. Prevalence and clinical implications of testosterone deficiency in men with end-stage renal disease. Nephrol Dial Transplant. 2011;26(1):184–90. https://doi.org/10.1093/ndt/gfq397.
46. Cigarran S, Pousa M, Castro MJ, Gonzalez B, Martinez A, Barril G, Aguilera A, Coronel F, Stenvinkel P, Carrero JJ. Endogenous testosterone, muscle strength, and fat-free mass in men with chronic kidney disease. J Ren Nutr. 2013;23(5):e89–95. https://doi.org/10.1053/j.jrn.2012.08.007.
47. Cobo G, Cordeiro AC, Amparo FC, Amodeo C, Lindholm B, Carrero JJ. Visceral adipose tissue and leptin hyperproduction are associated with hypogonadism in men with chronic kidney disease. J Ren Nutr. 2017;27(4):243–8. https://doi.org/10.1053/j.jrn.2017.01.023.
48. Muller MJ, Enderle J, Pourhassan M, Braun W, Eggeling B, Lagerpusch M, Gluer CC, Kehayias JJ, Kiosz D, Bosy-Westphal A. Metabolic adaptation to caloric restriction and subsequent refeeding: the Minnesota Starvation Experiment revisited. Am J Clin Nutr. 2015;102(4):807–19. https://doi.org/10.3945/ajcn.115.109173.
49. Khurana KK, Navaneethan SD, Arrigain S, Schold JD, Nally JV Jr, Shoskes DA. Serum testosterone levels and mortality in men with CKD stages 3-4. Am J Kidney Dis. 2014;64(3):367–74. https://doi.org/10.1053/j.ajkd.2014.03.010.
50. Carrero JJ, Qureshi AR, Parini P, Arver S, Lindholm B, Barany P, Heimburger O, Stenvinkel P. Low serum testosterone increases mortality risk among male dialysis patients. J Am Soc Nephrol. 2009;20(3):613–20. https://doi.org/10.1681/ASN.2008060664.
51. Johansen KL, Mulligan K, Schambelan M. Anabolic effects of nandrolone decanoate in patients receiving dialysis: a randomized controlled trial. JAMA. 1999;281(14):1275–81.
52. Macdonald JH, Marcora SM, Jibani MM, Kumwenda MJ, Ahmed W, Lemmey AB. Nandrolone decanoate as anabolic therapy in chronic kidney disease: a randomized phase II dose-finding study. Nephron Clin Pract. 2007;106(3):c125–35. https://doi.org/10.1159/000103000.
53. Eiam-Ong S, Buranaosot S, Eiam-Ong S, Wathanavaha A, Pansin P. Nutritional effect of nandrolone decanoate in predialysis patients with chronic kidney disease. J Ren Nutr. 2007;17(3):173–8. https://doi.org/10.1053/j.jrn.2007.01.001.
54. Hu Z, Wang H, Lee IH, Du J, Mitch WE. Endogenous glucocorticoids and impaired insulin signaling are both required to stimulate muscle wasting under pathophysiological conditions in mice. J Clin Invest. 2009;119(10):3059–69. https://doi.org/10.1172/JCI38770.
55. Marinovic AC, Zheng B, Mitch WE, Price SR. Tissue-specific regulation of ubiquitin (UbC) transcription by glucocorticoids: in vivo and in vitro analyses. Am J Physiol Renal Physiol. 2007;292(2):F660–6. https://doi.org/10.1152/ajprenal.00178.2006.
56. Lane NE, Yao W. Glucocorticoid-induced bone fragility. Ann N Y Acad Sci. 2010;1192:81–3. https://doi.org/10.1111/j.1749-6632.2009.05228.x.
57. Mauras N. Can growth hormone counteract the catabolic effects of steroids? Horm Res. 2009;72(Suppl 1):48–54. https://doi.org/10.1159/000229764.
58. Roelfsema V, Clark RG. The growth hormone and insulin-like growth factor axis: its manipulation for the benefit of growth disorders in renal failure. J Am Soc Nephrol. 2001;12(6):1297–306.
59. Kopchick JJ. Growth hormone. In: Degroot LJ, Jameson JL, editors. Endocrinology part III basic physiology. 4th ed. Philadelphia: Saunders; 2001.
60. Moller N, Copeland KC, Nair KS. Growth hormone effects on protein metabolism. Endocrinol Metab Clin N Am. 2007;36(1):89–100. https://doi.org/10.1016/j.ecl.2006.11.001.
61. Djurhuus CB, Gravholt CH, Nielsen S, Pedersen SB, Moller N, Schmitz O. Additive effects of cortisol and growth hormone on regional and systemic lipolysis in humans. Am J Phys Endocrinol Metab. 2004;286(3):E488–94. https://doi.org/10.1152/ajpendo.00199.2003.
62. Kopple JD, Massry SG. Kopple and Massry's nutritional management of renal disease. 2nd ed. Philadelphia: Lippincott Williams & Wilkins; 2004.
63. Hirschberg R, Adler S. Insulin-like growth factor system and the kidney: physiology, pathophysiology, and therapeutic implications. Am J Kidney Dis. 1998;31(6):901–19. https://doi.org/10.1053/ajkd.1998.v31.pm9631833.
64. Daughaday W. Growth hormone, normal synthesis, secretion, control, and mechanisms of action. Edition ed. In: Degroot LJ, Larry Jameson J, editors. Endocrinology. Philadelpthiia: Saunders; 1989.
65. Fouque D, Peng SC, Kopple JD. Impaired metabolic response to recombinant insulin-like growth factor-1 in dialysis patients. Kidney Int. 1995;47(3):876–83.
66. Ding H, Gao XL, Hirschberg R, Vadgama JV, Kopple JD. Impaired actions of insulin-like growth factor 1 on protein synthesis and degradation in skeletal muscle of rats with chronic renal failure. Evidence for a postreceptor defect. J Clin Invest. 1996;97(4):1064–75. https://doi.org/10.1172/JCI118499.
67. Yap J, Tsao T, Fawcett J, Fielder PJ, Keller GA, Rabkin R. Effect of insulin-like growth factor binding proteins on the response of proximal tubular cells to insulin-like growth factor-I. Kidney Int. 1997;52(5):1216–23.
68. Tonshoff B, Blum WF, Mehls O. Insulin-like growth factors (IGF) and IGF binding proteins in children with chronic renal failure. Prog Growth Factor Res. 1995;6(2–4):481–91.

69. Tonshoff B, Eden S, Weiser E, Carlsson B, Robinson IC, Blum WF, Mehls O. Reduced hepatic growth hormone (GH) receptor gene expression and increased plasma GH binding protein in experimental uremia. Kidney Int. 1994;45(4):1085–92.
70. Schaefer F, Chen Y, Tsao T, Nouri P, Rabkin R. Impaired JAK-STAT signal transduction contributes to growth hormone resistance in chronic uremia. J Clin Invest. 2001;108(3):467–75. https://doi.org/10.1172/JCI11895.
71. Palmblad J, Levi L, Burger A, Melander A, Westgren U, von Schenck H, Skude G. Effects of total energy withdrawal (fasting) on thelevels of growth hormone, thyrotropin, cortisol, adrenaline, noradrenaline, T4, T3, and rT3 in healthy males. Acta Med Scand. 1977;201(1–2):15–22.
72. Rabkin R. Nutrient regulation of insulin-like growth factor-I. Miner Electrolyte Metab. 1997;23(3–6):157–60.
73. Ziegler TR, Lazarus JM, Young LS, Hakim R, Wilmore DW. Effects of recombinant human growth hormone in adults receiving maintenance hemodialysis. J Am Soc Nephrol. 1991;2(6):1130–5.
74. Schulman G, Wingard RL, Hutchison RL, Lawrence P, Hakim RM. The effects of recombinant human growth hormone and intradialytic parenteral nutrition in malnourished hemodialysis patients. Am J Kidney Dis. 1993;21(5):527–34.
75. Ikizler TA, Wingard RL, Breyer JA, Schulman G, Parker RA, Hakim RM. Short-term effects of recombinant human growth hormone in CAPD patients. Kidney Int. 1994;46(4):1178–83.
76. Garibotto G, Barreca A, Russo R, Sofia A, Araghi P, Cesarone A, Malaspina M, Fiorini F, Minuto F, Tizianello A. Effects of recombinant human growth hormone on muscle protein turnover in malnourished hemodialysis patients. J Clin Invest. 1997;99(1):97–105. https://doi.org/10.1172/JCI119139.
77. Iglesias P, Diez JJ, Fernandez-Reyes MJ, Aguilera A, Burgues S, Martinez-Ara J, Miguel JL, Gomez-Pan A, Selgas R. Recombinant human growth hormone therapy in malnourished dialysis patients: a randomized controlled study. Am J Kidney Dis. 1998;32(3):454–63.
78. Pupim LB, Kent P, Caglar K, Shyr Y, Hakim RM, Ikizler TA. Improvement in nutritional parameters after initiation of chronic hemodialysis. Am J Kidney Dis. 2002;40(1):143–51. https://doi.org/10.1053/ajkd.2002.33923.
79. Kopple JD, Brunori G, Leiserowitz M, Fouque D. Growth hormone induces anabolism in malnourished maintenance haemodialysis patients. Nephrol Dial Transplant. 2005;20(5):952–8. https://doi.org/10.1093/ndt/gfh731.
80. Hansen TB, Gram J, Jensen PB, Kristiansen JH, Ekelund B, Christiansen JS, Pedersen FB. Influence of growth hormone on whole body and regional soft tissue composition in adult patients on hemodialysis. A double-blind, randomized, placebo-controlled study. Clin Nephrol. 2000;53(2):99–107.
81. Feldt-Rasmussen B, Lange M, Sulowicz W, Gafter U, Lai KN, Wiedemann J, Christiansen JS, El Nahas M. Growth hormone treatment during hemodialysis in a randomized trial improves nutrition, quality of life, and cardiovascular risk. J Am Soc Nephrol. 2007;18(7):2161–71. https://doi.org/10.1681/ASN.2006111207.
82. Kopple JD, Cheung AK, Christiansen JS, Djurhuus CB, El Nahas M, Feldt-Rasmussen B, Mitch WE, Wanner C, Gothberg M, Ikizler TA. OPPORTUNITY™: a large-scale randomized clinical trial of growth hormone in hemodialysis patients. Nephrol Dial Transplant. 2011;26(12):4095–103. https://doi.org/10.1093/ndt/gfr363.
83. Fouque D, Peng SC, Shamir E, Kopple JD. Recombinant human insulin-like growth factor-1 induces an anabolic response in malnourished CAPD patients. Kidney Int. 2000;57(2):646–54. https://doi.org/10.1046/j.1523-1755.2000.00886.x.
84. Nilsson E, Carrero JJ, Heimburger O, Hellberg O, Lindholm B, Stenvinkel P. A cohort study of insulin-like growth factor 1 and mortality in haemodialysis patients. Clin Kidney J. 2016;9(1):148–52. https://doi.org/10.1093/ckj/sfv118.
85. Pupim LB, Heimburger O, Qureshi AR, Ikizler TA, Stenvinkel P. Accelerated lean body mass loss in incident chronic dialysis patients with diabetes mellitus. Kidney Int. 2005;68(5):2368–74. https://doi.org/10.1111/j.1523-1755.2005.00699.x.
86. Spoto B, Pisano A, Zoccali C. Insulin resistance in chronic kidney disease: a systematic review. Am J Physiol Renal Physiol. 2016;311(6):F1087–F108. https://doi.org/10.1152/ajprenal.00340.2016.
87. Guarnieri G, Zanetti M, Vinci P, Cattin MR, Barazzoni R. Insulin resistance in chronic uremia. J Ren Nutr. 2009;19(1):20–4. https://doi.org/10.1053/j.jrn.2008.11.014.
88. Shoelson SE, Herrero L, Naaz A. Obesity, inflammation, and insulin resistance. Gastroenterology. 2007;132(6):2169–80. https://doi.org/10.1053/j.gastro.2007.03.059.
89. Kurella M, Lo JC, Chertow GM. Metabolic syndrome and the risk for chronic kidney disease among nondiabetic adults. J Am Soc Nephrol. 2005;16(7):2134–40. https://doi.org/10.1681/ASN.2005010106.
90. Siew ED, Pupim LB, Majchrzak KM, Shintani A, Flakoll PJ, Ikizler TA. Insulin resistance is associated with skeletal muscle protein breakdown in non-diabetic chronic hemodialysis patients. Kidney Int. 2007;71(2):146–52. https://doi.org/10.1038/sj.ki.5001984.
91. Bailey JL. Insulin resistance and muscle metabolism in chronic kidney disease. ISRN Endocrinol. 2013;2013:329606. https://doi.org/10.1155/2013/329606.
92. Price SR, Gooch JL, Donaldson SK, Roberts-Wilson TK. Muscle atrophy in chronic kidney disease results from abnormalities in insulin signaling. J Ren Nutr. 2010;20(5 Suppl):S24–8. https://doi.org/10.1053/j.jrn.2010.05.007.

93. Cianciaruso B, Brunori G, Traverso G, Panarello G, Enia G, Strippoli P, de Vecchi A, Querques M, Viglino E, Vonesh E, et al. Nutritional status in the elderly patient with uraemia. Nephrol Dial Transplant. 1995;10(Suppl 6):65–8.
94. Kojima M, Hosoda H, Date Y, Nakazato M, Matsuo H, Kangawa K. Ghrelin is a growth-hormone-releasing acylated peptide from stomach. Nature. 1999;402(6762):656–60. https://doi.org/10.1038/45230.
95. Kojima M, Kangawa K. Ghrelin: structure and function. Physiol Rev. 2005;85(2):495–522. https://doi.org/10.1152/physrev.00012.2004.
96. Nakazato M, Murakami N, Date Y, Kojima M, Matsuo H, Kangawa K, Matsukura S. A role for ghrelin in the central regulation of feeding. Nature. 2001;409(6817):194–8. https://doi.org/10.1038/35051587.
97. Marzullo P, Caumo A, Savia G, Verti B, Walker GE, Maestrini S, Tagliaferri A, Di Blasio AM, Liuzzi A. Predictors of postabsorptive ghrelin secretion after intake of different macronutrients. J Clin Endocrinol Metab. 2006;91(10):4124–30. https://doi.org/10.1210/jc.2006-0270.
98. Baldelli R, Bellone S, Castellino N, Petri A, Rapa A, Vivenza D, Bellone J, Broglio F, Ghigo E, Bona G. Oral glucose load inhibits circulating ghrelin levels to the same extent in normal and obese children. Clin Endocrinol. 2006;64(3):255–9. https://doi.org/10.1111/j.1365-2265.2006.02441.x.
99. Mafra D, Guebre-Egziabher F, Fouque D. Endocrine role of stomach in appetite regulation in chronic kidney disease: about ghrelin and obestatin. J Ren Nutr. 2010;20(2):68–73. https://doi.org/10.1053/j.jrn.2009.08.002.
100. Shiiya T, Nakazato M, Mizuta M, Date Y, Mondal MS, Tanaka M, Nozoe S, Hosoda H, Kangawa K, Matsukura S. Plasma ghrelin levels in lean and obese humans and the effect of glucose on ghrelin secretion. J Clin Endocrinol Metab. 2002;87(1):240–4. https://doi.org/10.1210/jcem.87.1.8129.
101. Tschop M, Weyer C, Tataranni PA, Devanarayan V, Ravussin E, Heiman ML. Circulating ghrelin levels are decreased in human obesity. Diabetes. 2001;50(4):707–9.
102. Cowley MA, Smith RG, Diano S, Tschop M, Pronchuk N, Grove KL, Strasburger CJ, Bidlingmaier M, Esterman M, Heiman ML, et al. The distribution and mechanism of action of ghrelin in the CNS demonstrates a novel hypothalamic circuit regulating energy homeostasis. Neuron. 2003;37(4):649–61.
103. Lanfranco F, Motta G, Baldi M, Gasco V, Grottoli S, Benso A, Broglio F, Ghigo E. Ghrelin and anterior pituitary function. Front Horm Res. 2010;38:206–11. https://doi.org/10.1159/000318512.
104. Inhoff T, Monnikes H, Noetzel S, Stengel A, Goebel M, Dinh QT, Riedl A, Bannert N, Wisser AS, Wiedenmann B, et al. Desacyl ghrelin inhibits the orexigenic effect of peripherally injected ghrelin in rats. Peptides. 2008;29(12):2159–68. https://doi.org/10.1016/j.peptides.2008.09.014.
105. Mak RH, Cheung W, Purnell J. Ghrelin in chronic kidney disease: too much or too little? Perit Dial Int. 2007;27(1):51–5.
106. Buscher AK, Buscher R, Hauffa BP, Hoyer PF. Alterations in appetite-regulating hormones influence protein-energy wasting in pediatric patients with chronic kidney disease. Pediatr Nephrol. 2010;25(11):2295–301. https://doi.org/10.1007/s00467-010-1588-9.
107. Borges N, Moraes C, Barros AF, Carraro-Eduardo JC, Fouque D, Mafra D. Acyl-ghrelin and obestatin plasma levels in different stages of chronic kidney disease. J Ren Nutr. 2014;24(2):100–4. https://doi.org/10.1053/j.jrn.2013.11.005.
108. Iglesias P, Diez JJ, Fernandez-Reyes MJ, Codoceo R, Alvarez-Fidalgo P, Bajo MA, Aguilera A, Selgas R. Serum ghrelin concentrations in patients with chronic renal failure undergoing dialysis. Clin Endocrinol. 2006;64(1):68–73. https://doi.org/10.1111/j.1365-2265.2005.02418.x.
109. Yoshimoto A, Mori K, Sugawara A, Mukoyama M, Yahata K, Suganami T, Takaya K, Hosoda H, Kojima M, Kangawa K, et al. Plasma ghrelin and desacyl ghrelin concentrations in renal failure. J Am Soc Nephrol. 2002;13(11):2748–52.
110. Barazzoni R, Gortan Cappellari G, Zanetti M, Guarnieri G. Ghrelin and muscle metabolism in chronic uremia. J Ren Nutr. 2012;22(1):171–5. https://doi.org/10.1053/j.jrn.2011.10.017.
111. Deboer MD, Zhu X, Levasseur PR, Inui A, Hu Z, Han G, Mitch WE, Taylor JE, Halem HA, Dong JZ, et al. Ghrelin treatment of chronic kidney disease: improvements in lean body mass and cytokine profile. Endocrinology. 2008;149(2):827–35. https://doi.org/10.1210/en.2007-1046.
112. Wynne K, Giannitsopoulou K, Small CJ, Patterson M, Frost G, Ghatei MA, Brown EA, Bloom SR, Choi P. Subcutaneous ghrelin enhances acute food intake in malnourished patients who receive maintenance peritoneal dialysis: a randomized, placebo-controlled trial. J Am Soc Nephrol. 2005;16(7):2111–8. https://doi.org/10.1681/ASN.2005010039.
113. Zhang JV, Ren PG, Avsian-Kretchmer O, Luo CW, Rauch R, Klein C, Hsueh AJ. Obestatin, a peptide encoded by the ghrelin gene, opposes ghrelin's effects on food intake. Science. 2005;310(5750):996–9. https://doi.org/10.1126/science.1117255.
114. Lagaud GJ, Young A, Acena A, Morton MF, Barrett TD, Shankley NP. Obestatin reduces food intake and suppresses body weight gain in rodents. Biochem Biophys Res Commun. 2007;357(1):264–9. https://doi.org/10.1016/j.bbrc.2007.03.138.
115. Oner-Iyidogan Y, Gurdol F, Kocak H, Oner P, Cetinalp-Demircan P, Caliskan Y, Kocak T, Turkmen A. Appetite-regulating hormones in chronic kidney disease patients. J Ren Nutr. 2011;21(4):316–21. https://doi.org/10.1053/j.jrn.2010.07.005.

116. Moraes-Vieira PM, Bassi EJ, Araujo RC, Camara NO. Leptin as a link between the immune system and kidney-related diseases: leading actor or just a coadjuvant? Obes Rev. 2012;13(8):733–43. https://doi.org/10.1111/j.1467-789X.2012.00997.x.
117. Kara E, Ahbap E, Sahutoglu T, Sakaci T, Basturk T, Koc Y, Sevinc M, Akgol C, Ucar ZA, Kayalar AO, et al. Elevated serum leptin levels are associated with good nutritional status in non-obese chronic hemodialysis patients. Clin Nephrol. 2015;83(3):147–53. https://doi.org/10.5414/CN108409.
118. Lee CT, Lee CH, Su Y, Chuang YC, Tsai TL, Cheni JB. The relationship between inflammatory markers, leptin and adiponectin in chronic hemodialysis patients. Int J Artif Organs. 2004;27(10):835–41.
119. Kadowaki T, Yamauchi T. Adiponectin and adiponectin receptors. Endocr Rev. 2005;26(3):439–51. https://doi.org/10.1210/er.2005-0005.
120. Ebinc H, Ozkurt ZN, Ebinc FA, Yilmaz M, Caglayan O. Adiponectin and insulin resistance in obesity-related diseases. J Int Med Res. 2008;36(1):71–9. https://doi.org/10.1177/147323000803600110.
121. Kuczera P, Adamczak M, Wiecek A. Endocrine abnormalities in patients with chronic kidney disease. Prilozi. 2015;36(2):109–18. https://doi.org/10.1515/prilozi-2015-0059.
122. Hyun YY, Lee KB, Oh KH, Ahn C, Park SK, Chae DW, Yoo TH, Cho KH, Kim YS, Hwang YH. Serum adiponectin and protein-energy wasting in predialysis chronic kidney disease. Nutrition. 2017;33:254–60. https://doi.org/10.1016/j.nut.2016.06.014.
123. Kalantar-Zadeh K, Rhee CM, Chou J, Ahmadi SF, Park J, Chen JL, Amin AN. The obesity paradox in kidney disease: how to reconcile it with obesity management. Kidney Int Rep. 2017;2(2):271–81. https://doi.org/10.1016/j.ekir.2017.01.009.
124. Cheng SY, Leonard JL, Davis PJ. Molecular aspects of thyroid hormone actions. Endocr Rev. 2010;31(2):139–70. https://doi.org/10.1210/er.2009-0007.
125. Liu YY, Brent GA. Thyroid hormone crosstalk with nuclear receptor signaling in metabolic regulation. Trends Endocrinol Metab. 2010;21(3):166–73. https://doi.org/10.1016/j.tem.2009.11.004.
126. Boelen A, Wiersinga WM, Fliers E. Fasting-induced changes in the hypothalamus-pituitary-thyroid axis. Thyroid. 2008;18(2):123–9. https://doi.org/10.1089/thy.2007.0253.
127. Ribeiro MO, Carvalho SD, Schultz JJ, Chiellini G, Scanlan TS, Bianco AC, Brent GA. Thyroid hormone – sympathetic interaction and adaptive thermogenesis are thyroid hormone receptor isoform – specific. J Clin Invest. 2001;108(1):97–105. https://doi.org/10.1172/JCI12584.
128. Fliers E, Klieverik LP, Kalsbeek A. Novel neural pathways for metabolic effects of thyroid hormone. Trends Endocrinol Metab. 2010;21(4):230–6. https://doi.org/10.1016/j.tem.2009.11.008.
129. Potenza M, Via MA, Yanagisawa RT. Excess thyroid hormone and carbohydrate metabolism. Endocr Prac. 2009;15(3):254–62. https://doi.org/10.4158/EP.15.3.254.
130. Sanai T, Okamura K, Rikitake S, Fukuda M, Onozawa K, Sanematsu M, Takashima T, Miyazono M, Ikeda Y. The high prevalence of reversible subclinical hypothyroidism with elevated serum thyroglobulin levels in chronic kidney disease patients. Clin Nephrol. 2017;87(5):237–44. https://doi.org/10.5414/CN109008.
131. Disthabanchong S, Treeruttanawanich A. Oral sodium bicarbonate improves thyroid function in predialysis chronic kidney disease. Am J Nephrol. 2010;32(6):549–56. https://doi.org/10.1159/000321461.
132. Rhee CM. The interaction between thyroid and kidney disease: an overview of the evidence. Curr Opin Endocrinol Diabetes Obes. 2016;23(5):407–15. https://doi.org/10.1097/MED.0000000000000275.

Index

C. M. Rhee et al. (eds.), *Endocrine Disorders in Kidney Disease*,
https://doi.org/10.1007/978-3-319-97765-2

MIX
Papier aus verantwortungsvollen Quellen
Paper from responsible sources
FSC® C105338

If you have any concerns about our products,
you can contact us on
ProductSafety@springernature.com

In case Publisher is established outside the EU,
the EU authorized representative is:
Springer Nature Customer Service Center GmbH
Europaplatz 3, 69115 Heidelberg, Germany

Printed by Libri Plureos GmbH
in Hamburg, Germany